Pharmaceutical Dosage Forms
and
Drug Delivery Systems

I am a Pharmacist

I am a specialist in medications

    I supply medicines and pharmaceuticals to those who need them.

    I prepare and compound special dosage forms.

    I control the storage and preservation of all medications in my care.

I am a custodian of medical information

    My library is a ready source of drug knowledge.

    My files contain thousands of specific drug names and tens of thousands of facts about them.

    My records include the medication and health history of entire families.

    My journals and meetings report advances in pharmacy from around the world.

I am a companion of the physician

    I am a partner in the case of every patient who takes any kind of medication.

    I am a consultant on the merits of different therapeutic agents.

    I am the connecting link between physician and patient and the final check on the safety of medicines.

I am a counselor to the patient

    I help the patient understand the proper use of prescription medication.

    I assist in the patient's choice of nonprescription drugs or in the decision to consult a physician.

    I advise the patient on matters of prescription storage and potency.

I am a guardian of the public health

    My pharmacy is a center for health-care information.

    I encourage and promote sound personal health practices.

    My services are available to all at all times.

This is my calling · This is my pride

Pharmaceutical Dosage Forms
and
Drug Delivery Systems

HOWARD C. ANSEL, Ph.D.

Professor and Dean, College of Pharmacy
The University of Georgia

NICHOLAS G. POPOVICH, Ph.D.

Professor, School of Pharmacy and Pharmacal Sciences
Purdue University

FIFTH EDITION

Lea & Febiger • *Philadelphia* • *London*

1990

Lea & Febiger
200 Chesterfield Parkway
Malvern, Pennsylvania   19355
U.S.A.
1-800-444-1785

Lea & Febiger (UK) Ltd.
145a Croydon Road
Beckenham, Kent BR3 3RB
U.K.

Library of Congress Cataloging-in-Publication Data

Ansel, Howard C., 1933–
    Pharmaceutical dosage forms and drug delivery systems / Howard C.
Ansel with contribution by Nicholas G. Popovich.—5th ed.
    p.   cm.
    Rev. ed of: Introduction to pharmaceutical dosage forms, 4th ed.
1985.
    Includes bibliographies and index.
    ISBN 0-8121-1255-5
    1. Drugs—Dosage forms. 2. Drug delivery systems. I. Popovich,
Nicholas G. II. Ansel, Howard C., 1933–   Introduction to
pharmaceutical dosage forms. III. Title.
    [DNLM: 1. Dosage Forms. 2. Drugs—administration & dosage. QV
785 A618i]
RS200.A57 1990
615′.1—dc20
DNLM/DLC
for Library of Congress
                                                                                89–8299
                                                                                CIP

1st Edition, 1969
Reprinted, 1972
2nd Edition, 1976
Reprinted, 1978
3rd Edition, 1981
Reprinted, 1982
4th Edition, 1985
Reprinted, 1987, 1988
5th Edition, 1990

Reprints of chapters may be purchased from Lea & Febiger in quantities of 100 or more.

The use of portions of the text of USPXXII-NFXVII is by permission of the USP Convention. The Convention
is not responsible for any inaccuracy of quotation or for any false or misleading implication that may arise
from separation of excerpts from the original context or by obsolescence resulting from publication of a
supplement.

PRINTED IN THE UNITED STATES OF AMERICA

Print No.   4   3   2   1

Preface

The title *Pharmaceutical Dosage Forms and Drug Delivery Systems*, represents the fifth edition of *Introduction to Pharmaceutical Dosage Forms*. The revised title reflects the purpose of the text in covering traditional pharmaceutical dosage forms as well as drug delivery systems resulting from new technology. As in the past, the text is intended to introduce beginning pharmacy students to medicinal and pharmaceutical substances, their formulation into discrete dosage forms and drug delivery systems, and their utilization in patient care.

This new edition also represents the introduction of Nicholas G. Popovich, Ph.D., as a contributor. Dr. Popovich brings to the text an expertise in the application of dosage forms and drug delivery systems in pharmacy practice and patient care. Accordingly, there is a new emphasis in the text on drug product selection and dosage form utilization to help the student understand how to improve patient outcomes and compliance with these systems.

As in previous editions, appropriate consideration is given in initial chapters to such topics as the heritage of pharmacy, historic development of the official compendia, pharmaceutical research and the discovery of drug substances, biopharmaceutic considerations in dosage form design, drug product regulation and control, current good manufacturing practices, clinical studies, and the pharmacist's role in professional practice.

The organization of the text, according to routes of administration and related dosage forms and drug delivery systems, has gained widespread acceptance and has been continued. New sections have been added on transdermal drug delivery systems, products of the new biotechnology, and principles of clinical pharmacokinetics. Other sections have been expanded including that on controlled-release dosage forms. The appendix chapter on systems and techniques of measurement has been continued, and the chapter containing definitions of selected drug categories has been completely revised to contain the newer categories of today's therapeutic agents.

Appreciation is extended to colleagues and students who have shared their thoughts regarding the content and format of this text. Special gratitude is extended to H. Douglas Johnson, Ph.D. for the appendix chapter on definitions of drug categories, to Glen J. Sperandio, Ph.D. for the inspiring "I Am A Pharmacist" which appers at the front of the book, to Mrs. Sue Foley for secretarial assistance, to Suzanne Ansel for proofreading, and Mr. George H. Mundorff of Lea & Febiger for editorial support.

Athens, Georgia　　　　　HOWARD C. ANSEL

Contents

1 | *Introduction to Drugs and Pharmacy*

A DRUG may be defined as an agent intended for use in the diagnosis, mitigation, treatment, cure, or prevention of disease in man or in other animals. One of the most astounding qualities of drugs is the diversity of their actions and effects on the body. Drugs categorized as ecbolics or oxytocics stimulate the activity of the uterine muscle, but other drugs act as uterine muscle relaxants. Some drugs selectively stimulate the cardiac muscle, the smooth muscles, or the skeletal muscles; other drugs have the opposite effect. Mydriatic drugs dilate the pupil of the eye; miotics constrict or diminish pupillary size. Drugs can render blood more coagulable or less coagulable; they can increase the hemoglobin content of the erythrocytes or expand blood volume.

Drugs termed emetics induce vomiting, whereas antiemetic drugs have the opposite effect. Diuretic drugs increase the flow of urine, expectorant drugs increase respiratory tract fluid, and cathartics or laxatives promote the evacuation of the bowel. Other drugs may decrease the flow of urine, diminish body secretions, or induce constipation.

Drugs can be employed to reduce pain, fever, thyroid activity, rhinitis, insomnia, gastric acidity, motion sickness, and mental depression. Drugs can elevate the mood, the blood pressure, or the activity of the endocrine glands. Drugs can combat infectious disease, destroy intestinal worms, or act as antidotes against the poisoning effects of other drugs. Antineoplastic drugs provide one means of attacking the cancerous process; radioactive pharmaceuticals provide another.

Drugs may be used to diagnose diabetes, liver malfunction, tuberculosis, or pregnancy, or they may be employed to replenish a body deficient in antibodies, vitamins, hormones, electrolytes, protein, enzymes, or blood. Drugs may be used to prevent measles, poliomyelitis, or pregnancy or to assist the maintenance of pregnancy or to extend life itself.

Certainly the vast array of effective medicinal agents available today represents one of man's greatest scientific accomplishments. It would be frightening to conceive of our civilization devoid of these remarkable and beneficial agents. Through their use, many of the diseases which have plagued mankind throughout history, as smallpox and poliomyelitis, are now virtually extinct. Illnesses such as diabetes, hypertension, and mental depression are now effectively controlled with modern drugs. Today's surgical procedures would be virtually impossible without the benefit of general anesthetics, analgesics, antibiotics, blood transfusions, and intravenous fluids and nutrients.

The process of drug discovery and development is complex. It involves the collective contributions of many scientific specialists including organic, physical, and analytical chemists, biochemists, bacteriologists, physiologists, pharmacologists, toxicologists, hematologists, immunologists, endocrinologists, pathologists, biostatisticians, pharmaceutical scientists, clinical physicians and many others.

After a potential new drug substance is discovered and has undergone definitive chemical and physical characterization, a great deal of biological information must be gathered. The basic *pharmacology* or the nature and mechanism of action of the drug on the biological system must be determined including toxicologic features. A study must be made of the drug's site and rate of absorption, its pattern of distribution and concentration within the body, its duration of action, and the method and rate of its elimination or excretion. Information must be obtained on the drug's metabolic degradation and the activity of any of its metabolites. A comprehensive study must be made of the drug's short term and long term effects on various body cells, tissues, and organs. Highly specific information may be obtained, as the effect of the drug on the fetus of a pregnant animal or its ability to pass to a nursing baby through the breast milk of its mother. Many a promising new drug has been abandoned because of its potential to cause excessive or hazardous adverse effects.

A new drug's most effective routes of administration (e.g., oral, rectal, parenteral) must be determined and guidelines established concerning the dosage recommended for persons of varying ages, weights, and states of illness. To facilitate administration of the drug by the selected routes, appropriate *dosage forms* as tablets, capsules, injections, suppositories, ointments, aerosols, and others are formulated and prepared. Each of these dosage units is designed to contain a specified quantity of medication for ease and accuracy of dosage administration. These dosage forms are highly sophisticated pharmaceutical drug delivery systems. Their design, development, production, and use are a prime example of the application of the pharmaceutical sciences—the blending of the basic, applied, and clinical sciences with pharmaceutical technology.

Each particular pharmaceutical product is a formulation unique unto itself. In addition to the active therapeutic ingredients, a pharmaceutical formulation also contains a number of nontherapeutic agents. These agents are generally referred to as *pharmaceutical adjuncts, excipients* or *necessities,* and it is through their use that a formulation achieves its unique composition and characteristic physical appearance. Included are such materials as fillers, thickeners, vehicles, suspending agents, tablet disintegrants, stabilizing agents, antimicrobial preservatives, flavors, colorants, and sweeteners.

In order to assure the stability of a drug in a formulation and the continued effectiveness of the drug product throughout its usual shelf life,[1] the principles of chemistry, physical pharmacy, microbiology, and pharmaceutical technology must be applied. The formulation must be such that all components are physically and chemically compatible, including the active therapeutic agents, the pharmaceutical ingredients and the packaging materials. The formulation must be preserved against decomposition due to chemical degradation and protected from microbial contamination and the destructive influences of excessive heat, light, and moisture. The therapeutic ingredients must be released from the dosage form in the proper amount and in such a manner that the onset and duration of the drug's action is that which is desired. The

pharmaceutical product must lend itself to efficient administration and must possess attractive features of flavor, odor, color, and texture that enhance patient acceptance. Finally, the product must be effectively packaged and clearly and completely labeled according to existing legal regulations.

Once prepared, the pharmaceutical product must be properly administered if the patient is to receive maximum benefit. The medication must be taken in sufficient quantity, at specified intervals, and for an indicated duration of time. The effectiveness of the medication in achieving the prescriber's objectives should be reevaluated at regular intervals and necessary adjustments made in the dosage, *dosage regimen* or dosage schedule, dosage form, or indeed, in the choice of the drug administered. Patient expressions of disappointment in his rate of progress or complaints of side effects to the prescribed drug should be evaluated upon report and decisions made as to the continuance, minor adjustment, or major change in drug therapy. Prior to initially taking a medication, a patient should be warned of any expected minor side effects, and of foods, beverages, and/or other drugs which may interfere with the effectiveness of the medication or with the course of therapy.

Through professional interaction and communication with other health professionals the pharmacist is able to contribute greatly to patient care. The pharmacist's intimate knowledge of drug actions, drug therapy, dosage form design and utilization, available pharmaceutical products, and drug information sources makes him or her a vital member of the health care team. The pharmacist is entrusted with the legal responsibility for the procurement, storage, control and distribution of effective pharmaceutical products and for the compounding and filling of prescription orders. Utilizing extensive training and knowledge, the pharmacist serves the patient as an advisor on drugs and encourages their safe and proper utilization. The pharmacist delivers pharmaceutical services in a variety of community and institutional health care environments and effectively utilizes record-keeping and monitoring techniques in safeguarding the public health.

To appreciate the progress that has been made in drug discovery and development in recent years and to provide some background for the study of modern drugs and pharmaceutical dosage forms, it is important to examine pharmacy's heritage.

The Heritage of Pharmacy

Drugs, in the form of vegetation and minerals, have existed longer than man himself. Human disease and man's instinct to survive have, through the ages, led to their discovery. The use of drugs, crude though they may have been, undoubtedly dates back long prior to recorded history, for the instinct of primitive man to relieve the pain of a wound by bathing it in cool water or by soothing it with a fresh leaf or protecting it with mud is within the realm of belief. From experience primitive man would learn that certain therapy was more effective than others, and from these beginnings the practice of drug therapy began.

Among many early races, disease was believed to be caused by the entrance of demons or evil spirits into the body. The treatment quite naturally involved ridding the body of the supernatural intruders. From the earliest records of history it is evident that the primary methods of doing so were through the use of spiritual incantations, the application of noisome materials, and the administration of specific herbs or plants.

The First Apothecary

Before the days of the priestcraft, the wise man or woman of the tribe, whose knowledge of the healing qualities of plants had been gathered through experience or handed down by word of mouth, was called upon to attend to the sick or wounded and prepare the remedy. It was in the preparation of the medicinal materials that the art of the apothecary originated.

The art of the apothecary has always been associated with the mysterious, and its practitioners were believed to have connection with the world of spirits and thus performed as intermediaries between the seen and the unseen. The belief that a drug had magical associations meant that its action, for good or for evil, did not depend upon its natural qualities alone. The compassion of a god, the observance of ceremonies, the absence of evil spirits, and the healing intent of the dispenser were individually and collectively needed to make the drug therapeutically effective. Because of this, the tribal apothecary was one to be feared, respected, trusted, sometimes mistrusted, worshipped,

and revered, for it was through his potions that spiritual contact was made and upon which the cures or failures depended. Throughout history the knowledge of drugs and their application to disease has always meant power. In the Homeric epics, the term *pharmakon* (Gr.) from which our word *pharmacy* was derived connotes a charm or a drug that can be used for good or for evil purposes. Many of the tribal apothecary's failures were doubtless due to impotent medicines, inappropriate medicines, underdosage, overdosage, and even poisoning. His successes may be attributed to an appropriate drug based on his experience, coincidence of proper therapy, inconsequential effect of the therapy for an individual with a nonfatal illness, or *placebo effects,* that is, successful treatment due to psychologic rather than therapeutic effects. Even today, placebo therapy with nonpotent or inconsequential chemicals is successfully employed in the treatment of individual patients and is a routine practice in the clinical evaluation of new drugs where subjects' responses to the effects of the actual drug and the placebo are compared and evaluated.

As time passed, the art of the apothecary became combined with priestly functions, and among the early civilizations the priest-magician or priest-physician became the healer of the body as well as of the soul. Pharmacy and medicine are indistinguishable in their early history, since their practice was generally the. function of the tribal religious leaders.

Early Drugs

Due to the patience and intellect of the archeologist, the types and the specific drugs employed in the early history of drug therapy are not as indefinable as one might suspect. Numerous ancient tablets, scrolls, and other relics dating as far back as 3000 B.C. have been uncovered and deciphered by archeologic scholars to the delight of historians of both medicine and pharmacy, for contained in these ancient documents are specific associations with our common heritage (Fig. 1–1).

Perhaps the most famous of these surviving memorials is the *Papyrus Ebers,* a continuous scroll some 60 feet long and a foot wide dating back to the 16th century before Christ. This document, which is now preserved at the University of Leipzig, is named for the noted German Egyptologist, Georg Ebers, who discovered it in the tomb of a mummy and partly translated

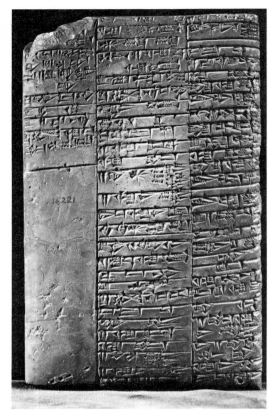

Fig. 1–1. *Sumerian clay tablet from the third millennium* B.C. *on which are believed to be the world's oldest written prescriptions. Among them are a preparation of the seed of "carpenter plant," gum resin of markhazi, and thyme, all pulverized and dissolved in beer, and a combination of powdered roots of "Moon plant," and white pear tree, also dissolved in beer. (Courtesy of the University Museum, University of Pennsylvania.)*

it during the last half of the nineteenth century. Since that time, many scholars have participated in the translation of the document's challenging hieroglyphics, and although they are not unanimous in their interpretations there is little doubt that by 1550 B.C. the Egyptians were using some drugs and dosage forms still employed today.

The text of the Ebers Papyrus is dominated by drug formulas, with more than 800 formulas or prescriptions being described and over 700 different drugs being mentioned. The drugs referred to are chiefly botanic, although mineral and animal drugs are also noted. Such botanic substances as acacia, castor bean (from which we express castor oil), and fennel are mentioned along with apparent references to such minerals as iron oxide, sodium carbonate, sodium chloride, and sulfur. Animal excrements were also employed in drug therapy.

The formulative vehicles of the day were beer, wine, milk, and honey. Many of the pharmaceutical formulas employed two dozen or more different medicinal agents, a type of preparation later referred to as a "polypharmacal." Mortars, hand mills, sieves, and balances were commonly used by the Egyptians in their compounding of suppositories, gargles, pills, inhalations, troches, lotions, ointments, plasters, and enemas.

Introduction of the Scientific Viewpoint

Throughout history many individuals have contributed to the advancement of the health sciences. Notable among those whose genius and creativeness had a revolutionary influence on the development of pharmacy and medicine were Hippocrates (ca. 460–377 B.C.), Dioscorides (1st century A.D.), Galen (ca. 130–200 A.D.), and Paracelsus (1493–1541 A.D.).

Hippocrates was a Greek physician who is credited with the introduction of scientific pharmacy and medicine. He rationalized medicine, systematized medical knowledge, and put the practice of medicine on a high ethical plane. His thinking on the ethics and science of medicine dominated the medical writings of his and successive generations, and his concepts and precepts are embodied into the now renowned Hippocratic oath of ethical behavior for the healing professions. His works included the descriptions of hundreds of drugs, and it was during this period that the term *pharmakon* came to mean a purifying remedy for good only, transcending the previous connotation of a charm or drug for good or for evil purposes. Because of his pioneering work in medical science and his inspirational teachings and advanced philosophies that have become a part of modern medicine, Hippocrates is honored by being called the "Father of Medicine."

Dioscorides, a Greek physician and botanist, was the first to deal with botany as an applied science of pharmacy. His work, *De Materia Medica*, is considered a milestone in the development of pharmaceutical botany and in the study of naturally occurring medicinal materials. This area of study is today known as pharmacognosy, a term formed from two Greek words, *pharmakon*, drug, and *gnōsis*, knowledge. Some of the drugs described by Dioscorides, as opium, ergot, and hyoscyamus, continue to have use in medicine. His descriptions of the art of identifying and collecting natural drug products, the methods of their proper storage, and the means of detecting adulterants or contaminants were the standards of the period and established the need for additional work and the guidelines for future investigators.

Claudius Galen, a Greek pharmacist-physician who attained Roman citizenship, aimed to create a perfect system of physiology, pathology, and treatment and formulated doctrines that were followed for 1500 years. He was one of the most prolific authors of his or any other era, having been credited with 500 treatises on medicine and some 250 others on subjects of philosophy, law, and grammar. His medical writings include descriptions of numerous drugs of natural origin with a profusion of drug formulas and methods of compounding. He originated so many preparations of vegetable drugs by mixing or melting the individual ingredients that the area of pharmaceutical preparations has been commonly referred to as "Galenic pharmacy." Perhaps the most famous of his formulas is one for a cold cream, called Galen's Cerate, which is remarkably similar in formulation to some in use today.

Pharmacy remained a function of medicine until the increasing variety of drugs and the growing complexity of compounding demanded specialists who could devote full attention to the art. Pharmacy was officially separated from medicine for the first time in 1240 A.D. when a decree of the German Emperor Frederick II regulated the practice of pharmacy within that part of his kingdom called the Two Sicilies. His edict separating the two professions acknowledged that pharmacy required special knowledge, skill, initiative, and responsibility if adequate care to the medical needs of the people was to be guaranteed. Pharmacists were obligated by oath to prepare reliable drugs of uniform quality according to their art. Any exploitation of the patient through business relations between the pharmacist and the physician was strictly forbidden. Between that time and the evolution of chemistry as an exact science, pharmacy and chemistry became united somewhat as pharmacy and medicine had been.

Perhaps no person in history exercised such a revolutionary influence on pharmacy and medicine as did Aureolus Philippus Theophrastus Bombastus von Hohenheim, a Swiss physician and chemist who called himself Paracelsus. He influenced the transformation of pharmacy from a profession based primarily on botanic science to one based on chemical science. Some of his chemical observations were astounding for his time and for their anticipation of later discoveries. He believed that it was possible to prepare a specific medicinal agent for use in combating each specific disease and introduced a host of chemical substances to internal therapy.

Early Research

As the knowledge of the basic sciences increased, so did their application to pharmacy. The opportunity was presented for the investigation of medicinal materials on a firm scientific basis, and the challenge was accepted by numerous pharmacists who conducted their research in the backrooms and basements of their pharmacies. Noteworthy among them was Karl Wilhelm Scheele (1742–1786), a Swedish pharmacist who is perhaps the most famous of all pharmacists because of his scientific genius and dramatic discoveries. Among his discoveries were the chemicals lactic acid, citric acid, oxalic acid, tartaric acid, and arsenic acid. He identified glycerin, invented new methods of preparing calomel and benzoic acid, and discovered oxygen a year prior to Priestley.

The isolation of morphine from opium by the German pharmacist Friedrich Sertürner (1783–1841) in 1805 prompted a series of isolations of other active materials from medicinal plants by a score of French pharmacists. Joseph Caventou (1795–1877) and Joseph Pelletier (1788–1842) combined their talents and isolated quinine and cinchonine from cinchona, and strychnine and brucine from nux vomica. Pelletier together with Pierre Robiquet (1780–1840) isolated caffeine, and Robiquet independently separated codeine from opium. Methodically one chemical after another was isolated from plant drugs and identified as an agent responsible for the plants' medicinal activity. Today we are still engaged in this fascinating activity as we probe nature for more useful and more specific therapeutic agents.

Throughout Europe during the late 18th century and the beginning of the 19th century, pharmacists like Pelletier and Sertürner were held in great esteem by their communities because of their intellect and technical abilities.

They applied the art and the science of pharmacy to the preparation of drug products that were of the highest standards of purity, uniformity, and efficacy possible at that time. The extraction and isolation of various active constituents from crude or unprocessed drugs were major breakthroughs in the development of concentrated dosage forms of uniform strength containing singly effective therapeutic agents of natural origin. Many pharmacists of the period began to manufacture quality pharmaceutical products on a small but steadily increasing scale to meet the growing drug needs of their communities. Some of today's gigantic pharmaceutical manufacturing companies developed from these progressive prescription laboratories of almost two centuries ago.

Although many of the drugs indigenous to America and first used by the American Indian were adopted by the settlers, the vast majority of drugs needed in this country before the 19th century were imported from Europe, either as the raw materials or as finished pharmaceutical products. With the Revolutionary War, however, it became more difficult to import drugs, and the American pharmacist was stimulated to acquire the scientific and technologic expertise of his European contemporary. From this period until the Civil War, pharmaceutical manufacture was in its infancy in this country, but some of the pharmaceutical firms established during that period are still in existence. Three firms are known to have been established before 1826, with 22 additional ones having their origin in the subsequent half century. In 1821, Philadelphia College of Pharmacy was established as the nation's first school of pharmacy.

The United States Pharmacopeia and the National Formulary

The term *pharmacopeia* comes from the Greek, *pharmakon*, meaning "drug," and *poiein*, meaning "make," and the combination indicates any recipe or formula or other standards required to make or prepare a drug. The term was first used in 1580 in connection with a local book of drug standards in Bergamo, Italy. From that time on there were countless city, state, and national pharmacopeias published by various European pharmaceutical societies. As time passed, the value of a uniform set of national drug standards became apparent. In England, for example, three city pharmacopeias—the London, the Edinburgh, and the Dublin—were

official throughout the kingdom until 1864, when they were replaced by the British Pharmacopoeia (BP).

In the United States drug standards were first provided on a national basis in 1820, when the first *United States Pharmacopeia* (USP) was published. The need for drug standards was recognized, however, in this country long before the first USP was published. For convenience and because of their familiarity with them, colonial physicians and apothecaries used the pharmacopeias and other references of their various homelands. The first American pharmacopeia was the so-called "Lititz Pharmacopeia," published in 1778 at Lititz, Pennsylvania, for use by the Military Hospital of the United States Army. It was a 32-page booklet containing information on 84 internal and 16 external drugs and preparations.

During the last decade of the 18th century, several attempts were made by various local medical societies to collate drug information, set appropriate standards, and prepare an extensive American pharmacopeia of the drugs in use at that time. In 1808 the Massachusetts Medical Society published a 272-page pharmacopeia containing information or monographs on 536 drugs and pharmaceutical preparations. Included were monographs on many drugs indigenous to America, which were not described in the European pharmacopeias of the day.

On January 6, 1817, Dr. Lyman Spalding, a physician from New York City, submitted a plan to the Medical Society of the County of New York for the creation of a national pharmacopeia. Dr. Spalding's efforts were later to result in his being recognized as the "Father of the United States Pharmacopeia." He proposed dividing the United States as then known into four geographical districts—Northern, Middle, Southern, and Western. The plan provided for calling a convention in each of these districts, to be composed of delegates from all medical societies and medical schools within them. Where there was as yet no incorporated medical society or medical school, voluntary associations of physicians and surgeons were invited to assist in the undertaking. Each district's convention was to draft a pharmacopeia and appoint delegates to a general convention to be held later in Washington, D.C. At the general convention, the four district pharmacopeias were to be compiled into a single national pharmacopeia.

Draft pharmacopeias were submitted to the convention by only the Northern and Middle districts. These were reviewed, consolidated, and adopted by the first United States Pharmacopeial Convention assembled in Washington, D.C., on January 1, 1820. The first *United States Pharmacopeia* was published on December 15, 1820, in English and also in Latin, then the international language of medicine, to render the book more intelligible to physicians and pharmacists of any nationality. Within its 272 pages were listed 217 drugs considered worthy of recognition, many of them taken from the Massachusetts Pharmacopeia, which is considered by some to be the precursor to the USP. The objective of the first USP was clearly stated in its preface and remains important. It reads in part:

"It is the objective of a Pharmacopeia to select from among substances which possess medicinal power, those, the utility of which is most fully established and best understood; and to form from them preparations and compositions, in which their powers may be exerted to the greatest advantage. It should likewise distinguish those articles by convenient and definite names, such as may prevent trouble or uncertainty in the intercourse of physicians and apothecaries."

Before adjourning, the Convention adopted a Constitution and Bylaws, with provisions for subsequent meetings of the Convention leading to a revised *United States Pharmacopeia* every 10 years. As many new drugs entered into drug therapy, the need for more frequent issuance of standards became increasingly apparent. In 1900, the Pharmacopeial Convention granted authority to issue supplements to the currently official USP whenever necessary to maintain satisfactory standards. At the 1940 meeting of the Convention, it was decided to revise the Pharmacopeia every 5 years while maintaining the use of periodic supplements. The *United States Pharmacopeia* was last revised in 1990, with the issuance of the USP XXII.

The first United States Pharmacopeial Convention was composed exclusively of physicians. In 1830, and again in 1840, prominent pharmacists were invited to assist in the revision, and recognition of their contributions pharmacists were awarded full membership in the Convention of 1850 and have participated regularly ever since. Indeed, by 1870 the *Pharmacopeia* was so nearly in the hands of pharmacists that vigorous efforts were required to revive interest in it among physicians. The present Bylaws provide that of the 6 elected members of the Board of Trustees, at least 2 shall be representative of the medical sciences and at least 2 members representative of the pharmaceutical sciences. The General Committee on Revision has a membership of 60 persons, of whom 20 shall be qualified in medical sciences and 40 in pharmaceutical and allied sciences.

After the appearance of the first USP, the art and science of both pharmacy and medicine changed remarkably. Prior to 1820, the drugs employed in the treatment of disease had been much the same for centuries. The *Pharmacopeia* of 1820 reflected the fact that the apothecary of that day was competent at collecting and identifying botanic drugs and preparing from them the mixtures and preparations required by the physician. The individual pharmacist seemed quite fulfilled as he applied his total art to the creation of elegant pharmaceutical preparations from crude botanic materials. It was a time that would never be seen again because of the impending upsurge in technologic capabilities and the steady development of the basic sciences, particularly synthetic organic chemistry.

The second half of the 19th century brought great and far-reaching changes. The United States was now under the full impact of the industrial revolution. The steam engine, which used water power to turn mills that powdered crude botanic drugs, was replaced by the gas, diesel, or electric motor. New machinery was substituted for the old whenever possible, and often machinery from other industries was adapted to the special needs of pharmaceutical manufacturing. Mixers from the baking industry, centrifugal machines from the laundry industry, and sugarcoating pans from the candy industry were a few examples of the type of improvisations made. Production increased rapidly, but the new industry had to wait for the scientific revolution before it could claim newer and better drugs for mankind. A symbiosis was needed between science and the advancing technology.

By 1880, the industrial manufacture of chemicals and pharmaceutical products had become well established in this country, and the pharmacist was relying heavily upon commercial sources for his drug supply. Synthetic organic chemistry began to have its influence on drug therapy. The isolations of some active constituents of plant drugs had led to knowledge of their chemical structure. From this arose methods of synthetically duplicating the same structures, as well as manipulating molecular structure to produce organic chemicals yet undiscovered in nature. In 1872 the synthesis of salicylic acid from phenol inaugurated the synthesis of a group of analgesic compounds. Other new chemicals synthesized for the first time were phenolphthalein, a laxative, and sleep-producing derivatives of barbituric acid called "barbiturates." A new source of drugs, synthetic organic chemistry, welcomed the turn into the 20th century.

Until this time, drugs created through the genius of the synthetic organic chemist relieved a host of maladies, but none had been found to be curative—none, that is, until 1910, when arsphenamine, a specific agent against syphilis, was introduced to medical science. This was the start of an era of *chemotherapy*, an era in which the diseases of mankind became curable through the use of specific chemical agents. The concepts, discoveries, and inspirational work that led mankind to this glorious period are credited to Paul Ehrlich, the German bacteriologist who together with a Japanese colleague, Sahachiro Hata, discovered arsphenamine. Today most of our new drugs, whether they be curative or palliative, originate in the flask of the synthetic organic chemist.

The advancement of science, both basic and applied, led to drugs of a more complex nature and to more of them. The drug standards advanced by the USP were more than ever needed to protect the public by insuring the purity and uniformity of the drugs administered.

When the American Pharmaceutical Association was organized in 1852, the only authoritative and generally recognized book of drug standards available was the third revision of the *United States Pharmacopeia*. In order to serve as a therapeutic guide to the medical profession, its scope, then as now, was restricted to drugs of established therapeutic merit. Because of this policy of strict selectivity, many drugs and formulas that were widely accepted and used by the medical profession were not granted admission to early revisions of the *Pharmacopeia*. As a type of a protest, and in keeping with the original objectives of the American Pharmaceutical Association to establish standardization of drugs and formulas, certain pharmacists, with the sanction of their national organization, prepared a formulary containing many of the popular drugs and formulas denied admission to the *Pharmacopeia*. The first edition was published in 1888 under the title *National Formulary of Unofficial Preparations*. The designation *Unofficial Preparations* reflected the protest mood of the authors, since the *Pharmacopeia* had earlier adopted the term "official" as applying to the drugs for which it provided standards. The title was changed to *National Formulary* on June 30, 1906 when President Theodore Roosevelt signed into law the first federal Pure Food and Drug Act, designating both the USP and NF as establishing legal standards for medicinal and pharmaceutic substances. Thus the two publications became *official compendia*. Among other things, the law required that whenever the designations "USP" or "NF" were used or implied on drug labeling that the products must conform to the physical and chemical standards set forth in the compendium monograph.

The early editions of the *National Formulary* served mainly as a convenience to practicing pharmacists by providing uniform names of drugs and preparations and working directions for the small-scale manufacture of popular pharmaceutical preparations prescribed by physicians. Prior to 1940, the NF, as the USP, was revised every 10 years. After that date, new editions appeared every 5 years, with supplements issued periodically as necessary.

In 1975, the United States Pharmacopeial Convention, Inc. purchased the National Formulary, unifying the official compendia and thereby provided the mechanism for a single, national compendium.

The first combined compendium, representing the USPXX and the NFXV became official on July 1, 1980. All monographs on therapeutically active drug substances appeared in the USP section of the volume, whereas all monographs on pharmaceutic agents appeared in the NF section.

The standards advanced by the *United States Pharmacopeia* and the *National Formulary* are put to active use by all members of the health care industry who share the responsibility and enjoy the public's trust for assuring the availability of quality drugs and pharmaceutical products. Included in this group are pharmacists, physicians, dentists, veterinarians, nurses, producers and suppliers of bulk chemicals for use in drug production, large and small manufacturers of pharmaceutical products, drug procurement officers of various private and public health agencies and institutions, drug regulatory and enforcement agencies, and many others.

The USP Drug Research and Testing Laboratory provides direct laboratory assistance to the *United States Pharmacopeia* and the *National Formulary*. The Laboratory's main functions are to develop specifications for new drugs, check new drug specifications proposed by others, assist in the development of official monographs, improve existing compendia monographs through the incorporation of more sophisticated analytical procedures, develop and evaluate new analytical methods which may be employed in the analysis of drugs in their basic state or in dosage forms, participate in collaborative studies with other laboratories with regard to drug standards, and to provide laboratory services regarding special problems relating to drugs and dosage forms.

As an aid to persons dispensing or administering drugs, The United States Pharmacopeial Convention, Inc. published in 1979, the first edition of the reference book, *USP Dispensing Information* (USP DI). Included were drug monographs containing information on category of use, precautions to use, side effects, dosing information and patient consultation guidelines.

Beginning in 1983, the *USP DI* was published as a two volume set: *Drug Information for the Health Care Provider*, for the health professional, and, *Advice for the Patient*, containing drug information readily understood by the layman. These volumes serve the health provider as a resource in patient consultation activities. The books also provide the basis for a program of Patient Medication Instruction (PMI). Through this program, patients receive drug-use information leaflets on the medications they are taking.

Other Pharmacopeias and Drug Standards

In addition to the USP and the NF, other references of drug standards such as the *Homeopathic Pharmacopeia of the United States* and the *International Pharmacopoeia* (IP) provide additional guidelines for drug quality required by certain practitioners and agencies. The *Homeopathic Pharmacopeia* is employed by a dwindling number of pharmacists and homeopathists and by law enforcement agencies which must insure the quality of homeopathic drugs. The term *homeopathy* was coined by Samuel Hahnemann (1755–1843) from the Greek *homoios*, meaning

similar, and *pathos*, meaning disease. In essence, the philosophy of homeopathy is that like cures like: that is, a drug that produces in healthy persons the effects or set of symptoms of the illness present will cure the disease. Embodied in the homeopathic approach are (1) the testing of a drug on healthy persons to find the drug's effects so that it may be employed against the same symptoms manifesting a disease in an ill person, (2) the use of only minute doses of drugs in therapy, (3) the administration of not more than one drug at a time, and (4) the treatment of the entire symptom complex of the patient, not just one symptom. The *Homeopathic Pharmacopeia* is essential for pharmacists who prepare drugs to be used in the practice of homeopathy.

The *Pharmacopoeia Internationalis*, or *International Pharmacopoeia*, is published by the World Health Organization (WHO) of the United Nations with the cooperation of member countries. It is intended as a recommendation to national pharmacopeial revision committees to modify their respective pharmacopeias according to the international standards adopted. It has no legal authority, only the mutual respect and recognition accorded it by the participating countries in their joint effort to provide acceptable drug standards on an international basis. The first volume of the *Pharmacopoeia Internationalis* was published in 1951. It has been revised periodically since that time.

A number of countries publish their own pharmacopeias, including Great Britain, France, Italy, Japan, India, East Germany, Norway, and the Union of Soviet Socialist Republics. Many of these pharmacopeias are utilized by multinational companies who develop and market products on an international basis. Countries not having a national pharmacopeia frequently adopt one of another country for their use in setting and regulating drug standards. The pharmacopeia selected is usually one based on geographic proximity, a common heritage or language, or a similarity of drugs and pharmaceutical products used.

In the United States, in addition to the official compendia, important drug standards are provided by means of the specifications set forth in individual New Drug and Antibiotic Applications approved by the Food and Drug Administration. The approved standards for individually marketed drugs must be rigidly adhered to by the manufacturer thereby maintaining the established quality of the product.

The Development of New Drugs

In the broad sense, the pharmaceutical industry encompasses all persons involved or required between the time a drug is first envisioned in the mind of a scientist to the time it is consumed by the patient. In the narrow sense, it refers to the pharmaceutical research and manufacturing companies providing pharmacists with medicines in prefabricated or ready-to-take form. Some firms specialize in manufacturing *proprietary* drug products, or those sold over-the-counter and advertised and promoted directly to the public. Other firms limit their activities to the production of *ethical* pharmaceuticals, or those products that may be prescription drugs or over-the-counter drugs but are promoted directly to the medical and pharmaceutical practitioner and not to the general public. Many of the large companies manufacture both categories of pharmaceuticals with some having subsidiary companies to specialize in either of the two functions.

The pharmaceutical industry in the United States grew phenomenally during World War II and in the years immediately following. The upsurge in the domestic production of drugs and pharmaceutical products stemmed in part from the wartime hazards and consequent undependability of overseas shipping, the unavailability of drugs from former sources in the enemy camp or control, and the increased need for drugs of all kinds, especially those of life-saving capabilities. One such drug is penicillin, which became commercially available in 1944, some 15 years after serendipitous discovery in England by Sir Alexander Fleming. The delay in the development of penicillin was in part due to a poor appreciation for its potential, and thus for many years it was not investigated with the required vigor.

After the war, other antibiotics were developed and today there is a host of them, some effective against limited types of microorganisms with others having a broad range of activity against pathogens. The postwar boom in drug discovery continued and has provided many drugs important to the conquest of disease. Vaccines, such as those effective in preventing poliomyelitis, measles, and influenza, have been as beneficial to mankind in preventing disease as have the antibiotic drugs in curing disease. New pharmacologic categories of drugs were developed in this period, including oral hypoglycemic drugs effective against certain types of diabetes mellitus, antineoplastic drugs active against the cancerous process, immunosuppressive agents which assist the body's acceptance of organ transplants, oral contraceptives, which prevent pregnancy, and a host of tranquilizers and antidepressant drugs that provide assistance to the emotionally distraught or distressed.

Most of the basic and applied research leading to the development of new drugs and ethical pharmaceuticals is performed by the major drug companies, which comprise the membership of the Pharmaceutical Manufacturers Association (the PMA), an organization founded in 1958 as the successor to the American Pharmaceutical Manufacturers Association and the American Drug Manufacturers Association. It is generally regarded as the spokesman for the prescription-drug manufacturers in matters of medical and pharmaceutical science, technologic advancements in drug manufacturing methods, and drug marketing matters. Its member companies and their domestic and international subsidiaries have provided world-wide leadership in the creation and development of new drugs and pharmaceutical products. New drugs are also being created in the laboratories of research scientists employed by academic and nonprofit research institutions; however, they too are ultimately supplied as finished drug products to the community pharmacist by the industrial pharmaceutical manufacturing firms.

Sources of New Drugs

New drugs may be discovered from a variety of natural sources or created synthetically in the laboratory. They may be found quite by accident or as the result of many years of tireless pursuit.

Throughout history, plant materials have served as a reservoir of potential new drugs. Only a small portion of the plant species thus far identified have been investigated for medicinal agents. Certain major contributions to modern drug therapy may be attributed to the successful conversion of botanic folklore remedies into modern wonder drugs. The chemical reserpine, a tranquilizer and hypotensive agent, is an example of a medicinal chemical isolated by design from the folklore remedy *Rauwolfia serpentina*. Another plant drug, periwinkle or

Vinca rosea, was scientifically investigated as a result of its reputation in folklore as an agent useful in the treatment of diabetes mellitus. Plant extractives yielded two potent drugs, which when screened for pharmacologic activity surprisingly exhibited antitumor capabilities. These two materials, vinblastine and vincristine, since have been used successfully in prolonging life and reducing the suffering of patients afflicted with certain types of cancer. After the isolation and structural identification of active plant constituents, organic chemists may recreate them by total synthesis in the laboratory or more importantly use the natural chemical as the starting material in the creation of slightly different chemical structures through molecule manipulation procedures. The new structures, termed semisynthetic drugs, may have a slightly or vastly different pharmacologic activity than the starting substance, depending upon the nature and extent of chemical alteration. Other plant constituents which in themselves may be inactive or rather unimportant therapeutically may be employed in the semisynthetic process to yield important drugs with profound pharmacologic activity. For example, the various species of *Dioscorea,* popularly known as Mexican yams, are rich in a chemical nucleus called the "steroid" structure from which hormonal chemicals like cortisone and estrogens, the female sex hormones, are semisynthetically produced.

Animals have served man in his search for drugs in a number of ways. They not only have yielded to drug testing and biologic assay procedures but also have provided drugs fashioned from their own tissues or through their biologic processes. Hormonal substances such as thyroid extract, insulin, and pituitary hormone obtained from the endocrine glands of cattle, sheep, and swine are lifesaving drugs employed daily as replacement therapy in the human body. The urine of pregnant mares is a rich source of estrogens. Knowledge of the structural architecture of the individual hormonal substances has led to the production of a variety of synthetic and semisynthetic compounds with hormone-like activity. The synthetic chemicals in oral contraceptive agents are a notable example. The use of animals in the production of various biologic products, including serums, antitoxins, and vaccines, has been of lifesaving significance ever since the pioneering work of Dr. Edward Jenner on the smallpox vaccine in England in 1796. Today, the poliomyelitis vaccine is prepared in cultures of minced monkey tissue, the mumps and influenza vaccines in fluids of the chick embryo, the rubella (German measles) vaccine in duck embryo and the smallpox vaccine in chick embryonic fluid or from the lymph of calves inoculated with vaccinia virus. Tomorrow, vaccines for diseases as AIDS and cancer may be developed through the utilization of cell and tissue cultures.

Today we are witnessing a new era in the development of pharmaceutical products due to the advent of genetic engineering, the sub-microscopic manipulation of the "double helix," the spiral DNA chain of life. And with this process, will come less expensive, more abundant, and vastly purer antibiotics, vaccines, and yet unknown chemical and biological products to combat human disease.[2]

There are two basic technologies that drive the genetic field of drug development; they are, recombinant DNA and monoclonal antibody production. Common to each technique is the ability to manipulate and produce proteins, the building blocks of living matter. Proteins represent an almost infinite source of drugs. Made up of long chains of amino acids, their sequence and spatial configuration offer a staggering number of possibilities. Both recombinant DNA and monoclonal antibody production techniques influence cells in their ability to produce proteins.

The more fundamental of the two techniques is recombinant DNA. It can potentially produce almost any protein. It is possible to transplant genetic material from higher species such as man into a lowly bacterium. This so-called "gene splicing" can induce the lower organism to make proteins it would not otherwise have made. Such drug products as human insulin, human growth hormone, and interferon may be produced in this manner. Recombinant techniques are also capable of producing new and extremely pure vaccines and other biological products.

Whereas recombinant DNA techniques involve the manipulation of proteins within the cells of lower animals, monoclonal antibody production is conducted entirely within the cells of higher animals, including the patient. The technique exploits the ability of cells that have the potential to produce a desired antibody and stimulates an unending stream of pure antibody production. These antibodies then have the capacity to combat the specific target.

Monoclonal antibodies have an enormous potential to change the face of medicine and pharmacy in the next decade and applications for their use are already in progress. Diagnostically, for example, monoclonal antibodies are used in home pregnancy testing products. Their use ensures that a woman can perform the test easily, in a short period of time, with high reproducibility, and in an inexpensive manner. In these tests, the monoclonal antibody is highly sensitive to binding upon one site on the human chorionic gonadotropin (HCG) molecule, a specific marker to pregnancy because in healthy women, HCG is synthesized exclusively by the placenta. In medicine, monoclonal antibodies are being used to stage and to localize malignant cells of cancer, and it is anticipated that they will be used in the future to combat disease such as lupus erythematosus, juvenile-onset diabetes, and myasthenia gravis.

However, today's most usual source of potential drugs is the flask of the synthetic organic chemist. Through his art he creates not only chemical modifications of known structures but also totally new synthetic organic compounds. These new chemical entities may resemble older drugs in both chemical structure and pharmacologic activity and, indeed, may be synthesized for that very reason. The modern sophisticated computer assists the process through the use of software packages on molecular modeling.

A drug need not be a new chemical entity to be considered a "new drug" by the Food and Drug Administration and therefore subject to the aforementioned requirements for proof of safety and efficacy. A well-known chemical formulated in a new manner with different excipients, coatings, solvents, vehicles, or other formulative materials results in a pharmaceutical product that has not been examined for safety and efficacy and therefore is a "new drug" under the law. It is well recognized that different methods of manufacture or different formulative additives can considerably alter the therapeutic efficacy of a product through chemical or physical interference with the therapeutic agents. A new combination of two or more old drugs or a change in the usual proportions of drugs in an established combination product can be considered "new" if a question of safety or efficacy is introduced by the alteration. A proposed new use for an old drug, a new dosage schedule or regimen, a proposed new route of administration, or a new dosage form can cause an old drug to be reconsidered for safety and efficacy.

A classic example of the need to evaluate safety and efficacy after reformulation is the emerging liposome technology. This technology may rescue some drugs, e.g., amphotericin B, doxorubicin HCl, whose use now is limited by dose-related toxicity. Basically, the drug is trapped within phospholipid vesicles which have the potential to adsorb to many body cell types to be endocytosed and release their contents. Future research will involve linking the liposomes to antigen-specific antibodies to specific target organs within the body to enhance the efficacy of the entrapped drug. Lastly, an old drug also may be considered "new" if the proposed manufacturer of it has never before received FDA approval for marketing the product even though his competitors have.

Drug Product Development and Marketing

As depicted in Figure 1–2, drug product development activities begin during the early stages of the investigation of a new drug and continue through the actual manufacturing or production of the product.

The new drug substance, which may be produced by organic synthesis, fermentation, or extraction, must be prepared in sufficient quantity to meet the projected large scale production of the dosage form. This scale-up work is generally performed by the organic chemists and chemical engineers of the process research and development group. Similarly, the product development scientists who developed the initial drug formulation in pilot plant work, collaborate with the technical people in the production area, engineers, machinists, and quality control specialists in developing the capability for the large scale production of the dosage form. Once in actual production, the mechanics, electricians, plumbers, and other maintenance personnel ensure continued function of the complex machinery. In-plant information systems and control procedures are developed to conform with established good manufacturing practice. Double check systems and methods of electronic data processing are integrated into the quality control procedures.

Throughout the developmental stages, exten-

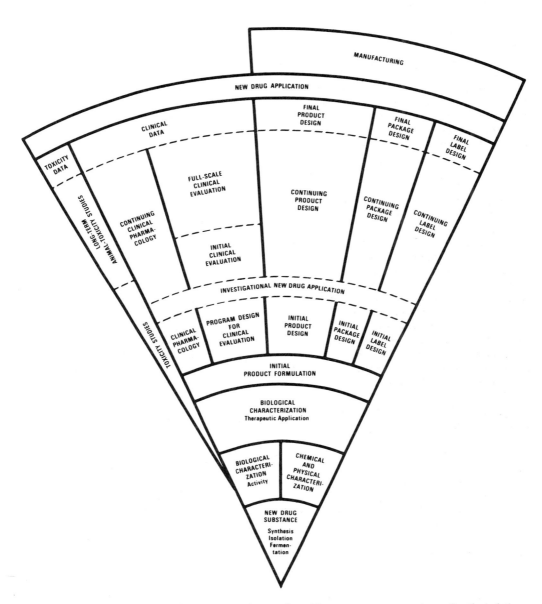

Fig. 1–2. *Schematic representation of development of a new drug. Five years or more may elapse after the isolation or synthesis of a new drug substance before it becomes available as a pharmaceutical product. During this period each new substance is subjected to intensive testing and study, first to characterize its activity and then to determine its safety and effectiveness. (Courtesy of Eli Lilly and Company.)*

sive testing must be undertaken to ensure the chemical and physical stability of the product. Drug stability in proposed packaging materials must be tested as well as stability under various conditions of storage.

The legal department is active in the development of patent protection for the new drug and for the assignment of a trademark name. Together with the medical department, they work to develop product literature, labeling, and promotion materials. This work involves interaction with literature scientists, the art and printing departments, and the plastics, glass, paper, or other container and packaging suppliers. Marketing analysts, the financial department, and sales personnel become involved in the upcoming promotion of the product to the prescribing practitioner.

As the drug is first advertised and promoted to the medical profession through professional journals, direct mailing, and personal visits by the manufacturer's professional representatives, the drug products are being shipped to the wholesale drug firms, hospitals, and community pharmacies throughout the nation. With the writing of the first prescription for the product by the physician, the filling of the order by the community or institutional pharmacist, and the taking of the drug by the patient, the product joins the armamentarium of drug therapy. Typically a pharmaceutical manufacturer prepares the drug substance into a number of dosage forms each having a special purpose.

The Need for Standards for Safety and Efficacy

The importance of drug standards, even among the nontherapeutic pharmaceutical necessities employed in product formulations, was tragically demonstrated in 1938. The then-new wonder drug, sulfanilamide, which was not soluble in most commonly used pharmaceutical solvents of the day, was prepared and distributed by a reputable manufacturer as an elixir, solubilized with diethylene glycol. Before the product could be removed from the market, over 100 persons had lost their lives due to the toxic effects of the formulation's solvent, diethylene glycol. The necessity for proper product formulation and for thorough pharmacologic testing of the therapeutic agent and of the completed pharmaceutical product was painfully recognized. Congress responded with the Federal Food, Drug, and Cosmetic Act of 1938 and

the creation of the Food and Drug Administration (FDA) to administer and enforce it. Included in the Act is a provision that prohibits the use of any new drug without the prior filing of a New Drug Application (NDA) with the Food and Drug Administration. The officials of the FDA grant or deny permission to distribute a new product after reviewing the applicant's filed data on the product's ingredients, manufacturing processes, toxicologic studies on animals, therapeutic claims, and clinical trials on human beings. Although the Act of 1938 required pharmaceutical products to be safe for human use, it should be noted that it did not require them to be efficacious.

By its nature, medical progress involves risk, for no drug is guaranteed completely safe and no drug is completely understood. This lack of understanding resulted in a major drug tragedy in 1960.[3] A new synthetic drug, called thalidomide, recommended as a sedative and tranquilizer, was being sold in Europe without the requirement of a physician's prescription. It was a drug of especial interest due to its apparent lack of toxicity even at extreme dosage levels. It was hoped that it would replace the barbiturates in popularity as a sedative and therefore prevent the frequent deaths caused from accidental and intentional overdosage with barbiturates. An American firm was awaiting FDA approval for marketing in this country when reports of a strange effect of the drug's use began to filter in from Europe. Thalidomide given to women during pregnancy produced phocomelia or an arrested development of the limbs of the newborn infant. Thousands of children were affected to various extents. Some were born with neither arms nor legs; others, with partially formed limbs. The more fortunate were born with only disfigurations of the nose, eyes, and ears. Those more severely afflicted died, the result of internal malformation of the heart or gastrointestinal tract. This drug catastrophe, which for the most part did not affect American citizens, spurred Congress to strengthen the existing laws regarding new drugs. Without dissent, on October 10, 1962, the Kefauver-Harris Drug Amendments to the Food, Drug, and Cosmetic Act of 1938 were passed by both houses of Congress. The purpose of the enactment was to insure a greater amount of safety in the drugs made available to our citizens, and for the first time the manufacturer was required to prove the drug efficacious before it would be granted FDA approval for marketing.

Preclinical (Animal) Studies and the Clinical (Human) Testing of New Drugs

Under the Food, Drug and Cosmetic Act as amended, the sponsor of a new drug (usually a drug manufacturer, but occasionally a research institution, an individual or a group of medical researchers) is required to file with the FDA a "Notice of Claimed Investigational Exemption for a New Drug" (IND) before the drug can be clinically tested on human beings. After submission of such a notice, the investigator must delay use of the drug in human subjects for a period of not less than 30 days from the date the FDA acknowledges receipt of the IND. This 30-day period may be waived or extended by the FDA upon a showing of good cause.

Among the items included in the IND are the following: the name and address of the sponsor of the drug; the name and chemical description of the drug substance to be investigated; a quantitative list of the active and inactive components of the dosage form to be administered; the source or supplier and method of preparation of the drug to be administered; a statement relating to the methods, facilities, and controls employed in the manufacture, processing, packaging and labeling of the new drug to assure appropriate standards of identity, strength, quality, and purity; a thorough presentation of all preclinical (animal) studies of the drug including the names and qualifications of the investigators and the names and locations of the laboratories in which the work was performed; the relation between the preclinical studies and the proposed clinical studies; information on any clinical studies performed in other countries and any related bibliography of publications on the new drug; if the new drug is a combination of previously investigated components, a complete preclinical and clinical summary of these components when administered singly and any data or expectations relating to the effect when combined; copies of labeling and other pertinent information to be distributed to the proposed clinical investigators of the drug; the names and summaries of the training and experience of the proposed clinical investigators; the name of the persons following the progress of the study and collating and evaluating the data received from the investigators; a description of the facilities in which the drug will be investigated; and a complete protocol on the methodology to be employed in the clinical investigation, including the method of selection of subjects for the investigation, the method and route of drug administration, the studies to be performed in the evaluation of the safety and effectiveness of the new drug, and the assurance of the safety and protection of the human subjects participating in the investigation (Fig. 1–3).

The human subjects participating in these clinical investigations do so at their own choosing. The sponsor of the investigation must certify that each person who will receive the drug during the investigational period will give his *informed consent*; that is, he will be informed of the purpose and nature of the investigation and the potential risks involved, and will give his written consent to participate. Appropriate consent forms are used for this purpose.

The Investigational Drug Branch of the FDA is charged with the responsibility of reviewing and evaluating the applications for clinical testing. A sponsor of a new drug will usually be permitted to proceed with his clinical investigation if the IND submitted is complete and the Agency is satisfied with the preclinical data and the entire protocol of the planned investigation. There are currently four "phases" to the clinical investigation of a drug, with each one entered into only after the successful completion of the preceding phase (Table 1–1).

Phase 1 of clinical testing generally involves a small number (20 to 100) of carefully chosen, *healthy volunteers*. The initial dose of the drug administered is usually quite low, based on the prior experience with animal studies. If the first dose is well tolerated, the investigation is continued with the administration of additional and carefully scheduled doses. Throughout the investigation, the subjects are closely observed and examined by expert clinicians. Among the basic data collected during this phase include the rate of the drug's absorption; the rate and level of its concentration in the blood; its rate and method of elimination from the body, and toxicological effect, if any, in body tissues and major organs; and changes in the blood forming organs or in the normal physiologic processes of the body. The subjects' ability to tolerate the drug are observed and any unpleasant effects of the drug are recorded. If Phase 1 is successful in demonstrating sufficient tolerance to the drug and if the order of toxicity remains low,

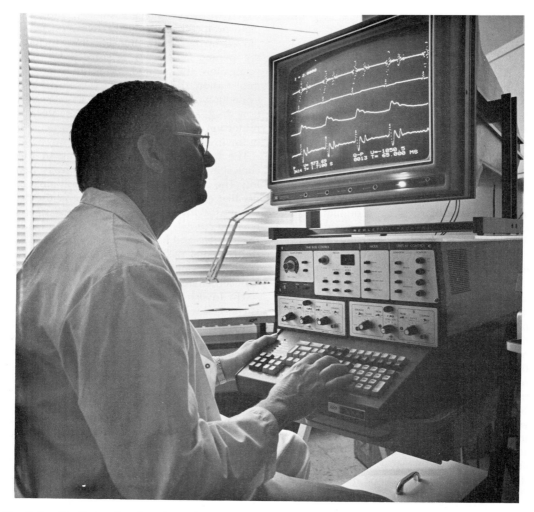

Fig. 1–3. *Monitoring the effects for cardiac function of an investigational drug as a part of its clinical evaluation. (Courtesy of Eli Lilly and Company.)*

Phase 2 of clinical testing is begun utilizing up to several hundred patients.

Patients suffering from a malady against which the new drug indicated promise through its pharmacological activity are treated in limited numbers and under close observation during *Phase 2* of clinical testing. The main purpose of Phase 2 is to determine the efficacy of the new drug in treating the disease against which it is being tested and to detect side effects or toxicity symptoms not manifest in the animal studies or in studies with healthy volunteers.

Clinicians familiar with the disease being treated with the investigational drug are utilized during Phase 2 studies. During this phase, ad-

ditional data are collected relating to the drug's patterns of absorption, distribution, and excretion, and drug metabolites which may be formed are identified. Each patient is monitored for the appearance of side effects while the dose of the drug is carefully increased to determine the minimal effective dose. Following this determination, the dose is extended beyond the minimally effective dose to ascertain the dosage level at which a patient reveals extremely undesirable or intolerable toxic or adverse effects from the drug. The greater the range between the amount of drug determined to be minimally effective and that determined to cause severe side effects, the greater is the safety margin of

Table 1–1. Phases of Clinical Testing

	Number of Patients	Length	Purpose	Percent of Drugs Successfully Completing*
Phase 1:	20–100	Several months	Mainly safety	67%
Phase 2:	Up to several hundred	Several months to 2 years	Some short-term safety, but mainly effectiveness	45%
Phase 3:	Several hundred to several thousand	1–4 years	Safety, effectiveness, dosage	5–10%

*For example, of 20 drugs entering clinical testing, 13 or 14 will successfully complete phase 1 trials and go on to phase 2; about nine will complete phase 2 and go to phase 3; only one or two will clear phase 3 and, on average, about one of the original 20 will ultimately be approved for marketing. (Reference: *FDA Consumer*, 21:12, 1987.)

the drug and the greater the promise for effective use in drug therapy.

If the clinical results of Phase 2 indicate continued promise for the new drug and if the margin of safety appears to be good, *Phase 3* may be embarked upon. In this phase, private practitioners of varying backgrounds and experiences are brought into the investigations by the more experienced clinicians. The objective is to determine the usefulness of the new drug in the hands of the community practitioner. Depending upon the nature of the drug and the disease for which it is recommended, this phase may involve a thousand or more patients. During this phase, the participating practitioners report on their findings to the principal investigator of the new drug and he relays the information and his evaluation to the Food and Drug Administration. Information about possible adverse effects due to the drug are evaluated upon receipt and the information disseminated to all participating practitioners. Should the data warrant it, a clinical investigation may be terminated at any point during the clinical trials.

If during these three phases of clinical testing the drug demonstrates sufficient safety and significant therapeutic effect, the sponsor of the drug may file a New Drug Application (NDA) with the Food and Drug Administration. The application contains a highly organized and complete presentation of all of the preclinical and clinical data that the sponsor has obtained during his investigation of the drug. In addition, the sponsor presents drug stability data and precise information regarding dosage form composition, method of manufacture, docu-

mentation of product uniformity as obtained from pilot plant studies, and proposed product labeling. This application is studied by the Food and Drug Administration, which decides whether to allow the sponsor to market the drug, to disallow marketing, or to require additional data before rendering a judgment. Should the sponsor of the drug be accorded a favorable decision, the FDA continues to require good manufacturing procedures, adequate scientific control over these procedures, continued receipt of information pertinent to the drug's side effects and toxicity, fairness in promotion and advertising, and above all the right to remove the drug from the market, temporarily or permanently, should further study later be justified. The time course from the initial synthesis of a new drug compound to approval for marketing by the FDA is shown in Figure 1–4. On average, approximately 8 to 9 years are required for this research and evaluation process.

Currently only a small proportion of the drugs that enter human testing reach the market. The others are dropped from consideration because they have unacceptable toxicity, they fail to produce the desired therapeutic effects, or the potential market for sales has been determined to be insufficient to justify continued developmental expense.[4]

The receipt of marketing status for a new drug product does not terminate a company's investigation of the activity of the drug. Continued clinical investigations, often referred to as *Phase 4* studies, add to the understanding of the mechanism of the drug's actions and frequently

New Drug Development

Pre-Clinical Research and Development	Clinical Research and Development	NDA Review	Post-Marketing Surveillance
Initial Synthesis and Characterization	Phase 1 → Phase 2 → Phase 3 →		Adverse Reaction Reporting Surveys / Sampling Testing
Animal Testing Short-Term → Long-Term →			Inspections
Range: 1-3 Years Average: 18 Months	Range: 2-10 Years Average: 5 Years	Range: 2 Months-7 Years Average: 24 Months	

FDA 30-Day Safety Review   NDA Submitted   NDA Approved

|← Average of Approx. 100 months from initial synthesis to approval of NDA →|

Fig. 1–4. *Time course for the development of a new drug. (Adapted from FDA Consumer, 21:5, 1987.)*

reveal new therapeutic applications or indications for the drug. Should the drug demonstrate usefulness in treating patients with diseases or illnesses other than that for which the drug was originally approved, the drug's sponsor can apply to the FDA for permission to promote and market the drug for the "new indication." The FDA would once again evaluate the new clinical data and make a determination. Postmarketing studies may continue as long as useful information is gathered on the safety and effectiveness of the product. As additional experience is gained with the drug, newly revealed adverse effects may also be generated and new cautions or restrictions to the use of the drug imposed.

In 1980, the Joint Commission on Prescription Drug Use, Inc. issued its final report on prescription drug use. The report encouraged and recommended that the FDA, drug product manufacturers and health professionals work together on post-marketing surveillance (PMS). This process systematically and comprehensively monitors the patterns of use and the ben-

eficial or harmful effects of prescription drugs as they are used in medical practice (or over-the-counter drugs as they are used by the consumer).

Additional Standards for Safety and Effectiveness

Following the full implementation of the procedures required for the evaluation of new drugs, the FDA turned its attention to the examination of products which had entered the marketplace between 1938 and 1962 and thus were never reviewed and "approved" under the same criteria for safety and efficacy as were the drugs marketed after 1962. The FDA initiated this Drug Efficacy Study in 1966 through an agreement reached with the National Academy of Sciences-National Research Council (NAS/NRC) for the review for safety and efficacy of some 4000 drug products then on the market. The NAS/NRC review was conducted by 30 panels of physicians, all experts in their fields. The drug products reviewed were primarily prescription drugs; however, over 400 nonprescription drugs were included in the study. In 1969, upon receipt of the NAS/NRC findings, a special task force of the FDA's Bureau of Drugs, called the Drug Efficacy Study Implementation (DESI) Project Office, began reviewing the NAS/NRC recommendations, preparing FDA findings, and setting up the necessary procedures for implementation through regulation. The products that were found to comply with the statutory requirements for safety and efficacy and bore correct labeling were allowed to remain on the market. Those that did not comply were either removed from the market by regulatory action or required to make the necessary changes in labeling, formulation, or submission of suitable additional data as was considered necessary to conform to the regulatory requirements. Through a 1970 FDA regulation, the opportunity for a drug sponsor to submit an Abbreviated New Drug Application (ANDA) was established. It provides an expeditious review and approval process for those drug products that were initially marketed in the period 1938–1962 and for which the FDA has information on the drug substance/product on file. The ANDA enables the manufacturer to expeditiously market a new dosage form of the approved drug or alter its formulation. Generally, the clinical investigations are not required to be repeated.

Changes to speed up the process of approval of ANDAs for generic drugs were a major component of the Drug Price Competition and Patent Restoration Act of 1984. Under the provisions of the legislation, generic copies of a pioneer drug (originally approved drug) can be approved if the generic is identical to the original drug, or, so similar that the FDA determines that the differences do not require additional tests for safety or efficacy. The legislation also provides an extension of patent-life for patented drugs, equal to the time required for NDA approval, plus half the time spent in the testing phase, for a maximum of 5 years.

An outgrowth of the NAS/NRC Drug Efficacy Study was the review by the FDA of "combination" prescription products; that is, products containing two or more medicinal agents in a fixed dosage unit as a tablet, capsule or teaspoonful. Among the disadvantages cited in the use of fixed combination products include the lack of flexibility in adjusting the dosage of each

therapeutic component to meet an individual patient's needs, the exposure of patients to additional and unnecessary drugs when perhaps a single drug would meet the therapeutic requirements, and the increased possibility of adverse drug reactions through the administration of multiple drugs, perhaps without increasing efficacy. The advantages cited for the use of fixed combination products include the likelihood of greater adherence to a therapeutic regimen by the patient, and greater patient convenience and economy than if each of the therapeutic ingredients was given separately but concurrently.

The essence of the Agency regulations, issued in October, 1971, held that combination products must offer to the patient a therapeutic advantage over any of the components administered separately. Thus, when two or more medicinal agents are combined into a single dosage unit, each must effectively contribute to the therapeutic claims for the product. Further, the dosage of each component must be at a level which is both safe and effective for a significant number of patients who require concurrent therapy with the drugs in the combination product. It is also permitted to add a second drug to a first if the added drug enhances the safety or effectiveness of the principal ingredient or minimizes the potential for abuse of the principal ingredient.

Another major effort of the Food and Drug Administration in achieving the goals of the 1962 Drug Amendments involved the massive review of nonprescription drug products. This effort which began in 1972 involved the use of expert scientific panels to review the safety, effectiveness, and labeling of the various categories of nonprescription drugs. As was the case with prescription drugs, products not conforming to the established standards were to be removed from the market unless they were reformulated, relabeled or otherwise changed to meet the prevailing standards.

In another development related to drug product effectiveness, the Food and Drug Administration, the American Pharmaceutical Association, the Academy of Pharmaceutical Sciences, the USP, the NF, and other scientific and professional bodies, organizations, and agencies have become increasingly interested in drug *bioavailability* studies. Bioavailability has been defined as:[5]

"The extent and rate of absorption from a dosage form as reflected by a time-concentration curve of the administered drug in the systemic circulation."

It has become well established that the rate and extent to which a drug in a dosage form becomes available for biologic absorption or utilization depends in great measure upon the materials utilized in the formulation and also on the method of manufacture. Thus, the same drug when formulated in *different* dosage forms may be found to possess different bioavailability characteristics and thus exhibit different clinical effectiveness. Further, two seemingly "identical" or "equivalent" products, of the same drug, in the same dosage strength and in the *same* dosage form type, but differing in formulative materials or method of manufacture, may vary widely in bioavailability and thus in clinical effectiveness. The following terms may be used to define the type or level of "equivalency" between drug products.[5,6]

> *Pharmaceutical equivalents*—Drug products that contain the same amount of the same therapeutically active ingredient(s) in the same dosage form.
> *Biological equivalents* (bioequivalents)—Pharmaceutical equivalents which, when administered to the same individuals in the same dosage regimen, will result in comparable bioavailability.
> *Therapeutic equivalents*—Pharmaceutical equivalents which, when administered to the same individuals in the same dosage regimen, will provide essentially the same therapeutic effect.

The FDA, through its publication "Approved Drug Products with Therapeutic Equivalent Evaluations" commonly referred to as the "FDA Orange Book" because of its color, provides the pharmacist with information on multiple-source drugs that are deemed therapeutically equivalent or inequivalent.

Drug bioavailability is an important measure of the efficacy of dosage forms in acting as drug delivery systems. The various criteria for the design and development of effective dosage forms are discussed more thoroughly in Chapter 3.

Drug Listing Act

The Drug Listing Act of 1972 was enacted to provide the Food and Drug Administration with the legislative authority to compile a list of currently marketed drugs to assist the Agency in the enforcement of Federal laws requiring that drugs be safe and effective and not adulterated or misbranded. Under the regulations of the Act, each firm which manufactures or repackages drugs for ultimate sale or distribution to patients or consumers must register with the FDA and submit appropriate information for listing. All foreign drug manufacturing and distributing firms whose products are imported into the United States are also included in this regulation. Exempt from the registration and listing requirement are hospitals, clinics, and the various health practitioners who prepare pharmaceutical products for use in their respective institutions and practices. Also exempt are research and teaching institutions in which drug products are prepared for purposes other than sale. Each registrant is assigned a permanent registration number, following the format of the National Drug Code (NDC) numbering system. Under this system, the first 4 numeric characteristics of 10-character code identify the manufacturer or distributor and are referred to as the "Labeler Code." The last 6 numeric characters of the 10-character code identify the drug formulation and the trade package size and type. The segment which identifies the drug formulation is known as the "Product Code," and the segment which identifies the trade package size and type is called the "Package Code." The manufacturer or distributor determines the ratio of use of the last 6 digits for the two codes, as a 3-to-3 digit Product-Code-Package Code configuration (e.g. 542-112) or a 4-to-2 digit configuration (e.g. 5421-12). Only one such type of configuration may be selected for use by a manufacturer or distributor who then assigns a code number to each of his products to be included in the drug listing. A final code number is presented as the example: "NDC 0081-5421-12."

The FDA requests that the National Drug Code number appear on all drug labeling, including the label of any prescription drug container furnished to a consumer. In some instances, manufacturers imprint the NDC number directly on the dosage units, as capsules and tablets, for rapid and positive identification when the number is matched in the *National Drug Code Directory* or against a decoding list provided by the manufacturer. Once a number is assigned to a drug product it is a permanent assignment. Even in instances in which a drug manufacturer discontinues the manufacture and distribution of a product, the number may not be used again. If a drug product is substantially changed, as through an alteration in the active ingredients, dosage form, or product name, a new NDC number is assigned to the product by the registrant and the FDA advised accordingly.

The product information received by the FDA is processed and stored by computer to provide easy access to the following types of information:

1. A list of all drug products.
2. A list of all drug products broken down by labeled indications or pharmacologic category.
3. A list of all drug products, broken down by manufacturer.
4. A list of a drug product's active ingredients.
5. A list of a drug product's inactive ingredients.
6. A list of drug products containing a particular ingredient.
7. A list of drug products newly marketed or remarketed.
8. A list of drug products discontinued.
9. All labeling of drug products.
10. All advertising of drug products.

The drug listing program enables the FDA to monitor the quality of all drugs on the market in this country.

In a continuing effort to assure the standards for drug quality control, the Food and Drug Administration's regulations provide not only for the inspection and certification of pharmaceutical manufacturing procedures and facilities, but also for the field surveillance and assay of products obtained from the shelves of retail distributors.

In instances in which it is found that a manufacturer is not meeting the established standards for drug product quality, that manufacturer will be denied permission to continue to produce products for distribution until compliance with the standards is attained.

Classification of Drugs

Drugs approved for marketing by the Food and Drug Administration are categorized according to the manner in which they may be legally obtained by the patient. Drugs deemed safe enough for use by the layman in the self-treatment of simple conditions for which competent medical care is not generally sought are classified as "over-the-counter" (O.T.C.) drugs and may be sold without the requirement of a physician's prescription. This status assigned to a drug product by the FDA may be changed should more stringent control over the drug's distribution and use later be warranted. Other drugs that are considered useful only after expert diagnosis or too dangerous for use in self-medication are made available only on the prescription of a licensed practitioner. These drugs are referred to as "Legend" drugs, because it is a requirement of their labeling to bear the legend: "Caution: Federal Law Prohibits Dispensing Without Prescription," under the provisions of the Durham-Humphrey Amendment of 1952 to the Federal Food, Drug, and Cosmetic Act. Drugs so designated may also change legal status from time to time according to the judgments of the Food and Drug Administration and the firm that distributes the product. New drugs that have not been shown to be safe in self-medication are generally limited to prescription dispensing until such time that they are considered useful and safe enough for the layman to use at his discretion.

According to the Durham-Humphrey Amendment, prescriptions for Legend drugs may not be refilled (dispensed again after the initial filling of the prescription) without the express consent of the prescriber. The refill status of prescriptions for certain Legend drugs known to be subject to public abuse was further regulated with the passage of the Drug Abuse Control Amendments of 1965 and then by the Comprehensive Drug Abuse Prevention and Control Act of 1970.

The Comprehensive Drug Abuse Prevention and Control Act of 1970 served to consolidate and codify drug control authority into a single statute. Under its provisions, the Drug Abuse Control Amendments of 1965, the Harrison Narcotic Act of 1914, and other related laws governing stimulants, depressants, narcotics and hallucinogenics were repealed and replaced by regulatory framework administered by the Bureau of Narcotics and Dangerous Drugs (BNDD) of the Department of Justice. In 1973, under another reorganization plan, the Drug Enforcement Administration (DEA) was established in the Department of Justice and took over the functions of the Bureau of Narcotics and Dangerous Drugs (which was abolished) and also the drug intelligence, investigation, and enforcement roles of several other governmental agencies.

The Comprehensive Drug Abuse Prevention and Control Act of 1970 established five "Schedules" for the classification and control of drug substances which are subject to public abuse. These schedules, which continue in effect under the jurisdiction of the DEA, provide for decreasing levels of control from Schedule I drugs to those classified as Schedule V drugs. The drugs in the five Schedules may be described as follows:

Schedule I—Drugs with no accepted medical use, or other substances, with a high potential for abuse. In this category are heroin, LSD, and similar items, but virtually any non-medical substance that is being abused can be placed in this category.

Schedule II—Drugs with accepted medical uses and a high potential for abuse which, if abused, may lead to severe psychological or physical dependence.

Schedule III—Drugs with accepted medical uses and a potential for abuse less than those listed in Schedules I and II which, if abused, may lead to moderate psychological or physical dependence.

Schedule IV—Drugs with accepted medical uses and low potential for abuse relative to those in Schedule III which, if abused, may lead to limited physical dependence or psychological dependence relative to drugs in Schedule III.

Schedule V—Drugs with accepted medical uses and low potential for abuse relative to those in Schedule IV and which, if abused, may lead to limited physical dependence or psychological dependence relative to drugs in Schedule IV.

It should be noted that in all instances, local and state laws may strengthen the Federal drug laws but may not be used to weaken them.

Drug Product Recall

In instances in which it is found by the FDA or by a manufacturer that a marketed product presents a threat or a potential threat to consumer safety, that product may be "recalled" or sought for return to the manufacturer from its depth of distribution. The pharmaceutical manufacturer is legally bound to report serious unlabeled adverse reactions to the FDA within 15 working days of learning of an adverse drug reaction. The FDA/USP Drug Product Problem Reporting (DPPR) Program, which began in 1970, is designed as an aid in the protection of the public health, to the monitoring of manufacturer compliance with Current Good Manufacturing Practices (CGMP) and to detect problem products in the marketplace. The pharmacist can report a problem with any drug product or medical device by telephone or written report. Problems may include and are not limited to product adulteration, container leakage, improper labeling and/or unexpected reactions, among others.

A drug product recall may be initiated by the FDA or by the manufacturer, the latter case being termed a "voluntary recall." A numerical classification, as follows, indicates the degree of consumer hazards associated with the product being recalled.

Class I is a situation in which there is a reasonable probability that the use of, or exposure to, a violative product will cause serious, adverse health consequences or death.

Class II is a situation in which the use of, or exposure to, a violative product may cause temporary or medically reversible adverse health consequences or where the probability of serious adverse health consequences is remote.

Class III is a situation in which the use of, or exposure to, a violative product is not likely to cause adverse health consequences.

The "depth of recall," or the level of market removal or correction (as wholesaler, retailer, consumer), depends upon the nature of the product, the urgency of the situation, and depth to which the product has been distributed. The lot numbers of packaging control numbers on the containers or labels of the manufactured products help in identifying the specific lot or batch of product to be recalled.

Prescription Drug Marketing Act of 1987

The Prescription Drug Marketing Act of 1987, passed by Congress and signed into law by the President, became effective on July 21, 1988. The legislation, amending the Federal Food, Drug, and Cosmetic Act, established new safeguards on the integrity of the nation's supply of prescription drugs. Because of its author, Representative John Dingell, and its purpose to prevent drug diversion, the Act has often been referred to as the "Dingell Bill," and the "Drug Diversion Act." The Act is intended to reduce the risks of adulterated, misbranded, repackaged, or mislabeled drugs entering the legitimate marketplace through "secondary sources." The primary sections of the Act are summarized as follows:

1. *Reimportation.* Prohibits the reimportation of drug products manufactured in the United States except by the manufacturer of the product.

2. *Sales Restrictions.* Prohibits selling, trading, purchasing, or the offer to sell, trade or purchase a drug sample. It also prohibits resales by health care institutions of pharmaceuticals purchased explicitly for the use of the institution. Charitable institutions that receive drugs at reduced prices or no cost cannot resell the drugs.

3. *Distribution of Samples.* Samples may only be distributed to: (a) practitioners licensed to prescribe such drugs and, (b) at the written request of the practitioner, to pharmacies of hospitals or other health care institutions. Sample distribution must be made through mail or common carrier and not directly by employees or agents of the manufacturer.

4. *Wholesale Distributors.* Manufacturers are required to maintain a list of their authorized distributors. Wholesalers who desire to distribute a drug for which they are not authorized distributors must inform their wholesale customers, prior to the sale, the name of the person from whom they obtained the goods and all previous sales.

5. *Penalties.* Severe penalties are imposed for the violation of the Act.

Medicare Catastrophic Coverage Act of 1988

The Medicare Catastrophic Coverage Act of 1988 became law on July 1 of that year and provided the most extensive changes in Medicare since its inception in 1965. The Act provides Medicare recipients with expanded protection against the high costs associated with catastrophic injury and illness. Included in the law are prescription drug benefits including for the first time, *outpatient* prescription drug coverage. Included also are expanded inpatient hospital benefits, hospice care, skilled nursing facility care, and home health care benefits. Medications administered intravenously in the home, including antibiotics and other drugs deemed safe for home IV are covered by the law. Under the terms of the law, participating pharmacies engage in *drug utilization reviews*, to detect potential adverse drug reactions and inappropriate drug use, and in *patient counseling* to assure optimum medication benefit and patient compliance.

The Practice of Pharmacy

Pharmacists perform capably in numerous settings in which acquired knowledge and training within the pharmaceutical sciences are applied and intertwined with the professional aspects of pharmacy. A majority of pharmacists practice within a community or an ambulatory setting. In this setting the pharmacist plays an active role in the patient's use of prescription and nonprescription medication. The pharmacist assists the patient in his decision to self-medicate with an available OTC product, to institute nondrug measures to remedy the problem, or to consult a physician or other health-care practitioner. Because of accessibility, the pharmacist also exercises a vital health education role through community service and participation in public education forums and programs. By serving as a source of drug information to the physician and allied health professionals this allows the community/ambulatory practice pharmacist the opportunity to influence directly or indirectly the selection and use of a drug or drug product.

A significant number of pharmacists practice in institutional settings, including hospitals, extended care facilities, and Health Maintenance Organizations (HMO). Practice in these settings may include the provision of professional and clinical services, e.g., nuclear pharmacy, intravenous admixture services, patient monitoring, the provision of educational and technical services, e.g., drug information and poison control, and/or the provision of research and support services, e.g., pharmacokinetic consult service, investigational drug studies division. Newer standards require the pharmacist, for example, to assume greater responsibility and participation in long-term facility care. In addition to maintaining a safe drug distribution and control system, the pharmacist is asked to apply his knowledge in a variety of ways, including drug regimen review and participation on patient-care review committees.

Some graduate pharmacists participate in postgraduate *residency* and/or *fellowship* programs to enhance their practice and/or research skills. A pharmacy residency is defined as: *an organized, directed postgraduate training program in a defined area of practice.* The chief purpose of pharmacy residencies is to train pharmacists in professional practice and management skills. Residency programs are conducted primarily in institutional practice settings. A fellowship is focused toward developing competency in scientific research. It is defined as: *a directed, highly individualized postgraduate program designed to prepare the participant to become an independent researcher.* Both pharmacy residencies and fellowships generally last 12 months or longer and require the close direction of a qualified preceptor.

Pharmacists working for pharmaceutical research, manufacturing, and distributing firms become involved in virtually every phase of drug product development, clinical testing, production, marketing, and management functions. Their knowledge of the basic and pharmaceutical sciences, dosage form design, and the technical aspects of production fits well with this major function of industrial pharmacy firms. Pharmacists with advanced degrees in the basic or pharmaceutical sciences, or in other areas as health care administration, marketing, law, or medicine contribute to their industrial employers in their respective areas of expertise.

In addition to the areas of drug research, product development, and production, many pharmacists in industry work in such varied areas as drug materials procurement; in public, trade, or professional relations; as scientific, technical, or professional information specialists; in liaison work with governmental agencies, educational or research institutions, or professional organizations; or in marketing, advertising, promotion, or pharmaceutical sales work.

In government service, pharmacists perform professional and administrative functions, as in the development and implementation of health care programs in the design and enforcement of regulations involving drug quality standards, good manufacturing practices, and drug distribution and utilization practices. Pharmacists also practice their profession in government supported hospitals, clinics, and specialized health care institutions.

Career opportunities for pharmacists in government service at the Federal level include positions in the military service, in the Public Health Service, and in such Civil Service agencies as the Food and Drug Administration, Veterans Administration, Department of Health and Human Services, Drug Enforcement Administration of the Department of Justice, National Institutes of Health, and others. At the state and local level, many pharmacists find rewarding careers in developing programs for drug procurement, distribution and utilization in the various health departments, welfare departments or agencies, drug investigation and regulatory agencies, clinics and health-care institutions, and also with state boards of pharmacy.

A number of pharmacists serve their profession in positions with various professional organizations, as state and national pharmaceutical associations.

Schools of pharmacy utilize pharmacists, some with and some without advanced degrees, to teach in the professional curriculum, to conduct pharmaceutical research, and to participate in the service and continuing education functions of the school. Although most of the educators working full time for the school do so within the classrooms and laboratories of the academic institution, many others provide professional instruction in the practice or clinical setting. A good number of part-time pharmacist-educators also are employed by schools of pharmacy to provide professional instruction within the academic institution or in affiliated teaching hospitals, medical specialty clinics, hospital pharmacies, drug information centers, nursing homes and extended care facilities, drug abuse clinics, health departments, mental health hospitals or clinics, community pharmacies, and other places in which pharmaceutical services are delivered. Many community and institutional pharmacy practitioners are serving educational institutions as "preceptors," and provide pharmacy students with educational experiences within their own daily practice of pharmacy.

The Pharmacist's Clinical Role

In 1971, the National Center for Health Services Research and Development issued a Report of the "Task Force on the Pharmacist's Clinical Role."[7] The Report was based on professional "functions" of the pharmacist as they were required then and as they were expected to be required in the years immediately ahead. Although a few of these functions were recognized as requiring a change in the law for their legal implementation (as the pharmacist's treatment of minor illness), they were included in the report to reflect reasonable future functions of the pharmacist in terms of his training and in relation to the health care needs of the patient. The Report classified the clinical functions of the pharmacist into seven main categories and described each one as follows:

A. Dispensing and Administering Drugs

The responsibility for dispensing medication upon an order from a physician rests with the pharmacist and his staff. The physician has a legal right to dispense, although generally he does not do so. Exceptions are found in rural communities where a pharmacist is not available and in those few cases where the physician chooses to dispense. When the pharmacist performs the dispensing function, it is assumed that he has drugs available by both brand and established (generic) names in products which are of known and acceptable quality. Furthermore, it is assumed that he has the knowledge to exert a discriminating judgment in selecting a drug product when several products of the same therapeutic class are available that meet the needs of the patient. When generic-name drugs are dispensed, it is assumed that if there is a potential savings the patient will benefit.

1. The pharmacist receives and interprets the drug order and either supervises the dispensing function or performs it himself.
2. The pharmacist should consult with the physician when the latter prescribes products of suspected or known low quality, or when a question arises as to the appropriateness of a drug or drug product in light of the patient's condition.
3. The pharmacist has a responsibility for personally dispensing or supervising the filling of orders that require technical knowledge and skill, such as preparing and dispensing intravenous fluids, radiopharmaceuticals, and compounded prescriptions, etc.
4. The pharmacist's dispensing function in the hospital overlaps with the administration of drugs, an act performed traditionally by the nurse. This is manifest today or will be in the future through (a) administration of medicines by the pharmacist, (b) administration by a technician who works under the supervision of the pharmacist, or (c) administration by a nurse who is responsible for this act. In addition to the pharmacist's potential responsibility for administration of bedside medication, his responsibilities could include the starting of as well as sharing in the assessment of intravenous therapy, and administering drugs in special programs, i.e., cancer chemotherapy.
5. The pharmacist, wherever he practices, may administer biological products for immunizations, i.e., polio (oral or injectable) and smallpox vaccines.
6. The pharmacist's function in preparing the dispensing medication extends logically to inclusion of the function of administering drugs.

Combining these functions provides for improved drug-use control. If the pharmacist's function would include responsibility for administering drugs, he will require special training for such an expanded role.

B. Prescribing Drugs

The physician determines if drug therapy is indicated and usually chooses the drug to be used as part of his overall therapy.

1. Pharmacists, in reissuing prescriptions designated to be refilled at the request of the patient (p.r.n.) may be regarded as performing a prescribing function.
2. Pharmacists, in complying with "standing orders" of the physician, may be performing an independent prescribing function. "Standing orders" refers to a prearranged plan or understanding between the physician and the pharmacist which permits the latter to dispense medications under certain circumstances without the immediate concurrence of the physician.
3. Pharmacists and pharmacy residents often help medical students to plan drug regimens.
4. Physicians may share responsibility for prescribing with the pharmacist when the latter has demonstrated competence. This may include the selection of drugs, the dosage forms and frequency of use, based upon the physician's diagnosis.
5. Pharmacists select over-the-counter (OTC) drugs for patients. Also by recommending against the purchase and/or use of OTC

drugs, they enter into the prescribing function.

6. Pharmacists prescribe medications in emergency situations when it appears to be in the best interest of the patient.

7. Pharmacists, after consultation with the prescriber, may select and dispense a drug other than the one prescribed under the authority of the drug formulary system.

8. Pharmacists may be considered to be performing a prescribing function when they reply to inquiries from patients about continued use of medications previously prescribed.

C. Documenting Professional Activities

The pharmacist is required to keep certain records of his activities in order to meet legal requirements. These are largely operational in nature and pertain to the acquisition and dispensing of narcotics, dangerous drugs, and appliances. In addition to keeping legally-required records, the pharmacist should keep records to document his activities related to patient care. The following are reasonable functions for the pharmacist to perform:

1. The pharmacist should obtain a drug history by recording medications currently used (prescription and OTC) and idiosyncrasies to specific drugs. He notes the past history of drug and/or chemical intoxication and present exposure to industrial, domestic and/or environmental chemicals, etc. The pharmacist may be able to obtain a detailed drug history by using check-off forms. This history becomes the medication part of the patient profile record developed by the health care team. In the community the pharmacist may use a system designed to meet the limitations of both his and the patient's time. This may include the use of a self-administered questionnaire and of automated equipment to provide record linkage with other health care providers used by the patient.

2. The pharmacist should have a meeting with the patient for purposes of reviewing instructions and counseling for home use of medications (a) at time of discharge from the hospital or (b) at time of delivery of medication to him at his community pharmacy. These instructions include mode of administration, conditions of storage, time

of renewal, and signs of untoward reactions. The patient is advised in the event of an unanticipated drug reaction to contact the physician or, if the physician is unavailable, the pharmacist.

3. The pharmacist in the hospital or other health care facility has access to the patient's chart and has the obligation to notify the physician when real or potential drug problems arise, such as development of an adverse drug reaction. He also checks charts to determine if changes in drug therapy are properly recorded. In outpatient clinics, the pharmacist may dispense or administer medication directly from instructions in the chart order.

4. The pharmacist, among others, makes proper reporting of adverse drug reactions (ADR) to the FDA.

5. The pharmacist's records in the community indicate when patients should renew their prescriptions; and if they fail to do so, the pharmacist should contact them to assure continuity of care. This is a follow-up function, primarily applicable to, but not limited to, the chronically ill patient.

6. The pharmacist prepares adequate records to assure himself of a documented source of expanding clinical experience which enhances his services as a drug specialist and consultant. The pharmacist in the hospital should make rounds with the physician and others on the health care team, or independently as appropriate. In the community setting, his direct contact with patients and physicians permits him to acquire a body of experience through which he becomes a useful clinician in the total care of patients.

7. The pharmacist's function in reviewing chart orders and other documents is to focus on four questions: (a) Is use of these drugs or this drug necessary? (b) Are they the drugs of choice (best drugs for need)? (c) Is the monitoring effort directed to the desired effects? (d) Is the monitoring effort designed to identify adverse drug reactions?

8. The pharmacist in the community setting does not have, in all cases, the equivalent of the patient's hospital chart. He may have no data on the patient's diagnosis or condition; in fact, he may not know whether the physician is treating symptoms or a

specifically diagnosed disease. The pharmacist's record, therefore, becomes the historical record of drug utilization, which in time defines the pattern of prescribing of the physician and the pattern (rate, cost, etc.) of utilization by the patient. This permits a periodic review and control function by the pharmacist. The record permits him to monitor therapy for both under- and over-utilization and to identify patients procuring drugs from multiple sources unknown to the physician(s). It also provides an opportunity to acquire information upon which rates of clinical response to individual drugs can be determined by epidemiologic techniques. These data, in correlation with other health records, provide a basis for judgments in which a benefit-risk ratio can be established or, expressed otherwise, an index for predicting likely drug effectiveness.

D. Direct Patient Involvement

The pharmacist should have a direct contact with the patient when he enters or leaves either the hospital system or the community (non-hospital) system. The objective of this contact in either case is the same, but implementation is adapted to fulfill local needs. The pharmacist should be capable of performing the following functions:

1. Conduct an admission interview, or equivalent, to obtain the drug history.
2. Conduct a discharge interview, or equivalent, to review instructions and provide counsel for home use of medications.
3. Provide patient education in personal health matters, i.e., smoking, drug abuse, need for annual health checkup and other preventive measures.
4. Provide patient education and referral when patients are continually using laxatives, antacids, analgesics, etc., or when patients describe symptoms such as one of the cardinal signs of cancer.
5. Screen patients and direct them to sources of appropriate services—a triage function based on the pharmacist's knowledge of community resources, services and means for obtaining access to them.
6. Provide instructions for home use of medications; how and when to take, how to store, cautions in use, when to reorder, expiration date, when to see the physician.
7. Provide instructions for the home use of diagnostic devices and kits. The pharmacist should also be capable of helping the patient interpret the results.
8. Provide instructions in the use of appliances such as inhalers, colostomy bags, trusses, etc. Anatomical models and other demonstration equipment are useful. Special facilities to insure privacy are desirable.
9. Interpret physician's instructions as they relate to drug therapy as well as the total treatment regimen.
10. Conduct rounds in the hospital and develop a system in the community for following a patient's progress when under drug treatment. The monitoring of patients should determine if patients are taking their medicines.
11. Acquaint patients with the name of their pharmacist and how he can be reached. A pharmacist should make arrangements with other pharmacists to provide for the special needs of his patients when he is not available.

E. Reviewing Drug Utilization

Some functions in this section have been noted, in part, previously.

1. Demonstrating concern for the need for organized programs to review and control drug utilization.
2. Developing and/or promoting planned drug utilization review programs.
3. Developing techniques that will lead to identification of drug prescribing patterns by physicians and drug use patterns by patients.
4. Disseminating accurate information concerning the use of drugs to physicians, other members of the health care team, and the public.
5. Implementing a local formulary system of drug-use control in the hospital and in the community.

F. Education

Education refers to those ongoing activities that are designed to influence the prescribing, the dispensing and the use of drugs. The pharmacist's goal as a member of the health care team is to improve patient care by improving the use of drugs and lessening the degree of misuse. Specific functions include:

1. Participation in continuing education through self-directed study and other methods.
2. Organization of inservice and continuing education programs—seminars, lectures, etc., for hospital staffs, group medical practices and professional societies.
3. Participation in the health education of the patient.
4. Participation in public information programs to promote respect for drugs as agents of good health.
5. Participation in the activity of the Pharmacy and Therapeutics Committee or its equivalent organization.
6. Organization of drug information service for physicians and other clinicians.
7. Participation in special programs in the hospital, such as grand rounds, teaching rounds, nursing conferences, medical staff meetings, etc.

G. Consultation

The pharmacist should exert a consultative function by being available to the physician and other clinicians and to the patient for advice and guidance. Although his role as consultant is based primarily on his role as a drug specialist, it is based also on his knowledge of personal and public health matters, community health resources, the treatment of minor illnesses, etc. The pharmacist exerts an *active* role when performing as a consultant. Particular consultations are carried out with the physician and patient concerning:

1. The screening process. For example, the pharmacist might perform certain screening procedures, i.e., determine blood pressure, and in consultation with a physician at some remote point decide what measures should be taken. This is part of the triage function.
2. The selection of drugs and monitoring of drug therapy.
3. The refusal to furnish medication when the best evidence supports this position.
4. The referral of patients to sources of competent medical care.

In 1983, the American Society of Hospital Pharmacists offered an independent study pro-

gram, *Basic Skills in Clinical Pharmacy Practice,* to assist pharmacists in developing their clinical skills and in implementing new clinical pharmacy services.[8] The following areas were delineated as those general clinical pharmacy functions and services now commonly provided in a variety of practice settings: (1) Providing Drug Information to Other Health Professionals; (2) Obtaining Patient Medication Histories and Using Patient Medication Profiles to Assure Proper Drug Utilization; (3) Monitoring Drug Therapy; (4) Providing Patient Education and Medication Counseling; (5) Providing Disease Screening, Monitoring, and Maintenance Care for Patients with Chronic Diseases; (6) Participation in the Management of Emergency Medical Care; (7) Serving as a Health Information and Education Source for the Public; (8) Participation in Drug Use Review and Patient Care Audits; and, (9) Providing Inservice Education for Physicians, Nurses, and Other Health Professionals.

It is the professional responsibility of the pharmacist to continue his education and be responsive to evolving and expanded practice roles particularly as these relate to patient involvement. In recent years there have been numerous certificate programs which have been developed to enhance the pharmacist's knowledge base and practice skills. These have been developed within a curricular-based approach to maximize learning and to allow the pharmacist to incorporate new knowledge and skills directly into his practice for the benefit of his patients.

Standards of Practice

In 1979, a joint effort by the American Pharmaceutical Association and the American Association of Colleges of Pharmacy resulted in the publication of a document titled "Standards of Practice for the Profession of Pharmacy."[9] This document was updated as "Competency Statements for Pharmacy Practice" in 1986.[10] The four major areas of responsibility for pharmacists may be summarized as follows:

General Management and Administration of the Pharmacy: Selects and supervises pharmacists and non-professionals for pharmacy staff; establishes a pricing structure for pharmaceutical services and products; administers budgets and negotiates with vendors; develops and maintains a purchasing and inventory system for all drugs and pharmaceutical supplies; initiates a formulary system. In general, establishes and administers pharmacy management, personnel and fiscal policy.

Activities Related to Processing the Prescription: Verifies prescription for legality, and physical and chemical compatibility; checks patient record before dispensing prescription; measures quantities needed to dispense prescription; performs final check of finished prescription; dispenses prescription.

Patient Care Functions: Clarifies patient's understanding of dosage; integrates drug-related with patient related information; advises patient of potential drug-related conditions; refers patient to other health care resources; monitors and evaluates therapeutic response of patient; reviews and/or seeks additional drug-related information.

Education of Health Care Professionals and Patients: Organizes, maintains and provides drug information to other health care professionals; organizes and/or participates in "in pharmacy"

education programs for other pharmacists; makes recommendations regarding drug therapy to physician or patient; develops and maintains system for drug distributions and quality control.

Each of the areas of responsibility were further broken down in the document with specific tasks reflecting the desired standards of practice.

The "Report of the Task Force in the Pharmacist's Clinical Role" the study program "Basic Skills in Clinical Pharmacy Practice," and the "Standards of Practice for the Profession of Pharmacy" capture the contemporary aspects of the professional practice of pharmacy. By definition, a profession is founded upon an art, built upon specialized intellectual training, and has as its primary objective the performing of a service. The principles upon which the professional practice of pharmacy is based are embodied in the Code of Ethics of the American Pharmaceutical Association.

Code of Ethics American Pharmaceutical Association*

Preamble

These principles of professional conduct are established to guide pharmacists in relationships with patients, fellow practitioners, other health professionals, and the public.

A PHARMACIST should hold the health and safety of patients to be of first consideration and should render to each patient the full measure of professional ability as an essential health practitioner.

A PHARMACIST should never knowingly condone the dispensing, promoting, or distributing of drugs or medical devices, or assist therein, that are not of good quality, that do not meet standards required by law, or that lack therapeutic value for the patient.

A PHARMACIST should always strive to perfect and enlarge professional knowledge. A pharmacist should utilize and make available this knowledge as may be required in accordance with the best professional judgment.

A PHARMACIST has the duty to observe the law, to uphold the dignity and honor of the profession, and to accept its ethical principles.

A pharmacist should not engage in any activity that will bring discredit to the profession and should expose, without fear or favor, illegal or unethical conduct in the profession.

A PHARMACIST should seek at all times only fair and reasonable remuneration for professional services. A pharmacist should never agree to, or participate in, transactions with practitioners of other health professions or any other person under which fees are divided or that may cause financial or other exploitation in connection with the rendering of professional services.

A PHARMACIST should respect the confidential and personal nature of professional records; except where the best interest of the patient requires or the law demands, a pharmacist should not disclose such information to anyone without proper patient authorization.

A PHARMACIST should strive to provide information to patients regarding professional services truthfully, accurately, and fully and should avoid misleading patients regarding the nature, cost, or value of these professional services.

A PHARMACIST should associate with organizations having for their objective the betterment of the profession of pharmacy and should contribute time and funds to carry on the work of these organizations.

Approved by APhA Active and Life members August, 1969; Amended December, 1975; Revised July, 1981

Selected Reading

Blake, M.I.: The Role of the Compendia in Drug Product Selection. *The Apothecary*, 90:16, 1978.

History of National Formulary, in *National Formulary*. 17th Ed., Rockville, MD., United States Pharmacopeial Convention, Inc., 1990.

History of the Pharmacopeia of the United States, in *United States Pharmacopeia*, 22nd revision, Rockville, MD., United States Pharmacopeial Convention, Inc., 1990.

Hussey, J.M.: How to Monitor Adverse Drug Reactions. *US Pharmacist*, 12(1):16, 1987.

Kalman, S.H. and Schlegel, J.F.: Standards of Practice for the Profession of Pharmacy, *Am. Pharm.*, NS19:21–35, 1979.

Moore, R.C., Stonecipher, B.F., and Reynolds, C.T.: The FDA/USP Product Problem Reporting Program. *US Pharmacist*, 11(1):35–41, 1986.

Pharmacists for the Future: The Report of the Study Commission on Pharmacy. Ann Arbor, Health Administration Press, 1975.

Sonnedecker, G.: *Kremer's and Urdang's History of Pharmacy*. 4th Ed., Philadelphia, J.B. Lippincott Co., 1976.

Notes

1. The term "shelf life" refers to the length of time a drug product may remain on the (pharmacist's) shelf, in the original package and under usual environmental conditions, and retain an acceptable level of its original potency and overall quality. In most instances solid dosage forms, as tablets and capsules, have a shelf life of 5 years from the date of manufacture. Usually liquid dosage forms, disperse systems as aerosols and emulsions, and semisolid forms as ointments and suppositories have shorter shelf lives. However, a great deal depends upon the individual chemical and physical characteristics of the active ingredients, the formulative materials, and the packaging employed. Poor storage conditions, with extremes of temperature, humidity, and light can adversely affect the stability of pharmaceutical products. Federal Good Manufacturing Practice regulations require expiration dating on the labels of all prescription-only and on most nonprescription pharmaceutical products to assure standards of strength, quality and purity. The expiration date for each product is determined by appropriate stability testing.

2. Drugs of the Future through Genetic Engineering, *Am. Pharm.*, NS 21, 11–20, 1981.

3. The Thalidomide Tragedy—25 Years Ago. *FDA Consumer*, 21(1):14–17, 1987.

4. In January, 1983, President Ronald Reagan signed into law the Orphan Drug Act. This Act provides incentives for sponsors of drugs useful in the treatment of rare diseases. There are many diseases and conditions, such as Huntington's Disease, myoclonus, ALS (Lou Gehrig's disease), Tourette syndrome, and muscular dystrophy which affect such small numbers of individuals residing in the United States that the diseases and conditions are considered rare in this country. Drugs for these rare diseases and conditions are commonly referred to as "orphan drugs." Adequate drugs for these and other such diseases and conditions were not being produced because a pharmaceutical company which developed an orphan drug would expect to generate such small sales in comparison to the cost of development, that it became a financial disincentive.

   Under the provisions of the Orphan Drug Act, sponsors of orphan drugs may receive tax credits for the clinical testing portion of orphan drug research, provided that the drug is officially designated as an "orphan" by the FDA. The bill also permits FDA approval of the orphan drug based on clinical studies that are fewer in number and scope (and thus less costly) than required for non-orphan drugs. As of April 1988, fifty-eight products were given orphan designation by the FDA including nine drugs related to the treatment of AIDS.

5. *Drug Bioequivalence*. A Report of the Office of Technology Assessment, Drug Bioequivalence Study Panel, Congress of the United States, Washington, D.C. 1974.

6. *Approved Drug Products*. Food and Drug Administration, January, 1979.

7. "Report of Task Force on the Pharmacist's Clinical Role," National Center for Health Services Research and Development, Department of Health, Education, and Welfare, Public Health Service, Health Services and Mental Health Administration, *HSRD Briefs*, No. 4, 1971.

8. Ray, M.D. (Ed.): *Basic Skills in Clinical Pharmacy Practice*, American Society of Hospital Pharmacists, 1983.

9. Kalman, S.H. and Schlegel, J.F.: Standards of Practice for the Profession of Pharmacy. *Am. Pharm.*, NS19:21–35, 1979.

10. Pancorbo, S.A., Campagna, K.D., Davenport, J.K., Garnett, W.R., and Littlefield, L.C.: Task Force Report of Competency Statements for Pharmacy Practice. *Am. J. Pharm. Ed.*, 51:196–206, 1987.

2 | *Drug Substances*

As DEFINED in Chapter 1, drug substances are physiologically active agents used in the diagnosis, prevention, treatment or cure of disease in man or animal. Drug substances may be of natural origin obtained from mineral, plant, or animal sources, or, they may be products of organic chemical synthesis or biosynthesis. Drug substances are combined with physiologically inactive pharmaceutic ingredients in preparing the various dosage forms in use today.

The *United States Pharmacopeia* and the *National Formulary* adopt standards for drug substances, pharmaceutic ingredients, and dosage forms reflecting the best in the current practices of medicine and pharmacy and provide suitable tests and assay procedures for demonstrating compliance with these standards. In fulfilling this function, the compendia become legal documents, every statement of which must be of a high degree of clarity and specificity.

The *United States Pharmacopeia* includes detailed monographs on drug substances and dosage forms, whereas the *National Formulary* contains monographs on pharmaceutic ingredients. These monographs represent the established standards and constitute the basis for maintaining quality.

It should be noted that many pharmaceutical products on the market, especially those which are combinations of therapeutic ingredients, are not represented by formulation or dosage form monographs in the official compendia. However, the individual components in these products are either represented by monographs in the compendia or are otherwise approved as a part of the manufacturer's drug applications and listings with the Food and Drug Administration and thus together with the approved product meet the designated standards.

An example of a typical monograph for a drug substance appearing in the *United States Pharmacopeia* is that for the therapeutic agent chlorambucil. This monograph, reproduced in Figure 2–1, reveals the type of information generally appearing for organic medicinal agents.

Following the official title or name of the chemical, its graphic or structural formula is presented along with empirical formula, molecular weight, established chemical names and the drug's Chemical Abstracts Service (CAS) Registry Number. The CAS Registry Number identifies each compound uniquely in the CAS computer-oriented information retrieval system. Appearing next in the monograph is a statement of chemical purity, a cautionary statement which reflects the toxic nature of the agent, packaging and storage recommendations, and chemical and physical tests and the prescribed method of assay to substantiate the identification and purity of the chemical.

In each monograph, the standards set forth are specific for the individual therapeutic agent, pharmaceutical necessity, or dosage form and vary with the particular requirements to insure purity, potency, and overall quality.

Nomenclature

The initial part of each drug monograph consists of the official title or name of the drug, pharmaceutic agent or preparation. The official titles for preparations contain the name of the primary or most distinguishing component(s) and the type of dosage form, as: *Chlorambucil Tablets*.

Drugs or agents of zoological or botanic origin are named according to the rules set forth by the International Botanical Congress and the International Zoological Congress. The inorganic salts are named according to the established precedent of a cation-anion order, as sodium chloride. It is in the area of naming pure organic chemicals of synthetic or natural origin that most of the current efforts in drug nomenclature are directed, since this group represents today's most prolific source of new drugs.

The official title for a drug substance is referred to as the drug's *nonproprietary* generic, or *public* name, in contrast to the *proprietary* or brand or trademark names given the chemical substance by specific manufacturers or distrib-

Chlorambucil

$(ClCH_2CH_2)_2N$—◯—$CH_2CH_2CH_2COOH$

$C_{14}H_{19}Cl_2NO_2$ 304.22 Benzenebutanoic acid, 4-[bis(2-chloroethyl)amino]-4-[*p*[Bis(2-chloroethyl)amino]phenyl]butyric acid [*305-03-3*].

▶ Chlorambucil contains not less than 98.0% and not more than 101.0% of $C_{14}H_{19}Cl_2NO_2$, calculated on the anhydrous basis.

Caution—Great care should be taken to prevent inhaling particles of Chlorambucil and exposing the skin to it.

Packaging and storage—Preserve in tight, light-resistant containers.

Reference standard—*USP Chlorambucil Reference*

Standard—[Caution—Avoid contact]—Dry over silica gel for 24 hours before using.

Identification—

A: The infrared absorption spectrum of a 1 in 125 solution in carbon disulfide, in a 1-mm cell, exhibits maxima only at the same wavelengths as that of a similar solution of USP Chlorambucil RS.

B: Dissolve 50 mg in 5 mL of acetone, and dilute with water to 10 mL. Add 1 drop of 2 N sulfuric acid, then add 4 drops of silver nitrate TS: no opalescence is observed immediately *(absence of chloride ion)*. Warm the solution on a steam bath: opalescence develops *(presence of ionizable chlorine)*.

Melting range (741): between 65° and 69°.

Water, *Method I* (921): not more than 0.5%.

Assay—Dissolve about 200 mg of Chlorambucil, accurately weighed, in 10 mL of acetone, add 10 mL of water, and titrate with 0.1 N sodium hydroxide VS, using phenolphthalein TS as the indicator. Each mL of 0.1 N sodium hydroxide is equivalent to 30.42 mg of $C_{14}H_{19}Cl_2NO_2$.

Fig. 2–1. Chlorambucil

utors of the drug.[1] The value of designating each drug by a single nonproprietary name is obvious in terms of achieving simplicity and uniformity in drug nomenclature. The nonproprietary name of a drug may be used without restriction in contrast to the brand name, which may be registered as a trademark with the United States Patent Office for the exclusive use of the registrant. If the drug is protected by a patent, this information is indicated in the USP monograph. Such a drug substance may be produced only by the patent holder unless he choses to license others to manufacture and distribute the drug. When a chemical agent is not protected with a patent, any drug manufacturer may coin a brand name, obtain a trademark, and manufacture and distribute the drug. Many manufacturers may engage in this activity for a single chemical compound, each promoting his product under a different name. For clarity and identification, it is required by law to include also the nonproprietary name whenever the brand name is used in drug advertising, promotion, and labeling.

As a result of the implementation of the Drug Price Competition and Patent Term Restoration Act of 1984, many more drugs became available in generic form than previously. Under the 1984 act, to gain approval for marketing by the fed-

eral Food and Drug Administration, a generic drug product must:

1. Contain the same active ingredients as the pioneer (brand name) drug product. Inert ingredients may vary.
2. Be identical in strength, dosage form, and route of administration.
3. Have the same indications for use, precautions, and other labeling instructions.
4. Be bioequivalent. That is, show the same rate and extent of absorption without significant difference from that of the pioneer drug when administered at the same molar dose of the therapeutic ingredient under the same experimental conditions. (Note: the allowed statistical variability of ±20% is the basis for evaluation of bioequivalency in blood level studies. According to the FDA, the average observed difference in absorption between generic and pioneer products has been about ±3%.)
5. Meet the same batch-to-batch requirements for identity, strength, purity, and quality.
6. Be manufactured under the same strict standards of FDAs Good Manufacturing Practice regulations as required for pioneer products.

Naming a Drug

The selection of a single nonproprietary name for older organic chemicals has been mostly a matter of accepting the name most widely accepted scientifically through the years. The early selection of a single nonproprietary name for a newly synthesized or discovered chemical is important to reduce the likelihood of its being referred to by several different names in the chemical, drug, and medical literature. Even so, a newly found organic chemical is normally referred to by a minimum of three and often four different names on its way to a recognized place in therapeutics.

When first synthesized, or identified from a natural source, an organic compound is represented by an *empirical formula,* as $C_{14}H_{19}Cl_2NO_2$ for chlorambucil, which indicates the number and the relationship of the atoms comprising the molecule. As knowledge of the relative locations of these atoms is gained, the compound receives a *systematic chemical name,* as 4-[bis(2-chloroethyl)amino] - 4 - [*p*-[Bis(2-chloroethyl)amino]phenyl]butyric acid. To be adequate and fully specific, the name must reveal every part of the compound's molecular structure, so that it describes only the compound concerned and no other. The systematic name is generally so formidable that it soon is replaced in scientific communication by a condensed name, which, although less descriptive chemically, is understood to refer only to that chemical compound. This new name may be the first attempt at assigning the nonproprietary name, or it may be an intermediate designation as a *code number,* which generally stays with the compound through its initial laboratory investigation for pharmacologic activity and through the human clinical trials. The practice of using code numbers for test substances was made famous over a half century ago when Paul Ehrlich numbered the compounds employed in his search for the "magic bullet" to cure syphilis. His compound "606" (the 606th compound he tested) became more famous than the chemical's other names of arsphenamine and Salvarsan. Today many companies give their new compounds code numbers prior to the assignment of a nonproprietary name. These code numbers generally take the form of an identifying prefix letter or letters that identify the drug's sponsor, followed by a number that further identifies the test compound.

When the results of testing indicate that a compound has sufficient promise, the inventor or discoverer of the new compound may propose a *nonproprietary* name and apply to the U.S. Patent Office (and foreign agencies as well) for a *proprietary* or trademark name. Should the drug receive recognition in an official compendium, the nonproprietary name established during the period of the drug's early usage is generally adopted. It should be pointed out that nonproprietary names are issued only for single agents whereas proprietary or trademark names may be associated with a single chemical entity or with a mixture of chemicals comprising a specific proprietary product.

The USAN Council

Today the task of designating appropriate nonproprietary names for chemical agents rests primarily with the United States Adopted Names Council (USAN Council). This organized effort at coining nonproprietary names for drugs was inagurated in 1961 as a joint project of the American Medical Association and the United States Pharmacopeial Convention. They were joined in 1964 by the American Pharmaceutical Association to form the USAN Council; in 1967, the Food and Drug Administration was invited to take part in the work of the Council and to place a voting member on it. Financial support for the Council programs is contributed by the three nongovernmental organizations, with the American Medical Association maintaining the secretariat and the USP Convention publishing the United States Adopted Names (USAN) in cumulative form each year.

The United States Pharmacopeial Convention publishes the *USAN* and the *USP Dictionary of Drug Names.* In addition to listing the US Adopted Names, the reference also includes brand names of research-oriented firms, investigational drug code designations, official names of USP and NF articles with their chemical names and graphic formulas, and international nonproprietary names (INN) published by the World Health Organization (WHO). This reference of drug names now includes over 18,000 entries.

A proposal for a USAN usually originates from a firm or an individual who has developed a substance of potential therapeutic usefulness to the point where there is a distinct possibility of its being marketed in the United States. Occasionally, the initiative is taken by the USAN Council in the form of a request to parties interested in a substance for which a nonproprietary name appears to be lacking. Proposals are expected to conform to the Council's guidelines for coining nonproprietary names. In general, the name should (1) be short and distinctive in sound and spelling and not be such that it is easily confused with existing names, (2) indicate the general pharmacologic or therapeutic class into which the substance falls or the general chemical nature of the substance if the latter is associated with the specific pharmacologic activity, (3) embody the syllable or syllables characteristic of a related group of compounds. It is recommended that drugs of the categories listed in Table 2–1 bear the appropriate syllable in their nonproprietary names.

When general agreement on a name has been reached between the Council and the drug's sponsor, it is announced as a "Proposed USAN." This indicates the Council's intention to adopt the name and serves notice on those who wish to protest the selection. The tentatively adopted USAN is then submitted for consideration by various American and foreign drug regulatory agencies, including the World Health Organization, the British Pharmaco-poeia Commission, the French Codex, the Nordic Pharmacopeia, the United States Pharmacopeia and National Formulary, and the U.S. Food and Drug Administration. Under the 1962 Drug Amendments, the Secretary of the Department of Health and Human Services has authority to designate the nonproprietary name for any drug in the interest of usefulness or simplicity. The authority is generally delegated to the Commissioner of the Food and Drug Administration within the Department. If no objections are raised, adoption is considered final, and the USAN is published in the various literature of the medical and pharmaceutical professions. With the creation of the USAN Council and the cooperation of the interested parties on a worldwide basis, nonproprietary drug nomenclature has been standardized.

Chemical and Physical Characteristics

Each drug substance has its own chemical and physical characteristics which make it

Table 2–1. Some USAN Recommended Prefixes and Suffixes for the Construction of Nonproprietary Names of Drugs

anabolic steroids	bol-; or -bol-
androgens	-andr-; or
	-stan-; or
	-ster-
anesthetics, local	-caine
anorexics	-orex
anti-adrenergics (beta receptor)	-olol
antibiotics (cefazolin type)	cef-
antibiotics produced by *Streptomyces* strains	-mycin
antibiotics (tetracycline derivatives)	-cycline
anticoagulants (coumarin type)	-arol
anti-inflammatory substances (ibuprofen type)	-profen
anti-inflammatory substances (indomethacin type)	-methacin
antimicrobial sulfonamides	sulfa-
bronchodilators (phenethylamine derivatives)	-terol
corticotropins, synthetic	-actide
cortisone derivatives	-cort-
diuretics (thiazide derivatives)	-thiazide
estrogens	-estr-
hypoglycemics, oral { guanidine	-formin
{ sulfonamide	gli-
imipramine type compounds	-pramine
iodine-containing contrast media	io-
morphinan derivatives that are narcotic antagonists or agonists	-orphan
normorphone derivatives that are narcotic antagonists	nal-
penicillins	-cillin
progestins	-gest-
prostaglandin derivatives	-prost-
steroids that are acetal derivatives	-onide
tranquilizers (diazepam type)	-azepam

ferent reagents and resulting in different impurities. These processes include the use of lead oxide, chlorine gas, animal fats and oils, and beet sugar molasses; contaminants resulting from these processes are heavy metals, chlorinated compounds, fatty acids and esters, and glucose. The limits to which each of these may be present in official glycerin is provided in the monograph.

The unique chemical and physical characteristics of a drug substance determine not only the analytical tests and methods employed for its identification and assay, but also have a bearing on the formulation of a stable, effective and safe dosage form. The drug substance should remain stable for the intended shelf-life of the product, it should be chemically and physically compatible with all other formulation components and should maintain its intended biological activity. Among the physicochemical properties of drug substances which are considered in formulating dosage forms are the following.

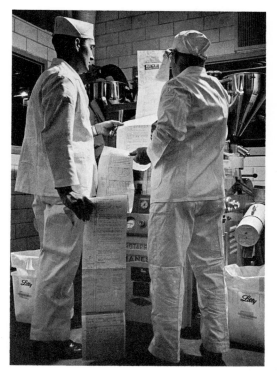

Fig. 2–2. *Quality control in the manufacture of tablets. The manufacturing ticket lists the ingredients of a given item, describes how they are to be combined, and specifies the checks and tests necessary for safety and purity. (Courtesy of Eli Lilly and Company.)*

unique. These characteristics are used in setting standards for the identification of the substance and for its assay. For each drug substance and for related dosage forms, the official monographs set forth the appropriate chemical and physical standards, tests, and assay procedures which must be met (Figs. 2–2 and 2–3).

Each test and standard noted in the monograph must be satisfied before the drug substance may be called "USP Quality." Each batch, lot, or container of a drug substance (or pharmaceutic ingredient) must pass the required quality standards before it may be utilized in the preparation of a drug product. The tests and limits for impurities are for those chemicals most likely to be present as contaminants. The impurities generally are due to processes of chemical manufacture or to the drug's deterioration. Glycerin, for example, a solvent used in many liquid pharmaceuticals, may be prepared in a number of different ways, each utilizing a different starting material and dif-

Solubility

A drug substance administered by any route of administration must possess some aqueous solubility for therapeutic efficacy. Relatively insoluble compounds may exhibit either incomplete or erratic absorption and thus produce minimal therapeutic response. Enhanced aqueous solubility of these compounds may be achieved through the preparation of more soluble derivatives, as salts or esters, or through techniques as micronization of the drug particles or through complexation.

Consideration of solubility after administration is also important. For example, if a drug is administered as a solution but precipitates into an insoluble form in the gastrointestinal fluids, its absorption and biological availability to the body could be substantially affected. pH solubility profiles (curves) must be determined to understand the solubility characteristics of the drug substance over the pH range of the biological fluids encountered. In some instances it may be desirable to achieve a lower aqueous solubility, for the purpose of masking the taste of a liquid preparation (through reduced contact of the drug with the taste buds) or to slow the rate of absorption of the drug substance to enhance its duration of action. This may be achieved by the preparation of slowly soluble salts or esters of the drugs.

In solubility studies, the lipid solubility of the

Fig. 2–3. *Scene of a portion of a quality control laboratory. (Courtesy of Eli Lilly and Company.)*

drug and the common ion effect are also considered. For example, hydrochloride salts of a drug substance can be appreciably less soluble in biological fluids containing sodium chloride and hydrochloric acid than other salt forms of the drug which may be prepared.

Partition Coefficient and pKa

To produce a pharmacological response, a drug molecule must first cross a biological membrane. The membrane, consisting of protein and lipid material, acts as a lipophilic barrier to the passage of many drugs. The resistance of this barrier to drug transfer is related to the lipophilic nature of the molecule being transported.

The oil/water partition coefficient is a measure of a molecule's lipophilic character; that is, its preference for the hydrophilic or lipophilic phase.

The partition coefficient should be considered in developing a drug substance into a dosage form. The partition coefficient (P) represents the ratio of the drug distribution in a two-phase system of organic solvent and aqueous phase. Using octanol-water as an example, it is defined as:

$$P = \frac{[\text{Conc. of drug in octanol}]}{[\text{Conc. of drug in water}]}$$

P is dependent on the drug concentration only if the drug molecules have a tendency to associate in solution. For an ionizable drug, the following equation is applicable:

$$P = \frac{[\text{Conc. of drug in octanol}]}{(1 - \alpha)\,[\text{Conc. of drug in water}]}$$

where α equals the degree of ionization.

The determination of the dissociation constant, pKa, is important because it may be an indication of a drug substance's absorption characteristics. This will be discussed in Chapter 3, where drug absorption is considered more thoroughly.

Drug Form and Dissolution Rate

The *rate* at which a drug substance dissolves in medium is referred to as its *dissolution rate.* Dissolution rate data, when considered along with data on the drug's solubility, partition characteristics, and dissolution constant, can provide an indication of the drug's absorption potential following administration. For a chemical entity, the acid, base or salt forms may produce substantial differences in the dissolution rate. In addition, the drug's particle size, crystal form and surface properties may also affect the dissolution rate. Factors of drug dissolution as they relate to drug absorption are considered further in Chapter 3.

Stability

The chemical and physical stability of the drug substance alone and together with formulation ingredients is a most important criterion for a successful drug product. The drug must be studied for stability over time at a variety of storage temperatures (as 50°, 60°, 70°C) and, in the presence of moisture, light, oxygen and other potentially destructive influences. Drug stability studies with a variety of pharmaceutic ingredients are also necessary to determine chemical and physical stability and compatibility prior to formulation into dosage forms.

For certain drugs, one crystal form or polymorph may be more stable than another and may be preferred. It is essential that the drug be pure before any stability tests are initiated. An impurity may catalyze the breakdown of a drug, or it might be unstable itself, altering the physical appearance of a perfectly stable drug substance.

Mechanism of Drug Action

Different drug substances, because of their unique chemical structures, exert their own individual effects on the biological system. Some drug substances are chemically related to others and exert similar effects. The chemical modification of an existing drug substance may yield a new compound with therapeutic advantages over the parent compound. Thus, a series of compounds may be synthetically prepared from a basic pharmacologically-active structure to obtain improved drug substances within the same family of compounds (e.g., benzodiazepines). The compounds with advantages over the others would be preferentially developed and used.

In general, drugs exert their effects by one of three means: (1) by exerting a physical action, such as the protective effects of ointments and lotions upon topical application; (2) by reacting chemically outside of the body's cells—for example, antacids to counteract excess acidity in the stomach or antibiotics to act against invading pathogenic microorganisms; or (3) by modifying the metabolic activity of the body's cells— for example antimetabolites used for chemotherapy of neoplastic diseases. These are chemically similar to endogenous metabolites in that they enter the same metabolic system but differ enough to disrupt normal metabolic pathways. The majority of drugs in use today act in the third manner by affecting the specialized cells of the brain, liver, heart, blood vessels, kidneys,

nerve ganglia or endings, and other tissues. The processes of life and metabolism within the body's cells involve intricate enzymatic reactions. Each component of these complex enzyme systems is vital to the normal functioning of the cell. The vitamins, for example, are indispensable to life because they are necessary components of essential enzyme systems. On the other hand, many poisons, including drugs in overdosage, exert their toxic effects by inactivating life-sustaining enzyme systems. Drugs modify the metabolism of cells by (1) adsorption on the cell membrane or surface, (2) penetration of the cell membrane, or (3) chemical combination with cellular components. Any of these actions alters the function of the cell and initiates a series of biochemical and physiological changes that result in the drug's effects and provide the basis for its categorization. The initial drug-cell interaction is appropriately termed the drug's "action"; the resulting events are properly referred to as its "effects."

The action of most drugs takes place at the molecular level with the drug molecules interacting with the molecules of the cell structure or its contents (Fig. 2–4).

The selectivity and specificity of drugs for a certain body tissue—for example, drugs that act primarily on the nerves, heart, or kidney—are related to specific sites on or within the cells, receptive only to chemicals of a particular chemical structure and configuration. The cellular component directly involved in the action of a drug is termed its *receptor*. The chemical groups that participate in the drug-receptor combination and the adjacent portions of the receptor that favor or hinder access of the drug to these active groups are known as *receptor groups* or *receptor sites*. Although receptors for most drugs have yet to be identified, they, like the active centers of enzymes, are thought to be carboxyl, amino, sulfhydryl, phosphate, and similar reactive groups oriented on or in the cell in a pattern complementary to that of the drugs with which they react. The binding of a drug to the receptor is thought to be accomplished mainly by ionic and other relatively weak reversible bonds. Occasionally, firm covalent bonding is involved, and the drug effect is then very slowly reversible. Because receptor sites bind chemicals with specific chemical groupings and orientation, many chemicals that are but slight modifications of an initial or parent compound possess the same pharmacologic effect. Thus,

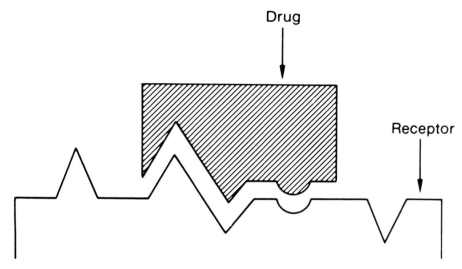

Fig. 2–4. *Schematic drawing of receptor site and substrate (drug). (From "How Modern Medicines are Discovered," Frank H. Clark, Ed., Courtesy of Futura Publishing Company, Inc.)*

based on the knowledge of the receptor size, shape, stereospecificity and arrangements of reactive groups, a drug can be redesigned to improve specificity and selectivity. This is exemplified by the development of prazosin, the first in a new class of adrenoreceptor antagonists with a high selectivity for the alpha$_1$-adrenoreceptor. Basically, the structure of a chemical compound affects two properties that are closely interrelated to its biological activity—its physical characteristics and its chemical reactivity. Such properties determine, for example, whether the molecule can permeate the various barriers between the external medium and the site of biochemical action within the cell and arrive at that site in adequate concentration. Modifications in a chemical's structure can alter the speed of drug action, the duration of the effects, and toxic or undesirable side effects. There are numerous derivatives of barbituric acid, including pentobarbital; each is a sedative, but each differs in its degree of activity and its onset and duration of action. Certain cells within the body are capable of receiving drug substances without eliciting a drug effect. These cells are important in the transport of drugs throughout the body, in their detoxification by metabolism or chemical breakdown, and in their ultimate elimination from the body.

Drugs may act by influencing any of the steps involved in the maintenance of normal cell function. Thus they may act individually to enhance or prevent cell metabolism. The effects of drug action may be described as either stimulation, depression, or irritation. An increased activity of specialized cells due to the presence of drugs is referred to as "stimulation" (e.g., sulfonylurea drugs stimulate the release of insulin from the beta cells of the pancreas). A decrease in cellular activity is called "depression." Pentobarbital is a depressant to the cells of the central nervous system. The degree of activity of depressants can usually be governed by the size of the dose; thus pentobarbital in greater than sedative doses may be employed as a hypnotic, or a drug that induces sleep. Stimulant drugs may stimulate cells to a point of inactivity resembling the effects of depressant drugs but comparable to physiological fatigue. This type of overstimulation is reversible and is only temporary, with the cells returning to normal activity as the drug is removed from the body through the metabolic process. Irritant drugs are useful in provoking idle cells to normal activity, but if used for extended periods of time or in excessive concentration they may result in cellular destruction.

Drug Category

Each drug substance in use today is categorized by one or more means as follows:

(1) Classification according to the anatomical site of action.

(2) Classification according to therapeutic activity or application.

(3) Classification according to the pharmacological mechanism of action.

(4) Classification according to the source of origin or the chemical and pharmacological properties of the drug.

Under these schemes, for example, diphenhydramine could be classified respectively as: (1) a drug acting upon histamine H_1 receptors, (2) an antihistamine, (3) a histamine H_1 receptor antagonist, and (4) a derivative of ethylamine. Generally, there is an overlapping of the methods used in categorizing drugs.

Definitions of selected drug categories and examples of representative drug substances are presented in Appendix I.

Drug Substance Selection and Utilization

Rational drug therapy is the goal of all concerned in the prescribing, dispensing and administration of medications. Included in this concept are the following:

1. the most appropriate drug substance is selected on the basis of an accurate diagnosis, cost effectiveness to desired outcome and provided to the patient according to a well-designed treatment plan;
2. the prescriber and pharmacist have a thorough understanding of the pharmacology of the drug substance including both the benefits and risks involved in its use;
3. the drug substance is provided in the appropriate chemical form (salt, ester, etc.) and administered by the most advantageous dosage form, at the correct dosage and dosage intervals throughout the course of treatment;
4. the patient (or the patient's family member) is provided instruction on the proper use of the medication, with emphasis placed on patient compliance and the need to report signs of drug ineffectiveness;
5. the drug substance is compatible with all foods and other medications taken concomitantly by the patient;
6. the drug's effects are monitored and the patient assessed at appropriate times during therapy to determine the effectiveness of the medication.

Pharmacists are playing an increasingly important role in assuring rational drug therapy. Through their professional practice activities, pharmacists participate in drug product selection (both prescription-only and OTC), the design of drug-therapy plans, securing and disseminating drug information, patient drug education, and patient monitoring for drug efficacy, drug interactions, adverse drug effects and review for appropriate utilization.

The therapeutic effectiveness of a drug product depends on a number of factors in three broad categories:

1. *Prescribing Factors*—generally comprised of those items embracing *rational drug therapy;* i.e., the correct drug, dosage, and dosage form, administered properly, with appropriate patient guidance and drug-effect monitoring.
2. *Patient Factors*—including the following which have a bearing on the drug dosage, drug absorption, drug metabolism, drug effectiveness:

    Age and General Health
    Status of Organ Systems (e.g. liver, kidney)
    Metabolic Disorders
    Diet and Nutrition
    Drug Sensitivities
    Multiple Disease State
    Multiple Drug Therapy
    (Concomitant Medication Taken)
    Psychological Health
    Attitude toward Compliance
    Interest in Own Health Status
    Support of Family Members
    Economic Ability (or Assistance Provided) to Obtain Required Medications
    Knowledge on Proper Use of Prescribed Medications
3. *Pharmaceutical Factors*—which relate to dosage form design and manufacture, the drug's biological availability after administration, packaging, labeling, distribution, storage, and dispensing, and include:

    Pharmaceutic Ingredients (as binders, coatings, disintegrators, buffers)
    Drug Substance Form (crystal, amorphous, particle size)
    Dissolution Rate
    Esthetic Factors (flavor, color, odor, etc.)

Drug Stability
Product Uniformity
Product Strength and Purity
Product Age and Potency on Dispensing
Appropriate Packaging for Stability, Safety, and Utility
Appropriate Labeling and Directions for Safe and Effective Use

Many of these factors are discussed in detail in subsequent chapters.

Adverse Drug Effects

There are no harmless medications; all are potentially toxic to some extent and must be prescribed and used with proper precaution. However, the hazards of medication can be greatly reduced through adherence to high quality drug standards, the application of rational drug therapy, and proper patient drug utilization.

Since the enactment of the Drug Amendments of 1962, the FDA has been more stringent in the required use of warnings regarding the use of drug products. Appropriate cautionary statements are required to be prominently displayed in a drug product's package insert as well as in all related advertising and promotional material. These statements are of the following types: *Contraindications, Warnings, Precautions,* and *Adverse Reactions.*

Contraindications.—A contraindication would preclude a particular drug from being used in a particular patient. The contraindication may be due to a patient's disease state, hypersensitivity to the drug, or interaction with another drug substance being administered. Use of the contraindicated drug in the circumstances stated could result in serious consequences to the patient, including possible death.

An example of a contraindication is as follows, for the drug ampicillin:

> **Contraindication:** Ampicillin is contraindicated in patients with a history of hypersensitivity to the penicillins.

Warnings.—Warning statements must be included in the product literature for drug substances that may be particularly dangerous to the patient under certain conditions. They are used for agents that have special toxic potential due to the inherent nature of the drug substance, or due to possible drug sensitivities, cumulative drug effects, effects on prolonged use, effects on a pregnant patient or upon the fetus, or for other reasons. The warnings do not necessarily preclude the use of the drug, but direct the prescriber to utilize the agent with great caution and with appropriate diligence.

An example of a warning is as follows, for the drug methotrexate:

> *Warning:* METHOTREXATE MUST BE USED ONLY BY PHYSICIANS EXPERIENCED IN ANTIMETABOLITE CHEMOTHERAPY.
>
> BECAUSE OF THE POSSIBILITY OF FATAL OR SEVERE TOXIC REACTIONS THE PATIENT SHOULD BE FULLY INFORMED BY THE PHYSICIAN OF THE RISKS INVOLVED AND SHOULD BE UNDER HIS CONSTANT SUPERVISION.
>
> DEATHS HAVE BEEN REPORTED WITH THE USE OF METHOTREXATE IN THE TREATMENT OF PSORIASIS. IN THE TREATMENT OF PSORIASIS METHOTREXATE SHOULD BE RESTRICTED TO SEVERE, RECALCITRANT, DISABLING, PSORIASIS WHICH IS NOT ADEQUATELY RESPONSIVE TO OTHER FORMS OF THERAPY, BUT ONLY WHEN THE DIAGNOSIS HAS BEEN ESTABLISHED, AS BY BIOPSY AND/OR AFTER DERMATOLOGIC CONSULTATION.
>
> 1. Methotrexate may produce marked depression of bone marrow, anemia, leukopenia, thrombocytopenia and bleeding.
> 2. Methotrexate may be hepatotoxic, particularly at high dosage or with prolonged therapy. Liver atrophy, necrosis, cirrhosis, fatty changes, and periportal fibrosis have been reported.
> 3. Methotrexate has caused fetal death and/or congenital anomalies, therefore, it is not recommended in women of childbearing potential unless there is appropriate medical evidence that the benefits can be expected to outweigh the considered risks. Pregnant psoriatic patients should not receive Methotrexate.

4. Impaired renal function is usually a contraindication.
5. Diarrhea and ulcerative stomatitis are frequent toxic effects and require interruption of therapy; otherwise hemorrhagic enteritis and death from intestinal perforation may occur.

Precautions.—These statements inform prescribers to be cautious in the use of the drug under certain circumstances related to the patient's condition, dosage levels, prolonged use, concomitant drug therapy, and other situations. A precautionary statement emphasizes special caution, beyond that which is normally heeded in the prescribing of any drug substance.

An example of a precaution is as follows, for the drug propranolol:

Precautions: Propranolol should be used with caution in patients with impaired liver function. Reduced metabolic capabilities in many elderly patients may require dosage reduction.

Caution is essential when the drug is administered in the presence of diabetes mellitus. Propranolol may blunt premonitory signs and symptoms (e.g., tachycardia, blood pressure changes) of acute hypoglycemia.

Propranolol may mask the clinical signs, e.g., tachycardia, of developing or continuing hyperthyroidism. Abrupt withdrawal may exacerbate symptoms of hyperthyroidism, including thyroid storm; therefore, slowly withdraw the drug.

Drug Interactions: The hypoglycemic effects of insulin may be prolonged by propranolol. The cardiostimulating and bronchodilating effects of sympathomimetics are antagonized by propranolol. Smoking may reduce serum levels and increase the clearance of propranolol in patients who take it on a chronic basis.

Nursing mothers: Problems in breast-feeding mothers maintained on propranolol have not been documented. However, risk-benefit must be considered because propranolol is excreted in breast milk in small quantities

Adverse Reactions.—These statements report undesired effects which may occur in pa-

tients taking a particular medication. Some of these undesired effects may be predictable and expected to occur in a given percentage of patients taking the medication whereas other effects may be unexpected. The unexpected effects may be due to patient hypersensitivity to the medication, patient idiosyncrasies, or other factors. Some adverse effects may be serious, as anaphylactic reactions of blood dyscrasias, and may require the discontinuance of the medication. Other adverse effects may be relatively minor, as constipation or dry skin, and may be tolerated by the patient. Each adverse effect must be promptly reported by the patient and evaluated for its seriousness and implication. Frequently, minor undesired drug effects may be modified by changing the dosage, the dosage form and route of administration, or by taking with or without food or at certain time intervals. Occasionally a second drug may be used to modify the adverse effects of the primary drug. Patients frequently refer to the undesired effects of a drug as *side effects* (as the drowsiness experienced with antihistamines).

For a given drug substance, the known adverse effects may be few in number or extensive. Glucocorticoids represent a good example of a drug group that has the potential to produce a wide range of adverse effects. Risk/benefit decisions must be made on an individual patient case basis when such reactions occur.

The following are some adverse effects associated with long-term use of glucocorticoids and indicating a need for medical attention (possible cause in parentheses where appropriate—not necessarily inclusive)

Acne or other skin problems
Back or rib pain (osteoporosis)
Black and/or tarry stools (gastrointestinal bleeding)
Impaired wound healing
Increased susceptibility to infections
Irregular heartbeat, muscle cramps or pain, and/or unusual tiredness or weakness (potassium depletion)
Menstrual problems (endocrine imbalance)

> Mental depression (psychic changes)
> Moon face (Cushing's syndrome)
> Stomach pain or burning (peptic ulcer, pancreatitis)
> Swelling of feet or lower legs (sodium and fluid retention)

Drug Dosage

There are various terms in use regarding the dose of drug substances. The *usual dose* of a drug may be defined as that amount which may be expected to produce, in adults, the medicinal effect for which it is indicated. It serves as a guide to physicians who then may vary the dose depending upon the particular requirements of the patient. The *usual dosage range* for a drug indicates the quantitative range or amounts of the drug that may be prescribed within the framework of usual medical practice. Doses falling outside of the usual dosage range may be questioned by the pharmacist as being either underdosage or overdosage, and subject to further scrutiny and consultation with the prescriber. For drugs which may be administered to children, a *usual pediatric dose* is generally included in the literature.

The schedule of dosage, or the *dosage regimen,* is frequently given in the drug literature. For instance, some drugs are best taken at specific intervals (e.g., every 8 hours) or at specific times (e.g., at bedtime, before meals, or on arising in the morning). Single doses are given for some drugs and daily doses for others, depending upon the drug substance, the dosage form, and the condition being treated. When a drug is taken for an extended period of time, as aspirin for arthritis, a daily dose is appropriate. When aspirin is taken occasionally as for a headache, a single dose is more appropriate.

For certain drugs, an *initial, priming,* or *loading* dose may be required to attain the desired concentration of the drug in the blood or tissues, which may then be maintained through the subsequent administration of regularly scheduled *maintenance doses.* Digoxin, a cardiotonic agent, is a good example of a drug which is administered in this way. The initial goal of digoxin therapy is to achieve the desired *digoxin level* in the patient through the initial administration of the drug four or more times a day. Then a single daily dose may be given to maintain the desired blood level of the drug.

For drugs like pentobarbital that produce more than one effect, depending upon the dose administered, the dose for each of the effects is provided in the literature. In doses of 20 mg, pentobarbital usually produces sedation in the adult patient, whereas in doses of 100 mg, the drug produces a hypnotic effect.

Pharmaceutical preparations are generally formulated so that the usual dose is provided in a convenient unit of the dosage form—as in one tablet, capsule, or suppository or in one teaspoonful (5 mL) or tablespoonful (15 mL) of a liquid preparation.[2] Doses of drug substances may vary depending upon the route of administration (e.g. oral, rectal, injection). This is largely due to a variation in the degree of drug absorption and subsequent action following administration by the various routes.

Certain biological products, as Tetanus Immune Globulin, may have two different usual doses, one the *prophylactic dose,* or that amount administered to protect the patient from contracting the illness, and the second, the *therapeutic dose* which is administered to a patient after exposure or contraction of the illness. The recommended doses of vaccines and other biological products including antibiotics and endocrine products are sometimes expressed in *units of activity* rather than in specific quantitative amounts of the drug substance. Units of activity derived from biological assay methods reflect a drug's potency and become necessary when suitable chemical assay methods are unavailable for a particular drug. Drugs from natural sources, with unknown or varying complex chemical composition, may vary in potency, one batch to another, even though the same quantitative amount of material is present. Biological assays are useful in determining relative potencies of different batches of the same drug and in their standardization. The potency of a given drug is based on the comparison with an international reference standard of that drug. Insulin injection, for example, is prepared to contain 40, 100, or 500 Insulin units of activity in each milliliter of injection to meet all dosage requirements in a convenient amount of injection. These units of activity reflect the relative potency of the different preparations in terms of biological activity and are uniform on an international basis. Since the biological activities of different products, such as penicillin, poliomyelitis vaccine, and insulin, are so varied, the units of activity for each is specific for each drug

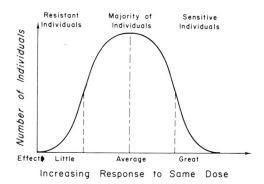

Fig. 2–5. *Drug effect in a population sample.*

and has no relation between the units of activity for another drug.

Today drug dosage is expressed almost exclusively in the metric system. Systems of weights and measures applicable to pharmacy are presented in Appendix II.

Factors Affecting Drug Dosage

The dose of a drug has been appropriately described as an amount which is "enough but not too much," the idea being to produce the drug's optimum therapeutic effect in a particular patient with the lowest possible dose. The dose of a given drug is specific to the patient, with many factors contributing to its size and effectiveness. The correct dose of aspirin to relieve the pain of a headache would vary from individual to individual and, indeed, within the same individual from one occasion to another. The familiar bell-shaped curve, presented in Figure 2–5 shows that in a normal distribution of patients, a drug's usual dose will provide what might be called an average effect in the majority of individuals. In a portion of the patients, however, the drug will produce little effect, whereas in another group of similar size, the drug will produce an effect greater than the average effect. The amount of drug that will generally produce the desired effect in the majority of patients is considered the drug's usual dose and would likely be the initial dose for an individual taking the drug for the first time. From this initial dose the physician may, if necessary, increase or decrease subsequent doses to meet the particular requirements of the patient.

In order for a drug to provide systemic effects, it must be absorbed from its route of administration at a suitable rate, be distributed in ad-

equate concentration to the receptor sites, and remain there for a sufficient duration of time. One measure of a drug's absorption characteristics is the determination of its blood serum concentration at various time intervals following administration. For systemic drugs, a correlation can be made between their blood serum concentration and the presentation of drug effects. An average blood serum concentration of a drug can be determined that represents the minimum concentration that can be expected to produce the drug's desired effects in a patient. This concentration is referred to as the *Minimum Effective Concentration* (MEC). As shown in Figure 2–6, for a hypothetical drug, the serum concentration of the drug reaches the MEC 2 hours following its administration, achieves a peak concentration in 4 hours and decreases below the MEC in 10 hours. If it would be desired to maintain the drug serum concentration above the MEC for a longer period of time, a second dose of the drug would be required at approximately the 8-hour time frame. The time-blood level curve presented in Figure 2–6 is an example. In practice, the curve would vary, depending on the nature of the drug substance, its chemical and physical characteristics, the dosage form administered as well as pathological state of the patient, dietary and smoking habits, concomitant drug therapy, and other considerations. Factors of dosage form design affecting the biological availability of a drug for absorption will be considered more extensively in Chapter 3. The second level of blood serum concentration of drug labeled MTC in Figure 2–6 refers to the *Minimum Toxic Concentration*. Drug serum concentrations above this level would produce dose-related toxic effects in the average individual and perhaps would negate the desirable effects of the drug, compromising the safety of the patient. Ideally, the serum drug concentration in a well-dosed patient would be maintained between the MEC and the MTC (the "therapeutic window" for the drug) for the period that drug effects are desired. Table 2–2 presents examples of therapeutic, toxic, and lethal concentrations for some drug substances.

The *median effective dose* of a drug is that amount which will produce the desired intensity of effect in 50% of the individuals tested. The *median toxic dose* is that amount which will produce a defined toxic effect in 50% of the individuals tested. The relationship between the desired and undesired effects of a drug is

Fig. 2–6. *Example of a blood level curve for a hypothetical drug as a function of time following oral administration. MEC stands for* minimum effective concentration *and MTC for* minimum toxic concentration.

commonly expressed as the *therapeutic index* and is defined as the ratio between a drug's median toxic dose and its median effective dose, TD50/ED50. Thus, a drug with a therapeutic index of 15 would be expected to have a greater margin of safety in its use than a drug with a therapeutic index of 5. For certain drugs, the therapeutic index may be as low as 2 and extreme caution must be exercised in the administration of agents such as these. Table 2–3 presents the therapeutic indices of various drugs.

The therapeutic index must be viewed as a general guide to the margin of safety of a drug, with each patient considered separately. The therapeutic index does not take into account

individual patient idiosyncrasy. Further, because the criteria for determining the therapeutic index involve the use of median figures and intentionally narrow definitions of "effectiveness" and "toxicity," the index does not reflect extremes of the population sample and, depending upon the definitions of effectiveness and toxicity used, a number of therapeutic indices may be determined for a single drug. For instance, the median effective dose for aspirin can be determined for simple headache, arthritic pain, fever, or other conditions and a different ED50 and therapeutic index calculated. Factors that can influence the proper dose of a drug for a given patient include the patient's

Table 2–2. Examples of Therapeutic and Toxic Blood Level Concentrations of Some Drug Substances*

Drug Substance	Drug Substance Concentration, mg/liter		
	Therapeutic	Toxic	Lethal
Acetaminophen	10–20	400	1500
Amitriptyline	0.5–0.20	0.4	10–20
Barbiturates:			
short acting	1	7	10
intermediate acting	1–5	10–30	30
long acting	~10	40–60	80–150
Dextropropoxyphene	0.05–0.2	5–10	57
Diazepam	0.5–2.5	5–20	>50
Digoxin	0.0006–0.0013	0.002–0.009	—
Imipramine	0.05–0.16	0.7	2
Lidocaine	1.2–5.0	6	—
Lithium	4.2–8.3	13.9	13.9–34.7
Meperidine	0.6–0.65	5	30
Morphine	0.1	—	0.05–4
Phenytoin	5–22	50	100
Quinidine	3–6	10	30–50
Theophylline	20–100	—	—

*Adapted from Winek, C.L.: *Clin. Chem.* 22:832, 1976, and Goth, A.: *Medical Pharmacology*, 11th ed, St. Louis, C.V. Mosby Co., 1984, pp. 757–759.

Table 2–3. **Examples of Therapeutic Indices for Various Drug Substances**[1]

Drug Substances with Therapeutic Indices		
Less than 5	Between 5 and 10	Greater than 10
Amitriptyline	Barbiturates	Acetaminophen
Chlordiazepoxide	Diazepam	Bromide
Diphenhydramine	Digoxin	Chloral hydrate
Ethchlorvynol	Imipramine	Glutethimide
Lidocaine	Meperidine	Meprobamate
Methadone	Paraldehyde	Nortriptyline
Procainamide	Primodone	Pentazocine
Quinidine	Thioridazine	Propoxyphene

[1]From Niazi, S.: *Textbook of Biopharmaceutics and Clinical Pharmacokinetics,* New York, Appleton-Century-Crofts, 1979, p. 254.

age, weight, sex, pathological state, his tolerance to the drug, the time of the drug's administration, the nature of the dosage form and the route of administration, the concurrent administration of other drugs, and a variety of physiologic and psychologic factors. Some of these factors are considered briefly here.

1. AGE. The age of the patient is a consideration in the determination of drug dosage. It is particularly true in treating neonatal, pediatric and geriatric patients. Newborn infants, particularly those born prematurely, are abnormally sensitive to certain drugs because of the immature state of their hepatic and renal function by which drugs are normally inactivated and eliminated from the body. Failure to detoxify and eliminate drugs results in their accumulation in the tissues to a toxic level.

Before there was an understanding of the physiologic differences between adult and pediatric patients, the latter were treated with drugs as if they were merely miniature adults. Various rules of dosage in which the pediatric dose was a fraction of the adult dose, based on relative age, were created for youngsters. Today these rules are not in general use because age alone is no longer considered to be a singularly valid criterion for use in the determination of children's dosage, especially when calculated from a *usual* adult dose which itself provides wide clinical variations in response. Instead, the *usual pediatric dose,* determined for specific drugs and dosage forms by clinical evaluation, is most commonly utilized. These pediatric doses are included in drug literature and in pharmaceutical product labeling and are used as guidelines to be considered with other factors in the dosage determination for a specific pediatric patient. In instances in which dosage for a pediatric patient

is calculated, methods using body weight and body surface area are most used (see below). Administering the drug at the proper dosing interval (e.g., every 4 hours) is also important to assure therapeutic efficacy.

The number and proportion of persons over age 65 in the United States have increased steadily during this century. In 1900, only 3.1 million people, comprising 4% of the population, were over the age of 65. Today, about 12% of the population has reached that age, and projections indicate that this figure will double by the year 2030.[3,4] By that date, there are expected to be approximately 55 million persons over the age of 65, comprising 20% of the population in this country. The number of persons over the age of 85 is expected to triple.

As a group, persons over the age of 65 utilize more health services and products, including prescription and non-prescription medications, than any other age group. They also present unique therapeutic problems which require the special attention, skill, and understanding of health practitioners. It is essential that physicians and pharmacists recognize the physiologic changes that may occur with age. Most physiologic functions begin to diminish in adults following their third decade of life. For example, cardiac output declines approximately 1% per year from age 20 to age 80. Glomerular filtration rate also falls progressively until at age 80, it may be only half of what it was at age 20. There is also a decrease in vital capacity, immune capacity and liver microsomal enzyme function.[3]

The decline in renal and hepatic function in the elderly may slow drug clearance and increases the possibility of drug accumulation in the body and subsequent toxicity. Dosing of medication in the elderly must include this consideration. Elderly persons may also respond differently to drugs than younger patients because of changes in drug-receptor sensitivity or because of age-related alterations in target tissues or organs.[4]

Chronic conditions have largely replaced acute illnesses as the leading causes of death in the elderly population. Frequently, acute illnesses represent the terminal episode of a progressively debilitating chronic disorder. The chronic disorders present in the majority of geriatric patients include cardiovascular disease, cerebrovascular disease, malignant neoplasms, diabetes, and rheumatic disease. Frequently in the elderly patient, there are multiple medical problems which require concomitant treatment. An acute illness may present itself along with one or more chronic conditions, complicating drug therapy and raising the possibility of drug-drug interactions, adverse drug effects, and even therapeutic failure. The elderly patient, taking multiple medications frequently faces difficulty in taking each one according to the prescribed schedule. The elderly have special problems in complying with therapeutic regimens. The hearing and sight of the elderly are frequently diminished. Because of these physical impairments, their ability to communicate is often affected. The pharmacist can be of special assistance in achieving patient compliance with medications through careful communications, skillful drug packaging and labeling techniques and patient monitoring.

2. BODY WEIGHT. The *usual doses* for drugs are considered generally suitable for 70 kg (150 pound) individuals. The ratio between the amount of drug administered and the size of the body influences the drug concentration at its site of action. Therefore, drug dosage may require adjustment from the usual adult dose for abnormally lean or obese patients. The determination of drug dosage for youngsters on the basis of body weight is considered more dependable than that based strictly on age.

For some drug substances, a pediatric dose may be based on a combination of age and weight. For example, the recommended dose for iron replacement in deficiency states is:

6 months to 2 years of age—up to 6 mg/kg/day
2 years to 12 years of age—3 mg/kg/day

For maintenance following institution of iron therapy, generally 6 months of oral iron therapy is required to reverse uncomplicated iron defi-ciency anemia, or approximately 2 to 4 months beyond the time the anemia is reversed as indicated by laboratory blood analysis.

As indicated above, when dosage is based on body weight, it is frequently expressed on a *milligram* (drug) *per kilogram* (body weight) basis. Occasionally, a literature reference may express the dose of a drug based on a *milligram per pound* of body weight.

3. BODY SURFACE AREA. Other methods of determining drug dosage have been proposed in preference to those based solely on age or weight. One such method has as its basis the recognition that a close correlation exists between a large number of physiological processes and body surface area (BSA). A formula for the determination of a child's dose based on relative body surface area and the adult dose is:

$$\frac{\text{Surface of child's body}}{\text{Surface area adult's body}}$$

$$\times \text{ Adult Usual Dose}$$

$$= \text{ Approximate Child's Dose}$$

The surface area of individuals may be determined from a nomogram composed of scales of height, weight, and surface area. Two such nomograms are presented in Fig. 2–7. Surface area is indicated where a straight line drawn to connect the height and weight of an individual intersects the surface area column. The administration of a total adult dose is considered appropriate when the body surface area reaches 1.7 square meters, thus this figure may be employed in the denominator of the just-mentioned formula.

For some drug substances, the dose may be indicated in terms of *milligrams per square meter*. For instance, the usual pediatric dose of chlorambucil based in BSA is 4.5 mg per square meter per day as a single dose or in divided doses. Using the nomogram for calculating the BSA of children and using the example of a child weighing 15 kg and measuring 100 cm in height, the surface area would be 0.64 square meter. Thus, the dose of chlorambucil for this child would be: 4.5 mg $\times$ 0.64 = 2.88 mg once a day or in divided daily doses.

4. SEX. Women are thought to be more susceptible to the effects of certain drugs than are men, and in some instances this difference is considered sufficient to necessitate reduction in

Nomogram for Calculating the Body Surface Area of Children[1]

Nomogram for Calculating the Body Surface Area of Adults[1]

[1] From the formula of Du Bois and Du Bois, *Arch. intern. Med.* **17**, 863, 1916: $S = W^{0.425} \times H^{0.725} \times 71.84$, or $\log S = 0.425 \log W + 0.725 \log H + 1.8564$, where S = body surface area in square centimeters, W = weight in kilograms, H = height in centimeters

Fig. 2–7. *Nomograms for calculating body surface area. (From* Documenta Geigy Scientific Tables, *6th ed., pp. 632–633. By permission of R.J. Geigy S.A.)*

dosage. During pregnancy, caution is necessary in the administration of drugs that might affect the uterus or fetus. A number of drugs have been shown to be readily transported from the maternal to the fetal circulation including such agents as: alcohol, anesthetic gases, barbiturates, narcotic and non-narcotic analgesics, anticoagulants, anti-infective agents, and many others.[5,6] Fetal exposure to agents such as these has resulted in adverse effects to the fetus, sometimes resulting in death *in utero* or in congenital damage to the neonate. The fetus is apparently more sensitive to the effects of certain drugs than is the mother. For instance, respiration in the fetus may be halted at a level of general anesthesia that does not impair maternal respiration. Also, because of the undeveloped and thus ineffective drug detoxication and excretion mechanisms present in the fetus, concentrations of drugs may actually reach a higher level in the fetus than in the maternal circulation. The addiction of newborn infants to narcotic drugs as heroin and morphine due to the maternal use of these agents during pregnancy is not an uncommon occurrence. The same result occurs when an infant is breast-fed by a narcotic-dependent mother. The transfer of drugs from the mother to the nursing infant through human milk may occur with a wide variety of drugs with the drug effects becoming manifest in the infant.[7,8] Thus, pregnant women and nursing mothers should use medications only with the advice and under the guidance of their physician. In an effort to protect pregnant/nursing women, the Food and Drug Administration instituted in 1983, the following labeling requirement on *non*prescription drug products:

As with any drug, if you are pregnant or nursing a baby, seek the advice of a health professional before using this product.

5. PATHOLOGIC STATE. The effects of certain drugs may be modified by the pathologic condition of the patient and must be considered in determining the drug to use as well as its proper dose. For example, if tetracycline HCl is used in the presence of renal impairment, it may lead to the excessive systemic accumulation of the drug and possible liver toxicity. Under such conditions, lower than usual doses are indicated, and if therapy is prolonged, blood serum levels of the drug should be taken and the patient monitored at regular intervals to assure the maintenance of non-toxic levels of the drug.

Also, liver function tests may be performed to detect possible liver damage. Drugs having a high danger potential in a given therapeutic situation should be used only when the possible benefit to the patient exceeds the possible risk and when no other suitable drug with a lesser toxicity is available.

6. TOLERANCE. The ability to endure the influence of a drug, particularly when acquired by a continued use of the substance, is referred to as drug *tolerance*. It is usually developed to a specific drug or to its chemical congeners; in the latter instance it is referred to as *cross-tolerance*. The effect of drug tolerance is that the drug dosage must be increased to maintain a given therapeutic response. Tolerance occurs commonly to the use of such drugs as antihistaminics, narcotic analgesics, and barbiturates. After the development of tolerance to a certain drug or type of drug, normal sensitivity may be regained only by suspending the drug's administration for a period of time. For most drugs, the development of tolerance can be minimized by initiating therapy with the lowest effective dose and by avoiding prolonged administration.

7. CONCOMITANT DRUG THERAPY. The effects of a drug may be modified by the prior or concurrent administration of another drug. Such interferences between drugs are referred to as *drug-drug interactions* and are due to the chemical or physical interaction between the drugs or to an alteration of the absorption, distribution, metabolism, or excretion patterns of one of the drugs. The effects of drug-drug interactions may be desirable and beneficial to the patient or they may be detrimental. An example of a beneficial interaction involves the drugs probenecid and penicillin or its derivatives. Given concomitantly, probenecid causes the prolongation of penicillin serum levels, enabling a reduction in the total dose of penicillin required as well as in the frequency of its administration. This has the effect of reducing the incidence of missed dosage administration by patients.

A detrimental interaction between drugs may be exemplified by that between certain metal ions and the antibiotic tetracycline or its derivatives. Tetracyclines can combine with the metal ions calcium, magnesium, aluminum, and iron in the gastrointestinal tract to form complexes that are poorly absorbed. Many antacid drugs are particularly rich in calcium, magnesium, and aluminum and should be avoided during tetracycline administration. If offending antacids and tetracycline are both required in a patient, they should be given alternately according to a strict schedule which avoids their simultaneous presence during the period allowed for tetracycline absorption. Certain calcium-containing foods, as milk, cheese, and other dairy products must similarly be restricted during tetracycline administration.

Another example of drug-drug interaction which can alter the effectiveness of a given dose of drug involves the drug cimetidine and the anticoagulant drug warfarin. Cimetidine reduces liver microsomal enzymes which can result in the decreased rate of metabolism of a number of drugs including warfarin. Thus, a person stabilized on a specific dose of warfarin may require an decreased dosage level of that drug if cimetidine is subsequently added to the therapeutic regimen. Conversely, if a patient is stabilized on a level of warfarin while also being administered cimetidine, the dosage of the warfarin would likely need to be increased if the cimetidine therapy is discontinued.

A person's use of "social" agents may also interact with prescribed medications. Numerous studies have demonstrated that smoking can influence the rate of elimination of theophylline from the body. Cigarette and marijuana smoking stimulates the hepatic metabolism of theophylline and shortens its half-life, increases total body theophylline clearance, and reduces theophylline serum concentration levels. Smokers may require a 50 to 100% increase in theophylline dosage to accommodate this interaction and a period of time between 3 months to 2 years may be necessary to normalize the effects of smoking on theophylline kinetics. Interestingly, because of the smoking-induced reduction in serum theophylline levels smokers tend to encounter less adverse reactions to theophylline. When patients stop smoking, the smoking-induced metabolism of theophylline dissipates slowly over a period of time and downward adjustments in theophylline dosage are made accordingly. It has also been demonstrated that diabetic patients who smoke heavily may require insulin dosage one-third higher than normal. It is thought that this is due partly to the increased catecholamine and corticosteroid release caused by smoking. In addition, it has been demonstrated that smoking-induced peripheral vasoconstriction will reduce the rate of insulin absorption following subcutaneous injection.

The study of drug interactions is an important facet of drug therapy and pharmacy practice. A number of excellent reference sources are available in this area for student and practitioner use.

8. TIME OF ADMINISTRATION. The time at which a drug is administered sometimes influences dosage. This is especially true for oral therapy in relation to meals. Absorption proceeds more rapidly if the stomach and upper portions of the intestinal tract are free of food, and an amount of a drug that is effective when taken before a meal may be ineffective if administered during or after eating. On the other hand, irritating drugs are better tolerated by the patient if food is present in the stomach to dilute the drug's concentration.

The proper schedule of a drug's dosage (as "four times a day," or "every 8 hours") is a factor of the illness and the body drug level desired, the physicochemical nature of the drug itself, the dosage form design, and the degree and rate of the drug's absorption, distribution, metabolism and elimination from the body. These factors will be discussed in Chapter 4.

9. DOSAGE FORM AND ROUTE OF ADMINISTRATION. The dosage of a given drug may vary, depending upon the dosage form employed and the route of administration utilized. This is due to the different rates and extents of absorption resulting from the various means of administering drugs. Drugs administered intravenously enter the blood stream directly and thus the full amount administered is present in the blood. In contrast, drugs administered orally are rarely, if ever, fully absorbed due to the various physical, chemical, and biologic barriers to their absorption, including interactions with the gastric and intestinal contents. Thus in many instances, a lesser parenteral (injectable) dose of a drug is required than the oral dose to achieve the same blood levels of drug or clinical effects. This is not to say that adequate absorption cannot take place from the various body sites. Sufficient absorption of certain drugs can be achieved from the rectum, gastrointestinal tract, under the tongue, through the skin and from other sites. However, each drug has to be studied individually to determine the best routes of its administration and then suitable dosage forms and drug delivery systems designed to carry the necessary amount of drug to meet the desired clinical requirements.

Commercially prepared dosage forms contain fixed amounts of drugs designed to meet the *usual dosage* requirements of patients. The liquid dosage forms, as injections, syrups and elixirs, are flexible in that they permit the dosage administered to be easily adjusted simply by altering the volume of product used. Some tablets are *scored* or grooved to permit even breaking to facilitate the accurate administration of partial dosage units. However, some dosage forms as capsules and unscored tablets do not permit easy and accurate partial dosage unit administration. Thus, to provide greater flexibility in the selection and use of commercially prepared dosage forms, manufacturers generally prepare more than a single strength of a given drug product. For instance, phenobarbital tablets are commercially available containing 15, 30, 60, and 100 mg of phenobarbital. Information as to the available strengths of drug products is provided to the pharmacist by means of drug package inserts, drug literature, and reference books.

Selected Reading

Allan, F.M.: Standardization of Drug Names. *JAMA*, 229:541, 1974.

Cohen, H.J.: The Elderly Patient. A Challenge to the Art and Science of Medicine. *Drug Therapy*, 13:41, 1983.

Faich, G.A.: *Postmarketing Surveillance of Prescription Drugs: Current Status*. New York, Clinical Medicine Research Institute, 1986.

Griffiths, M.C. (ed.): *USAN and the USP Dictionary of Drug Names*. Rockville, MD., United States Pharmacopeial Convention, Inc., 1986.

Hansten, P.D., and Horn, J.R.: *Drug Interactions*. 6th Ed., Philadelphia, Lea & Febiger, 1989.

Leff, R.D., and Roberts, R.J.: Problems in Drug Therapy for Pediatric Patients. *Am. J. Hosp. Pharm.*, 44:865, 1987.

Sills, J.M., Tanner, L.A., and Milstein, J.B.: Food and Drug Administration Monitoring of Adverse Drug Reactions. *Am. J. Hosp. Pharm.*, 43:2764–2769, 1986.

Simonson, W.: The Pharmacist's Role in Geriatric Care. *Wellcome Trends in Pharmacy*, 9:8, 1987.

Stanasek, W.F. and Baker, D.: Drug Monitoring in the Geriatric Patient. *Am. Pharm.*, NS23:32, 1983.

Notes

1. Over the past few decades, concern over rising health care costs has led to attempts to reduce the drug-portion of these costs through the use of less expensive generic drug products. Initially, physicians were urged to write prescriptions for generic drugs. Subsequently, a number of states passed laws permitting or mandating the generic substitution of drugs by pharmacists. Then, in 1984, the Drug Price Competition and Patent Term Restoration Act was enacted which simplifies and expedites the process by which generic drug products are approved for marketing. Between 1981 and 1988, generic drug product sales quadrupled to a level of about 35% of the prescription drug market. (The "generic equivalency" of drug products is discussed in Chapter 3.)

2. Although the American National Standards Institute has established the volume of the American Standard Teaspoon to be 4.93 ± 0.24 mL and thus, for practical purposes, pharmacists utilize 5 mL, the actual volumes of household teaspoons and tablespoons may vary widely. A recent report noted that volumes of commonly used teaspoons may vary from 2.5 to 9.7 mL and tablespoons from 6.0 to 16.5 mL. In fact, the same spoon will deliver varying volumes depending upon the person measuring the medication and the nature of the medication itself. For accuracy of measurement, many pharmacists dispense a calibrated measuring spoon with liquid medication. (Kimminau, M.D.: Spoons Provide Potential for Dosing Errors. *American Pharmacy*, NS19, No. 12:25–27, 1979.)

3. Cohen, H.J.: The Elderly Patient, A Challenge to the Art and Science of Medicine, *Drug Therapy* 13:41, 1983.

4. Futerman Reses, S.S.: The Geriatric Patient—Pharmacy Care Can Make a Difference. *The Apothecary*, 94:34, 1982.

5. Martin, E.W.: *Hazards of Medication*. Philadelphia, J.B. Lippincott Co., 1972, pp. 274–280.

6. Richardson, E.R.: Drugs and Pregnancy, *Wellcome Trends in Pharmacy*, 7:4, 1983.

7. Goldberg, R.J. and Cutie, A.J.: Drug Excretion into Human Milk. *Pharmacy Times*, May, 1982, p. 60.

8. The Transfer of Drugs and Other Chemicals Into Human Breast Milk. *Am. Pharm.*, NS23:29–36, 1983.

3 | *Dosage Form Design: Biopharmaceutic Considerations*

THE BIOLOGIC response to a drug is the result of an interaction between the drug substance and functionally important molecules (receptors) in the living system. The response is due to an alteration in the biologic processes that were present prior to the drug's administration. The magnitude of the response is related to the concentration of the drug achieved at the site of its action. This drug concentration depends upon the dosage of the drug administered, the extent of its absorption and distribution to the site, and the rate and extent of its elimination from the body. The physical and chemical constitution of the drug substance—particularly its lipid solubility, degree of ionization, and molecular size—determines to a great extent its ability to effect its biological activity. The area of study embracing this relationship between the physical, chemical, and biological sciences as they apply to drugs, dosage forms, and to drug action has been given the descriptive term *biopharmaceutics*.

In general, for a drug to exert its biologic effect, it must be transported by the body fluids, traverse the required biologic membrane barriers, escape widespread distribution to unwanted areas, endure metabolic attack, penetrate in adequate concentration to the sites of action, and interact in a specific fashion, causing an alteration of cellular function. A simplified diagram of this complex series of events between a drug's administration and its elimination is presented in Figure 3–1.

The absorption, distribution, biotransformation (metabolism), and elimination of a drug from the body are dynamic processes that continue from the time a drug is taken until all of the drug has been removed from the body. The *rates* at which these processes occur affect the onset, intensity, and the duration of the drug's activity within the body. The area of study which elucidates the time course of drug concentration in the blood and tissues is termed *pharmacokinetics*. It is the study of the kinetics

of absorption, distribution, metabolism and excretion of drugs and their corresponding pharmacologic, therapeutic, or toxic response in animals and man.[1] Further, since one drug may alter the absorption, distribution, metabolism or excretion of another drug, pharmacokinetics also may be applied in the study of interactions between drugs.

Once a drug is administered and drug absorption begins, the drug does not remain in a single body location, but rather is distributed throughout the body until its ultimate elimination. For instance, following the oral administration of a drug and its entry into the gastrointestinal tract, a portion of the drug is absorbed into the circulatory system from which it is distributed to the various other body fluids, tissues, and organs. From these sites the drug may return to the circulatory system and be excreted through the kidney as such or the drug may be metabolized by the liver or other cellular sites and be excreted as metabolites. As shown in Figure 3–1, drugs administered by intravenous injection are placed directly into the circulatory system, thereby avoiding the absorption process which is required from all other routes of administration for systemic effects.

The various body locations to which a drug travels may be viewed as separate compartments, each containing some fraction of the administered dose of drug. The transfer of drug from the blood to other body locations is generally a rapid process and is reversible; that is, the drug may diffuse back into the circulation. The drug in the blood therefore exists in equilibrium with the drug in the other compartments. However, in this equilibrium state, the concentration of the drug in the blood may be quite different (greater or lesser) than the concentration of the drug in the other compartments. This is due largely to the physiochemical properties of the drug and its resultant ability to leave the blood and traverse the biological membranes. Certain drugs may leave the cir-

51

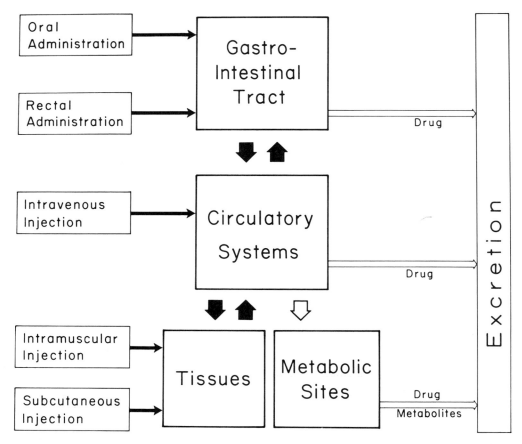

Fig. 3–1. *Schematic representation of events of absorption, metabolism, and excretion of drugs after their administration by various routes.*

culatory system rapidly and completely, whereas other drugs may do so slowly and with difficulty. A number of drugs become bound to blood proteins, particularly the albumins, and only a small fraction of the drug administered may actually be found at locations outside of the circulatory system at a given time. The transfer of drug from one compartment to another is mathematically associated with a specific rate constant describing that particular transfer. Generally, the rate of transfer of a drug from one compartment to another is proportional to the concentration of the drug in the compartment from which it exits; the greater the concentration, the greater is the amount of drug transfer.

Metabolism is the major process by which foreign substances, including drugs are eliminated from the body. In the process of metab-

olism a drug substance may be biotransformed into pharmacologically active or inactive metabolites. Often, both the drug substance and its metabolite(s) are active and exert pharmacologic effects. For example, desmethyldiazepam is an active metabolite common to halazepam, prazepam and diazepam. In some instances a pharmacologically inactive drug (termed a *prodrug* in this instance) may be administered for the known effects of its active metabolites. Dipivefrin, for example, is a prodrug of epinephrine formed by the esterification of epinephrine and pivalic acid. This enhances the lipophilic character of the drug, and as a consequence its penetration into the anterior chamber of the eye is 17 times that of epinephrine. Within the eye, dipivefrin HCl is converted by enzymatic hydrolysis to epinephrine.

The metabolism of a drug to inactive products

is usually an irreversible process which culminates in the excretion of the drug from the body, usually via the urine. The pharmacokineticist may calculate an elimination rate constant (termed k_{el}) for a drug to describe its rate of elimination from the body. The term *elimination* refers to both metabolism and excretion. For drugs which are administered intravenously, and therefore involve no absorption process, the task is much less complex than for drugs administered orally or by other routes. In the latter instances, drug absorption and drug elimination are occurring simultaneously but at different rates.

General Principles of Drug Absorption

Before an administered drug can arrive at its site of action in effective concentrations, it must surmount a number of barriers. These barriers are chiefly a succession of biologic membranes such as those of the gastrointestinal epithelium, lungs, blood, and brain. Body membranes are generally classified as three main types: (a) those composed of several layers of cells, as the skin; (b) those composed of a single layer of cells, as the intestinal epithelium; and (c) those of less than one cell in thickness, as the membrane of a single cell. In most instances a drug substance must pass more than one of these membrane types before it reaches its site of action. For instance, a drug taken orally must first traverse the gastrointestinal membranes (stomach, small and large intestine), gain entrance into the general circulation, pass to the organ or tissue with which it has affinity, gain entrance into that tissue, and then enter into its individual cells.

Although the chemistry of body membranes differs one from another, the membranes may be viewed in general as a bimolecular lipoid (fat-containing) layer attached on both sides to a protein layer. Drugs are thought to penetrate these biologic membranes in two general ways: (1) by passive diffusion and (2) through specialized transport mechanisms. Within each of these main categories, more clearly defined processes have been ascribed to drug transfer.

Passive Diffusion

The term *passive diffusion* is used to describe the passage of (drug) molecules through a membrane which behaves inertly in that it does not actively participate in the process. Drugs absorbed according to this method are said to be *passively absorbed*. The absorption process is driven by the concentration gradient (i.e., the differences in concentration) existing across the membrane, with the passage of drug molecules occurring primarily from the side of high drug concentration to the side of lower drug concentration. Most drugs pass through biologic membranes by diffusion.

Passive diffusion is described by *Fick's first law*, which states that the rate of diffusion or transport across a membrane (dc/dt) is proportional to the difference in drug concentration on both sides of the membrane:

$$-\frac{dc}{dt} = P\,(C_1 - C_2)$$

in which C_1 and C_2 refer to the drug concentrations on each side of the membrane and P is a permeability coefficient or constant. The term C_1 is customarily used to represent the compartment with the greater concentration of drug and thus the transport of drug proceeds from compartment one (e.g., absorption site) to compartment two (e.g., blood).

Because the concentration of drug at the site of absorption (C_1) is usually much greater than on the other side of the membrane, due to the rapid dilution of the drug in the blood and its subsequent distribution to the tissues, for practical purposes the value of $C_1 - C_2$ may be taken simply as that of C_1 and the equation written in the standard form for a first order rate equation:

$$-\frac{dc}{dt} = P\,C_1$$

The gastrointestinal absorption of most drugs from solution occurs in this manner in accordance with *first order kinetics* in which the rate is dependent upon drug concentration i.e., doubling the dose doubles the transfer rate. The magnitude of the permeability constant, depends on the diffusion coefficient of the drug, the thickness and area of the absorbing membrane, and the permeability of the membrane to the particular drug.

Because of the lipoid nature of the cell membrane, it is highly permeable to lipid soluble substances. The rate of diffusion of a drug across the membrane depends not only upon its concentration but also upon the relative extent of its affinity for lipid and rejection of water (a high lipid partition coefficient[2]). The greater its affinity for lipid and the more hydrophobic it is, the faster will be its rate of penetration into the lipid-rich membrane. Erythromycin base, for example, possesses a higher partition coefficient than other erythromycin compounds, e.g., estolate, gluceptate. Consequently, the base is the preferred agent for the topical treatment of acne where penetration into the skin is desired.

Because biologic cells are also permeated by water and lipid-insoluble substances, it is thought that the membrane also contains water-filled pores or channels that permit the passage of these types of substances. As water passes in bulk across a porous membrane, any dissolved solute molecularly small enough to traverse the pores passes in by *filtration*. Aqueous pores vary in size from membrane to membrane and thus in their individual permeability characteristics for certain drugs and other substances.

The majority of drugs today are weak organic acids or bases. Knowledge of their individual ionization or dissociation characteristics is important, because their absorption is governed to a large extent by their degrees of ionization as they are presented to the membrane barriers. Cell membranes are more permeable to the unionized forms of drugs than to their ionized forms, mainly because of the greater lipid solubility of the unionized forms and to the highly charged nature of the cell membrane which results in the binding or repelling of the ionized drug and thereby decreases cell penetration. Also, ions become hydrated through association with water molecules, resulting in larger particles than the undissociated molecule and again decreased penetrating capability.

The degree of a drug's ionization depends both on the pH of the solution in which it is presented to the biologic membrane and on the pK_a, or dissociation constant, of the drug (whether an acid or a base). The concept of pK_a is derived from the Henderson-Hasselbalch equation and is:

For an acid:

$$pH = pK_a + \log \frac{\text{ionized conc. (salt)}}{\text{unionized conc. (acid)}}$$

For a base:

$$pH = pK_a + \log \frac{\text{unionized conc. (base)}}{\text{ionized conc. (salt)}}$$

Since the pH of body fluids varies (stomach, $\simeq$ pH 1; lumen of the intestine, $\simeq$ pH 6.6; blood plasma, $\simeq$ pH 7.4), the absorption of a drug from various body fluids will differ and may dictate to some extent the type of dosage form and the route of administration preferred for a given drug.

By rearranging the equation for an acid:

$$pK_a - pH$$

$$= \log \frac{\text{unionized concentration (acid)}}{\text{ionized concentration (salt)}}$$

one can theoretically determine the relative extent to which a drug remains unionized under various conditions of pH. This is particularly useful when applied to conditions of body fluids. For instance, if a weak acid having a pK_a of 4 is assumed to be in an environment of gastric juice with a pH of 1, the left side of the equation would yield the number 3, which would mean that the ratio of unionized to ionized drug particles would be about 1000 to 1, and gastric absorption would be excellent. At the pH of plasma the reverse would be true, and in the blood the drug would be largely in the ionized form. Table 3–1 presents the effect of pH on the ionization of weak electrolytes and Table 3–2 offers some representative pK values of common drug substances.

From the equation and from Table 3–1 it may be seen that a drug substance is half ionized at a pH value which is equal to its pKₐ. Thus pKₐ may be defined as the pH at which a drug is 50% ionized. For example, phenobarbital has a pKₐ value of about 7.4 and in the small intestine it is present as ionized and unionized forms in equal amounts. However, a drug substance cannot reach the blood plasma for distribution throughout the body unless it is placed there directly through intravenous injection or is favorably absorbed from a site along the route of entry, as the gastrointestinal tract, and is able to pass into the general circulation. Utilizing Table 3–2 it may be easily seen that phenobarbital, a weak acid, with a pKₐ of 7.4 would be largely undissociated in the gastric environment

Table 3–1. The Effect of pH on the Ionization of Weak Electrolytes*

	% Unionized	
pK_a-pH	If weak acid	If weak base
−3.0	0.100	99.9
−2.0	0.990	99.0
−1.0	9.09	90.9
−0.7	16.6	83.4
−0.5	24.0	76.0
−0.2	38.7	61.3
0	50.0	50.0
+0.2	61.3	38.7
+0.5	76.0	24.0
+0.7	83.4	16.6
+1.0	90.9	9.09
+2.0	99.0	0.99
+3.0	99.9	0.100

*From Doluisio, J.T., and Swintosky, J.V.; *Amer. J. Pharm.*, 137:149, 1965.

of pH 1, and would likely be well absorbed. A drug may enter the circulation rapidly and at high concentrations if membrane penetration is easily accomplished or at a low rate and low level if the drug is not readily absorbed from its route of entry. The pH of the drug's current environment influences the rate and the degree of its further distribution, since it becomes more or less unionized and therefore more or less lipid-penetrating under some condition of pH than under another. If an unionized molecule is able to diffuse through the lipid barrier and

Table 3–2. pK$_a$ Values for Some Acidic and Basic Drugs

		pK_a
Acids:	Acetylsalicylic acid	3.5
	Barbital	7.9
	Benzylpenicillin	2.8
	Boric acid	9.2
	Phenobarbital	7.4
	Theophylline	9.0
	Thiopental	7.6
	Tolbutamide	5.5
	Warfarin	4.8
Bases:	Amphetamine	10.0
	Apomorphine	7.0
	Atropine	9.7
	Cocaine	8.4
	Codeine	7.9
	Guanethidine	11.8
	Procaine	8.8
	Quinine	8.4
	Reserpine	6.6

remain unionized in the new environment, it may return to its former location or go on to a new one. However, if in the new environment it is greatly ionized due to the influence of the pH of the second fluid, it likely will be unable to cross the membrane with its former ability. Thus a concentration gradient of a drug usually is reached at equilibrium on each side of a membrane due to different degrees of ionization occurring on each side.

Absorption from the various sites can be facilitated in certain instances by an adjustment of the pH at the absorbing surface. This may be accomplished by building into the pharmaceutical formulation buffering agents that have the capacity to maintain a certain pH. Buffering agents are frequently added to ophthalmic preparations and on occasion to orally administered drugs. Under proper guidance, a patient may be instructed to take an antacid along with certain medication in order to increase drug absorption (particularly for weak bases).

It is often possible for pharmaceutical scientists to make structural modifications in organic drugs and thereby favorably alter their lipid solubility, partition coefficients, and dissociation constants while maintaining the same basic pharmacologic activity. These efforts frequently result in increased absorption, better therapeutic response, and lower dosage.

Specialized Transport Mechanisms

In contrast to the passive transfer of drugs and other substances across a biologic membrane, certain substances, including some drugs and biologic metabolites, are conducted across a membrane through one of several postulated *specialized transport* mechanisms. This type of transfer seems to account for those substances, many naturally occurring as amino acids and glucose, that are too lipid-insoluble to dissolve in the boundary and too large to flow or filter through the pores. This type of transport is thought to involve membrane components that may be enzymes or some other type of agent capable of forming a complex with the drug (or other agent) at the surface membrane, after which the complex moves across the membrane where the drug is released, with the carrier returning to the original surface. Figure 3–2 presents the simplified scheme of this process. Specialized transport may be differentiated from passive transfer in that the former process may become "saturated" as the amount of car-

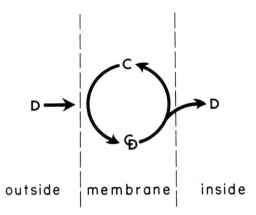

Fig. 3–2. *Active transport mechanism. D represents a drug molecule; C represents the carrier in the membrane. (After O'Reilly, W.J.: Aust. J. Pharm., 47:568, 1966.)*

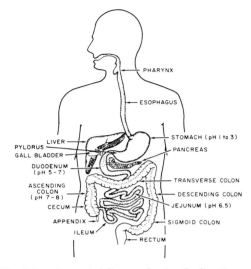

Fig. 3–3. *Anatomical diagram showing the digestive system including the locations involved in drug absorption and their respective pHs.*

rier present for a given substance becomes completely bound with that substance resulting in a delay in the "ferrying" or transport process. Other features of specialized transport include the specificity by a carrier for a particular type of chemical structure so that if two substances are transported by the same mechanism one will competitively inhibit the transport of the other. Further, the transport mechanism is inhibited in general by substances that interfere with cell metabolism. The term *active transport*, as a subclassification of specialized transport, denotes a process with the additional feature of the solute or drug being moved across the membrane against a concentration gradient, that is, from a solution of lower concentration to one of a higher concentration or, if the solute is an ion, against an electrochemical potential gradient. In contrast to active transport, *facilitated diffusion* is a specialized transport mechanism having all of the above characteristics except that the solute is not transferred against a concentration gradient and may attain the same concentration inside the cell as that on the outside.

Many body nutrients, as sugars and amino acids, are transported across the membranes of the gastrointestinal tract by carrier processes. Certain vitamins, as thiamine, niacin, riboflavin and vitamin B_6, and drug substances as methyldopa and 5-fluorouracil, require active transport mechanisms for their absorption.

Dissolution and Drug Absorption

In order for a drug to be absorbed, it must first be dissolved in the fluid at the absorption site. For instance, a drug administered orally in tablet or capsule form cannot be absorbed until the drug particles are dissolved by the fluids at some point within the gastrointestinal tract. In instances in which the solubility of a drug is dependent upon either an acidic or basic medium, the drug would be dissolved in the stomach or intestines respectively (Fig. 3–3). The process by which a drug particle dissolves is termed *dissolution*.

As a drug particle undergoes dissolution, the drug molecules on the surface are the first to enter into solution creating a saturated layer of drug-solution which envelops the surface of the solid drug particle. This layer of solution is referred to as the *diffusion layer*. From this diffusion layer, the drug molecules pass throughout the dissolving fluid and make contact with the biologic membranes and absorption ensues. As the molecules of drug continue to leave the diffusion layer, the layer is replenished with dissolved drug from the surface of the drug particle and the process of absorption continues.

If the process of dissolution for a given drug particle is rapid, or if the drug is administered as a solution and remains present in the body as such, the rate at which the drug becomes absorbed would be primarily dependent upon its ability to traverse the membrane barrier. However, if the rate of dissolution for a drug particle is slow, as may be due to the physiochemical characteristics of the drug substance or the dosage form, the dissolution process itself would be a rate-limiting step in the absorption process. Slowly soluble drugs such as digoxin, may not only be absorbed at a slow rate, they may be incompletely absorbed, or, in some cases largely unabsorbed following oral administration, due to the natural limitation of time that they may remain within the stomach or the intestinal tract. Thus, poorly soluble drugs or poorly formulated drug products may result in a drug's incomplete absorption and its passage, unchanged, out of the system via the feces. Under normal circumstances a drug may be expected to remain in the stomach for 2 to 4 hours (*gastric emptying time*) and in the small intestines for 4 to 10 hours. The gastric emptying time for a drug is most rapid with a fasting stomach, becoming slower as the food content is increased. Changes in gastric emptying time and/or in intestinal motility can affect drug transit time and thus the opportunity for drug dissolution and absorption.

These changes can be effected by drugs the patient may be taking. Certain drugs with anticholinergic properties, e.g., dicyclomine HCl, amitriptyline HCl, have the ability to slow down gastric emptying. This can enhance the rate of absorption of drugs normally absorbed from the stomach, and reduce the rate of absorption of drugs that are primarily absorbed from the small intestine. Alternatively, drugs which enhance gastric motility, e.g., laxatives, may cause some drugs to move so quickly through the gastrointestinal system and past their absorptive site at such a rate to reduce the amount of drug actually absorbed. This effect has been demonstrated with digoxin, whose absorption is significantly decreased by accelerating gastrointestinal motility.

The aging process itself may also influence gastrointestinal absorption. In the elderly, gastric acidity, the number of absorptive cells, intestinal blood flow, the rate of gastric emptying and intestinal motility are all decreased. It appears, however, that drugs whose absorption is dependent upon passive processes are not affected by these factors as much as those who are dependent upon active transport mechanisms, e.g., calcium, iron, thiamine, sugars. A decrease in gastric emptying time would be ad-

vantageous for those drugs that are absorbed from the stomach but disadvantageous for those drugs which are prone to acid degradation, e.g., penicillins, erythromycin, or inactivated by stomach enzymes, e.g., L-dopa.

The dissolution of a substance may be described by the modified Noyes-Whitney equation[3]:

$$\frac{dc}{dt} = kS(c_s - c_t)$$

in which dc/dt is the rate of dissolution, k is the dissolution rate constant, S is the surface area of the dissolving solid, c_s is the saturation concentration of drug in the diffusion layer (which may be approximated by the maximum solubility of the drug in the solvent since the diffusion layer is considered saturated), and c_t is the concentration of the drug in the dissolution medium at time t ($c_s - c_t$ is the concentration gradient). The rate of dissolution is governed by the rate of diffusion of solute molecules through the diffusion layer into the body of the solution. The equation reveals that the dissolution rate of a drug may be increased by increasing the surface area (reducing the particle size) of the drug, by increasing the solubility of the drug in the diffusion layer, and by factors embodied in the dissolution rate constant, k, including the intensity of agitation of the solvent and the diffusion coefficient of the dissolving drug. For a given drug, the diffusion coefficient and usually the concentration of the drug in the diffusion layer will increase with increasing temperature. Also, increasing the rate of agitation of the dissolving medium will increase the rate of dissolution. A reduction in the viscosity of the solvent employed is another means which may be used to enhance the dissolution rate of a drug. Changes in the pH or the nature of the solvent which influence the solubility of the drug may be used to advantage in increasing dissolution rate. Effervescent, buffered aspirin tablet formulations use some of these principles to their advantage. Due to the alkaline adjuvants in the tablet, the solubility of the aspirin is enhanced within the diffusional layer and the evolution of carbon dioxide agitates the solvent system, i.e., gastric juices. Consequently, the rate of aspirin absorbed into the bloodstream is faster than that achieved from a conventional aspirin tablet formulation. If this dosage form is acceptable to the patient, it provides a quicker means for the patient to gain relief from a troublesome headache. Many manufacturers will utilize a particular amorphous, crystalline, salt or ester form of a drug that will exhibit the solubility characteristics needed to achieve the desired dissolution characteristics when administered. Some of these factors which affect drug dissolution will be briefly discussed in the following paragraphs, whereas others will be brought into the discussions of succeeding chapters in which they are relevant.

Surface Area

When a drug particle is reduced to a larger number of smaller particles, the total surface area created is increased. For drug substances that are poorly or slowly soluble, this generally results in an increase in the *rate* of dissolution. The actual solubility of a pure drug remains the same.

Increased therapeutic response to orally administered drugs due to smaller particle size has been reported for a number of drugs, among them theophylline, a xanthine derivative used to treat bronchial asthma; griseofulvin, an antibiotic with antifungal activity; sulfisoxazole, an anti-infective sulfonamide, and nitrofurantoin, a urinary anti-infective drug. To achieve increased surface area, pharmaceutical manufacturers frequently use *micronized* powders in their solid dosage form products. Micronized powders consist of drug particles reduced in size to about 5 microns and smaller. The use of micronized drugs is not confined to oral preparations. For example, ophthalmic ointments and topical ointments utilize micronized drugs for their preferred release characteristics after application.

Due to the different rates and degrees of absorption obtainable from drugs of various particle size, it is conceivable that products of the same drug substance prepared by two or more reliable pharmaceutical manufacturers may result in different degrees of therapeutic response in the same individual. A classic example of this occurs with phenytoin sodium capsules where there are two distinct forms. The first is the rapid-release type, i.e., Prompt Sodium Phenytoin Capsules, and the second is the slow-dissolution type, i.e., Extended Sodium Phenytoin Capsules. The former has a dissolution rate of not less than 85% in 30 minutes and is recommended for patient use 3 to 4 times per day.

The latter has a slower dissolution rate, e.g., 15 to 35% in 30 minutes, which lends itself for use in patients who could be dosed on a once-a-day schedule. Because this difference in formulation exists with some drugs, including phenytoin sodium capsules, it is generally advisable for a person to continue taking the same brand of medication, provided it produces the desired therapeutic effect. Patients who are stabilized on one brand of drug should not be switched to another unless necessary. However, when a change is necessary, appropriate blood or plasma concentrations of the drug should be monitored until the patient is stablized on the new product.

Occasionally, a rapid rate of drug absorption is not desired in a pharmaceutical preparation. Research pharmacists, in providing sustained rather than rapid action in certain preparations, may employ agents of varying particle size to provide a controlled dissolution and absorption process.

Crystal or Amorphous Drug Form

Solid drug materials may occur as pure crystalline substances of definite identifiable shape or as amorphous particles without definite structure. The amorphous or crystalline character of a drug substance may be of considerable importance to its ease of formulation and handling, its chemical stability, and, as has been recently shown, even its biological activity. Certain medicinal agents may be produced to exist in either a crystalline or an amorphous state. Since the amorphous form of a chemical is usually more soluble than the crystalline form, different extents of drug absorption may result with consequent differences in the degree of pharmacologic activity obtained from each. Experiences with two antibiotic substances, novobiocin and chloramphenicol palmitate, have revealed that these materials are essentially inactive when administered in crystalline form, but when they are administered in the amorphous form, absorption from the gastrointestinal tract proceeds rapidly with good therapeutic response. In other instances, crystalline forms of drugs may be used because of greater stability than the corresponding amorphous forms. For example, the crystalline forms of Penicillin G as either the potassium or sodium salt are considerably more stable than the analogous amorphous forms. Thus, in formulation work involving Penicillin G, the crystalline forms are preferred and result in excellent therapeutic response.

The hormonal substance insulin presents another striking example of the different degree of activity that may result from the use of different physical forms of the same medicinal agent. Insulin is the active principle of the pancreas gland and is vital to the body's metabolism of glucose. The hormone is produced by two means. The first is by extraction procedures from either beef or pork pancreas. The second process involves a biosynthetic process with strains of *Escherichia coli,* i.e., recombinant DNA. Insulin is used by man as replacement therapy, by injection, when his body's production of the hormone is insufficient. Insulin is a protein, which, when combined with zinc in the presence of acetate buffer, forms an extremely insoluble zinc-insulin complex. Depending upon the pH of the acetate buffer solution, the complex may be an amorphous precipitate or a crystalline material. Each type is produced commercially to take advantage of their unique absorption characteristics.

The amorphous form, referred to as *semilente insulin* or Prompt Insulin Zinc Suspension, USP, is rapidly absorbed upon intramuscular or subcutaneous (under the skin) injection. The larger crystalline material, called *ultralente insulin* or Extended Insulin Zinc Suspension, USP, is more slowly absorbed with a resultant longer duration of action. By combining the two types in various proportions, a physician is able to provide his patients with intermediate acting insulin of varying degrees of onset and duration of action. A physical mixture of 70% of the crystalline form and 30% of the amorphous form, called *lente insulin* or Insulin Zinc Suspension, USP, is commercially available and provides an intermediate acting insulin preparation that meets the requirements of many diabetics.

Some medicinal chemicals that exist in crystalline form are capable of forming different types of crystals, depending upon the conditions (temperature, solvent, time) under which crystallization is induced. This property, whereby a single chemical substance may exist in more than one crystalline form, is known as "polymorphism." It is known that only one form of a pure drug substance is stable at a given temperature and pressure with the other forms, called metastable forms, converting in time to the stable crystalline form. It is therefore not unusual for a metastable form of a medicinal agent to change form even when present in a completed pharmaceutical preparation, although the time required for a complete change may exceed the normal shelf-life of the product itself. However, from a pharmaceutical point of view, any change in the crystal structure of a medicinal agent may critically affect the stability and even the therapeutic efficacy of the product in which the conversion takes place.

The various polymorphic forms of the same chemical generally differ in many physical properties, including their solubility and dissolution characteristics, which are of prime importance to the rate and extent of drug absorption into the body's system. These differences are manifest so long as the drug is in the solid state. Once solution is effected, the different forms are indistinguishable one from another. Therefore, differences in drug action, pharmaceutically and therapeutically, can be expected from polymorphs contained in solid dosage forms as well as in liquid suspension. The use of metastable forms generally results in higher solubility and dissolution rates than the respective stable crystal forms of the same drug. If all other factors remain constant, more rapid and complete drug absorption will likely result from the metastable forms than from the stable form of the same drug. On the other hand, the stable polymorph is generally more resistant to chemical degradation and because of its lower solubility is frequently preferred in pharmaceutical suspensions of insoluble drugs. If metastable forms are employed in the preparation of suspensions, their gradual conversion to the stable form may be accompanied by an alteration in the consistency of the suspension itself, thereby affecting its permanency. In all instances, the advantages of the metastable crystalline forms in terms of increased physiologic availability of the drug must be balanced against the increased product stability when stable polymorphs are employed. Sulfur and cortisone acetate are two examples of drugs that exist in more than one crystalline form and are frequently prepared in pharmaceutical suspensions. In fact, cortisone acetate is reported to exist in at least five different crystalline forms. It is possible for the commercial products of two manufacturers to differ in stability and in therapeutic effect, depending upon the crystalline form of the drug used in the formulation.

Salt Forms

The dissolution rate of a salt form of a drug is generally quite different from that of the parent compound. Sodium and potassium salts of weak organic acids and hydrochloride salts of weak organic bases dissolve much more readily than do the respective free acids or bases. The result is a more rapid saturation of the diffusion layer surrounding the dissolving particle and the consequent more rapid diffusion of the drug to the absorption sites.

Numerous examples could be cited to demonstrate the increased rate of drug dissolution due to the use of the salt form of the drug rather than the free acid or base, but the following will suffice: the addition of the ethylenediamine moiety to theophylline increases the water solubility of theophylline 5-fold. The use of the ethylenediamine salt of theophylline has allowed the development of oral aqueous solutions of theophylline and diminished the need to use hydroalcoholic mixtures, e.g., elixirs. This has resulted in increased patient acceptance of liquid theophylline formulations without the problem of patient intoxication associated with elixir use.

Other Factors

The *state of hydration* of a drug molecule can affect its solubility and pattern of absorption. Usually the anhydrous form of an organic molecule is more readily soluble than the hydrated form. This characteristic has been demonstrated recently with the drug ampicillin, when the anhydrous form was shown to have a greater rate of solubility than the trihydrate form.[4] It was also shown in the same study that the rate of absorption for the anhydrous form was greater than that for the trihydrate form of the drug.

Once swallowed, a drug is placed in the gastrointestinal tract where its solubility can be affected not only by the pH of the environment, but by the normal components of the tract and the foodstuffs which may be present. A drug may interact with one of the other agents present to form a chemical complex which may result in reduced drug solubility and decreased drug absorption. The classic example of this complexation phenomenon is that which occurs between tetracycline analogues and certain cations, e.g., calcium, magnesium, aluminum, resulting in a decreased absorption of the tetracycline derivative. Also, if the drug becomes adsorbed onto insoluble material in the tract, its availabiltiy for absorption may be correspondingly reduced.

Concept of Bioavailability

The term *bioavailability* describes the *rate* and *extent* to which an active drug ingredient or therapeutic moiety is absorbed from a drug product and becomes available at the site of drug action. The term *bioequivalence* refers to the *comparison* of bioavailabilities of different formulations, drug products, or batches of the same drug product.

The availability to the biologic system of a drug substance formulated into a pharmaceutical product is integral to the goals of dosage form design and paramount to the effectiveness of the medication. The study of a drug's bioavailability depends upon the drug's absorption or entry into the systemic circulation, and studying the pharmacokinetic profile of the drug or its metabolite(s) over time in the appropriate biologic system, e.g., blood, plasma, urine. Graphically, bioavailability of a drug is portrayed by a concentration-time curve of the administered drug in an appropriate tissue system, e.g., plasma (Fig. 3–4). Bioavailability data are used to determine: (1) the amount or proportion of drug absorbed from a formulation or dosage form; (2) the rate at which the drug was absorbed; (3) the duration of the drug's presence in the biologic fluid or tissue; and, when correlated with patient response, (4) the relationship between drug blood levels and clinical efficacy and toxicity.

During the product development stages of a proposed drug product, pharmaceutical manufacturers may employ bioavailability studies to compare different formulations of the drug substance to ascertain the one which allows the most desirable absorption pattern. Later, bioavailability studies may be used to compare the availability of the drug substance from different production batches of the product. They may also be used to compare the availability of the drug substance from different dosage forms (as tablets, capsules, elixir, etc.), or from the same dosage form produced by different (competing) manufacturers.

Most of the bioavailability studies have been applied to drugs contained in solid dosage forms intended to be administered orally for systemic effects. The emphasis in this direction has been primarily due to the proliferation of competing products on the market in recent years, particularly the nonproprietary (generic) capsules and tablets, and the scientific revelation that certain drug entities when formulated and manufactured differently into solid dosage forms are particularly prone to variations in biologic availability. Thus, the present discussions will be centered around the solid dosage form product. However, this is not to imply that systemic drug absorption is not intended from other routes of administration or other dosage forms, or that bioavailability problems may not exist from these products as well. Indeed, drug absorption from other routes is affected by the physicochemcial properties of the drug and the formulative and manufacturing aspects of the dosage form design.

Blood (or Serum or Plasma) Concentration-Time Curve

Following the oral administration of a medication, if blood samples are drawn from the patient at specific time intervals and analyzed for drug content, the resulting data may be plotted on ordinary graph paper to yield the type of drug blood level curve presented in Figure 3–4. The vertical axis of this type of plot characteristically presents the concentration of drug present in the blood (or serum or plasma) and the horizontal axis presents the time the samples were obtained following the administration

of the drug. When the drug is first administered (time zero), the blood concentration of the drug should also be zero. As the drug passes into the stomach and/or intestine, it is released from the dosage form, eventually dissolves, and is absorbed. As the sampling and analysis continue, the blood samples reveal increasing concentrations of drug until the maximum (peak) concentration (C_{max}) is reached. Then, the blood level of the drug progressively decreases and, if no additional dose is given, eventually falls to zero. The diminished blood level of drug after the peak height is reached indicates that the rate of drug elimination from the blood stream is greater than the rate of drug absorption into the circulatory system. It should be understood that drug absorption does not terminate after the peak blood level is reached, but may continue for some time. Similarly the process of drug elimination is a continuous one. It begins as soon as the drug first appears in the blood stream and continues until all of the drug has been eliminated. When the drug leaves the blood it may be found in various body tissues and cells for which it has an affinity until ultimately it is excreted as such or as drug metabolites in the urine or via some other route (see Fig. 3–5). An urinalysis for the drug or its metabolites may be used to indicate the extent of drug absorption and/or the rate of drug elimination from the body.

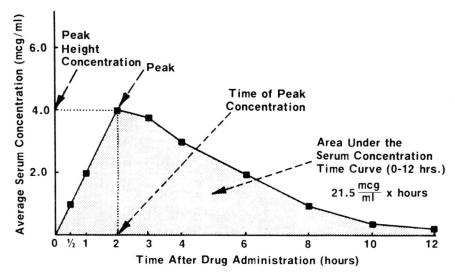

Fig. 3–4. *Serum concentration-time curve showing peak height concentration, time of peak concentration, and area under the curve. (Courtesy of D.J. Chodos and A.R. DiSanto, The Upjohn Company.)*

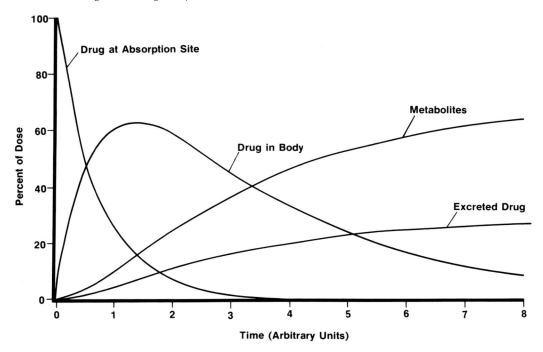

Fig. 3–5. *Time course of drug in the body. (From Rowland, M., and Tozer, T.N.:* Clinical Pharmacokinetics. *2nd Ed., Philadelphia, Lea & Febiger, 1989.)*

Parameters for Assessment and Comparison of Bioavailability

In discussing the important parameters to be considered in the comparative evaluation of the blood level curves following the oral administration of single doses of two formulations of the same drug entity, Chodos and DiSanto[5] list the following:

1. The Peak Height Concentration (C_{max})
2. The Time of the Peak Concentration (T_{max})
3. The Area Under the Blood (or serum or plasma) Concentration-Time Curve (AUC)

Using Figure 3–4 as an example, the height of the peak concentration is equivalent ot 4.0 mcg/mL of drug in the serum; the time of the peak concentration is 2 hours following administration; and the area under the curve from 0 to 12 hours is calculated as 21.5 mcg/mL × hours. The meaning and use of these parameters are further explained as follows.

PEAK HEIGHT. Peak height concentration is the maximum drug concentration (C_{max}) observed in the blood plasma or serum following a dose of the drug. For conventional dosage forms, as tablets and capsules, the C_{max} will usually occur

at only a single time point, referred to as T_{max}. The amount of drug is usually expressed in terms of its concentration in relation to a specific volume of blood, serum, or plasma. For example, the concentration may be expressed as g/100 mL, mcg/mL or mg% (mg/100 mL). Figure 3–6 depicts concentration-time curves showing different peak height concentrations for *equal* amounts of drug from two different formulations following oral administation. The horizontal line drawn across the figure indicates that the minimum effective concentration (MEC) for the drug substance is 4.0 mcg/mL. This means that in order for the patient to exhibit an adequate response to the drug, this concentration in the blood must be achieved. Comparing the blood levels of drug achieved after the oral administration of equal doses of formulations "A" and "B" in Figure 3–6, it is apparent that formulation "A" will achieve the required blood levels of drug to produce the desired pharmacologic effect whereas the administration of formulation "B" will not. On the other hand, if the minimum effective concentration for the drug was 2.0 mcg/mL and the minimum toxic concentration (MTC) was 4.0 mcg/mL as depicted in Figure 3–7, equal doses

Fig. 3–6. *Serum concentration-time curve showing different peak height concentrations for equal amounts of drug from two different formulations following oral administration. (Courtesy of D.J. Chodos and A.R. DiSanto, The Upjohn Company.)*

Fig. 3–7. *Serum concentration-time curve showing peak height concentrations, peak height times, times to reach minimum effective concentration (MEC) and areas under the curves for equal amounts of drug from two different formulations following oral administration. (Courtesy of D.I. Chodos and A.R. DiSanto, The Upjohn Company.)*

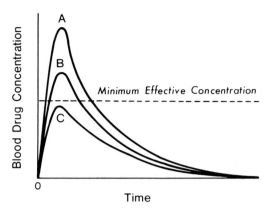

Fig. 3–8. *The influence of dose size on the resultant blood drug concentration-time curves when three different doses of the same drug are administered and the rates of drug absorption and elimination are equal after the three doses. A = 100 mg, B = 80 mg, C = 50 mg. (From C.T. Ueda, "Concepts in Clinical Pharmacology. Essentials of Bioavailability and Bioequivalence," 1979, The Upjohn Company, Reproduced with permission.)*

of the two formulations would result in toxic effects produced by formulation "A" but only desired effects by formulation "B." The objective in the individual dosing of a patient is to achieve the MEC but not the MTC.

The *size* of the dose administered influences the blood level concentration and C_{max} for that drug substance. Figure 3–8 depicts the influence of dose on the blood level time curve for a hypothetical drug administered by the same route and in the same dosage form. In this example, it is assumed that all doses are completely absorbed and eliminated at the same rates. It is evident that as the dose increases, the C_{max} is proportionately higher and the area-under-the-curve (AUC) proportionately greater. The peak time, T_{max}, is the same for each dose.

TIME OF PEAK. The second parameter of importance in assessing the comparative bioavailability of two formulations is the time required to achieve the maximum level of drug in the blood (T_{max}). In Figure 3–6, the time required to achieve the peak serum concentration of drug is 1 hour for formulation "A" and 4 hours for formulation "B." This parameter reflects the *rate* of drug absorption from a formulation. It is the rate of drug absorption that determines the time needed for the minimum effective concentration to be reached and thus for the initiation of the desired pharmacologic effect. The rate of drug absorption also influences the period of

time over which the drug enters the blood stream and therefore affects the duration of time that the drug is maintained in the blood. Looking at Figure 3–7, formulation "A" allows the drug to reach the MEC within 30 minutes following administration and a peak concentration in 1 hour. Formulation "B" has a slower rate of drug release. Drug from this formulation reached the MEC 2 hours after administration and its peak concentration 4 hours after administration. Thus formulation "A" permits the greater rate of drug absorption; it allows drug to reach both the MEC and its peak height sooner than drug formulation "B." On the other hand, formulation "B" provides the greater duration of time for drug concentrations maintained above the MEC, 8 hours (from 2 to 10 hours following administration) to 5½ hours (from 30 minutes to 6 hours following administration) for formulation "A". Thus, if a rapid onset of action is desired, a formulation similar to "A" would be preferred, but, if a longer duration of action is desired rather than a rapid onset of action, a formulation similar to "B" would be preferred.

In sum, changes in the *rate* of drug absorption will result in changes in the values of both C_{max} and T_{max}. Each product has its own characteristic rate of absorption. When the *rate* of absorption is decreased, the C_{max} is lowered and the T_{max} occurs at a later time. If the doses of the drugs are the same and presumed completely absorbed, as in Figure 3–7, the AUC for each is essentially the same.

AREA UNDER THE SERUM CONCENTRATION-TIME CURVE. The area under the curve (AUC) of a concentration-time plot (Fig. 3–4) is considered representative of the total amount of drug absorbed into the circulation following the administration of a single dose of that drug. Equivalent doses of a drug, when fully absorbed, would produce the same AUC. Thus, two curves much unlike in terms of peak height and time of peak, as those in Figure 3–7, may be much alike in terms of area under the curve, and thus in the amount of drug absorbed. As indicated in Figure 3–7, the area under the curve for formulation

"A" is 34.4 $\frac{mcg}{mL}$ × hours and for formulation

"B" is 34.2 $\frac{mcg}{mL}$ × hours, essentially the same.

If equivalent doses of drug in different formulation produce *different* AUC values, differences exist in the *extent* of absorption between the formulations. Figure 3–9 depicts concentration-time curves for three different formulations of equal amounts of drug with greatly different areas under the curve. In this example, formulation "A" delivers much greater amount of drug to the circulatory system than do the other two formulations. In general, the smaller the AUC, the less drug absorbed.

The area under the curve may be measured mathematically, using a technique known as the trapezoidal rule, and is reported in $\dfrac{\text{amount of drug}}{\text{volume of fluid}} \times \text{time}$ (e.g., $\dfrac{\text{mcg}}{\text{mL}} \times$ hours; $\dfrac{\text{g}}{100} \times$ hours; etc.)

According to the trapezoidal rule, the area beneath a drug concentration-time curve can be estimated through the assumption that the AUC can be represented by a series of trapezoids (quadrilateral planes having two parallel and two nonparallel sides). The total AUC would be the sum of the areas of the individual trapezoids. The area of each trapezoid is calculated taking $\frac{1}{2}(C_{n-1} + C_n)(t_n - t_{n-1})$, where C_n and t_n are drug concentrations in the blood, plasma, or serum, and time, respectively. Ueda[6] demonstrates the use of the trapezoid by the data reproduced in Table 3–3 and plotted into a plasma drug concentration-time curve as shown in Figure 3–10.

The fraction (F) (or bioavailability) of an orally administered drug may be calculated by comparison of the AUC after oral administration with that obtained after intravenous administration:

$$F = (AUC)_{oral}/(AUC)_{intravenous}$$

Bioequivalence of Drug Products

A great deal of discussion and scientific investigation has been devoted recently to the problem of determining the equivalence between drug products of competing manufacturers. Differences in bioavailability have been demonstrated for a number of products involving the following and other drugs: tetracycline, chloramphenicol, digoxin, phenylbutazone, warfarin, diazepam, levodopa, and oxytetracycline. Not only has bio*in*equivalence been shown to exist in products of different manufacturers but there have also been variations in the bioavailability of different batches of drug products from the same manufacturer. Variations in the bioavailability of certain drug products have resulted in some therapeutic failures in patients who have taken two inequivalent drug products in the course of their therapy.

The most common experimental plan to compare the bioavailability of two drug products is the simple *crossover design study*. In this method, each of the 12 to 24 individuals in the group of carefully matched subjects (usually healthy

Fig. 3–9. *Serum concentration-time curve showing peak height concentrations, peak height times, and areas under the curves for equal amounts of drugs from three different formulations following oral administration. (Courtesy of D.J. Chodos and A.R. DiSanto, The Upjohn Company.)*

Table 3–3.   Determination of AUC Using the Trapezoidal Rule for the Following Plasma Drug Concentration-Time Data*

Sample (n)	Time (hr)	Plasma Concentration (μg/mL)	AUC/t_nt_{n-1} (μg/mL × hr)
1	0	0	½(0+ 1)(0.5− 0) = 0.25
2	0.5	1	½(1+11)(1 − 0.5)= 3.00
3	1.0	11	½(11+28)(1.5− 1) = 9.75
4	1.5	28	½(28+30)(2 − 1.5)= 14.50
5	2	30	½(30+21)(3 − 2) = 25.50
6	3	21	½(21+17)(4 − 3) = 19.00
7	4	17	½(17+ 9)(6 − 4) = 26.00
8	6	9	½(9+ 4)(8 − 6) = 13.00
9	8	4	½(4+ 2)(10 − 8) = 6.00
10	10	2	½(2+ 1)(12 −10) = 3.00
11	12	1	½(1+ 0)(18 −12) = 3.00
12	18	0	

AUC = 123.00

*(From C.T. Ueda, "Concepts in Clinical Pharmacology. Essentials of Bioavailability and Bioequivalence," 1979, The Upjohn Company, Reproduced with permission.)

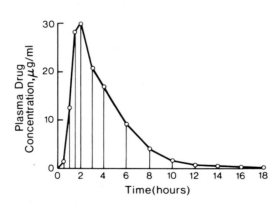

Fig. 3–10.   *Estimation of area under the drug concentration-time curve using the trapezoidal rule (see Table 4–3 for raw data). (From C.T. Ueda, "Concepts in Clinical Pharmacology. Essentials of Bioavailability and Bioequivalence," 1979, The Upjohn Company, Reproduced with permission.)*

adult males between 18 and 40 years of age of similar height and weight) is administered both products under fasting conditions and essentially serves as his own control. To avoid bias of the test results, each test subject is randomly assigned one of the two products for the first phase of the study. Once the first assigned product is administered, samples of blood or plasma are drawn from the subjects at predetermined times and analyzed for drug concentration. The same procedure is then repeated (*crossover*) with the second product after an appropriate interval of time, i.e., a washout period to ensure that there is no residual amount of drug from the first administered product that would artificially inflate the test results of the second administered product. Afterward, the patient population data is tabulated and the parameters used to assess and compare bioavailability, i.e., C_{max}, T_{max}, AUC, are then analyzed with statistical procedures. Statistical differences in bioavailability parameters may not always be clinically significant in therapeutic outcome.

It should be recognized that there are inherent differences in individuals which result in different patterns of drug absorption, metabolism and excretion. These differences must be statistically analyzed to separate them from the factors of bioavailability related to the products themselves. The value in the crossover-designed experiment is that each individual serves as his own control by taking each of the products. Thus, inherent differences as mentioned between individuals is minimized.

Absolute bioequivalency between drug products rarely, if ever, occurs. Such absolute equivalency would yield serum concentration-time curves for the products involved that would be exactly superimposable. This simply is not expected of products which are made at different times, in different batches, or indeed by different manufacturers. However, some expectations of bioequivalency are expected of products which are considered to be of equivalent merit for therapy.

In most studies of bioavailability, the originally marketed product (frequently referred to as the "prototype," "pioneer," or "innovator" drug product) is recognized as the established product of the drug and is utilized as the standard for the bioavailability comparative studies.

As a result of the implementation of the Drug Price Competition and Patent Term Restoration Act of 1984, many additional drugs became available in generic form. Prior to the 1984 act, only those drugs marketed before 1962 could be processed by an Abbreviated New Drug Application (ANDA). The ANDA process does not require the sponsor to repeat costly clinical research on active ingredients already found to be safe and effective. The 1984 act extended the eligibility for ANDA processing to drugs first marketed after 1962, making generic versions immediately possible for about 150 drugs previously available only as brand name (pioneer) drugs.

According to the FDA, a generic drug is considered bioequivalent if the rate and extent of absorption do not show a significant difference from that of the pioneer drug when administered at the same molar dose of the therapeutic ingredient under the same experimental conditions.[7] Because, in the case of a systemically absorbed drug, blood levels even if from an identical product may vary in different subjects, in bioequivalence studies each subject receives both the pioneer and the test drug and thus serves as his own control.

Under the 1984 act, to gain FDA approval a generic drug product must:
-Contain the same active ingredients as the pioneer drug (inert ingredients may vary)
-Be identical in strength, dosage form, and route of administration
-Have the same indications and precautions for use and other labeling instructions
-Be bioequivalent
-Meet the same batch-to-batch requirements for identity, strength, purity, and quality
-Be manufactured under the same strict standards of FDA's Good Manufacturing Practice regulations as required for pioneer products.

In the design and evaluation of bioequivalence students, the FDA employs the "80/20 rule." This rule requires that a study be large enough to provide an 80% probability to detect a 20% difference in average bioavailability. The allowance of a statistical variability of $\pm 20\%$ in bioequivalence applies to both reformulated pioneer drugs and generics. Pioneer manufacturers often reformulate their products after they conduct clinical trials to demonstrate the safety and effectiveness of the active ingredient(s). To gain FDA approval of the subsequent formulations they are required to perform the same type of bioequivalence test required of generic manufacturers.

The FDA recommends generic substitution only among products that it has evaluated to be therapeutically equivalent. Since 1980, the Agency has published an annual *Approved Drug Products with Therapeutic Equivalence Evaluations* (also known as the "Orange Book"). This publication is updated monthly and contains information on more than 8,000 approved prescription drug products. Of these, about 6,000 are available from more than one manufacturer. Of the latter, more than 80% are evaluated by the FDA as therapeutically equivalent. The remaining 20% of listed products are not therapeutically equivalent. For example, the FDA rates all conjugated estrogens and esterified estrogen products as "not therapeutically equivalent," because no manufacturer to date has submitted an acceptable *in vivo* bioequivalence study. Therefore, the FDA does not recommend that these products be substituted for each other.

The differences in bioavailability between drug products of the same therapeutic agent may be due to differences in the formulative ingredients employed, the methods of product manufacture utilized, the rigor of in-process

Table 3–4. Some Factors Which Can Influence the Bioavailability of Orally Administered Drugs

I. *Drug Substance Physiochemical Properties*
 A. Particle Size
 B. Crystalline or Amorphous Form
 C. Salt Form
 D. Hydration
 E. Lipid/Water Solubility
 F. pH and pK$_a$

II. *Pharmaceutic Ingredients and Dosage Form Characteristics*
 A. Pharmaceutic Ingredients
  1. Fillers
  2. Binders
  3. Coatings
  4. Disintegrating Agents
  5. Lubricants
  6. Suspending Agents
  7. Surface Active Agents
  8. Flavoring Agents
  9. Coloring Agents
  10. Preservative Agents
  11. Stabilizing Agents
 B. Disintegration Rate (Tablets)
 C. Dissolution Time of Drug in Dosage Form
 D. Product Age and Storage Conditions

III. *Physiologic Factors and Patient Characteristics*
 A. Gastric Emptying Time
 B. Intestinal Transit Time
 C. Gastrointestinal Abnormality or Pathologic Condition
 D. Gastric Contents
  1. Other drugs
  2. Food
  3. Fluids
 E. Gastrointestinal pH
 F. Drug Metabolism (Gut and during first passage through liver).

quality control procedures, and even the methods of handling, packaging, and storage. The variables which can contribute to the differences between products are many (Table 3–4). For instance in the manufacture of a tablet, different materials or amounts of such formulative components as fillers, disintegrating agents, binders, lubricants, colorants, flavorants and coatings may be used. The particle size or crystalline form of a therapeutic or pharmaceutic component may vary between formulations. The tablet may vary in shape, size, and hardness depending upon the punches and dies selected for use by the manufacturer and the compression forces utilized in the process. During packaging, shipping and storage the integrity of the tablets may be altered by physical impact, or changes in conditions of humidity, temperature, or through interactions with the components of the container. Each of the factors noted may have an effect on the rates of tablet disintegration, drug dissolution, and consequently on the rate and extent of drug absorption. Although the bioequivalency problems are perhaps greater among tablets than for other dosage forms because of the multiplicity of variables, the same types of problems exist for the other dosage forms and must be considered in bioequivalency evaluations.

There are situations in which even therapeutically equivalent drugs may not be equally suitable for a particular patient. For example, a patient may be sensitive to an inert ingredient in one product (brand name or generic) that another product does not contain. Or a psychiatric patient may become confused or belligerent if the color, flavor, shape, or packaging varies from that to which he or she has become accustomed. Switching among brand name drugs or among generic drugs can product problems and thus pharmacists need to be prudent in both initial product selection and in product interchange.

Routes of Drug Administration

The absorption of drug substances is a most important factor in the selection of the appropriate route of administation, in the design of the most efficacious dosage forms, and therefore, in drug therapy. Some of these factors specific to certain dosage forms or routes of administration are briefly introduced in this section. The various routes of drug administration and applicable dosage forms are presented in Tables 3–5 and 3–6.

An individual drug substance may be formulated into multiple dosage forms which result in different drug absorption rates and times of onset, peak, and duration of action. This is demonstrated by Figure 3–11 and Table 3–7, for the drug nitroglycerin in various dosage forms. The sublingual, intravenous, and buccal forms present extremely rapid onsets of action whereas the oral (swallowed), topical ointment and topical disc present slower onsets of action but greater durations of action. The disc provides the longest duration of action, up to 24 hours following application of a single patch to the skin. The transdermal nitroglycerin disc allows a single daily dose, whereas the other

Table 3–5. Routes of Drug Administration

Term	Site
oral	mouth
peroral (per os[1])	gastrointestinal tract via mouth
sublingual	under the tongue
parenteral	other than the gastro-intestinal tract (by injection)
intravenous	vein
intraarterial	artery
intracardiac	heart
intraspinal or intrathecal	spine
intraosseous	bone
intraarticular	joint
intrasynovial	joint-fluid area
intracutaneous or intradermal	skin
subcutaneous	beneath the skin
intramuscular	muscle
epicutaneous (topical)	skin surface
transdermal	skin surface
conjunctival	conjunctiva
intraocular	eye
intranasal	nose
aural	ear
intrarespiratory	lung
rectal	rectum
vaginal	vagina
urethral	urethra

[1]The abbreviation "p.o." is commonly employed on prescriptions to indicate to be swallowed.

Table 3–6. Dosage Form/Drug Delivery System Application

Route of Administration	Primary Dosage Forms
oral	tablets
	capsules
	solutions
	syrups
	elixirs
	suspensions
	magmas
	gels
	powders
sublingual	tablets
	troches or lozenges
parenteral	solutions
	suspensions
epicutaneous/transdermal	ointments
	creams
	infusion pumps
	pastes
	plasters
	powders
	aerosols
	lotions
	transdermal patches, discs, solutions
conjunctival	contact lens inserts
	ointments
intraocular/intraaural	solutions
	suspensions
intranasal	solutions
	sprays
	inhalants
	ointments
intrarespiratory	aerosols
rectal	solutions
	ointments
	suppositories
vaginal	solutions
	ointments
	emulsion foams
	tablets
	inserts, suppositories, sponge
urethral	solutions
	suppositories

forms require multiple dosing to maintain drug levels within the therapeutic window.

The difference in drug absorption between dosage forms is a function of the formulation itself and the route of administration. For example, a problem associated with the oral administration of a drug is that once absorbed through the lumen of the gastrointestinal tract into the portal vein, the drug may pass directly to the liver and undergo the *first-pass effect*. In essence a portion or all of the drug may be metabolized by the liver. This phenomenon occurs only that drugs which are cleared or metabolized by the liver and are administered by a first-pass route, e.g., oral administration. Consequently, as the drug is extracted by the liver, its bioavailability to the body is decreased. Thus, the bioavailable fraction of a drug that is administered orally, for example, is determined by the fraction of drug that is absorbed and the fraction that escapes metabolism during its first

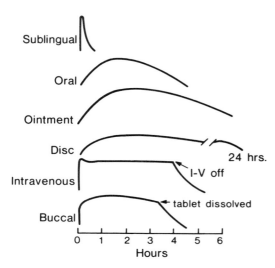

Fig. 3–11. *Blood-level curves of nitroglycerin following administration of dosage forms by various routes. (From Abrams, J.: Nitroglycerin and Long-Acting Nitrates in Clinical Practice.* The American Journal of Medicine, Proceedings of a Symposium: First North American Conference on Nitroglycerin Therapy, June 27, 1983. Reprinted with Permission.)

pass through the liver. The bioavailable fraction (*f*) is the product of these two fractions as follows:

f = Fraction of drug absorbed

   × Fraction escaping first-pass metabolism

The bioavailability is lowest, then, for those drugs that undergo a significant first-pass effect. For these drugs, a hepatic extraction ratio, or the fraction of drug metabolized, *E,* is cal-

culated. The fraction of drug that enters the system circulation and is ultimately available to exert its effect then is equal to the quantity (1 − E). Table 3–8 lists some drugs according to their pharmacologic class that undergo a significant first-pass effect when administered by the oral route.

To compensate for this marked effect, the drug manufacturer may consider other routes of drug administration, e.g., intravenous, intramuscular, sublingual, that avoid the first-pass effect. With these routes there will be a corresponding decrease in the dosage required when compared to oral administration. A good example of this is with nitroglycerin, which when administered sublingually is absorbed directly into the superior vena cava to exert its beneficial effects. However, some of these routes, e.g., intravenous, may not be practical for use in the general population. Thus, the manufacturer may consider preparing an oral dosage form with a higher amount of drug that will compensate for the amount of drug lost through the liver. This, however, may not be feasible, as is the case of lidocaine, because of the high liver extraction associated with this drug.

Another difficulty centers around the metabolites themselves, and whether they are pharmacologically active or inactive. If they are inactive, a larger oral dose will be required to attain the desired therapeutic effect when compared to a lower dosage in a nonfirst-pass effect route. The classic example of drug that exhibits this effect is propranolol. If, on the other hand, the metabolites are the active species, the oral dosage must be carefully tailored to the desired therapeutic effect. First-pass metabolism in this

Table 3–7.   Dosage and Kinetics of Nitroglycerin in Various Dosage Forms[1]

Nitroglycerin, Dosage Form	Usual Recommended Dosage (mg)	Onset of Action (Minutes)	Peak Action (Minutes)	Duration (Minutes/hours)
Sublingual	0.3–0.8	2–5	4–8	10–30 minutes
Buccal	1–3	2–5	4–10	30–300 minutes[a]
Oral	6.5–19.5	20–45	45–120	2–6 hours[n]
Ointment (2%)	½–2 inches	15–60	30–120	3–8 hours
Discs	5–10	30–60	60–180	Up to 24 hours

[a]Effect persists so long as tablet is intact.
[n]Some short-term dosing studies have demonstrated effects to 8 hours.

[1]From Abrams, J.: Nitroglycerin and Long-Acting Nitrates in Clinical Practice. *The American Journal of Medicine,* Proceedings of a Symposium: First North American Conference of Nitroglycerin Therapy, June 27, 1983, p. 88.

Table 3–8. **Examples of Drugs that Undergo Significant Liver Metabolism and Exhibit Low Bioavailability when Administered by First-pass Routes**

Drug Class	Examples
Analgesics	Aspirin, meperidine, penta-zocine, propoxyphene
Antianginal	Nitroglycerin
Antiarrhythmics	Lidocaine
Beta-adrenergic blockers	Labetolol, metoprolol, propranolol
Calcium channel blockers	Verapamil
Sympathomimetic amines	Isoproterenol
Tricyclic antidepressants	Desipramine, imipramine, nortripyline

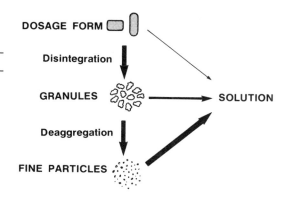

Fig. 3–12. *Schematic drawing showing disintegration of a tablet dosage form and direct availability of the contents in a capsule dosage form for dissolution and drug absorption after oral administration.* (From Rowland, M., and Rozer, T.N.: Clinical Pharmacokinetics. *2nd Ed., Philadelphia, Lea & Febiger, 1989.*)

case will result in a quicker therapeutic response than that achieved by a nonfirst-pass effect route.

One must remember also that the flow of blood through the liver can be decreased under certain conditions. Consequently, the bioavailability of those drugs that undergo a first-pass effect then would be expected to increase. For example, during cirrhosis the blood flow to the kidney is dramatically decreased and efficient hepatic extraction by enzymes responsible for a drug's metabolism also falls off. Consequently, in cirrhotic patients the dosage of drug that undergoes a first-pass effect from oral administration will have to be reduced to avoid toxicity.

Drugs intended to provide localized effects are applied directly to the site of their intended action. This includes most of the products utilized in the eye, ear, nose, throat, as well as those applied to the skin or placed in the vagina or rectum or swallowed for localized effects within the gastrointestinal tract.

Oral Route

Drugs are most frequently taken by oral administration. Although a few drugs taken orally are intended to be dissolved within the mouth, the vast majority of drugs taken orally are swallowed. Of these, the majority are taken for the *systemic* drug effects that result after absorption from the various surfaces along the gastrointestinal tract. A few drugs are swallowed for their local action within the confines of the gastrointestinal tract, made possible by their insolubility and/or poor absorbability from this route.

Compared with alternate routes, the oral route is considered the most natural, uncomplicated, convenient, and safe means of administering drugs. Disadvantages of the oral route include slow drug response (when compared with parenterally administered drugs); chance of irregular absorption of drugs, depending upon such factors as constitutional make-up, the amount or type of food present within the gastrointestinal tract; and the destruction of certain drugs by the acid reaction of the stomach or by gastrointestinal enzymes.

DOSAGE FORMS APPLICABLE. Drugs are administered by the oral route in a variety of pharmaceutical forms, each with inherent therapeutic advantages that result in their selective use by physicians. The most popular forms are tablets, capsules, suspensions, and various pharmaceutical solutions. Briefly, *tablets* are solid dosage forms prepared by compression or molding and contain medicinal substances with or without suitable diluents, disintegrants, coatings, colorants, and other pharmaceutical adjuncts. Diluents are necessary in preparing tablets of the proper size and consistency. Disintegrants are used when rapid separation of the tablet's compressed ingredients is desired. This ensures prompt exposure of drug particles to the dissolution process thereby enhancing drug absorption, as shown in Figure 3–12. Tablet coatings are of several types and for several different purposes. Some called *enteric coatings* are employed to permit safe passage of a tablet through the acid environment of the stomach where certain drugs may be destroyed, to the more suitable juices of the intestines where tablet dissolution safely takes place. Other coatings are employed to protect the drug substance from the destructive influences of moisture, light, and air throughout their period of storage or to conceal a bad or bitter taste from the taste buds of a patient. Commercial tablets, because of their distinctive shapes, colors, and frequently employed monograms of company symbols and code numbers facilitate identification by persons trained in their use and serve as an added protection to public health.

Capsules are solid dosage forms in which the drug substance and appropriate pharmaceutical adjuncts as fillers are enclosed in either a hard or a soft "shell," which is generally composed of a form of gelatin. Capsules vary in size, depending upon the amount of drug to be administered, and are of distinctive shapes and colors when produced commercially. Generally, drug materials are released from capsules faster than from tablets. Capsules of gelatin, a protein, are rapidly disfigured within the gastrointestinal tract, permitting the gastric juices to permeate and reach the contents. Unfortunately, however, capsules are prone to tampering by unscrupulous individuals. Thus, capsule-shaped and coated tablets, called "caplets," are increasingly utilized. These are easily swallowed but their contents are sealed and protected from tampering like tablets.

Suspensions are preparations of finely divided drugs held in suspension throughout a suitable vehicle. Suspensions taken orally generally employ an aqueous vehicle, whereas those employed for other purposes may utilize a different vehicle. Suspensions of certain drugs to be used for intramuscular injection, for instance, may be maintained in a suitable oil. To be suspended, the drug particles must be insoluble in the vehicle in which they are placed. Nearly all suspensions must be shaken before use because they tend to settle. This ensures not only uniformity of the preparation but more importantly the administration of the proper dosage. Suspensions are a useful means to administer large amounts of solid drugs that would be inconveniently taken in tablet or capsule form. In addition, suspensions have the advantage over solid dosage forms in that they are presented to the body in fine particle size, ready for the dissolution process immediately upon administration. However, not all oral suspensions are intended to be dissolved and absorbed by the body. For instance, Kaolin Mixture with Pectin an antidiarrheal preparation, contains suspended kaolin, which acts in the intestinal tract by adsorbing excessive intestinal fluid on the large surface area of its particles.

Drugs administered in aqueous solution are generally absorbed much more rapidly than those administered in solid form, because the processes of disintegration and dissolution are not required. Pharmaceutical solutions may differ in the type of solvent employed and therefore in their fluidity characteristics. Several of the solutions frequently administered orally are *elixirs*, which are solutions in a sweetened hydroalcoholic vehicle and are generally more mobile than water; *syrups*, which generally utilize sucrose solutions as the sweet vehicle resulting in a viscous preparation; and *solutions* themselves, which officially are preparations in which the drug substance is dissolved predominantly in an aqueous vehicle and do not for reasons of their method of preparation (e.g., injections, which must be sterilized) fall into another category of pharmaceutical preparations.

ABSORPTION. Absorption of drugs after oral administration may occur at the various body sites between the mouth and rectum. In general, the higher up a drug is absorbed along the length of the alimentary tract, the more rapid will be its action, a desirable feature in most instances. Because of the differences in the chemical and physical nature among drug substances, a given drug may be better absorbed from the environment of one position than from another within the alimentary tract.

The oral cavity is used on certain occasions as the absorption site for certain drugs. Physically, the oral absorption of drugs is managed by allowing the drug substance to be dissolved (if not presented as a solution) and withheld in the oral cavity with infrequent or no swallowing until the taste of the drug has dissipated. This process is accommodated pharmaceutically by providing the drug in a dissolved state (impregnated on a cotton swab, for instance) or as extremely soluble and rapidly dissolving uncoated tablets. Drugs capable of being absorbed in the mouth may present themselves to the absorbing surface in a much more concentrated form than when swallowed, since drugs become progressively more diluted with gastro-intestinal secretions and contents as they pass along the alimentary tract.

Currently the oral or *sublingual* (beneath the tongue) administration of drugs is regularly employed for only a few drugs, with nitroglycerin and certain steroid sex hormones being the best examples. Nitroglycerin, a coronary vasodilator used in the prophylaxis and treatment of angina pectoris, is available in the form of tiny tablets which are allowed to dissolve under the tongue, producing therapeutic effects in a few minutes after administration. The dose of nitroglycerin is so small (usually 400 mcg) that if it were swallowed the resulting dilute gastrointestinal concentration may not result in reliable and sufficient drug absorption. Even more important, however, is the fact that nitroglycerin is rapidly destroyed by the liver, thereby further reducing its chances of reaching its site of action. Many sex hormones have been shown to be absorbed materially better from sublingual administration than when swallowed. Although the sublingual route is probably an effective absorption route for many other drugs, it has not been extensively studied primarily because other routes have proven satisfactory and more convenient for the patient. Retaining drug substances in the mouth presents a psychological barrier to some, is unattractive to others because of the bitter taste of most drugs, and would be difficult to manage with certain patients, as children.

Drugs may be altered within the gastrointestinal tract into forms that render them less or more slowly available for absorption. This alteration may be the result of the drug's association with or binding to some other agent, which may be a normal constituent of the gastrointestinal tract or a foodstuff or even another drug. For instance, the absorption of the tetracycline group of antibiotics is greatly interfered with by the simultaneous presence of calcium. Because of this, tetracycline drugs must not be taken with milk or other calcium-containing foods. It is also of vital concern that the pharmaceutical adjuncts, such as the fillers and diluents employed in the preparation of the dosage forms, do not interfere with the therapeutic efficacy of the drug. It is the responsibility of the research pharmacist to assess carefully the total compatibility of all formulative materials prior to production.

In some instances it is the intent of the pharmacist to prepare a formulation that releases the drug slowly over an extended period of time. There are many commercial and patented methods by which slow release is accomplished, including the complexation or combination of the medicinal agent with another material, the combination of which is only slowly released from the dosage form, or only slowly soluble or absorbable once released. A good example of this is the slow-release waxy matrix potassium chloride tablets. These are designed to release their contents gradually as they are shunted through the gastrointestinal tract. Because their contents are leached out gradually there is less incidence of adverse side effects encountered by the patient and comparable bioavailability to other potassium chloride dosage forms is achieved.

Whether or not a drug truly interacts with food present in stomach, the intermingling of food and drug generally results in delayed absorption for the latter, although there are instances in which food enhances the absorption of drugs, e.g., benzodiazepines and griseofulvin. The stomach contents tend to dilute the drug concentration, with a greater dilution and decreased absorption resulting from an increased proportion of food present. Since most drugs are absorbed more effectively from the intestines than from the stomach, when rapid absorption is intended, it is generally desirable to have the drug pass from the stomach into the intestines as rapidly as possible. Therefore, gastric emptying time is an important factor in effecting drug action dependent upon intestinal absorption. Also, slow gastric emptying time is especially detrimental to drugs that may be destroyed by the gastric environment if permitted lengthy exposure. Gastric emptying time may be increased by a number of factors, including the presence of fatty foods (more effect than proteins, which in turn have more effect than carbohydrates), lying on the back when bedridden (lying on the right side facilitates passage in many instances), and the presence of drugs (for example, morphine) that have a quieting effect on the movements of the gastrointestinal tract. If a drug is administered in the form of a solution, it may be expected to pass into the intestines more rapidly than drugs administered in solid form. However, it should be borne in mind that drugs even when administered in solution may precipitate from solution in the stomach, in which case drug absorption may not be as rapid as would be otherwise expected.

As a rule, large volumes of water taken with medication facilitate gastric emptying and passage into the intestines.

The pH of the gastrointestinal tract increases progressively along its length from a pH of about 1 in the stomach to approximately pH 8 at the far end of the intestines. pH has a definite bearing on the degree of ionization of most drugs, and this in turn affects lipid solubility, membrane permeability and absorption. Because most drugs are absorbed by passive diffusion through the lipoid barrier, the lipid/water partition coefficient and the pK$_a$ of the drugs are of prime importance to both their degree and site of absorption within the gastrointestinal tract. As a general rule, weak acids are largely *un*ionized in the stomach and are absorbed fairly well from this site, whereas weak bases are highly ionized in the stomach and are not significantly absorbed from the gastric surface. Alkalinization of the gastric environment by artificial means (simultaneous administration of alkaline or antacid drugs) would be expected to decrease the gastric absorption of weak acids and to increase that of weak bases. Strong acids and bases are generally poorly absorbed due to their high degrees of ionization.

The small intestine serves as the major absorption pathway for drugs because of its suitable pH and the great surface area available for drug absorption within its approximate 20-foot length extending from the pylorus at the base of the stomach to the junction with the large intestine at the cecum. The pH of the lumen of the intestine is about 6.5 (see Fig. 3–3) and both weakly acidic and weakly basic drugs are well absorbed from the intestinal surface, which behaves in the ionization and distribution of drugs between it and the plasma on the other side of the membrane as though its pH were about 5.3.

Rectal Route

Drugs are frequently administered rectally for their local effects and less frequently for their systemic effects. Drugs given rectally are generally administered as solutions, suppositories, or ointments. *Suppositories* are defined as solid bodies of various weights and shapes intended for introduction into a body orifice (usually rectal, vaginal, or urethral) where they soften or melt, release their medication, and exert their drug effects. These effects simply may be the promotion of laxation (as with glycerin suppositories), the soothing of inflamed tissues (as with various commercial suppositories used to relieve the discomfort of hemorrhoids), or the promotion of systemic effects (as antinausea or antimotion sickness). The composition of the suppository base, or carrier of the medication, can greatly influence the degree and rate of drug release and should be selected on an individual basis for each drug to be prepared into a suppository. The use of rectal ointments is generally limited to the treatment of local conditions. Rectal solutions are usually employed as enemas or cleansing solutions.

The rectum and the colon are capable of absorbing many soluble drugs, and administration rectally for drugs intended for systemic action may be preferred for those drugs destroyed or inactivated by the environments of the stomach and intestines. The administration of drugs by the rectal route may also be indicated when the oral route is precluded because of vomiting or when the patient is unconscious or incapable of swallowing drugs safely without choking. It is estimated that about 50% of a dose of drug absorbed from rectal administration is likely to bypass the liver, an important factor when considering those orally administered drugs that are rapidly destroyed in the liver by the first-pass effect. On the negative side, compared with oral administration, rectal administration of drugs is inconvenient, and the absorption of drugs from the rectum is frequently irregular and difficult to predict (e.g., theophylline suppositories).

Parenteral Route

The term *parenteral* is derived from the Greek words *para*, meaning beside, and *enteron*, meaning intestine, which together indicate something done outside of the intestine and not by way of the alimentary tract. A drug administered parenterally is one injected through the hollow of a fine needle into the body at various sites and to various depths. The three primary routes of parenteral administration are subcutaneous, intramuscular (i.m.), and intravenous (i.v.) although there are others such as intracardiac and intraspinal.

Drugs destroyed or inactivated in the gastrointestinal tract or too poorly absorbed to provide satisfactory response may be parenterally administered. The parenteral route is also preferred when rapid absorption is essential, as in emergency situations. Absorption by the parenteral route is not only faster than after oral administration, but the blood levels of drug that result are far more predictable, because little is lost after subcutaneous or intramuscular injection, and virtually none by intravenous injection; this also generally permits the administration of smaller doses. The parenteral route of administration is especially useful in treating patients who are uncooperative, unconscious, or otherwise unable to accept oral medication.

One disadvantage of parenteral administration is that once the drug is injected, there is no retreat. That is, once the substance is within the tissues or is placed directly into the blood stream, removal of the drug warranted by an untoward or toxic effect or an inadvertent overdose is most difficult. By other means of administration, there is more time between drug administration and drug absorption, which in essence becomes a safety factor by allowing for the extraction of unabsorbed drug (as by the induction of vomiting after an orally administered drug). Also, because of the strict sterility requirements for all injections, they are generally more expensive than other dosage forms and require competent trained personnel for their proper administration.

DOSAGE FORMS APPLICABLE. Pharmaceutically, injectable preparations are usually either sterile suspensions or solutions of a drug substance in water or in a suitable vegetable oil. In general, drugs in solution act faster than drugs in suspension, with an aqueous vehicle providing faster action in each instance than an oleaginous vehicle. As in other instances of drug absorption, a drug must be in solution to be absorbed, and a suspended drug must first submit to the dissolution process. Also, because body fluids are aqueous, they are more receptive to drugs in an aqueous vehicle than those in an oily one. For these reasons, the rate of drug absorption can be varied in parenteral products by selective combinations of drug state and supporting vehicle. For instance, a suspension of a drug in a vegetable oil likely would be much more slowly absorbed than an aqueous solution of the same drug. Slow absorption generally means prolonged drug action, and when this is achieved through pharmaceutical means, the resulting preparation is referred to as a *depot* or *repository* injection, because it represents a storage reservoir of the drug substance within the body from which it is slowly removed into the systemic circulation. In this regard, even more sustained drug action may be achieved through the use of subcutaneous implantation of compressed tablets, termed pellets which are only slowly dissolved from their site of implantation, releasing their medication at a rather constant rate over a period of several weeks to many months. The repository type of injection is mainly limited to the intramuscular type. It is obvious that drugs injected intravenously do not encounter absorption barriers and thus produce only rapid drug effects. From a pharmaceutical standpoint, preparations for intravenous injection must not interfere in any way with the blood components or with circulation and therefore are limited largely to aqueous solutions of drugs.

SUBCUTANEOUS INJECTIONS. The subcutaneous (hypodermic) administration of drugs involves their injection through the layers of skin into the loose subcutaneous tissue. Generally, subcutaneous injections are prepared as aqueous solutions or as suspensions and are administered in relatively small volumes of 2 mL or less. Insulin is an example of a drug administered by the subcutaneous route. Subcutaneous injections are generally given in the forearm, upper arm, thigh, or nates. If the patient is to receive frequent injections, it is best to alternate injection sites to reduce tissue irritation. After injection, the drug comes into the immediate vicinity of blood capillaries and permeates them by diffusion or filtration. The capillary wall is an example of a membrane that behaves as a lipid pore barrier, with lipid-soluble substances penetrating the membrane at rates varying with their oil/water partition coefficients. Lipid-insoluble (generally more water-soluble) drugs penetrate the capillary membrane at rates which appear to be inversely related to their molecular size, with smaller molecules penetrating much more rapidly than larger ones. All substances, whether lipid-soluble or not, cross the capillary membrane at rates that are much more rapid than the rates of their transfer across other body membranes. The blood supply to the site of injection is an important factor in considering the rate of drug absorption, consequently the more proximal capillaries are to the site of injection, the more prompt will be the drug's entrance into the circulation. Also, the more capillaries, the more surface area for absorption, and the faster the rate of absorption. Some substances have the capability of modifying the rate of drug absorption from a subcutaneous site of injection. The addition of a vasoconstrictor to the injection formulation (or its prior injection) will generally diminish the rate of drug absorption by causing constriction of the blood vessels in the area of injection and thereby reducing blood flow and the capacity for absorption. This principle is frequently utilized in the administration of local anesthetics by employing the vasoconstrictor epinephrine, which is additionally effective in delaying drug absorption because of its own resistance to destruction after injection. Conversely, vasodilators may be employed to enhance subcutaneous absorption by increasing blood flow to the area. Physical exercise can also influence the bioavailability of drug from an injection site. Diabetic patients who rotate subcutaneous injection sites and then do physical exercise, e.g., jogging, must realize the onset of insulin activity might be influenced by the selected site of administration. Because of the movement of the leg and blood circulation to it during running, the absorption of insulin from a thigh injection site would be expected to be faster than that from an abdominal injection site.

INTRAMUSCULAR INJECTIONS. Intramuscular injections are performed deep into the skeletal muscles, generally the gluteal or lumbar muscles. The site is selected where the danger of hitting a nerve or blood vessel is minimal. Aqueous or oleaginous solutions or suspensions may be used intramuscularly with rapid effects or depot activity selected to meet the requirements of the patient. Certain drugs, because of their inherent low solubilities, provide sustained drug action after an intramuscular injection of a suspension of the drug. For instance, one deep intramuscular injection of a suspension of penicillin G benzathine results in effective blood levels of the drug for seven to ten days.

Drugs which are irritating to subcutaneous tissue are often administered intramuscularly. Also, greater volumes (2 to 5 mL) may be administered intramuscularly than subcutaneously. When a volume greater than 5 mL is to be injected, it is frequently administered in divided doses using two injection sites. Injection sites are also rotated when a patient is receiving repeated injections over a period of time.

INTRAVENOUS INJECTIONS. In the intravenous administration of drugs, an aqueous solution is injected directly into the vein at a rate commensurate with efficiency, safety, comfort to the patient, and the desired duration of drug response. The latter point refers mainly to drugs administered as a slow drip during intravenous feeding of nutrients and drugs to a patient after surgery. Intravenous injections are usually made into the veins of the forearm and are especially useful in emergency situations where immediate drug response is desired. It is essential that the drug be maintained in solution after injection and not be precipitated within the circulatory system, an event that might produce emboli. Because of a fear of the development of pulmonary embolism, oleaginous bases are not usually intravenously administered. However, an intravenous fat emulsion is used therapeutically as a caloric source for patients receiving parenteral nutrition whose caloric requirements cannot be met by glucose. It may be administered either through a peripheral vein or a central venous catheter at a distinct rate to help prevent the occurrence of untoward reactions. After intravenous injection, the optimum blood level of the drug may be obtained with an accuracy and immediacy not possible by any other means. However, when an immediate drug effect is not required, another route of parenteral administration is preferred.

INTRADERMAL INJECTIONS. These injections are administered into the corium of the skin, usually in volumes of about a tenth of a milliliter. Common sites for the injection are the arm and the back. The injections are frequently performed as diagnostic measures, as in tuberculin and allergy testing.

Epicutaneous Route

Drugs are administered topically, or applied to the skin, chiefly for their action at the site of application or for systemic drug effects.

In general, drug absorption via the skin is enhanced if the drug substance is in solution, if it has a favorable lipid/water partition coefficient, and if it is a nonelectrolyte. Drugs that are absorbed enter the skin by way of the pores, sweat glands, hair follicles, sebaceous glands, and other anatomic structures of the skin's surface. Because blood capillaries are present just below the epidermal cells, a drug that penetrates the skin and is able to traverse the capillary wall finds ready access to the general circulation.

Among the few drugs currently employed topically to the skin surface for percutaneous absorption and systemic action are nitroglycerin and scopolamine. Each of these drugs is available for use in the form of transdermal delivery systems fabricated as an adhesive disc or patch which slowly releases the medication for percutaneous absorption. Additionally, nitroglycerin is available in an ointment form for application to the skin's surface for systemic absorption. Nitroglycerin is employed therapeutically for ischemic heart disease, with the transdermal dosage forms becoming increasingly popular because of the benefit in patient compliance through their long-acting (24 hours) characteristics. The nitroglycerin patch is generally applied to the arm or chest, preferably in a hair-free or shaven area. The transdermal scopolamine system is also in the form of a patch to be applied to the skin; in this case, behind the ear. The drug system is indicated for the prevention of nausea and vomiting associated with motion sickness. The commercially available product is applied to the postauricular area several hours before need (as prior to an air or sea trip) where it releases its medication over a period of 3 days. The concepts of transdermal therapeutic systems are discussed further in Chapter 9.

For the most part, pharmaceutical preparations applied to the skin are intended to serve some local action and as such are formulated to provide prolonged local contact with minimal absorption. Drugs applied to the skin for their local action include antiseptics, antifungal agents, anti-inflammatory agents, local anesthetic agents, skin emollients, and protectants, against environmental conditions, as the effects of the sun, wind, pests, and chemical irritants. For these purposes drugs are most commonly administered in the form of ointments and related semisolid preparations such as creams and pastes, as solid dry powders, aerosol sprays or as liquid preparations such as solutions and lotions.

Pharmaceutically, ointments, creams, and pastes are semisolid preparations in which the drug is contained in a suitable base (ointment base) which is itself semisolid and either hydrophilic or hydrophobic in character. These bases play an important role in the proper formulation of semisolid preparations, and there is no single base universally suitable as a carrier of all drug substances or for all therapeutic indications. The proper base for a drug must be determined individually to provide the desired drug release rate, staying qualities after application, and texture. Briefly, *ointments* are simple mixtures of drug substances in an ointment base, whereas *creams* are semisolid emulsions and are generally less viscid and lighter than ointments. Creams are considered to have greater esthetic appeal due to their nongreasy character and their ability to "vanish" into the skin upon rubbing. *Pastes* contain more solid materials than do ointments and are therefore stiffer and less penetrating. Pastes are usually employed for their protective action and for their ability to absorb serous discharges from skin lesions. Thus when protective rather than therapeutic action is desired, the formulation pharmacist will favor a paste, but when therapeutic action is required, he will prefer ointments and creams. Commercially, many therapeutic agents are prepared in both ointment and cream form and are dispensed and used according to the particular preference of the patient and the prescribing practitioner. Even though these dosage forms may have the same strength of active ingredient, the pharmacist must realize that these dosage forms are not interchangeable by virtue of their differing therapeutic intent for use and topical effect.

Medicinal powders are intimate mixtures of medicinal substances usually in an inert base like talcum powder. Depending upon the particle size of the resulting blend, the powder will have varying dusting and covering capabilities. In any case, the particle size should be small enough to ensure against grittiness and consequent skin irritation. Powders are most frequently applied topically to relieve such conditions as diaper rash, chafing, and athlete's foot.

When topical application is desired in liquid form other than solution, lotions are most frequently employed. *Lotions* are generally suspensions of solid materials in an aqueous vehicle, although certain emulsions and even some true solutions have been designated as lotions because of either their appearance or application. Lotions may be preferred over semisolid preparations because of their nongreasy character and their increased spreadability over large areas of skin.

Ocular, Oral, and Nasal Routes

Drugs are frequently applied topically to the eye, ear, and the mucous membranes of the nose. In these instances, ointments, suspensions, and solutions are generally employed. Ophthalmic solutions and suspensions are sterile aqueous preparations with other qualities essential to the safety and comfort of the patient. Ophthalmic ointments must be sterile, and also free of grittiness. Innovative new delivery systems for ophthalmic drugs continue to be investigated. One dosage form, the Ocusert, already available for patient use is an elliptically-shaped unit designed for continuous release of pilocarpine following its placement into the cul-de-sac of the eye. Further, case reports of the ability of soft contact lenses to absorb drug from the eye have spawned research interested in the development of soft contact lenses impregnated with drug for therapeutic application in the eye. Nasal preparations are usually solutions or suspensions administered by drops or as a fine mist from a nasal spray container. Currently, research is investigating the feasibility of the nasal administration of insulin for diabetes mellitus and leuprolide acetate for endometriosis. Otic, or ear preparations are usually viscid so that they have prolonged contact with the affected area. They may be employed simply to soften ear wax, to relieve an earache, or to combat an ear infection. Eye, ear, and nose preparations are not generally employed for systemic effects, and although ophthalmic and otic preparations are not usually absorbed to any great extent, nasal preparations *may* be absorbed, and systemic effects after the intranasal application of solution are not unusual.

Other Routes

The lungs provide an excellent absorbing surface for the administration of gases and for aerosol mists of very minute particles of liquids or solids. The gases employed are mainly oxygen and the common general anesthetic drugs administered to patients entering surgery. The rich capillary area of the alveoli of the lungs, which in man covers nearly a thousand square feet, provides rapid absorption and drug effects comparable in speed to those following an intravenous injection. In the case of drug particles, their size largely determines the depth to which they penetrate the alveolar regions; their solubility, the extent to which they are absorbed. After contact with the inner surface of the lungs, an insoluble drug particle is caught in the mucus and is moved up the pulmonary tree by ciliary action. Soluble drug particles that are approximately 0.5 to 1.0 micron in size reach the minute alveolar sacs and are most prompt and efficient in providing systemic effects. Particles that are smaller than 0.5 micron are expired to some

extent, and thus their absorption is not total but variable. Particles from 1 to 10 microns in size effectively reach the terminal bronchioles and to some extent the alveolar ducts and are favored for local therapy. Therefore, in the pharmaceutical manufacture of aerosol sprays for inhalation therapy, the manufacturers not only must attain the proper drug particle size but also must ensure their uniformity for consistent penetration of the pulmonary tree and uniform effects.

In certain instances and generally for local effects, drugs are inserted into the vagina and the urethra. Drugs are generally presented to the vagina in tablet form, as suppositories, ointments, emulsion foams, or solutions, and to the urethra as suppositories or solutions. Systemic drug effects, which may result after the vaginal or urethral application of drugs due to absorption of the drug from the mucous membranes of these sites, are generally undesired.

Fate of Drug after Absorption

After absorption into the general circulation from any route of administration, a drug may become bound to blood proteins and delayed in its passage into the surrounding tissues. Many drug substances may be highly bound to blood protein and others little-bound. For instance, when in the blood stream, naproxen is 99% bound to plasma proteins, penicillin G is 60% bound, and amoxicillin only 20% bound.

The degree of drug binding to plasma proteins is usually expressed as a percentage or as a fraction (termed *alpha*, or α) of the bound concentration (C_b) to the total concentration (C_t), bound plus unbound (C_u) drug:

$$\alpha = \frac{C_b}{C_u + C_b} = \frac{C_b}{C_t}$$

Thus, if one knows two of the three terms in the equation, the third may be calculated. Drugs having an alpha value of greater than 0.9 are considered highly bound (90%); those drugs with an alpha value of less than 0.2 are considered to be little (20% or less) protein bound. Table 3–9 presents approximate serum protein binding characteristics for representative drugs present in the blood under conditions associated with usual therapy. The drug-protein complex is reversible and generally involves albu-

Table 3–9.   Examples of Drug Binding to Plasma Proteins

Drug	Percent Bound*
Naproxen (Naprosyn, Syntex)	>99
Chlorambucil (Leukeran, B/W)	99
Phenylbutazone (Butazolidin, Geigy)	98
Warfarin (Coumadin, DuPont)	97
Reserpine (Serpasil, Ciba)	96
Cloxacillin (Tegopen, Bristol)	95
Ceftriaxone (Rocephin, Roche)	85–95
Cefoperazone (Cefobid, Roerig)	82–93
Cefonicid (Monocid, SKF)	>90
Indomethacin (Indocin, MSD)	90
Spironolactone (Aldactone, Searle)	90
Digitoxin (Crystodigin, Lilly)	90
Cyclosporine (Sandimmune, Sandoz)	90
Sulfisoxazole (Gantrisin, Roche)	85
Penicillin V (Veetids, Squibb)	75
Nitroglycerin (Nitrol, Rorer)	60
Penicillin G (Crysticillin, Squibb)	60
Methotrexate (Lederle)	50
Methicillin (Staphcillin, Bristol)	40
Ceftizoxime (Cefizox, SKF)	30
Captopril (Capozide, Squibb)	25–30
Digoxin (Lanoxin, B/W)	20–25
Ampicillin (Omnipen, Wyeth-Ayerst)	20
Amoxicillin (Amoxil, Beecham)	20
Metronidazole (Flagyl, Searle)	<20
Mercaptopurine (Purinethol, B/W)	19
Cephradine (Valosef, Squibb)	8–17
Ranitidine (Zantac, Glaxo)	15
Ceftazidime (Tazicef, SKF)	<10
Amidinocillin (Coactin, Roche)	5–10
Minoxidil (Loniten, Upjohn)	0

*Average literature values, based on conditions usually associated with drug therapy.

min, although globulins are also involved in the binding of drugs, particularly some of the hormones. The binding capacity of blood proteins is limited, and once they are saturated, additional drug absorbed into the blood stream remains unbound unless bound drug is released, creating a vacant site for another drug molecule to attach. However, once the binding proteins are saturated, there can be no additional net increase in bound drug, so the unbound portion of drug remains free to leave the blood and enter the surrounding tissues. Additional drug being absorbed into the blood stream must also remain free and may result in a sudden upsurge in the concentration of free or unbound drug in the blood.

Bound drug is neither exposed to the body's detoxication (metabolism) processes nor is it filtered through the renal glomeruli. Bound drug is therefore referred to as the *inactive* portion in the blood, and unbound drug, with its ability to penetrate cells, is termed the *active* blood portion. The bound portion of drug serves as a drug reservoir or a depot, from which the drug is released as the free form when the level of free drug in the blood no longer is adequate to insure protein saturation. The free drug may be only slowly released, thereby increasing the duration of the drug's stay in the body. For this reason a drug that is highly protein bound may remain in the body for longer periods of time and require less frequent dosage administration than another drug that may be only slightly protein bound and may remain in the body for only a short period of time. Evidence suggests that the concentration of serum albumin decreases about 20% in the elderly. This may be clinically significant for drugs that bind strongly to albumin, e.g., phenytoin, because if there is less albumin available to bind the drug there will be a corresponding increase of the free drug in the body. Without a downward dosage adjustment in an elderly patient there could be an increase incidence of adverse effects.

In addition to the normal complexities, drug binding to proteins is further complicated by the fact that certain drugs are capable of influencing the binding capabilities of other drugs to protein. Their simultaneous presence may result in drug effects or durations of drug action quite dissimilar to that found when each is administered alone. Salicylates, for instance, have the effect of decreasing the binding capacity of thyroxin, the thyroid hormone, to proteins. Phenylbutazone is an example of a drug that competitively displaces several other drugs from serum binding sites, including other anti-inflammatory drugs, oral anticoagulants, oral antidiabetics, and sulfonamides. Through this action, the displaced drugs become less protein bound and their activity and toxicity may be increased. The intensity of a drug's pharmacologic response is related to the ratio of the bound drug *versus* free, active drug, and the therapeutic index of the drug. Warfarin, an anticoagulant is 97% bound to plasma protein leaving 3% in free form to exert its effect. If a second drug, such as naproxen, which is strongly bound to plasma proteins is administered and results in only 90% of the warfarin being bound, this means that 10% of warfarin is now in the free form. Thus, the blood level of the free warfarin (3 to 10%) has tripled and could result in serious toxicity. The displacement of drugs from plasma protein sites is typical in the elderly who normally are maintained on numerous medicines. Coupled with the aforementioned decrease in serum protein through the aging process the addition of a highly protein-bound drug to an elderly patient's existing treatment regimen could pose significant problems if the patient is not monitored carefully for signs of toxicity.

In the same manner as they are bound to blood proteins, drugs may become bound to specific components of certain cells. Thus drugs are not distributed uniformly among all cells of the body, but rather tend to pass from the blood into the fluid bathing the tissues and may accumulate in certain cells according to their permeability capabilities and chemical and physical affinities. This affinity for certain body sites influences their action, for they may be brought into contact with reactive tissues (their *receptor*

sites) or deposited in places where they may be inactive. Many drugs, because of their affinity for and solubility in lipids, are found to be deposited in fatty body tissue, thereby creating a storage place or drug reservoir from which they are slowly released to other tissues.

Drug Metabolism (Biotransformation)

Although some drugs are excreted from the body in their original form, many drugs undergo biotransformation prior to excretion. Biotransformation is a term used to indicate the chemical changes that occur with drugs within the body as they are metabolized and altered by various biochemical mechanisms. Generally, the biotransformation of a drug results in its conversion to a compound that is more water soluble, more ionized, less capable of binding to proteins of the plasma and tissues, less capable of being stored in fat tissue, and less able to penetrate cell membranes, thereby resulting in a less active compound. Because of its new characteristics, a drug so transformed is rendered less toxic and is more readily excreted. It is for this reason that the process of biotransformation is also commonly referred to as the "detoxification" or "inactivation" process.

The exact metabolic processes (pathways) by which drugs are transformed represent an active area of biomedical research. Much work has been done with the processes of animal degradation of drugs and in many instances the biotransformation in the animal is thought to parallel that in man. There are four principal chemical reactions involved in the metabolism of drugs: oxidation, reduction, hydrolysis, and conjugation.

In recent years, much interest has been shown in the metabolites of drug biotransformation. It is known that certain metabolites may be as active or even more active pharmacologically than the original compound. Occasionally an active drug may be converted into an active metabolite, which must be excreted as such or undergo further biotransformation to an inactive metabolite, e.g., amitriptyline to nortriptyline. In other instances of drug therapy, an inactive parent compound, referred to as a *prodrug,* may be converted to an active therapeutic agent by chemical transformation in the body. The prodrug dipivefrin mentioned earlier in this chapter is a classic example of this phenomenon. The possible use of these active metabolites as "original" drugs represents a new area of drug investigation and a vast reservoir of potential therapeutic agents.

Several examples of biotransformations occurring within the body are as follows:

(1) Acetaminophen $\xrightarrow{\text{conjugation}}$ Acetaminophen glucuronide
　　　(active)　　　　　　　　　　　　(inactive)

(2) Amoxapine $\xrightarrow{\text{oxidation}}$ 8-hydroxy-amoxapine
　　　(active)　　　　　　　　(inactive)

(3) Procainamide $\xrightarrow{\text{hydrolysis}}$ p-Aminobenzoic acid
　　　(active)　　　　　　　　(inactive)

(4) Nitroglycerin $\xrightarrow{\text{reduction}}$ 1-2 and 1-3 dinitroglycerol
　　　(active)　　　　　　　　　(active)

Typically, biotransformation of a drug is from an active form to an inactive metabolite. However, in the case of nitroglycerin it is initially converted to an active dinitro-metabolite. Subsequently, this active metabolite is converted by reduction mechanisms to the inactive nitroglycerol.

It is relevant to mention that several factors influence drug metabolism. For example, there are marked differences between *species* in pathways of hepatic metabolism of a given drug, as well as differential rates of metabolism along the same chemical pathway in different animal species. Species differences make it extremely difficult to extrapolate from one species to another, e.g., laboratory animals to humans. Furthermore, there are many examples of *interindividual variations* in hepatic metabolism of drugs within one species. Genetic factors are involved in the determination of the basal activity of the drug-metabolizing enzyme systems. Thus, there can be marked intersubject variation in the rate at which certain individuals metabolically handle drugs. Because of this variation, a physician must individualize therapy to maximize the chances for a constructive therapeutic outcome with minimal toxicity. Studies in humans have demonstrated that these differences have occurred within the cytochrome P-450 genes codes for a family of isoenzymes responsible to drug metabolism.

Age of the patient is another significant factor that influences drug metabolism. Although pharmacokinetic calculations have not been able to develop a specific correlative relationship with age, it is known, for example, that the ability to metabolize drugs decreases at the extremes of the age scale, i.e., elderly, neonate. For example, the half-life of chlordiazepoxide increases from about 6 hours at age 20 to about 36 hours at age 80. Further, an immature hepatic system disallows the effective metabolism of drugs by the newborn or premature infant. As mentioned earlier, the half life of theophylline ranges between 14 to 58 hours in the premature infant to 2.5 to 5 hours in young children between the ages of 1 to 4 whose liver enzyme systems are mature.

Diet has also been demonstrated to modify the metabolism of some drugs. For example, the conversion of an asthmatic patient from a high to a low protein diet will increase the half life of theophylline. It has also been demonstrated that the production of polycyclic hydrocarbons by the charcoal broiling of beef enhances the hepatic metabolism and shortens the plasma half-life of theophylline. It is conceivable that this effect could also occur with drugs that are metabolized in similar fashion to theophylline. Diet type, e.g., starvation, certain vegetables (brussels sprouts, cabbage, broccoli), has been shown to influence the metabolism of certain drugs. Lastly, it is important to mention that exposure to other drugs or chemicals, e.g., pesticides, alcohol, nicotine, and the presence of disease states, e.g., hepatitis, have all demonstrated an influence on the drug metabolism and consequently the pharmacokinetic profile of certain drugs.

Excretion of Drugs

The excretion of drugs and their metabolites terminates their activity and presence in the body. They may be eliminated by various routes, with the kidney playing the dominant role by eliminating drugs via the urine. Drug excretion with the feces is also important, especially for drugs that are poorly absorbed and remain in the gastrointestinal tract after oral administration. Exit through the bile is significant only when the drug's reabsorption from the gastrointestinal tract is minimal. The lungs provide the exit for many volatile drugs through the expired breath. The sweat glands, saliva, and milk play only minor roles in drug elimination. However, it should be recognized that if a drug gains access to the milk of a mother during lactation, it could easily exert its drug effects in the nursing infant. Examples of drugs that do enter breast milk and may be passed on to nursing infants include theophylline, penicillin, reserpine, and thiazide diuretics. It is generally good practice for the mother to abstain from taking medication during the period of time she is nursing her infant. If she must take medication, she should abide by a dosage regimen and nursing schedule that permit her own therapy yet ensure the safety of her child. Not all drugs gain entrance into the milk; nevertheless, caution is advisable.

The unnecessary use of medications during the early stages of pregnancy is likewise being more strictly prohibited by physicians, because certain drugs are known to have the ability to cross the placental barrier and gain entrance to the tissues and blood of the fetus. Among the many drugs known to do so after administration to an expectant mother are all of the anesthetic gases, many barbiturates, sulfonamides, salicylates, and a number of other potent agents like quinine, meperidine, and morphine, the latter two drugs being narcotic analgesics with great addiction liabilities. In fact, it is not unusual for a newborn infant to be born an addict due to the narcotic addiction of its mother and the passage of the narcotic drugs across the placental barrier.

The kidney, as the main organ for the elimination of drugs from the body, must be functioning adequately if drugs are to be efficiently eliminated. For instance, elimination of digoxin occurs largely through the kidney according to first-order kinetics; that is, the quantity of digoxin eliminated at any time is proportional to the total body content. Renal excretion of digoxin is proportional to the glomerular filtration rate which when normal results in a digoxin half life that may range from 1.5 to 2.0 days. When the glomerular filtration rate becomes impaired or disrupted, however, as in an anuric patient, the elimination rate decreases. Consequently, the half life of digoxin may be between 4 to 6 days. Because of this prolongation of digoxin's half life, the dosage of the drug must be decreased or the dosage interval prolonged. Otherwise the patient will experience digoxin toxicity. The degree of impairment can be estimated by measurements of glomerular filtration rates, most often by creatinine clearance determination. Usually, however, this is not feasible and the patient's serum creatinine value is used within appropriate pharmacokinetic equations to help determine a drug's dosage regimen.

Some drugs may be reabsorbed from the renal tubule even after having been sent there for excretion. Because the rate of reabsorption is proportional to the concentration of drug in unionized form, it is possible to modify this rate by adjusting the pH of the urine. By acidifying the urine, as with the oral administration of ammonium chloride, or by alkalinizing it, as with the administration of sodium bicarbonate, one can increase or decrease the ionization of the drug and thereby alter its prospect of being reabsorbed. Alkalinization of the urine has been shown to enhance the urinary excretion of weak acids such as salicylates, sulfonamides, and phenobarbital. The opposite effect can be achieved by acidifying the urine. Thus, the duration of a drug's stay within the body may be markedly altered by changing the pH of the urine.

The urinary excretion of drugs may also be retarded by the concurrent administration of agents capable of inhibiting their tubular secretion. A well-known example is the use of probenecid to inhibit the tubular secretion of various types of penicillin, thereby reducing the frequency of dosage administrations usually necessary to maintain adequate therapeutic blood levels of the antibiotic drug. In this particular instance, the elevation of penicillin blood levels, by whatever route the antibiotic is administered, to twofold and even fourfold levels has been demonstrated by adjuvant therapy with probenecid. The effects are completely reversible upon withdrawal of the probenecid from concomitant therapy.

The fecal excretion of drugs appears to lag behind the rate of urinary excretion partly because a day or so elapses before the feces reach the rectum. It should be easily seen that drugs administered orally for local activity within the gastrointestinal tract and not absorbed will be eliminated completely via the feces. Unless the drug is particularly irritating to the gastrointestinal tract (in which case diarrhea or vomiting would likely occur), there is generally no urgency in removing unabsorbable drugs from the system by means other than the normal defecation process. Some drugs that are only partially absorbed after oral administration will naturally be partly eliminated by the rectum.

Pharmacokinetic Principles

This section introduces the concept of pharmacokinetics and how it interrelates the various processes that take place when one administers a drug to a patient, i.e., absorption, distribution, metabolism, excretion. It is not comprehensive, and for more in-depth information about the subject the reader is referred to other appropriate literature sources.

A problem encountered when one needs to determine a more accurate dosage of a drug or a more meaningful interpretation of a biologic response to a dose is the inability to determine the drug concentration at the active site in the body. Consequently, to solve this dilemma, the concept of compartmental analysis is used within the discipline of pharmacokinetics in an attempt to quantitatively define what has become of the drug as a function of time from the moment it is administered until it is no longer in the body. Pharmacokinetic analysis utilizes mathematical models to simplify or simulate the disposition of the drug in the body. The idea is to begin with a simple model and then modify as necessary. The principal assumption is that the human body may be represented by one or more *compartments* or pools in which a drug resides in a dynamic state for a short period of time. A compartment is a hypothetical space bound by an unspecified membrane across which drugs are transferred (Fig. 3–13). The transfer of drugs into and out of this compartment is indicated by arrows that point in the direction of drug movement into or out of the compartment. The rate at which a drug is transferred throughout the system is designated by a symbol that usually represents an exponential rate constant. Typically, the letter K or k with numerical or alpha-numerical subscripts is utilized.

There are several assumptions associated with modeling of drug behavior once in the body. It is assumed that the volume of each compartment remains constant. Thus, an equation that describes the time course of the amount of drug in the compartment can be converted to an equation that depicts the time course of the drug concentration in the compartment by dividing both sides of the equation by the volume of the compartment. Secondly, it is assumed that once a drug enters the compartment it is instantaneously and uniformly distributed throughout the entire compartment. Thus, it is assumed that a sampling of any one portion of the compartment will yield the drug concentration of the entire compartment.

In compartment models it is assumed that drug passes freely into and out of compartments. Thus, these compartmental systems are known as "open" systems. Typically, the process of drug transport between compartments

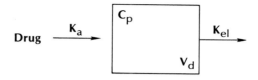

Where:
C_p is the drug concentration in plasma
V_d is the volume of the compartment or volume of distribution

Fig. 3–13. *Schematic of a one-compartment system.*

follows first-order kinetics, herein a constant fraction of drug present is eliminated per unit time, and can be described by ordinary differential equations. In these linear systems the time constants that describe the rate at which the plasma or blood concentration curve of a drug decays are independent of the dose of the drug, the volume of distribution of the drug and the route of administration.

The simplest pharmacokinetic model is the single compartment *open-model system* (Fig. 3–13). This model depicts the body as one compartment characterized by a certain volume of distribution (V_d) that remains constant. Each drug has its own distinct volume of distribution and this can be influenced by certain patient factors, e.g., age, disease state status. In this scheme a drug can be instantaneously introduced into the compartment, i.e., rapid intravenous administration, or gradually, e.g., oral administration. In the former example it is assumed that the drug distributes immediately to tissues with instantaneous attainment of equilibrium. In the latter example, the drug is absorbed at a certain rate and is characterized by the rate constant K_a. Lastly, the drug is eliminated from the compartment at a certain rate that is characterized by a rate constant K_{el}.

It is relevant at this point to consider the *volume of distribution*, V_d. The volume of distribution is a proportionality constant and is a term that refers to the volume into which the total amount of drug in the body would have to be uniformly distributed to provide the concentration of drug actually measured, e.g., in plasma, in blood. This term can be misleading because it does not represent a specific body fluid or volume. It is influenced by the plasma-protein binding and tissue binding characteristics of a drug. These then influence the distribution of

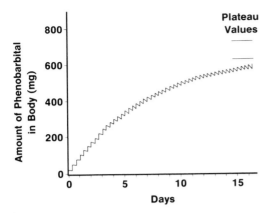

Fig. 3–14. *Semilogarithmic plot of the plasma concentration-time data. (From Rowland, M., and Tozer, T.N.: Clinical Pharmacokinetics. 2nd Ed., Philadelphia, Lea & Febiger, 1989.)*

the drug between plasma water, extracellular fluid, intracellular fluid and total body water. Further, because a drug can partition between fat and water according to its unique partition coefficient, this can also influence the volume of distribution. Because of these phenomena, pharmacokineticists find it convenient to describe a drug distribution in terms of compartment models.

To determine the rate of drug transfer into and out of the compartment, plasma, serum or blood samples are drawn at predetermined times after the drug is administered and analyzed for drug concentration. Once a sufficient number of experimental data points is determined, these are plotted on semi-logarithmic paper and an attempt is made to fit the experimental points with the smoothest curve to fit these points. Figure 3–14 depicts the plasma concentration *versus* time profile for a hypothetical drug following rapid intravenous injection of a bolus dose of the drug with instantaneous distribution. For drugs whose distribution follows first-order, one-compartment pharmacokinetics, a plot of the logarithm of the concentration of drug in the plasma (or blood) versus time will yield a straight line. The equation that describes the plasma decay curve is:

$$C_p = C_p^0 \, e^{-K_{el}t} \qquad \text{(Equation 3–1)}$$

where K_{el} is the first-order rate of elimination of the drug from the body, C_p is the concentra-

tion of the drug at a time equal to t, and C_p^0 is the concentration of drug at time equal to zero, when all of the drug administered has been absorbed but none has been removed from the body through elimination mechanisms, e.g., metabolism, renal excretion. The apparent first-order rate of elimination, K_{el}, is usually the sum of the rate constants of a number of individual processes, e.g., metabolic transformation, renal excretion.

For the purpose of pharmacokinetic calculation it is simpler to convert Equation 3–1 to natural logs:

$$\text{Ln } C_p = \text{Ln } C_p^0 - K_{el} (t) \qquad \text{(Equation 3–2)}$$

and then to log base₁₀:

$$\text{Log } C_p = \text{Log } C_p^0$$
$$- K_{el} (t)/2.303 \qquad \text{(Equation 3–3)}$$

Equation 3–3 is then thought of in terms of the Y-intercept form:

$$Y = b + m \, X$$

$$\text{Log } C_p = \text{Log } C_p^0 - K_{el}/2.303 \, (t)$$

and interpreted as such in the semi-logarithmic plot illustrated in Figure 3–14. Most drugs administered orally can be adequately described using a one-compartment model, whereas drugs administered by rapid intravenous infusion are usually best described by a two-compartment or three-compartment model system.

Assuming that a drug's volume of distribution, V_d, is constant within this system, the total amount of drug in the body (Q_b) can be calculated from the following equation:

$$Q_b = [C_p^0] \, [V_d] \qquad \text{(Equation 3–4)}$$

Usually, C_p^0 is determined by extrapolating the drug-concentration time plot back to time zero.

In this simple one compartment system it is assumed that the administered drug is confined to the plasma (or blood) and then excreted. Drugs that exhibit this behavior will have small volumes of distribution. For example, a drug such as warfarin which is extensively bound to plasma albumin will have a volume of distribution equivalent to that of plasma water, about

Drug

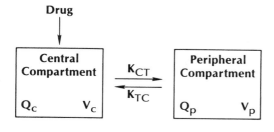

Where:
Q_c = Quantity of drug in central compartment
V_c = Volume of the central compartment
Q_p = Quantity of drug in peripheral compartment
V_p = Volume of the peripheral compartment

Fig. 3–15. *Schematic of a two-compartment system.*

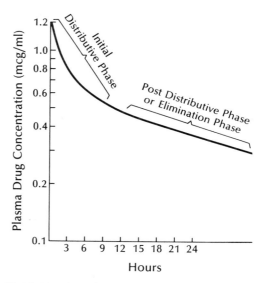

Fig. 3–16. *A semilogarithmic plasma concentration versus time plot of an intravenously administered drug that follows first order, two-compartment pharmacokinetics.*

2.8 liters in an average 70 kg adult. Some drugs, however, will initially be distributed at somewhat different rates in various fluids and tissues. Consequently, these drugs' kinetic behavior can best be illustrated by considering an expansion of the one-compartment system to the *two-compartment model* (Fig. 3–15).

In the two-compartment system, a drug enters into and is instantaneously distributed throughout the central compartment. Its subsequent distribution into the second or peripheral compartment is slower. For simplicity, on the basis of blood perfusion and tissue-plasma partition coefficients for a given drug, various tissues and organs are considered together and given the designation as central compartment or peripheral compartment. The central compartment is usually considered to include the blood, the extracellular space, and organs with good blood perfusion, e.g., lungs, liver, kidneys, heart. The peripheral compartment is usually constituted by those tissues and organs which are poorly perfused by blood, e.g., skin, bones, fat.

Figure 3–16 depicts the plasma-drug concentration versus time plot for a rapidly administered intravenous dose of a hypothetical drug which exhibits kinetic behavior exemplifying a two-compartment system. Note the initial steep decline of the plasma drug concentration curve. This typifies the distribution of the drug from the central compartment to the peripheral compartment. During this phase the drug concentration in the plasma will decrease more rapidly than in the post-distributive phase, i.e., elimination phase. Whether or not this distributive

phase is apparent will depend upon the timing of the plasma samples, particularly in the time immediately following administration. A distributive phase can be very short, a few minutes, or last for hours and even days.

A semi-logarithmic plot of the plasma concentration versus time after rapid intravenous injection of a drug which is best described by a two-compartment model system can often be resolved into two linear components. This procedure can be performed by the method of residuals (or feathering), Figure 3–17. In this procedure, a straight line is fitted through the tail of the original curve and extrapolated back to the Y-axis (the value obtained is B). A plot is then made of the absolute difference values of the original curve and the resultant extrapolated straight line. The slope of the feathered line ($-a/2.303$) and the extrapolated line ($-b/2.303$) and the intercepts, A and B, are determined. Then the following equation is constructed that describes a two-compartment system:

$$C_p = Ae^{-at} + Be^{-bt} \qquad \text{(Equation 3–5)}$$

This is a bi-exponential equation which describes the two-compartment system.

In this scheme, the slope of the line, i.e., $-a/2.303$, obtained from feathering yields the distributive rate of the drug. The slope of the ter-

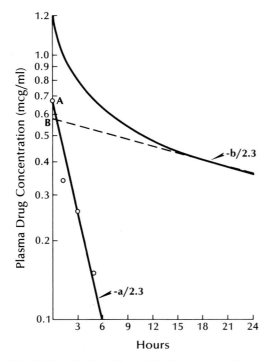

Fig. 3–17. *The logarithm of the drug concentration in plasma plotted versus time (solid line) after intravenous administration of a drug whose disposition can be described by a two-compartment model.*

minal linear phase or elimination phase, i.e., $-b/2.303$, describes the rate of loss of the drug from the body, and usually is considered to be a reflection of the metabolic processes and renal elimination from the body. Appropriate pharmacokinetic formulas allow the clinician to calculate the various volumes of distribution and rates of distribution and elimination for drugs whose pharmacokinetic behavior is exemplified by the two-compartment system.

Half-Life

The half-life $(T_{1/2})$ of a drug describes the time required for a drug's blood or plasma concentration to decrease by one half. This fall in drug concentration is a reflection of metabolic processes and/or excretion, e.g., renal, fecal. The biological half-life of a drug in the blood may be determined graphically off of a pharmacokinetic plot of a drug's blood-concentration time plot, typically after intravenous administration to a sample population. The amount of time required for the concentration of the drug to decrease by one half is considered its half-life.

The half-life can also be mathematically determined. Recall Equation 3–3 and rearrange the equation as follows:

$$\frac{K_{el}\, t}{2.303} = \text{Log } C_p^0 - \text{Log } C_p$$

$$= \text{Log } \frac{C_p^0}{C_p} \qquad \text{(Equation 3–6)}$$

Then, if it assumed that C_p is equal to one-half of C_p^0, the equation will become:

$$\frac{K_{el}\, t}{2.303} = \text{Log } \frac{C_p^0}{0.5\, C_p^0} = \text{Log } 2 \qquad \text{(Equation 3–7)}$$

Thus,

$$t_{1/2} = \frac{2.303 \text{ Log } 2}{K_{el}} = \frac{0.693}{K_{el}} \qquad \text{(Equation 3–8)}$$

If this latter equation is rearranged, the half-life finds utility in the determination of drug elimination from the body, provided of course that the drug follows first-order kinetics. Rearranging the prior equation:

$$K_{el} = \frac{0.693}{t_{1/2}} \qquad \text{(Equation 3–9)}$$

Elimination rate constants are reported in time^{-1}, e.g., minutes^{-1}, hours^{-1}. Thus, an elimination constant of a drug is 0.3 hr^1 indicates that 30% of the drug is eliminated per hour.

The half-life varies widely between drugs; for some drugs it may be a few minutes, whereas for other drugs it may be hours or even days (see Table 3–10). Data on a drug's biologic half-life are useful in determining the most appropriate dosage regimen to achieve and maintain the the desired blood level of drug. Such determinations usually result in such recommended dosage schedules for a drug, as the drug to be taken every 4 hours, 6 hours, 8 hours, etc. Although these types of recommendations generally suit the requirements of most patients, they do not suit all patients. The most exceptional patients are those with reduced or impaired ability to metabolize or excrete drugs. These patients, generally suffering from liver dysfunction or kidney disease, retain the administered drug in the blood or tissues for ex-

Table 3–10.   Some Elimination Half-Life Values

Drug Substance/Product	Elimination Half-Life* $(t_{1/2})$	
Acetaminophen (Tylenol, McNeil)	2– 3	hours
Amoxicillin (Polymox, Bristol)	1	hour
Butabarbital Sodium (Butisol Sodium, Wallace)	100	hours
Cimetidine (Tagamet, SKF)	2	hours
Digitoxin (Crystodigin, Lilly)	7– 9	days
Digoxin (Lanoxin, Burroughs Wellcome)	1.5– 2	days
Diltiazem (Cardizem, Marion)	3.5	hours
Ibuprofen (Motrin, Upjohn)	1.8– 2	hours
Indomethacin (Indocin, Merck, Sharp & Dohme)	4.5	hours
Lithium Carbonate (Lithane, Miles)	24	hours
Nitroglycerin (Tridil, American Critical Care)	1– 4	minutes†
Phenytoin Sodium (Dilantin, Parke-Davis)	22	hours
	(7–42	hours, range)
Pentobarbital Sodium (Nembutal Sodium, Abbott)	15–50	hours
Propoxyphene (Darvon, Lilly)	6–12	hours
Propranolol HCl (Inderal, Ayerst)	2– 4	hours
Ramitidine HCl (Zantac, Glaxo)	2.5– 3	hours
Theophylline (Theobid, Glaxo)	4– 9	hours
Tobramycin Sulfate (Nebcin, Dista)	2	hours
Tolbutamide (Orinase, Upjohn)	4.5– 6	hours

*Mean, average, or value ranges, taken from product information found in *Physicians' Desk Reference*, 41st ed., 1987, Medical Economics Co., Inc., Oradell, New Jersey. Half-life values may vary depending upon patient characteristics (age, liver or renal function, smoking habits, etc.), dose levels administered, and routes of administration.

†After intravenous infusion; nitroglycerin is rapidly metabolized to dinitrates and mononitrates.

tended periods of time due to their decreased ability to eliminate the drug. The resulting extended biologic half-life of the drug generally necessitates an individualized dosage regimen calling for less frequent drug administration than that called for in patients with normal processes of drug elimination, or a maintenance of the usual dosage schedule, but a decrease in the amount of drug administered.

The drug digoxin presents a good example of a drug having a half-life which is affected by the patient's pathologic condition. Digoxin is eliminated in the urine. Renal excretion of digoxin is proportional to glomerular filtration rate. In subjects with normal renal function, digoxin has a half-life of 1.5 to 2.0 days. In anuric patients (absence of urine formation), the half-life may be prolonged to 4 to 6 days. Theophylline also demonstrates differing half lives dependent upon certain patient populations. In premature infants with immature liver enzyme systems in the cytochrome P-450 family, the half life of theophylline ranges from 14 to 58 hours, whereas in young children between the ages of 1 to 4 whose liver enzyme systems are more mature the theophylline half life ranges be-

tween 2 to 5.5 hours. In adult nonsmokers, the half-life ranges from 6.1 to 12.8 hours, whereas in adult smokers the average half-life of theophylline is 4.3 hours. The increase in theophylline clearance from the body among smokers is believed to be due to an induction of the hepatic metabolism of theophylline. The half life of theophylline is decreased and total body clearance is enhanced to such a degree in smokers that these individuals may actually require a 50 to 100% increase in theophylline dosage to produce effective therapeutic results. Between 3 months and 2 years may actually be required to normalize the effect of smoking on theophylline metabolism in the body once the patient stops smoking. Because theophylline is metabolized in the liver, the half life of theophylline will be extended in liver disease. For example, in one study 9 patients with decompensated cirrhosis, the average theophylline half-life was 32 hours.

The half-life of a drug in the blood stream may also be affected by a change in the extent to which it is bound to blood protein or cellular components. Such a change in a drug's binding pattern may be brought about by the administration of a second drug having a greater affinity than the first drug for the same binding sites. The result is the displacement of the first drug from these sites by the second drug and the sudden availability of free (unbound) drug which may pass from the blood stream to other body sites, including those concerned with its elimination. It should be noted that the displacement of one drug from its binding sites by another is generally viewed as an undesired event, since the amount of free drug resulting is greater than the level normally achieved during single drug therapy and may result in untoward drug effects.

Concept of Clearance

The three main mechanisms by which a drug is removed or cleared from the body include (1) the hepatic metabolism, i.e., hepatic clearance, Cl_h, of a drug to either an active or inactive metabolite, (2) the renal excretion, i.e., renal clearance, Cl_r, of a drug unchanged in the urine, and (3) elimination of the drug into the bile and subsequently into the intestines for excretion in feces. An alternate way to express this removal or elimination from the body is to use total body clearance (Cl_B), which is defined as the fraction of the total volume of distribution that can be cleared per unit time. Because most drugs when administered will undergo one or more of these processes, the total body clearance, Cl_B, of a drug is the sum of these clearances, usually hepatic, Cl_h and renal clearances Cl_r. Clearance via the bile and feces is usually not significant for most drugs.

These processes of elimination within the body work together and consequently a drug that is eliminated by renal excretion and hepatic biotransformation will have an overall rate of elimination. K_{el}, that is the sum of the renal excretion, k_u, and hepatic biotransformation, k_m. In the one compartment model described earlier, total body clearance is the product of the volume of distribution, V_d, and the overall rate of elimination, k_{el} (Equation 3–10):

$$Cl_B = V_d \times k_{el} \qquad \text{(Equation 3–10)}$$

But, recall that k_{el} equals $0.693/t_{1/2}$. If this is substituted into Equation 3–10, and one solves for the half life, $t_{1/2}$, the following equation is obtained:

$$t_{1/2} = \frac{0.693\ V_d}{Cl_B} \qquad \text{(Equation 3–11)}$$

Recall that total body clearance is a function of one or more processes, thus if a drug were eliminated from the body through hepatic biotransformation and renal clearance, Equation 3–11 becomes:

$$t_{1/2} = \frac{0.693\ V_d}{Cl_h + Cl_r} \qquad \text{(Equation 3–12)}$$

Thus, a drug's half life is directly proportional to the volume of distribution and inversely proportional to the total body clearance which is comprised of hepatic and renal clearances. Illustratively, if one considers infants and children who exhibit larger volumes of distribution and have lower clearance values, drugs will usually have greater half-lives than that exhibited in adults.

A decrease in the hepatic or renal clearances will prolong the half life of a drug. This typically occurs for example in renal failure, and consequently, if one can estimate the percentage decrease in excretion due to renal failure one can use Equation 3–12 to calculate the new half life of the drug in the patient. Thus, an adjusted dosage regimen can then be calculated to decrease the chance of drug toxicity.

Dosage Regimen Considerations

In the previous chapter those factors that can influence the dosage of a drug were mentioned. The question of how much drug and how often to administer it for a desired therapeutic effect is not easily attainable. Basically, there are two approaches to the development of dosage regimens. The first is the *empirical approach*, which involves the administration of a drug in a certain quantity, noting the therapeutic response and then modifying the dosage of drug and the dosing interval accordingly. Unfortunately, experience with the administration of a drug usually starts with the first patient, and eventually a sufficient number of patients receive the drug so that a fairly accurate prediction can be made. Besides the desired therapeutic effect, consideration must also involve the occurrence and severity of side effects. Empirical therapy is usually employed when the drug concentration in serum or plasma does not reflect the concentration of drug at the receptor site in the body, or the pharmacodynamic effect of the drug is not related (or correlated) with the receptor site drug concentration. Empirical therapy, for example, is utilized for many anticancer drugs that demonstrate effects long after they have been excreted from the body. It is difficult to relate the serum level of these drugs with the desired therapeutic effect.

The second approach to the development of a dosage regimen is thorugh the use of pharmacokinetics or the *kinetic approach*. This approach is based on the assumption that the therapeutic and toxic effects of a drug are related to the amount of drug in the body or to the plasma (or serum) concentration of drug at the receptor site. Through careful pharmacokinetic evaluation of a drug's absorption, distribution, metabolism and excretion in the body from a single dose, the levels of drug attained from multiple dosing can be estimated. One can then determine the appropriateness of a dosage regimen to achieve a desired therapeutic concentration of drug in the body and evaluate the regimen based upon therapeutic response.

When one considers the development of a dosage regimen, pharmacokinetics is but one of a number of factors that should be considered. Table 3–11 illustrates a number of these. Certainly an important factor is the inherent activity, i.e., pharmacodynamics, and toxicity, i.e., toxicology of the drug. A second consideration is the pharmacokinetics of the drug, which are influenced by the dosage form in which the drug is administered to the patient, e.g., biopharmaceutical considerations. The third factor focuses upon the patient to whom the drug will be given and encompasses the clinical state of the patient and how the patient will be managed. Lastly, atypical factors may influence the dosage regimen. Collectively, all of these factors influence the dosage regimen.

The dosage regimen of a drug may simply involve the administration of a drug once for its desired therapeutic effect, e.g., pinworm medication, or encompass the administration of drug for a specific time through multiple doses. In the latter instance, the objective of pharmacokinetic dosing is to design a dosage regimen that will continually maintain a drug's therapeutic serum or plasma concentration within the drug's therapeutic index, i.e., above the minimum effective concentration but below the minimum toxic level.

Frequently drugs are administered between 1 to 4 times per day, most often in a fixed dose,

Table 3–11. Factors That Determine a Dosage Regimen*

Activity-Toxicity	Pharmacokinetics
Minimum therapeutic dose	Absorption
Toxic dose	Distribution
Therapeutic index	Metabolism
Side effects	Excretion
Dose-response relationships	

Dosage Regimen

Clinical Factors		Other Factors
Clinical state of patient	Management of therapy	Tolerance-dependence
Age, weight, urine pH	Multiple drug therapy	Pharmacogenetics-idiosyncrasy
Condition being treated	Convenience of regimen	Drug interactions
Existence of other disease states	Compliance of patient	

*(From Rowland, M. and Tozer, T.N.: *Clinical Pharmacokinetics.* 2nd Ed., Philadelphia, Lea & Febiger, 1989.)

e.g., 75 mg 3 times daily after meals. As mentioned earlier, after a drug is administered its level within the body varies because of the influence of all of the processes, e.g., absorption, distribution, metabolism and excretion. A drug will accumulate in the body when the dosing interval is less than the time needed for the body to eliminate a single dose. For example, Figure 3–18 illustrates the plasma concentration for a drug given by intravenous administration and oral administration. The 50 mg dose of this drug was given at a dosing interval of 8 hours. The drug has a elimination half life of 12 hours. As one can see with continued dosing the drug concentration reaches a *steady state* or *plateau* concentration. At this limit the amount of drug lost per interval is replenished when the drug is dosed again. Consequently the concentration of drug in the plasma or serum fluctuates between a minimum concentration and a maximum concentration. Thus for certain patient types it is optimal to target dosing so that the plateau concentration resides within the therapeutic index of a drug to maintain a minimum effective concentration of drug. For example, the asthmatic patient maintained on theophylline must have a serum concentration between 10 to 20 mcg/mL. Otherwise the patient may be susceptible to an asthmatic attack. Thus, when dosing the asthmatic patient it is preferable to give theophylline around the clock 4 times daily to sustain levels at least above the minimum effective concentration. If on the other hand this medicine is only administered every 4 hours during the waking hours, it is possible that the minimum concentration will fall below effective levels between the at-bedtime dose and the next morning dose. Consequently, the patient may awaken in the middle of the night and exhibit an asthmatic attack.

Patients can be monitored pharmacokinetically through appropriate plasma, serum or blood samples, and many hospital pharmacies have implemented pharmacokinetic dosing services. The intent is to maximize drug efficacy, minimize drug toxicity and keep health care costs at a minimum. Thus, for example, complications associated with overdose are controlled or drug interactions that are known to occur, e.g., smoking-theophylline, can be accommodated. In these services, for example, once the physician prescribes a certain amount of drug and monitors the clinical response, it is the clinical pharmacist who coordinates the ap-

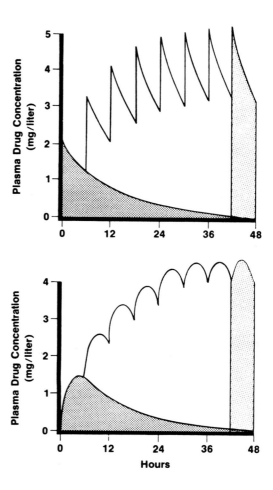

Fig. 3–18. *Plasma concentration of a drug given intravenously (top) and orally (bottom) on a fixed dose of 50 mg and fixed dosing interval of 8 hours. The half-life is 12 hours. Note that the area under the plasma concentration-time curve during a dosing interval at steady state is equal to the total area under the curve for a single dose. The fluctuation of the concentration is diminished when given orally (half-life of absorption is 1.4 hours) but the average steady-state concentration is the same as that after intravenous administration, since F = 1. (From Rowland, M. and Tozer, T.N.: Clinical Pharmacokinetics, Lea & Febiger, 1989.)*

propriate sample time to determine drug concentration in the appropriate body fluid. After the level of drug is attained, it is the clinical pharmacist who interprets the result, and consults with the physician regarding subsequent dosages.

Pharmacokinetic research has demonstrated that the determination of a patient's dosage regimen depends on numerous factors and daily dose formulas exist for a number of drugs that must be administered on a routine maintenance schedule, e.g., digoxin, procainamide, theophylline. For certain drugs such as digoxin, which are not highly lipid soluble, it is preferable to use a patient's lean body weight (LBW) rather than total body weight (TBW) to provide a better estimate of the patient's volume of distribution. Alternatively, even though pharmacokinetic dosing formulas may exist, one must be cognizant that patient factors may be more relevant. For example, with the geriatric patient it is advisable to begin drug therapy with the lowest possible dose and increase the dosage as necessary in small increments to optimize the patient's clinical response. Then the patient should be monitored for drug efficacy and re-evaluated periodically.

Selected Reading

Arnold, J.D. and Sice, J.: Biologic Availability and Therapeutic Equivalence. *J. Clin. Pharmacol.*, 16:546–549, 1976.

Garnett, W.R., and Barr, W.H.: *Geriatric Pharmacokinetics.* Kalamazoo, The Upjohn Company, 1984.

Niazi, S.: *Textbook of Biopharmaceutics and Clinical Pharmacokinetics.* New York, Appleton-Century-Crofts, 1979.

Rowland, M., and Tozer, T.N.: *Clinical Pharmacokinetics: Concepts and Applications.* 2nd Ed., Philadelphia, Lea & Febiger, 1989.

Skelly, J.P.: Bioavailability and Bioequivalence. *J. Clin. Pharmacol.*, 16:539–545, 1976.

Ueda, C.T.: *Concepts in Clinical Pharmacology. Essentials of Bioavailability and Bioequivalence.* Kalamazoo, The Upjohn Company, 1979.

Notes

1. *J. Pharmacokinet. Biopharm.*, 1(1):3, 1973.
2. Partition coefficients are determined by dissolving drugs in aqueous solution, shaking the solution with an organic solvent, and assaying each of the two phases for drug content. The partition coefficient is the organic solvent:water-drug concentration ratio.
3. Noyes, A.A., and Whitney, W.R., *J. Am. Chem. Soc.*, 19:930, 1897.
4. Poole, J.: *Curr. Therapeut. Res.*, 10:292–303, 1968.
5. Chodos, D.J., and DiSanto, A.R.: *Basics of Bioavailability*, Kalamazoo, The Upjohn Company, 1973.
6. Ueda, C.T.: *Concepts in Clinical Pharmacology. Essentials of Bioavailability and Bioequivalence.* Kalamazoo, The Upjohn Company, 1979, p. 11.
7. *FDA Drug Bulletin*, 16, No. 2, 1986, pp. 14–15.

4 | Dosage Form Design: Pharmaceutic Ingredients, Product Formulation, and Current Good Manufacturing Practice

DRUG SUBSTANCES are seldom administered alone, but rather as part of a formulation in combination with one or more nonmedical agents that serve varied and specialized pharmaceutical functions. Through selective use of these nonmedicinal agents, referred to as *pharmaceutic ingredients*, dosage forms of various types result. The pharmaceutic ingredients solubilize, suspend, thicken, dilute, emulsify, stabilize, preserve, color, flavor, and fashion medicinal agents into efficacious and appealing dosage forms. Each type of dosage form is unique in its physical and pharmaceutical characteristics. These varied preparations provide the manufacturing pharmacist with the challenges of formulation and the physician with the choice of drug and drug delivery system to prescribe. The general area of study concerned with the formulation, manufacture, stability, and effectiveness of pharmaceutical dosage forms is termed *pharmaceutics*.

The proper design and formulation of a dosage form requires consideration of the physical, chemical and biological characteristics of all of the drug substances and pharmaceutic ingredients to be used in fabricating the product. The drug and pharmaceutic materials utilized must be compatible with one another to produce a drug product that is stable, efficacious, attractive, easy to administer and safe. The product should be manufactured under appropriate measures of quality control and packaged in containers that contribute to product stability. The product should be labeled to promote correct use and be stored under conditions that contribute to maximum shelf life.

Methods for the preparation of specific types of dosage forms and drug delivery systems are described in subsequent chapters. This chapter presents some general considerations regarding pharmaceutic ingredients, drug product formulation, and standards for good manufacturing practice.

The Need for Dosage Forms

The potent nature and low dosage of most of the drugs in use today precludes any expectation that the general public could safely obtain the appropriate dose of a drug from the bulk material. The vast majority of drug substances are administered in milligram quantities, much too small to be weighed on anything but a sensitive laboratory balance. For instance, how could the layman accurately obtain the 325 mg or 5 gr of aspirin found in the common aspirin tablet from a bulk supply of aspirin? He couldn't. Yet, compared with many other drugs, the dose of aspirin is formidable (Table 4–1). For example, the dose of ethinyl estradiol, 0.05 mg, is 1/6500 the amount of aspirin in an aspirin tablet. To put it another way, 6500 ethinyl estradiol tablets, each containing 0.05 mg of drug, could be made from an amount of ethinyl estradiol equal to the amount of aspirin in just one 5 gr aspirin tablet. When the dose of the drug is minute, as that for ethinyl estradiol, solid dosage forms such as tablets and capsules must be prepared with fillers or diluents so that the size of the resultant dosage unit is large enough to pick up with the fingertips.

Besides providing the mechanism for the safe and convenient delivery of accurate dosage, dosage forms are needed for additional reasons:

Table 4–1. Examples of Some Drugs with Relatively Low Usual Doses

Drug	Usual Dose, mg	Category
Lithium Carbonate	300	Antidepressant
Ferrous Sulfate	300	Hematinic
Cimetidine	300	Antiulcer
Ibuprofen	300	Antinflammatory
Amoxicillin	250	Antibacterial
Erythromycin	250	Antibacterial
Nitrofurantoin	100	Antibacterial (urinary)
Propoxyphene HCl	65	Analgesic
Thyroid	60	Thyroid
Hydrochlorothiazide	50	Diuretic
Codeine Phosphate	30	Analgesic
Phenobarbital	30	Sedative
Chlorpromazine HCl	25	Tranquilizer
Diphenhydramine HCl	25	Antihistaminic
Morphine Sulfate	10	Narcotic analgesic
Prednisolone	5	Adrenocortical steroid
Chlorpheniramine maleate	4	Antihistaminic
Colchicine	0.5	Gout Supressant
Nitroglycerin	0.4	Antianginal
Digoxin	0.25	Cardiotonic (maintenance)
Levothyroxine	0.1	Thyroid
Ethinyl Estradiol	0.05	Estrogen

1. For the protection of a drug substance from the destructive influences of atmospheric oxygen or humidity (e.g., coated tablets, sealed ampuls).
2. For the protection of a drug substance from the destructive influence of gastric acid after oral administration (e.g., enteric-coated tablets).
3. To conceal the bitter, salty, or offensive taste or odor of a drug substance (e.g., capsules, coated tablets, flavored syrups).
4. To provide liquid preparations of substances that are either insoluble or unstable in the desired vehicle (e.g., suspensions).
5. To provide clear liquid dosage forms of substances (e.g., syrups, solutions).
6. To provide time-controlled drug action (e.g., various controlled-release tablets, capsules, and suspensions).
7. To provide optimal drug action from topical administration sites (e.g., ointments, creams, transdermal patches, ophthalmic, ear, and nasal preparations).
8. To provide for the insertion of a drug into one of the body's orifices (e.g., rectal or vaginal suppositories).
9. To provide for the placement of drugs directly into the bloodstream or into body tissues (e.g., injections).
10. To provide for optimal drug action through inhalation therapy (e.g., inhalants and inhalation aerosols).

There are many different forms into which a medicinal agent may be placed for the convenient and efficacious treatment of disease (Table 3–6). Most commonly, a pharmaceutical manufacturer prepares a drug substance in several dosage forms and strengths for the efficacious and convenient treatment of disease (Fig. 4–1). Before a medicinal agent is formulated into one or more dosage forms, among the factors considered are such therapeutic matters as: the nature of the illness, the manner in which it is generally treated, locally or through systemic action, and the age and anticipated condition of the patient.

If the medication is intended for systemic use and oral administration is desired, tablets and/or capsules are generally prepared. These dosage units are easily handled by the patient and are most convenient in the self-administration of medication. If a drug substance has application in an emergency situation in which the patient may be comatose or unable to take oral medication, an injectable form of the medication may also be prepared. Many other examples of therapeutic situations affecting dosage form design could be cited, including the preparation of agents for motion sickness, nausea, and vomiting into tablets and skin patches for prevention and suppositories and injections for treatment.

The age of the intended patient also plays a role in dosage form design. For infants and children under 5 years of age, pharmaceutical liquids rather than solid dosage forms are preferred for oral administration. These liquids, which are generally flavored aqueous solutions, syrups or suspensions, are usually administered directly into the infant's or child's mouth by drop, spoon, or oral dispenser (Fig. 4–2) or incorporated into the child's food. A single liquid pediatric preparation may be used for infants and children of all ages, with the dose of the drug varied by the volume administered. When an infant is in the throes of a vomiting

Fig. 4–1. *Examples of varied dosage forms of a drug substance marketed by a pharmaceutical manufacturer to meet the special requirements of the patient. (Courtesy of SK&F Lab Co.)*

crisis, is gagging, has a productive cough, or is simply rebellious, there may be some question as how much of the medicine administered is actually swallowed and how much is expectorated. In such instances, injections may be required. Infant size rectal suppositories may also be employed although drug absorption from the rectum is often erratic.

During childhood and even in adult years, a person may have difficulty swallowing solid dosage forms, especially uncoated tablets. For this reason, some medications are formulated as chewable tablets that can be broken up in the mouth before swallowing. Many of these tablets are comparable in texture to an after-dinner mint and break down into a pleasant tasting, creamy material. Capsules have been found by many to be more easily swallowed than whole tablets. If a capsule is allowed to become moist in the mouth before swallowing, it becomes slippery and slides down the throat more readily with a glass of water. In instances in which a person has difficulty swallowing a capsule, the contents may be emptied into a spoon, mixed with jam, honey, or other similar food to mask the taste of the medication and swallowed. Some older persons have difficulty in swallowing and thus tablets and capsules are frequently avoided. Medications intended for the elderly are commonly formulated into oral liquids or may be extemporaneously prepared into an oral liquid by the pharmacist.

Many patients, particularly the elderly, take multiple medications daily. The more distinctive the size, shape, and color of solid dosage forms, the easier is the proper identification of the medications. Frequent errors in taking medications among the elderly occur because of their multiple drug therapy and reduced eyesight. Dosage forms that allow reduced frequency of administration without sacrifice of efficiency are particularly advantageous.

Pharmaceutic Ingredients

In order to prepare a drug substance into a final dosage form, pharmaceutic ingredients are required. For example, in the preparation of

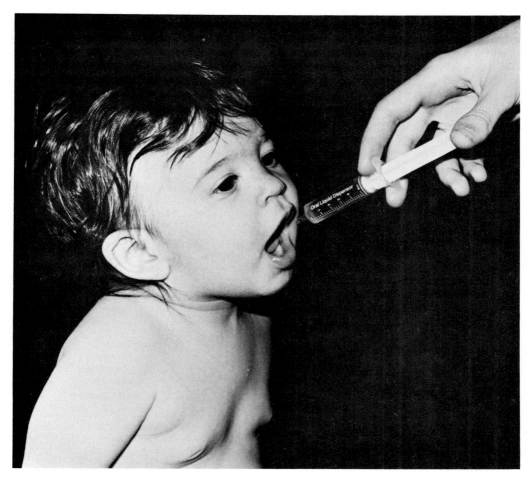

Fig. 4–2. *"Pee Dee Dose" brand of oral liquid dispenser used to administer measured volumes of liquid medication to youngsters. (Courtesy of Baxa Corporation)*

pharmaceutical solutions, one or more *solvents* are utilized to dissolve the drug substance, *preservatives* may be added to prevent microbial growth, *stabilizers* may be used to prevent drug decomposition, and *colorants* and *flavorants* added to enhance product appeal. In the preparation of tablets, *diluents* or *fillers* are commonly added to increase the bulk of the formulation, *binders* to cause the adhesion of the powdered drug and pharmaceutic substances, *antiadherents* or *lubricants* to assist the smooth tableting process, *disintegrating agents* to promote tablet break-up after administration, and coatings to improve stability, control disintegration, or to enhance appearance. Ointments, creams, and suppositories achieve their characteristic features due to the pharmaceutic *bases* which are

utilized. Thus, for each dosage form, the pharmaceutic ingredients establish the primary features of the product, and contribute to the physical form, texture, stability, taste and overall appearance.

Table 4–2 presents the principal categories of pharmaceutic ingredients, with examples of some of the official agents currently used.

General Considerations in Drug Product Formulation

In dealing with the problem of formulating a drug substance into a proper dosage form, research pharmacists employ knowledge that has been gained through experience with other chemically similar drugs and through the

Table 4–2. Examples of Pharmaceutic Ingredients

Ingredient Type	Definition	Examples
Acidifying Agent	Used in liquid preparations to provide acidic medium for product stability.	acetic acid hydrochloric acid nitric acid
Alkalinizing Agent	Used in liquid preparations to provide alkaline medium for product stability.	ammonia solution ammonium carbonate potassium hydroxide sodium borate sodium carbonate sodium hydroxide trolamine
Adsorbent	An agent capable of holding other molecules onto its surface by physical or chemical (chemisorption) means.	powdered cellulose activated charcoal
Aerosol Propellant	An agent responsible for developing the pressure within an aerosol container and expelling the product when the valve is opened.	dichlorodifluoromethane dichlorotetrafluoroethane trichloromonofluoromethane
Air Displacement	An agent which is employed to displace air in a hermetically sealed container to enhance product stability.	nitrogen
Antifungal Preservative	Used in liquid and semi-solid preparations to prevent the growth of fungi.	benzoic acid butylparaben ethylparaben methylparaben propylparaben sodium benzoate sodium propionate
Antimicrobial Preservative	Used in liquid and semi-solid preparations to prevent the growth of micro-organisms.	benzalkonium chloride benzethonium chloride benzyl alcohol cetylpyridinium chloride chlorobutanol phenol phenylethyl alcohol phenylmercuric nitrate thimerosal
Antioxidant	An agent which inhibits oxidation and thus is used to prevent the deterioration of preparations by the oxidative process.	ascorbyl palmitate butylated hydroxyanisole butylated hydroxytoluene hypophophorous acid monothioglycerol propyl gallate sodium bisulfite sodium formaldehyde sulfoxylate sodium metabisulfite
Buffering Agent	Used to resist change in pH upon dilution or addition of acid or alkali.	potassium metaphosphate potassium phosphate, monobasic sodium acetate
Chelating Agent	A substance that forms stable complexes with metals. Chelating agents are used in some liquid pharmaceuticals as stabilizers to complex heavy metals which might promote instability. In such use they are also called *sequestering* agents.	edetate disodium edetic acid

Table 4–2.   Continued

Ingredient Type	Definition	Examples
Colorant	Used to impart color to pharmaceutical preparations.	FD&C Red No. 3 FD&C Red No. 20 FD&C Yellow No. 6 FD&C Blue No. 2 D&C Green No. 5 D&C Orange No. 5 D&C Red No. 8 caramel ferric oxide, red
Emulsifying Agent	Used to promote and maintain the dispersion of finely subdivided particles of a liquid in a vehicle in which it is immiscible.	acacia sorbitan monooleate polyoxyethylene 50 stearate
Encapsulating Agent	Used to form thin shells for the purpose of enclosing a drug substance or drug formulation for ease of administration.	gelatin cellulose acetate phthalate
Flavorant	Used to impart a pleasant flavor and often odor to a pharmaceutical preparation.	anise oil cinnamon oil cocoa menthol orange oil peppermint oil vanillin
Humectant	Used to prevent the drying out of preparations—particulalry ointments and creams—due to the agent's ability to retain moisture.	glycerin propylene glycol sorbitol
Levigating Agent	A liquid used as an intervening agent to reduce the particle size of a drug powder by grinding together, usually in a mortar.	mineral oil glycerin
Ointment Base	The semisolid vehicle into which drug substances may be incorpoated in preparing medicated ointments.	lanolin hydrophilic ointment polyethylene glycol ointment petrolatum hydrophilic petrolatum white ointment yellow ointment rose water ointment
Solvent	An agent used to dissolve another pharmaceutic substance or a drug in the preparation of a solution.	alcohol isopropyl alcohol mineral oil oleic acid peanut oil purified water water for injection sterile water for injection sterile water for irrigation
Stiffening Agent	Used to increase the thickness or hardness of a pharmaceutical preparation, usually an ointment.	cetyl alcohol paraffin white wax yellow wax

Table 4–2.   Continued

Ingredient Type	Definition	Examples
Suppository Base	Used as a vehicle into which drug substances are incorporated in the preparation of suppositories.	cocoa butter polyethylene glycols (mixtures)
Surfactant (surface active agent)	Substances which adsorb to surfaces or interfaces to reduce surface or interfacial tension. May be used as wetting agents, detergents or emulsifying agents.	benzalkonium chloride nonoxynol 10 octoxynol 9 polysorbate 80 sodium lauryl sulfate sorbitan monopalmitate
Suspending Agent	A viscosity increasing agent used to reduce the rate of sedimentation of dispersed particles.	agar bentonite carboxymethylcellulose sodium hydroxypropyl methyl- cellulose methylcellulose tragacanth veegum
Sweetening Agent	Used to impart sweetness to a preparation.	aspartame saccharin sodium sucrose
Tablet Antiadherents	Agents which prevent the sticking of tablet formulation ingredients to punches and dies in a tableting machine during production.	magnesium stearate talc
Tablet Binders	Substances used to cause adhesion of powder particles in tablet granulations.	acacia ethylcellulose gelatin methylcellulose
Tablet and Capsule Diluent	Inert substances used as fillers to create the desired bulk, flow properties, and compression characteristics in the preparation of tablets and capsules.	microcrystalline cellulose lactose
Tablet Coating Agent	Used to coat a formed tablet for the purpose of protecting against drug decomposition by atmospheric oxygen or humidity, to provide a desired release pattern for the drug substance after administration, to mask the taste or odor of the drug substance, or for aesthetic purposes.	cellulose acetate phthalate sucrose pharmaceutical glaze (shellac in alcohol)
Tablet Disintegrant	Used in solid dosage forms to promote the disruption of the solid mass into smaller particles which are more readily dispersed or dissolved.	cornstarch sodium alginate
Tablet Glidant	Agents used in tablet and capsule formulations to improve the flow properties of the powder mixture.	colloidal silica cornstarch talc
Tablet Lubricant	Substances used in tablet formulations to reduce friction during tablet compression.	calcium stearate magnesium stearate stearic acid
Tablet Polishing Agent	Used to impart an attractive sheen to coated tablets.	carnauba wax white wax

Table 4–2.   Continued

Ingredient Type	Definition	Examples
Tonicity Agent	Used to render a solution similar in osmotic characteristics to physiologic fluids.	dextrose sodium chloride

Vehicle	A carrying agent for a drug substance.	*Flavored/Sweetened*
		  Acacia Syrup
		  Aromatic Elixir
		  Cherry Syrup
		  Cocoa Syrup
		  Orange Syrup
		  Syrup
		Oleaginous
		  Corn Oil
		  Mineral Oil
		  Peanut Oil
		  Sesame Oil
		Sterile
		  Bacteriostatic Sodium
		    Chloride Injection
		  Bacteriostatic Water
		    for Injection

proper utilization of the disciplines of the physical, chemical, and biologic and pharmaceutical sciences. The early stages of any new formulation involves studies to collect basic information on the physical and chemical characteristics of the drug substance to be prepared into pharmaceutical dosage forms. These basic studies comprise the *preformulation* work needed before actual product formulation begins.

Preformulation Studies[1]

Physical Description

It is important to have an understanding of the physical description of a drug substance prior to dosage form development. The majority of drug substances in use today occur as solid materials. Most of them are pure chemical compounds of either crystalline or amorphous constitution. Liquid drugs are used to a much lesser extent; gases, even less frequently.

Among the few liquid medicinal agents in use today are the following:

Amyl nitrite, vasodilator by inhalation
Castor oil, cathartic
Clofibrate, antihyperlipidemic
Dimercaprol, antidote for arsenic, gold, and mercury poisoning

Dimethylsulfoxide, analgesic in interstitial cystitis
Ethchlorvynol, hypnotic
Glycerin, cathartic in suppository form
Mineral oil, cathartic
Nitroglycerin (as tablets), anti-anginal
Paraldehyde, sedative-hypnotic
Paramethadione, anticonvulsant
Prochlorperazine, tranquilizer and antiemetic
Propylhexedrine, vasoconstrictor by nasal inhalation
Undecylenic acid, fungistatic agent

Liquid drugs pose an interesting problem in the design of dosage forms or drug delivery systems. Many of the liquids are volatile substances and as such must be physically sealed from the atmosphere to insure their continued presence. Amyl nitrite, for example, is a clear yellowish liquid that is volatile even at low temperatures and is also highly flammable. It is maintained for medicinal purposes in small sealed glass cylinders wrapped with gauze or another suitable material. When amyl nitrite is administered, the glass is broken between the fingertips and the liquid wets the gauze covering, producing vapors that are inhaled by the patient requiring vasodilation. Propylhexedrine provides another example of a volatile liquid drug that must be contained in a closed system to maintain its presence. This drug is used as a nasal inhalant for its vasoconstrictor action. A cylindrical roll of fibrous material is impregnated with propylhexedrine, and the saturated cylinder is placed in a suitable, generally plastic, sealed nasal inhaler. The inhaler's cap must be securely tightened each time it is used. Even then, the inhaler maintains its effectiveness for only a limited period of time due to the volatilization of the drug.

Another problem associated with liquid drugs is that those intended for oral administration cannot generally be formulated into tablet form, the most popular form of oral medication, without undertaking major chemical modification of the drug. An exception to this is the liquid drug nitroglycerin which is formulated into tablet triturates which disintegrate within seconds after placement under the tongue. However, because the drug is volatile, it has a tendency to escape from the tablets during storage and it is critical that the tablets be stored in tightly sealed glass containers. For the most part, when a liquid drug is to be administered orally and a solid dosage form is desired, two approaches are used. First, the liquid substance may be sealed in a soft gelatin capsule. Paramethadione and ethchlorvynol are examples of liquid drugs commercially available in capsule form.[2] Secondly, the liquid drug may be developed into a solid ester or salt form that will be suitable for tableting or drug encapsulating. For instance, scopolamine hydrobromide is a solid salt of the liquid drug scopolamine and is easily produced into tablets.

For certain liquid drugs, especially those employed orally in large doses or applied topically, their liquid nature may be of some advantage in therapy. For example, 15-mL doses of mineral oil may be administered conveniently as such. Also, the liquid nature of undecylenic acid certainly does not hinder but rather enhances its use topically in the treatment of fungus infections of the skin. However, for the most part, solid materials are preferred by pharmacists in formulation work because of their ease of preparation into tablets and capsules.

Formulation and stability difficulties arise less frequently with solid dosage forms than with liquid pharmaceutical preparations, and for this reason many new drugs first reach the market as tablets or dry-filled capsules. Later, when the pharmaceutical problems are resolved, a liquid form of the same drug may be marketed. This procedure, when practiced, is doubly advantageous, because for the most part physicians and patients alike prefer small, generally tasteless, accurately dosed tablets or capsules to the analogous liquid forms that may have an unpleasant taste and are likely to be measured by the patient with highly variable household spoons. Therefore, marketing a drug in solid form first is more practical for the manufacturer and also suits the majority of patients. It is estimated that tablets and capsules comprise the dosage form dispensed 70% of the time by community pharmacists, with tablets dispensed twice as frequently as capsules.

Microscopic Examination

Microscopic examination of the raw drug substance is an important step in preformulation work. It gives an indication of particle size and particle size range of the raw material as well as the crystal structure. Photomicrographs of the initial and subsequent batch lots of the drug substance can provide important information should problems arise in formulation processing attributable to changes in particle or crystal characteristics of the drug.

Particle Size

Certain physical and chemical properties of drug substances are affected by the particle size distribution, including drug dissolution rate, bioavailability, content uniformity, taste, texture, color, and stability. In addition, properties such as flow characteristics and sedimentation rates, among others, are also important factors related to particle size. It is essential to establish as early as possible how the particle size of the drug substance may affect formulation and product efficacy. Of special interest is the effect of particle size on the drug's absorption. Particle size has been shown to significantly influence the oral absorption profiles of certain drugs as griseofulvin, nitrofurantoin, spironolactone, and procaine penicillin.

Satisfactory content uniformity in solid dosage forms depends to a large degree on particle size and the equal distribution of the active ingredient throughout the formulation.

There are several methods available to evaluate particle size and distribution including sieving or screening, microscopy, sedimentation, and stream scanning. For powders in the range of approximately 44 microns and greater, sieving or screening is the most widely used method of size analysis. The difficulty with using this method early in the preformulation program is the requirement of a relatively large sample size. The main advantage of the sieve method is simplicity, both in technique and equipment requirements. Optical microscopy is frequently the first step in the determination of particle size and shape for the new drug substance. This is usually a qualitative assessment since quantitation by the microscope technique is tedious and time consuming. A key element in utilizing the microscope for particle size determination is preparation of the slide. It must be representative of the bulk of the material and be properly suspended and thoroughly dispersed in a suitable liquid phase. In order to do a quantitative particle size evaluation a minimum of 1000 of the particles should be counted.

Sedimentation techniques utilize the relationship between rate of fall of particles and their size. Techniques utilizing devices that continuously collect a settling suspension are used. These methods share the disadvantage of the microscope technique in that it is tedious to obtain the data. Also, proper dispersion, consistent sampling, temperature control, and other experimental variables must be carefully controlled in order to obtain consistent and reliable results.

Stream scanning is a valuable method for determining particle size distribution of powdered drug substances. This technique utilizes a fluid suspension of particles which pass the sensing zone where individual particles are sized, counted, and tabulated. Sensing units may be based on light scattering or transmission, as well as conductance. Two popular units in the pharmaceutical industry for this purpose are the Coulter Counter and Hiac Counter. Both units electronically size, count, and tabulate the individual particles that pass through the sensing zone. This technique has obvious advantages in that data can be generated in a relatively short time with reasonable accuracy. Thousands of particles can be counted in seconds and used to determine the size distribution curve. All stream scanning units convert the particles to effective diameter, and therefore, have the shortcoming of not providing information relative to particle shape. Nevertheless, stream scanning methods are powerful tools and can be used for evaluation of such parameters as crystal growth in suspension formulations.

Partition Coefficient and Dissociation Constant

As discussed in the previous chapter, in order to produce a biological response, the drug molecule must first cross a biological membrane. The biological membrane acts as a lipid barrier to most drugs and permits the absorption of lipid soluble substances by passive diffusion while lipid insoluble substances can diffuse across the barrier only with considerable difficulty, if at all. The interrelationship of the dissociation constant, lipid solubility, and pH at the absorption site and absorption characteristics of various drugs are the basis of the pH-partition theory. The determination of the degree of ionization or pKa value of the drug substance is an important physical-chemical characteristic relative to evaluation of possible effects on absorption from various sites of administration.

Dissociation constant or pKa is usually determined by potentiometric titration.

Polymorphism

An important factor on formulation is the crystal or amorphous form of the drug substance. Polymorphic forms usually exhibit different physical-chemical properties including melting point and solubility. The occurrence of polymorphic forms with drugs is relatively common and it has been estimated that polymorphism is exhibited by at least one-third of all organic compounds.

In addition to the polymorphic forms in which compounds may exist, they also can occur in non-crystalline or amorphous forms. The energy required for a molecule of drug to escape from a crystal is much greater than required to escape from an amorphous powder. Therefore, the amorphous form of a compound is always more soluble than a corresponding crystal form.

Evaluation of crystal structure, polymorphism, and solvate form is an important preformulation activity. The changes in crystal characteristics can influence bioavailability, chemical and physical stabiltiy, and have important implications in dosage form process functions. For example, it can be a significant factor relating to the tableting processes due to flow and compaction behaviors, among others.

Various techniques are used in determining crystal properties. The most widely used methods are hot stage microscopy, thermal analysis, infrared spectroscopy, and x-ray diffraction.

Solubility

An important physical-chemical property of a drug substance is solubility, especially aqueous system solubility. A drug must possess some aqueous solubility for therapeutic efficacy. In order for a drug to enter the systemic circulation to exert a therapeutic effect, it must first be in solution. Relatively insoluble compounds often exhibit incomplete or erratic absorption. If the solubility of the drug substance is less than desirable, consideration must be given to improve its solubility. The methods to accomplish this will depend on the chemical nature of the drug and the type of drug product under consideration. For example, if the drug substance is acidic or basic, solubility may be influenced by changes in pH.

However, there are many drug substances for which pH adjustment is not an effective means of improving solubility. Weak acidic or basic drugs may require extremes in pH that are outside accepted physiologic limits or may cause stability problems with formulation ingredients. Adjustment of pH usually has little effect on the solubility of non-electrolytes. In many cases, it is desirable to utilize co-solvents or other techniques such as complexation, micronization, or solid dispersion to improve aqueous solubility.

A drug's solubility is usually determined by the equilibrium solubility method, by which an excess of the drug is placed in a solvent and shaken at a constant temperature over a prolonged period of time until equilibrium is obtained. Chemical analysis of the drug content in solution is performed to determine degree of solubility.

Dissolution

Variations in the biological activity of a drug substance may be brought about by the rate at which it becomes available to the organism. In many instances, dissolution rate, or the time it takes for the drug to dissolve in the fluids at the absorption site, is the rate-limiting step in the absorption process. This is true for drugs administered orally in solid forms such as tablets, capsules or suspensions, as well as drugs administered intramuscularly in the form of pellets or suspensions. When the dissolution rate is the rate-limiting step, anything which affects it will also affect absorption. Consequently, dissolution rate can affect the onset, intensity, and duration of response, and control the overall bioavailability of the drug from the dosage form, as discussed in the previous chapter.

As discussed previously, the dissolution rate of drugs may be increased by increasing the drug's particle size. It may also be increased by increasing its solubility in the diffusion layer. The most effective means of obtaining higher dissolution rates is to use a highly water soluble salt of the parent substance. Although a soluble salt of a weak acid will subsequently precipitate as the free acid in the bulk phase of an acidic solution, such as gastric fluid, it will do so in the form of fine particles with a large surface area.

The dissolution rates of chemical compounds are generally determined by two methods: the constant surface method which provides the intrinsic dissolution rate of the agent, and particulate dissolution in which a suspension of the agent is added to a fixed amount of solvent without exact control of surface area.

The constant surface method utilizes a compressed disc of known area. This method eliminates surface area and surface electrical charges as dissolution variables. The dissolution rate obtained by this method is termed the *intrinsic dissolution rate*, and is characteristic of each solid compound and a given solvent under the fixed experimental conditions. The value is generally expressed as milligrams dissolved per minute centimeters squared ($mg/min/cm^2$). It has been suggested that this value is useful in predicting probable absorption problems due to dissolution rate. In particulate dissolution, a weighed amount of powdered sample is added to the dissolution medium in a constant agitation system. This method is frequently used to study the influence of particle size, surface area, and excipients upon the active agent. Occasionally, an inverse relationship of particle size to dissolution is noted due to the surface properties of the drug. In these instances, surface charge and/or agglomeration results in the reduced particle size form of the drug presenting a lower effective surface area to the solvent due to incomplete wetting or agglomeration.

Early studies should include the effects of pharmaceutic ingredients on the dissolution characteristics of the drug substance.

Membrane Permeability

Modern preformulation studies include an early assessment of passage of drug molecules across biological membranes.

Data obtained from the basic physical-chemical studies, specifically, pKa, solubility, and dissolution rate provide an indication of absorption expectations.

To enhance these data, a technique utilizing the "everted intestinal sac" may be used in evaluating absorption characteristics of drug substances. In this method, a piece of intestine is removed from an intact animal, everted, filled with a solution of the drug substance, and the degree and rate of passage of the drug through the membrane sac is determined. Through this method, both passive and active transport can be evaluated.

In the latter stages of preformulation testing or early formulation studies, animals and man must be studied to assess the absorption efficiency, pharmacokinetic parameters and to establish possible *in vitro/in vivo* correlation for dissolution and bioavailability.

Stability

One of the most important activities of preformulation work is the evaluation of the physical and chemical stability of the pure drug substance. It is essential that these initial studies be conducted using drug samples of known purity. The presence of impurities can lead to erroneous conclusions in such evaluations. Stability studies conducted in the preformulation phase include solid state stability of the drug alone, solution phase stability, and stability in the presence of expected excipients.

Initial investigation begins through knowledge of the drug's chemical structure which allows the preformulation scientist to anticipate the possible degradation reactions.

Chemical instability of medicinal agents may take many forms, because the drugs in use today are of such diverse chemical constitution. Chemically, drug substances are alcohols, phenols, aldehydes, ketones, esters, ethers, acids, salts, alkaloids, glycosides, and others, each with reactive chemical groups having different susceptibilities toward chemical instability. Chemically, the most frequently encountered destructive processes are hydrolysis and oxidation.

Hydrolysis is a solvolysis process in which (drug) molecules interact with water molecules to yield breakdown products of different chemical constitution. For example, aspirin or acetylsalicylic acid combines with a water molecule

and hydrolyzes into one molecule of salicylic acid and one molecule of acetic acid:

Aspirin   Salicylic Acid   Acetic Acid

The process of hydrolysis is probably the most important single cause of drug decomposition mainly because a great number of medicinal agents are esters or contain such other groupings as substituted amides, lactones, and lactams, which are susceptible to the hydrolytic process.

Another destructive process is oxidation. The oxidative process is destructive to many drug types, including aldehydes, alcohols, phenols, sugars, alkaloids, and unsaturated fats and oils.

Chemically, oxidation involves the loss of electrons from an atom or a molecule. Each electron lost is accepted by some other atom or molecule, thereby accomplishing the reduction of the recipient. In inorganic chemistry, oxidation is accompanied by an increase in the positive valence of an element—for example, ferrous ($+2$) oxidizing to ferric ($+3$). In organic chemistry, oxidation is frequently considered synonymous with the loss of hydrogen (dehydrogenation) from a molecule. The oxidative process frequently involves free chemical radicals, which are molecules or atoms containing one or more unpaired electrons, as molecular (atmospheric) oxygen (•O—O•) and free hydroxyl (•OH). These radicals tend to take electrons from other chemicals, thereby oxidizing the donor. Many of the oxidative changes in pharmaceutical preparations have the character of autoxidations. Autoxidations occur spontaneously under the initial influence of atmospheric oxygen and proceed slowly at first and then more rapidly as the process continues. The process has been described as a type of chain reaction commencing by the union of oxygen with the drug molecule and continuing with a free radical of this oxidized molecule participating in the destruction of other drug molecules and so forth.

In drug product formulation work, steps are taken to reduce or prevent the occurrence of drug substance deterioration due to hydrolysis, oxidation, and other processes. These techniques are discussed in the next section in this chapter.

Drug Product Stability

As indicated previously, many pharmaceutic ingredients may be utilized in preparing the desired dosage form of a drug substance. Some of these agents may be used to achieve the desired physical and chemical characteristics of the product or to enhance its appearance, odor, and taste. Other substances may be used to increase the stability of the drug substance, particularly against the hydrolytic and oxidative processes. In each instance, the added pharmaceutic ingredient must be compatible with and must not detract from the stability of the drug substance in the particular dosage form prepared.

There are several approaches to the stabilization of pharmaceutical preparations containing drugs subject to deterioration by hydrolysis. Perhaps the most obvious is the reduction, or better yet, the elimination of water from the pharmaceutical system. Even solid dosage forms containing water-labile drugs must be protected from the humidity of the atmosphere. This may be accomplished by applying a waterproof protective coating over tablets or by enclosing and maintaining the drug in tightly closed containers. It is not unusual to detect hydrolyzed aspirin by noticing an odor of acetic acid upon opening a bottle of aspirin tablets. In liquid preparations, water can frequently be replaced or reduced in the formulation through the use of substitute liquids such as glycerin, propylene glycol, and alcohol. In certain injectable products, anhydrous vegetable oils may be used as the drug's solvent to reduce the chance of hydrolytic decomposition.

Decomposition by hydrolysis may be prevented for other drugs to be administered in liquid form by suspending them in a non-aqueous vehicle rather than by dissolving them in an aqueous solvent. In still other instances, particularly for certain unstable antibiotic drugs, when an aqueous preparation is desired, the drug may be supplied to the pharmacist in a dry form for *reconstitution* by adding a specified volume of purified water just before dispensing. The dry powder supplied commercially is actually a mixture of the antibiotic, suspending agents, flavorants, and colorants, which, when reconstituted by the pharmacist, remains a stable suspension or solution of the drug for the time period in which the preparation is normally consumed. Storage under refrigeration is advisable for most preparations considered unstable due to hydrolytic causes. Together with temperature, pH is a major determinant in the stability of a drug prone to hydrolytic decomposition. The hydrolysis of most drugs is dependent upon the relative concentrations of the hydroxyl and hydronium ions, and a pH at which each drug is optimally stable can be easily determined. For most hydrolyzable drugs the pH of optimum stability is on the acid side, somewhere between pH 5 and 6. Therefore, through judicious use of buffering agents, the stability of otherwise unstable compounds can be increased.

Pharmaceutically, the oxidation of a susceptible drug substance is most likely to occur when it is maintained in other than the dry state in the presence of oxygen, exposed to light, or combined in formulation with other chemical agents without proper regard to their influence on the oxidation process. The oxidation of a chemical in a pharmaceutical preparation is usually attendant with an alteration in the color of that preparation. It may also result in precipitation or a change in the usual odor of a preparation.

The oxidative process is diverted, and the stability of the drug is preserved by agents called *antioxidants,* which react with one or more compounds in the drug to prevent progress of the chain reaction. In general, antioxidants act by providing electrons and easily available hydrogen atoms that are accepted more readily by the free radicals than are those of the drug being protected. Various antioxidants are employed in pharmacy. Among those more frequently used in aqueous preparations are sodium sulfite (Na_2SO_3), sodium bisulfite ($NaHSO_3$), hypophosphorous acid (H_3PO_2), and ascorbic acid. In oleaginous (oily or unctuous) preparations, alphatocopherol, butylhydroxyanisole, and ascorbyl palmitate find application.

In June, 1987 FDA labeling regulations went into effect requiring a warning about possible allergic-type reactions, including anaphylaxis in the package insert for prescription drugs to which sulfites have been added to the final dosage form. Sulfites are used as preservatives in many injectable drugs, such as antibiotics and local anesthetics. Some inhalants and ophthalmic preparations also contain sulfites, but relatively few oral drugs contain these chemicals.

The purpose of the regulation is to protect the estimated 0.2% of the population who suffer allergic reactions from the chemicals. Many of the sulfite-sensitive persons suffer from asthma or other allergic conditions. Previous to the regulations dealing with prescription medication, the FDA issued regulations for the use of sulfites in foods.[3] Asthmatics and other patients who may be sulfite-sensitive should be reminded to read the labels of packaged foods and medications to check for the presence of these agents.

The most frequent symptom of a sulfite reaction is difficulty breathing. Other symptoms include diarrhea, nausea and vomiting, abdominal pain and cramps, dizziness, wheezing, hives, itching, local swelling, rash, difficulty swallowing, headache, fainting, change in body temperature, chest pain, change in heart rate, unconsciousness and coma. Symptoms usually occur within minutes of ingesting or taking sulfited foods or drug products.

Sulfiting agents covered by the regulations are potassium bisulfite, potassium metabisulfite, sodium bisulfite, sodium metabisulfite, sodium sulfite and sulfur dioxide.

The labeling of drugs to which sulfites have been added to the final dosage form must contain the following statement in the ''Warnings'' section of the labeling:

"Contains (name of the sulfite), a sulfite that may cause allergic-type reactions including anaphylactic symptoms and life-threatening or less severe asthmatic episodes in certain susceptible people. The overall prevalence of sulfite sensitivity in the general population is unknown and probably low. Sulfite sensitivity is seen more frequently in asthmatic than nonasthmatic people."

Sulfite-containing epinephrine for injection for use in allergic emergencies must contain the following statement:

"Epinephrine is the preferred treatment for serious allergic or emergency situations even though this product contains (name of sulfite), a sulfite that may cause in other products cause allergic-type reactions including anaphylactic symptoms or life-threatening or less severe asthmatic episodes in certain susceptible persons. The alternatives to using epinephrine in a life-threatening situation may not be satisfactory. The presence of a sulfite(s) in this product should not deter the administration of the drug for treatment of serious allergic or other emergency situations."

The FDA decided to continue to permit the use of sulfites in prescription products, with the proper labeling, because there are no generally suitable substitutes for sulfites to maintain potency in certain medications.

The proper use of antioxidants involves their specific application only after appropriate biomedical and pharmaceutical studies. In certain instances other pharmaceutical additives have been found to inactivate a given antioxidant when used in the same formulation. In other cases certain antioxidants have been found to react chemically with the drugs they were intended to stabilize, without a noticeable change in the appearance of the preparation.

Because the stability of oxidizable drugs may be adversely affected by oxygen, certain pharmaceuticals may require an oxygen-free atmosphere during their preparation and storage. Oxygen may be present in pharmaceutical liquids in the airspace within the container or may be dissolved in the liquid vehicle. To avoid these exposures, oxygen-sensitive drugs may be prepared in the dry state and they, as well as liquid preparations, may be packaged in sealed containers with the air replaced by an inert gas such as nitrogen. This is common practice in the commercial production of vials and ampuls of easily oxidizable preparations intended for parenteral use.

Trace metals originating in the drug, solvent, container, or stopper are a constant source of difficulty in preparing stable solutions of oxidizable drugs. The rate of formation of color in epinephrine solutions, for instance, is greatly increased by the presence of ferric, ferrous, cupric, and chromic ions. Great care must be taken to eliminate these trace metals from labile preparations by thorough purification of the source of the contaminant or by chemically complexing or binding the metal through the use of specialized agents that make it chemically unavailable for participation in the oxidative process. These agents are referred to as *chelating agents* and are exemplified by calcium disodium edetate and ethylenediamine tetra-acetic acid (EDTA).

$$HOOC-CH_2 \qquad\qquad CH_2-COOH$$
$$\underset{HOOC-CH_2}{\diagdown} N-CH_2-CH_2-N \underset{CH_2-COOH}{\diagup} + Ca^{++} \rightarrow$$

EDTA

$$\left[\begin{array}{c} OOC-CH_2 \quad CH_2 \\ N \qquad C=O \\ CH_2 \qquad O \\ CH_2 \qquad Ca \\ N \qquad O \\ OOC-CH_2 \quad CH_2 \quad C=O \end{array}\right]^{2-}$$

Proposed calcium complex of EDTA

Light can also act as a catalyst to oxidation reactions. As a photocatalyst, light waves transfer their energy (photon) to drug molecules, making the latter more reactive through increased energy capability. As a precaution against the acceleration of the oxidative process, sensitive preparations are packaged in light-resistant colored glass or opaque containers.

Since most drug degradations proceed more rapidly with an advanced temperature, it is also advisable to maintain oxidizable drugs in a cool place. Another factor that could affect the stability of an oxidizable drug in solution is the pH of the preparation. Each drug must be maintained in solution at the pH most favorable to its stability. This, in fact, varies from preparation to preparation and must be determined on an individual basis for the drug in question.

Statements in the USP, as those in Table 4–3, warn of the oxidative decomposition of drugs and preparations. In some instances the specific agent to employ as a stabilizer is mentioned in the monograph, and in others the term "suitable stabilizer" is used. An example in which a particular agent is designated for use is in the monograph for Potassium Iodide Oral Solution, USP. Potassium iodide in solution is prone to photocatalyzed oxidation and the release of free iodine with a resultant brown discoloration of the solution. The use of light-resistant containers is essential to its stability. As a further precaution against decomposition if the solution is not to be used within a short time, the USP recommends the addition of 0.05% of sodium thiosulfate to the preparation. In the event free iodine is released during storage, the sodium thiosulfate converts it to colorless and soluble sodium iodide:

$$I_2 + 2Na_2S_2O_3 \rightarrow 2\ NaI + Na_2S_4O_6$$

In summary, for easily oxidizable drugs, the formulation pharmacist may stabilize the respective preparations by the selective exclusion from the system of oxygen, oxidizing agents, trace metals, light, heat, and other chemical catalysts to the oxidation process. He may add antioxidants, chelating agents, and buffering agents to create and maintain a favorable pH.

In addition to oxidation and hydrolysis, other destructive processes such as polymerization, chemical decarboxylation, and deamination may occur in pharmaceutical preparations. However, these processes occur less frequently and are peculiar to only small groups of chemical substances. Drug polymerization involves a reaction between two or more identical molecules with resultant formation of a new and generally larger molecule. Formaldehyde is an example of a drug capable of polymerization. In solution it may polymerize to paraformaldehyde $(CH_2O)_n$, a slowly soluble white crystalline substance that may cause the solution to become cloudy. The formation of paraformaldehyde is enhanced by cool storage temperatures, especially in solutions with high concentrations of formaldehyde. The official formaldehyde solution contains approximately 37% formaldehyde and according to the USP should be stored at temperatures greater than 15°C (59°F). If the solution becomes cloudy upon standing in a cool place, it generally may

Table 4–3. Examples of Some Official Drugs and Preparations Especially Subject to Chemical or Physical Deterioration

Preparation	Category	Monograph or Label Warning
Epinephrine Inhalation Solution, USP Epinephrine Injection, USP Epinephrine Nasal Solution, USP Epinephrine Ophthalmic Solution, USP	Adrenergic	Do not use the inhalation, injection, nasal or ophthalmic solution if it is brown or contains a precipitate.
Isoproterenol Sulfate Inhalation, Solution, USP	Adrenergic (bronchodilator)	Do not use the inhalation or injection if it is brown or contains a precipitate.
Nitroglycerin Tablets, USP	Antianginal	To prevent loss of potency, keep these tablets in the original container. Close tightly immediately after each use.
Paraldehyde, USP	Hypnotic	Paraldehyde is subject to oxidation to form acetic acid.

be cleared by gentle warming. Formaldehyde is prepared by the limited oxidation of methanol (methyl alcohol), and the USP permits a residual amount of this material to remain in the final product, since it has the ability to retard the formation of paraformaldehyde. Formaldehyde solution must be maintained in tight containers because oxidation of the formaldehyde yields formic acid.

$$CH_3OH \xrightarrow{(O)} HCHO \xrightarrow{(O)} HCOOH$$

methanol   formaldehyde   formic acid

Other organic drug molecules may be degraded through processes in which one or more of their active chemical groups are removed. These processes may involve various catalysts, including light and enzymes. Decarboxylation and deamination are examples of such processes, with the former involving the decomposition of an organic acid (R•COOH) and the consequent release of carbon dioxide gas and the latter involving the removal of the nitrogen-containing group from an organic amine. Organic amines are organic compounds formed by replacing one or more of the hydrogen atoms of ammonia (NH_3) with carbon-containing radicals. The resulting compounds are classified as primary amines ($R-NH_2$), secondary amines (R_2NH), and tertiary amines (R_3N).

Stability Testing

Drug instability in pharmaceutical formulations may be detected in some instances by a change in the physical appearance, color, odor, taste or texture of the formulation whereas in other instances chemical changes may occur which are not self-evident and may only be ascertained through chemical analysis. Scientific data pertaining to the stability of a formulation leads to the prediction of the expected shelf-life of the proposed product and, when necessary, to the redesign of the drug (e.g. into more stable salt or ester form) and to the reformulation of the dosage form. Obviously the *rate* or speed at which drug degradation occurs in a formulation is of prime importance. The study of the rate of chemical change and the way in which it is influenced by such factors as the concentration of the drug or reactant, the solvent employed, the conditions of temperature and pressure, and the presence of other chemical agents in the formulation is termed *reaction kinetics*.

In general a kinetic study begins by measuring the concentration of the drug being examined at given time intervals under a specific set of conditions including temperature, pH, ionic strength, light intensity, and drug concentration. The measurement of the drug's concentration at the various time intervals reveals the stability or instability of the drug under the specified conditions with the passage of time. From this starting point, each of the original conditions may be varied on an individual basis to determine the influence that such changes make on the drug's stability. For example, the pH of the solution may be changed, whereas the temperature, light intensity, and original drug concentration remain as they were in the original or baseline experiment.

The data collected may be presented graphically, by plotting the drug concentration as a function of time. From the experimental data, the reaction rate may be determined and a rate constant calculated. The rate constant describes the rate at which a drug is degrading under the conditions of the experiment and may be expressed as for example "2.6 mg/day," "0.1%/hour," or "0.155 g/liter/day."

The data also may be utilized in determining the experimental half-life of the drug. The *half-life* of a drug is defined as the time required for the drug to degrade to one-half of its original concentration. The half-life of a drug is expressed as its $t_{1/2}$ or t_{50}. Other expressions of drug remaining with reference to the original concentration may be used, as t_{90} and t_{95} indicating the drug remaining is 90 and 95% respectively of the original concentration.

The use of *exaggerated* conditions of temperature, humidity, light, and others, to test the stability of drug formulations is termed *accelerated stability testing*. Accelerated temperature stability studies, for example, are generally conducted at 37°, 50°, and 60°C (140°F), as well as at "room," refrigerator, and freezing temperatures. The use of short-term accelerated studies is for the purpose of determining the most stable of the proposed formulations for a drug product. Once the most stable formulation is ascertained, its long-term stability is predicted from the data generated from continuing stability studies. Depending upon the types and severity of conditions employed, it is not unusual to maintain samples under exaggerated conditions for periods of 1 month to 1 year. Such studies lead to the prediction of shelf-life for a drug product.

In addition to the accelerated stability studies, drug products are also stored under the usual conditions of transport and storage expected during product distribution. Samples maintained under these conditions may be retained for periods of 5 years or longer during which time they are observed for physical signs of deterioration and chemically assayed. These studies considered with the accelerated stability studies previously performed then lead to a more precise determination of drug product stability, actual shelf-life, and expiration dating.

Under usual circumstances, most manufactured products require a shelf-life of 2 or more years to insure their stability at the time of patient consumption. Commercial products must bear an appropriate expiration date. This date identifies the time during which the product may be expected to maintain its potency and remain stable under the designated storage conditions. The expiration date limits the time during which the product may be dispensed by the pharmacist or used by the patient.

Prescriptions requiring extemporaneous compounding by the pharmacist generally do not require the extended shelf-life that commercially manufactured and distributed products do because they are intended to be utilized immediately upon their receipt by the patient and used only during the immediate course of the prescribed treatment. However, these compounded prescriptions must remain stable and efficacious during the course of their use and the compounding pharmacist must employ formulative components and techniques which will result in a stable product. Thus, in the instance where an oral liquid preparation is made from an existing tablet or capsule formulation, the pharmacist should make up only at most a few days supply. Further, he must also dispense the medication in a container conducive to stability and use and must advise the patient of the proper method of use and conditions of storage of the medication.

In years past pharmacists were confronted primarily with innocuous, topical prescriptions that required extemporaneous formulation. However, in recent years with the advent of prescribing individualization there has been a need to compound other drug delivery systems as well, e.g., progesterone vaginal suppositories, oral suspensions, from existing tablets or capsules. When presented with a prescription that requires extemporaneous compounding, the pharmacist is confronted with a difficult situation because the potency and the stability of these prescriptions is a serious matter. Occasionally, the results of compatibility and stability studies on such prescriptions are published in scientific and professional journals. These are very useful, however, there are also prescriptions for which stability and compatability information is not readily available. In these instances it behooves the pharmacist to at least contact the drug manufacturer of the active ingredient(s) to solicit stability information. Alternatively, the pharmacist should use one's own personal network of professional associates to secure compounding procedure information. This latter approach by a group of hospital pharmacists lead to the eventual publication of the book titled, *Handbook of Extemporaneous Formulations*, by the American Society of Hospital Pharmacists. Finally, when compounding on the basis of extrapolated or less than concrete information it is best for the pharmacist to keep the formulation simple and not to shortcut but use the necessary pharmaceutical adjuvants to prepare the prescription.

Preservation Against Microbial Contamination

In addition to the stabilization of pharmaceutical preparations against chemical and physical degradation due to changed environmental conditions within a formulation, certain liquid and semisolid preparations also must be preserved against microbial contamination. Although some types of pharmaceutical products like ophthalmic and injectable preparations are sterilized by physical methods (autoclaving for 20 minutes at 15 pounds pressure and 120°C, dry heat at 170°C for 1 hour, or by bacterial filtration) during their manufacture, many of them additionally require the presence of an antimicrobial preservative to maintain their aseptic condition throughout the period of their storage and use. Other types of preparations that are not sterilized during their preparation but are particularly susceptible to microbial growth because of the nature of their ingredients are protected by the addition of an antimicrobial preservative. Preparations that provide excellent growth media for microbes are most aqueous preparations, especially syrups, emulsions, suspensions, and some semisolid preparations, particularly creams. Certain hydroalcoholic and most alcoholic preparations may not require the addition of a chemical preservative when the alcoholic content is sufficient to prevent microbial growth. Generally, 15% alcohol will prevent microbial growth in acid media and 18% in alkaline media. Most alcohol-containing pharmaceuticals such as elixirs, spirits, and tinctures are self-sterilizing and do not require additional preservation. The same would apply to other pharmaceuticals on an individual basis, which by virtue of their vehicles or other formulative agents, may not permit the growth of microorganisms.

Selection of Preservatives

When experience or shelf-storage experiments indicate that a preservative is required in a pharmaceutical preparation, its selection is based on many cross considerations including some of the following.

1. The preservative is effective in preventing the growth of the type of microorganisms considered the most likely contaminants of the preparation being formulated.
2. The preservative is soluble enough in water to achieve adequate concentrations in the aqueous phase of a two or more phase system.
3. The proportion of preservative remaining undissociated at the pH of the preparation makes it capable of penetrating the microorgansims and destroying its integrity.
4. The required concentration of the preservative does not affect the safety or comfort of the patient when the pharmaceutical preparation is administered by the usual or intended route; i.e., nonirritating, nonsensitizing, nontoxic.
5. The preservative has adequate stability and will not be reduced in concentration due to chemical decomposition or volatilization during the desired shelf-life of the preparation.
6. The preservative is completely compatible with all other formulative ingredients and does not interfere with them, nor do they interfere with the effectiveness of the preservative agent.
7. The preservative does not adversely affect the preparation's container or the closure.

General Considerations

Pharmaceutical preparations may be contaminated by molds, yeasts, or bacteria, with the latter generally favoring a slightly alkaline medium and the others an acid medium. Although few microorganisms can grow below a pH of 3 or above pH 9, most aqueous pharmaceutical preparations are within the favorable pH range and therefore must be protected against microbial growth. To be effective, a preservative agent must be dissolved in sufficient concentration in the aqueous phase of a preparation. Further, only the undissociated fraction or molecular form of a preservative possesses preservative capability, because the ionized portion is incapable of penetrating the microorganism. Thus the preservative selected must be largely undissociated at the pH of the formulation being prepared. Acidic preservatives like benzoic, boric, and sorbic acids are more undissociated and thus more effective as the medium is made more acid. Conversely, alkaline preservatives are less effective in acid or neutral media and more effective in alkaline media. Thus, it is meaningless to suggest preservative effectiveness at specific concentrations unless the pH of the system is mentioned and the undissociated concentration of the agent is calculated or otherwise determined. Also, if formulative materials interfere with the solubility or availability of the preservative agent, its chemical concentration may be misleading, because it may not be a true measure of the effective concentration. Many incompatible combinations of preservative agents and other pharmaceutical adjuncts have been discovered in recent years, and undoubtedly many more will be uncovered in the future as new preservatives, pharmaceutical adjuncts, and therapeutic agents are combined for the first time. Many of the recognized incompatible combinations that result in preservative inactivation involve macromolecules such as various cellulose derivatives, polyethylene glycols, and natural gums such as tragacanth, which have been shown to attract and hold preservative agents, such as the parabens and phenolic compounds, rendering them unavailable for their preservative function. It is essential for the research pharmacist to examine all formulative ingredients as one affects the other to assure himself that each agent is free to do the job for which it was included in the formulation. In addition, the preservative must not interact with a container such as a metal ointment tube or a plastic medication bottle or with an enclosure such as a rubber or plastic cap or liner. Such an interaction could result in the decomposition of the preservative or the container closure, or both, with resultant product decomposition and contamination. Appropriate tests should be devised and conducted to insure against this type of preservative interaction.

Mode of Action for Preservatives

Preservatives interfere with microbial growth, multiplication, and metabolism through one or more of the following mechanisms:

1. modification of cell membrane permeability and leakage of cell constituents (partial lysis)
2. lysis and cytoplasmic leakage
3. irreversible coagulation of cytoplasmic constituents (e.g., protein precipitation)
4. inhibition of cellular metabolism as through interference with enzyme systems or inhibition of cell wall synthesis
5. oxidation of cellular constituents
6. hydrolysis

A few of the commonly used pharmaceutical preservatives and their possible mode of action are presented in Table 4–4.

Preservative Utilization

Suitable substances may be added to a pharmaceutical preparation to enhance its permanency or usefulness. Such additives are suitable only if they are nontoxic and harmless in the amounts administered and do not interfere with the therapeutic efficacy or tests or assays of the preparation. Certain intravenous preparations given in large volumes as blood replenishers or as nutrients are not permitted to contain bacteriostatic additives, because the amounts required to preserve such large volumes would constitute a health hazard when administered to the patient. Thus preparations like Dextrose Injection, USP, and others commonly given as fluid and nutrient replenishers by intravenous injections in amounts of 500 to 1000 mL may not contain antibacterial preservatives. On the other hand, injectable preparations given in small volumes—for example, Morphine Sulfate Injection, USP, which provides a therapeutic amount of morphine sulfate in approximately a 1-mL volume—can be preserved with a suitable preservative without the danger of coadministering an excessive amount of the preservative to the patient.

Examples of the preservatives and their concentrations commonly employed in pharmaceutical preparations are: benzoic acid (0.1 to 0.2%), sodium benzoate (0.1 to 0.2%), alcohol (15 to 20%), phenylmercuric nitrate and acetate (0.002 to 0.01%), phenol (0.1 to 0.5%), cresol (0.1 to 0.5%), chlorobutanol (0.5%), benzalkonium chloride (0.002 to 0.01%), and combinations of methylparaben and propylparaben (0.1 to 0.2%), the latter being especially good against fungus. The required proportion would vary with the factors of pH, dissociation, and others already indicated as well with the presence of other formulative ingredients with inherent preservative capabilities that contribute to the preservation of the preparation and require less additional preservation assistance.

For each type of preparation to be preserved, the research pharmacist must consider the influence of the preservative on the comfort of the patient. For instance, it is apparent that a preservative in an ophthalmic preparation would have to have an extremely low degree of irritant qualities, which is characteristic of chlorobutanol, benzalkonium chloride, and phenylmer-

Table 4–4. Probable Mode of Action of Some Preservatives

Preservative	Probable Mode of Action
Benzoic acid, boric acid, and p-hydroxybenzoates	Denaturation of proteins
Phenols and chlorinated phenolic compounds	Lytic and denaturation action on cytoplasmic membranes and for chlorinated preservatives, also by oxidation of enzymes
Alcohols	Lytic and denaturation action on membranes
Quaternary compounds	Lytic action on membranes
Mercurials	Denaturation of enzymes by combining with thiol ($-SH$) groups

curic nitrate, frequently used preservatives in ophthalmic preparations. In all instances, the preserved preparation must be biologically tested to determine its safety and efficacy and shelf-tested to determine its stability for the intended shelf life of the product.

Appearance and Palatability

Although most drug substances in use today are unpalatable and unattractive in their natural state, modern pharmaceutical preparations present them to the patient as colorful, flavorful formulations attractive to the sight, smell, and taste. These qualities, which today are the rule rather than the exception, have virtually eliminated the natural reluctance of many patients to take medications because of their disagreeable odor or taste. In fact, the inherent attractiveness of today's pharmaceuticals has caused them to acquire the dubious distinction of being a major source of accidental poisonings in the home, particularly among children who are lured by their organoleptic appeal.

There is a great psychologic basis to drug therapy, and the odor, taste, and color of a pharmaceutical preparation can play their own peculiar part. Certain individuals consider a colorless or water-like preparation as being impotent, even though a pharmacist may advise to the contrary. To some, a black or purplish preparation may allude to the toxic or poisonous character of the medicine. Whatever the basis of belief, an appropriate drug will have its most beneficial effect when it is accepted, trusted, and believed in by the patient. The proper combination of flavor, fragrance, and color in a pharmaceutical product contributes to its acceptance.

Flavoring Pharmaceuticals

The flavoring of pharmaceuticals applies primarily to liquid dosage forms intended for oral administration. The 9000 taste buds of the mouth are located principally on the tongue and respond quickly and favorably or unfavorably to contact with medication. Medication in liquid form obviously comes into immediate and direct contact with these taste buds. By the addition of flavoring agents to liquid medication, the disagreeable taste of drugs may be successfully masked. Drugs placed in capsules or prepared as coated tablets may be easily swallowed with total avoidance of contact between the drug and

the taste buds. Tablets containing drugs that are not especially distasteful may remain uncoated and unflavored. Rapidly swallowing them with water usually is sufficient to avoid undesirable drug taste sensations. However, tablets of the chewable type as certain antacid and vitamin products, which are intended for mastication in the mouth usually *are* sweetened and flavored to receive better patient acceptance.

The flavor sensation of a food or pharmaceutical is actually a complex blend of taste and smell with lesser influences of texture, temperature, and even sight. In flavor formulating a pharmaceutical product, the pharmacist must give consideration to the color, odor, texture, and taste of the preparation. It would be incongruous, for example, to color a liquid pharmaceutical red, give it a banana taste, and a mint odor. The color of a pharmaceutical must have a psychogenic balance with the taste, and the odor must also enhance that taste. Odor greatly affects the flavor of a preparation or foodstuff. If one's sense of smell is impaired, as during a head cold, the usual flavor sensation of food is similarly diminished.

The medicinal chemist and the formulation pharmacist are well acquainted with the taste characteristic of certain chemical types of drugs and strive to mask effectively the unwanted taste through the appropriate use of flavoring agents. Although there are no dependable rules for unerringly predicting the taste sensation of a drug based upon its chemical constitution, experience permits the presentation of several observations. For instance, although we recognize and assume the salty taste of sodium chloride, the formulation pharmacist knows that all salts are not salty, but that their taste is a function of both the cation and anion. Whereas salty tastes are evoked by sodium, potassium, and ammonium chlorides and by sodium bromide, potassium and ammonium bromides elicit simultaneous bitter and salty sensations, and potassium iodide and magnesium sulfate (epsom salt) are predominantly bitter. In general, low molecular weight salts are salty, and higher molecular weight salts are bitter. With organic compounds, an increase in the number of hydroxyl groups (-OH) seems to increase the sweetness of the compound. Sucrose, which has eight hydroxyl groups, is sweeter than glycerin, another pharmaceutical sweetener, which has but three hydroxyl groups. In general, the organic esters, alcohols, and aldehydes are pleasant to the taste, and since many of them are volatile, they also contribute to the odor and thus the flavor of preparations in which they are used. Many nitrogen-containing compounds are extremely bitter, especially the plant alkaloids (as quinine), but certain other nitrogen-containing compounds are extremely sweet (as aspartame). The medicinal chemist recognizes that even the most simple structural change in an organic compound can alter its taste. D-glucose is sweet, but L-glucose has a slightly salty taste; saccharin is very sweet, but N-methyl-saccharin is tasteless:[4]

| Saccharin | N-Methylsaccharin |
| (Very sweet) | (Tasteless) |

Thus, the predictability of the taste characteristics of a new drug is only speculative. However, it is soon learned, and the formulation pharmacist is then put to the task of increasing the drug's palatability in the environment of other formulative agents. The proper selection of the appropriate flavoring agent depends upon several factors, but primarily upon the taste of the drug substance itself. Certain flavoring materials have been found through experience to be more effective than others in masking or disguising the particular bitter, salty, sour, or otherwise undesirable taste of medicinal agents. Although individuals' tastes and flavor preferences differ, cocoa-flavored vehicles are considered effective for masking the taste of bitter drugs. Fruit or citrus flavors are frequently used to combat sour or acid tasting drugs, and cinnamon, orange, raspberry, and other flavors have been successfully employed to make preparations of salty drugs more palatable.

The age of the intended patient should also be considered in the selection of the flavoring agent, because certain age groups seem to prefer certain flavors. Children prefer sweet, candy-like preparations with fruity flavors, but adults seem to prefer less sweet preparations with a tart rather than a fruit flavor, and geriatric patients may favor the refreshing taste of mint or of wine. Many natural and synthetic flavors are employed commercially to achieve the par-

ticular distinctive quality desired for a preparation by its manufacturer.

In addition to sucrose, a number of artificial sweetening agents have been utilized in foods and pharmaceuticals over the years. Some of these, as aspartame, saccharin and cyclamate, have faced challenges over their safety by the FDA and restrictions to their use and sale; in fact, the cyclamates were banned from use in the United States by the FDA in 1969.

The introduction of diet soft drinks in the 1950s provided the spark for the widespread use of artificial sweeteners today. Besides dieters, diabetics are regular users of artificial sweeteners. Over the years, each of the three artificial sweeteners has undergone long periods of review and debate. Critical to the evaluation of food additives are issues such as how the body uses a substance and metabolizes it down into other forms, and how the substance affects body functions. For example, almost none of the saccharin a person consumes is broken down by the body; it is excreted by the kidneys virtually unchanged. Cyclamate, on the other hand, is metabolized, or processed, in the digestive tract, and its byproducts are excreted by the kidneys. Aspartame breaks down in the body into three basic components: the amino acids phenylalanine and aspartic acid, and methanol. These three components, which also occur naturally in various foods, are in turn metabolized through regular pathways in the body. Because of its metabolism to phenylalanine, the use of aspartame by phenylketonurics is discouraged and diet foods and drinks must bear an appropriate label warning indicating that the particular foodstuff not be consumed by such individuals.

Passage in 1958 of the Food Additives Amendment to the Food, Drug, and Cosmetic Act produced a major change in how food additives would be regulated by the federal government. For one thing, no new food additive could be used if animal feeding studies or other appropriate tests showed that it caused cancer. This is the now-famous Delaney Clause. The *amount* of the substance one would have to consume to induce cancer is not of significance under the Delaney Clause.

Another critical feature of the 1958 amendment, however, was that it did not apply to additives that were generally recognized by experts as safe for their intended uses. Saccharin, cyclamate and a long list of other substances were being used in foods before the amendment's passage and were considered "generally recognized as safe"—or what is known today as GRAS. Aspartame, on the other hand, became the first artificial sweetener to fall under the 1958 amendment's requirement for premarketing proof of safety because the first petition to FDA for its approval was filed in 1973. In 1968, the Committee on Food Protection of the National Academy of Sciences issued an interim report on the safety of non-nutritive sweeteners, including saccharin. In the early 1970s, FDA began a major review of hundreds of food additives on the GRAS list to determine whether more current studies still justified their safe status. In 1972, with new studies under way, FDA decided to take saccharin off the GRAS and establish interim limits that would permit its continued use until additional studies were completed. (Previous studies indicated that male and female rats fed doses of saccharin developed a significant incidence of bladder tumors.) In November 1977, Congress passed the Saccharin Study and Labeling Act, which permitted saccharin's continued availability while mandating that warning labels be used to advise consumers that saccharin caused cancer in animals. The law also directed FDA to arrange further studies of carcinogens and toxic substances in foods.

Cyclamate was introduced into beverages and foods in the 1950s and dominated the artificial sweetener market in the 1960s. After much controversy regarding the substance's safety, the FDA issued a final ruling in 1980 stating that the agent's safety has not been demonstrated. Since that date, scientific studies have continued in order to conclusively support or refute the basis for the FDA decision. At question is the agent's possible carcinogenicity and its possible effects in causing genetic damage and testicular atrophy. The student is referred to the footnote reference for a review of the recent history of sweeteners including: saccharin, cyclamate, fructose, polyalcohols, sucrose, and aspartame.[5]

Table 4–5 compares three of the most used sweeteners in the food and drug industry.

Most large pharmaceutical manufacturers have special laboratories for the taste-testing of proposed formulations of their products. Panels of employees or interested community participants become involved in evaluating the various formulations and their assessments become the basis for the firm's flavoring decisions.

In flavoring liquid pharmaceutical products, the flavoring agent is added to the solvent or vehicle-component of the formulation in which it is most soluble or miscible. That is, water soluble flavorants are added to the aqueous component of a formulation and poorly water-soluble flavorants are added to the alcoholic or other non-aqueous solvent component of the formulation. In a hydroalcoholic or other multi-solvent system, care must be exercised to maintain the flavorant in solution. This is accomplished through experience in the order of mixing of the formulative components by constantly maintaining a sufficient level of solvent in which the flavorant is soluble.

Coloring Pharmaceuticals

The use of coloring agents in pharmaceutical preparations for purposes of esthetics, as sensory adjuncts to the flavors employed, and for purposes of product distinctiveness is important. A distinction should be made between agents that have inherent color and those agents which are employed as colorants. Certain agents—sulfur (yellow), cupric sulfate (blue), ferrous sulfate (bluish green), and red mercuric iodide (vivid red)—are not thought of as pharmaceutical colorants in the usual sense of the term.

Although most pharmaceutical colorants in use today are of synthetic origin, a few are obtained from natural mineral and plant sources. For example, red ferric oxide is mixed in small proportions with zinc oxide powder to prepare calamine, giving the latter its characteristic pink color intended to match the skin tone upon application.

The synthetic coloring agents used in pharmaceutical products were first prepared in the middle of the 19th century from principles of coal tar. Coal tar (*pix carbonis*), a thick, black, viscid liquid, is a by-product in the destructive distillation of coal. Its composition is extremely complex, and many of its constituents are separated from it by fractional distillation. Among the many products obtained from coal tar are anthracene, benzene, naphtha, creosote, phenol, and pitch. About 90% of the total dyes used in the products FDA regulates are synthesized from a single, colorless derivative of benzene, called aniline. These aniline dyes are also known as synthetic organic dyes or as "coal tar"

Table 4–5.   Comparison of Sweeteners

	Sucrose	Saccharin	Aspartame
Source:	sugar cane; sugar beet	chemical synthesis; phthalic anhydride, a petroleum product	chemical synthesis; methyl ester dipeptide of phenylalanine and aspartic acid
Relative Sweetness:	1	300	180–200
Bitterness:	none	moderate/strong	none
Aftertaste:	none	moderate/strong; sometimes metallic or bitter	none
Calories	4/g	0	4/g
Acid Stability:	good	excellent	fair
Heat Stability:	good	excellent	poor

dyes since aniline was originally obtained from bituminous coal. Aniline dyes today come mainly from petroleum.

Many coal-tar dyes were originally used indiscriminately in foods and beverages to enhance their appeal without regard to their toxic potential. It was only after careful scrutiny that some dyes were found to be hazardous to health due to either their own chemical nature or the impurities they carried. As more dyestuffs became available, it became apparent that some expert guidance and regulation was needed to insure the safety of the public. After passage of the Food and Drug Act in 1906, the United States Department of Agriculture established regulations by which a few colorants were *permitted* or *certified* for use in certain products. Today, the use of color additives in foods, drugs, and cosmetics is regulated by the Food and Drug Administration through the provisions of the Federal Food, Drug, and Cosmetic Act of 1938, as amended in 1960 with the Color Additive Amendments. A list of certified colors to be used as additives is maintained and made available by the Food and Drug Administration.[6] These approved color additives are classified into three groups: (1) FD&C dyes, which may be legally used in foods, drugs, and cosmetics; (2) D&C dyes, which may be legally used only in drugs and cosmetics; and (3) External D&C dyes, which may be legally used only to color externally applied drugs and cosmetics. The selection of a synthetic color additive for use in a pharmaceutical preparation to be used internally would have to be from among the certified colors of the first two categories. For each certification category there is a variety of basic colors with various choices within each

color group. One may select from a variety of FD&C, D&C, and External D&C reds, yellows, oranges, greens, blues, and even violets and blacks. By selective combinations of the colorants one can create unique colors (Table 4–6).

The certification status of the colorants is continuously reviewed, and changes are made in the list of certified colors in accordance with toxicologic findings. These changes may involve (1) the withdrawal of certification, (2) the transfer of a colorant from one certification category to another, or (3) the addition of new colors to the list. Before gaining certification, a color additive must be demonstrated to be safe. In the case of pharmaceutical preparations, color additives, like all additives, must not interfere with the therapeutic efficacy of the product in which they are used nor may they interfere with the prescribed assay procedure for that preparation.

In the 1970s, concern and scientific questioning of the safety of some color additives heightened. A color that drew particular attention was FD&C Red No. 2, because of its extensive use in foods, drugs and cosmetics. Researchers in Russia had reported that this color, also known as amaranth, caused cancer in rats. Although the FDA was never able to determine the purity of the amaranth tested in Russia, these reports led to FDA investigations and a series of tests that eventually resulted in withdrawal of FD&C Red No. 2 from the FDA certified list in 1976 because its sponsors were unable to prove safety. That year, the Agency also terminated approval for use of FD&C Red No. 4 in maraschino cherries and ingested drugs because of unresolved safety questions. FD&C Red No. 4

Table 4–6. Examples of Color Formulations*

Shade/Color	FD&C Dye	% of Blend
Orange	Yellow #6	100
	or	
	Yellow #5	95
	Red #40	5
Cherry	Red #40	100
	or	
	Red #40	99
	Blue #1	1
Strawberry	Red #40	100
	or	
	Red #40	95
	Red #3	5
Lemon	Yellow #5	100
Lime	Yellow #5	95
	Blue #1	5
Grape	Red #40	80
	Blue #1	20
Raspberry	Red #3	75
	Yellow #6	20
	Blue #1	5
Butterscotch	Yellow #5	74
	Red #40	24
	Blue #1	2
Chocolate	Red #40	52
	Yellow #5	40
	Blue #1	8
Caramel	Yellow #5	64
	Red #3	21
	Yellow #6	9
	Blue #1	6
Cinnamon	Yellow #5	60
	Red #40	35
	Blue #1	5

*From literature of Warner-Jenkinson Co., St. Louis, Mo.

is now permitted only in externally applied drugs and cosmetics.

The dye FD&C Yellow No. 5 (also known as tartrazine) can cause many people to have allergic-type reactions. People who are allergic to aspirin will also likely be allergic to this dye. As a result, the FDA requires the listing of this dye by name on the labels of foods and ingested drugs containing the substance. Persons allergic to this dye should be careful to look for it on product labels.

A colorant becomes an integral part of a pharmaceutical formulation, and its exact quantitative amount must be reproducible each time the formulation is prepared, or else the preparation would have a different appearance from batch to batch. This requires a high degree of pharmaceutical skill, for the amount of colorant generally added to liquid preparations ranges between 0.0005 and 0.001% depending upon the colorant and the depth of color desired. Because of their color potency, whenever possible dyes are added to pharmaceutical preparations in the form of diluted solutions rather than as concentrated dry powders. This permits greater accuracy in measurement and more consistent color production.

In addition to the use of liquid dyes in the coloring of pharmaceuticals, *Lake pigments* may also be used. Whereas a chemical material which exhibits coloring power or tinctorial strength when *dissolved*, pigment is an insoluble material which colors by dispersion. An FD&C Lake is a pigment consisting of a substratum of alumina hydrate on which the dye is absorbed or precipitated. Having aluminum hydroxide as the substrate, the Lakes are insoluble in nearly all solvents. FD&C Lakes are subject to certification and must be made from dyes which have been previously certified. Lakes do not have a specified dye content and range from 10 to 40% pure dye. By their very nature, Lakes are suitable for coloring products in which the moisture levels are low.

Lakes are commonly utilized in the form of fine dispersons or suspensions when coloring pharmaceuticals. The pigment particles may range in size from less than 1 μm up to 30 μm. The finer the particle, the less chance there would be for color speckling to occur in the finished product. Blends of various Lake pigments may be used to achieve a variety of colors and different vehicles may be employed to disperse the colorants, as glycerin, propylene glycol, and sucrose-based syrup.

In the preparation of capsules, various colored empty gelatin capsule shells may be used to hold the powdered drug mixture. Many commercial capsules are prepared with capsule bodies of one color and a different colored capsule cap, resulting in a two-colored capsule. This makes certain commercial products even more readily identifiable than solid colored capsules. For powdered drugs dispensed as such or compressed into tablets, a generally larger proportion of dye is required (about 0.1%) to achieve the desired hue than with liquid preparations.

Both dyes and Lakes have application in the coloring of sugar-coated tablets, film-coated tablets, direct-compression tablets, pharmaceutical suspensions and other dosage forms. Traditionally, sugar-coated tablets have been colored with syrup solutions containing varying amounts of the water-soluble dyes, starting with very dilute solutions, working up to concentrated color syrup solutions. As many as 30 to 60 coats are not uncommon. Using the FD&C Lakes, fewer color coats are used. Appealing tablets have been made with as few as 8 to 12 coats using Lakes dispersed in syrup. Water-soluble dyes in aqueous vehicles or Lakes dispersed in organic solvents may be effectively sprayed on tablets to achieve attractive film coatings. There is continued interest today in chewable tablets, due to the availability of many direct-compression materials such as dextrose, sucrose, mannitol, sorbitol, and spray-dried lactose. The direct-compression colored chewable tablets may be prepared utilizing 1 pound of Lake per 1000 pounds of tablet mix. For aqueous suspensions, FD&C water-soluble colors or Lakes may be satisfactory. In non-aqueous suspensions, FD&C Lakes are necessary. The Lakes, added either to the aqueous or non-aqueous phase, generally at a level of 1 pound of color per 1000 pounds of suspension, require homogenizing or mechanical blending to achieve uniform coloring.

For the most part, ointments, suppositories, and ophthalmic and parenteral products assume the color of their ingredients and do not contain color additives. Should a dye lose the certification status it held when a product was first formulated, manufactured, and marketed, the manufacturer must, within a reasonable length of time, reformulate, using only color additives certified at the new date of manufacture.

In addition to esthetics and the certification status of a dye, a formulation pharmacist must select the dyes to be used in a particular formula on the basis of the physical and chemical properties of the dyes available. Of prime importance is the solubility of a prospective dye in the vehicle to be used for a liquid formulation or in a solvent to be employed in conjunction with it during a pharmaceutical process, as when the dye is sprayed on a batch of tablets. In general, most dyes may be broadly grouped into those that are water-soluble and those that are oil-soluble; few, if any, dyes are both. Usually, a water-soluble dye is also adequately soluble in commonly used pharmaceutical liquids

like glycerin, alcohol, and glycol ethers. Oil-soluble dyes may overlap somewhat and also be soluble to some extent in these three liquids, as well as in liquid petrolatum (mineral oil), fatty acids, fixed oils, and waxes. It should be remembered that generally a great deal of solubility is not required, for the concentration of dye in a given preparation is rather minimal.

Another important consideration when selecting a dye for use in a liquid pharmaceutical is the pH and pH stability of the preparation to be colored. Dyes can change color with a change in pH, and a dye must be selected for a product so that any anticipated pH change will not alter the color during the usual shelf life. Needless to say, the dye must be chemically stable in the environment of the other formulative ingredients and must not interfere with the stability of the other agents. To maintain their original colors, FD&C dyes must be protected from oxidizing agents, reducing agents, (especially metals as iron, aluminum, zinc and tin), strong acids and alkalis, and excessive heating. Dyes must also be reasonably photostable; that is, they must not change color when exposed to light of reasonable intensities and wavelengths for a reasonable length of time. Here again, the product must be color stable under the usual conditions of shelf storage. Certain medicinal agents, particularly those prepared in liquid form, must be protected from light to maintain their chemical stability and their therapeutic effectiveness. These preparations are generally maintained and dispensed in dark amber or opaque containers, and the esthetic value of added coloring agents appears tenuous. However, it should be remembered that the patient will see the liquid medication upon its administration, and the value of the color in terms of balance with the flavor and product identification remains, even though the preparation does not reveal the color through its container. For solid dosage forms of photolabile drugs, a colored capsule shell (which may be prepared clear or opaque) may actually enhance the drug's stability by shielding out light rays.

Although the official compendia permit the use of color additives, few are official. The standards and regulations are provided by the federal Food and Drug Administration.

Packaging, Labeling, and Storage of Pharmaceuticals

The proper packaging and storage of pharmaceutical products are essential in maintaining product stability and efficacious use. Proper labeling of manufactured products and dispensed prescriptions is also vital to the appropriate use of medication. Standards for the packaging, labeling and storage of pharmaceutical products have been established by the USP and NF, the Food and Drug Administration, the Consumer Product Safety Commission, and state regulatory agencies, as Boards of Pharmacy, to ensure the safe and effective use of these products.

Containers

The official compendia terms applying to conditions of storage and types of containers have definite meaning and must not be loosely interpreted. According to the USP, a *container* is the device that holds a drug and is, or may be, in direct contact with the drug. The *immediate container* is that which is in direct contact with the drug at all times. The *closure* is part of the container. The container, including the closure, should be clean and dry prior to its being filled with the drug. The container must not interact physically or chemically with the drug placed in it so as to alter to any significant degree the strength, quality, or purity beyond the official requirements for that particular drug.

Containers may be classified according to their ability to protect their contents from external conditions. The minimally acceptable container is termed a *well-closed container.* It protects the contents from extraneous solids and from loss of the drug under ordinary conditions of handling, shipment, storage, and distribution. A *tight container* protects the contents from contamination by extraneous liquids, solids, or vapors, from loss of the drug, and from efflorescence, deliquescence, or evaporation under the usual conditions of handling, shipment, storage, and distribution. A tight container is capable of reclosure to its original capability after being opened. A *hermetic container* is impervious to air or any other gas under the ordinary or customary conditions of handling, shipment, storage, and distribution. Hermetic containers which are sterile are generally used to hold pharmaceutical preparations intended for injection or parenteral administration. These containers may be *single-dose containers* in which the quantity of sterile drug contained is intended as a single dose and which once opened cannot be resealed with assurance that sterility has been maintained. These containers include fusion-sealed ampuls, pre-filled syringes, dispos-

Fig. 4–3. *Examples of injectable products packaged in single-dose (ampuls) and multiple-dose (vials) containers and in unit-dose syringes.*

able syringes and cartridges. A *multiple-dose container* is a hermetic container which permits withdrawal of successive portions of the contents without changing the strength or endangering the quality or purity of the remaining portion. These containers are commonly referred to as vials. Examples of single-dose and multiple-dose products are shown in Figure 4–3.

Dosage forms, as tablets, capsules, and oral liquids, may be packaged in *single-unit* or *multiple-unit* containers. A single-unit container is one that is designed to hold a quantity of drug intended for administration as a single dose promptly after the container is opened. Multiple unit containers contain more than a single unit or dose of the medication. Examples of single-unit and multiple-unit packages are shown in Figure 4–4. A single-use package is termed a *unit-dose* package at the time a prescribing physician orders that particular amount of the drug for a specific patient. The single-unit packaging of drugs may be performed on a large scale by the industrial manufacturer or distributor or on a smaller in-house scale by the pharmacy actually dispensing the medication. In each instance, the single-unit package is appropriately labeled with the product identity, quality and/or strength, name of manufacturer, and lot number of product to insure the positive identification of the medication. Although single-unit packaging has particular usefulness in institutional settings as hospitals and extended care facilities it is not limited to such. Many

Fig. 4–4. *Examples of multiple-unit and single-unit packaging, including patient cup, unit dose of powder, blister packaging of single capsule, and strip packaging of tablets. (Courtesy of Philips Roxane Laboratories.)*

outpatients find single-unit packages a convenient and sanitary means of maintaining and utilizing their medication. Among the advantages cited for single-unit packaging and unit-dose dispensing are the following: positive identification of each dosage unit after it leaves the pharmacy or nursing station and the consequent reduction of medication errors, reduced contamination of the drug by virtue of its protective wrapping, reduced preparation and dispensing time, greater ease of inventory control in the pharmacy or nursing station, and elimination of waste through better medication management with less discarded medication.

Most hospitals with unit-dose systems use strip packaging equipment for the packaging of oral solids (Fig. 4–5). Such equipment seals solid dosage forms into four-sided pouches and imprints dose identification on each package at the same time. The equipment can be adjusted to produce individual single-cut packages or perforated strips or rolls of singly packaged dosage units. The packaging materials may be paper, foil, plastics or cellophane, alone or in combination. Some drugs must be packaged in foil-to-foil wrappings to prevent the deteriorating effects of light or the permeation of moisture. The packaging of solid dosage forms in clear

Fig. 4–5. *Strip packaging equipment capable of producing 50 packages per minute. Seals solid dosage units in a variety of wrapping materials and labels each package simultaneously. (Courtesy of Packaging Machinery Associates.)*

Fig. 4–6. *Components of Owens-Illinois' UNI-PAK System, including amber vials for oral liquids, aluminum closures, capper, and plastic hinged boxes for blister packaged solid dosage forms. Approximately 2,000 vials may be sealed per hour using the capper shown. (Courtesy of Owens-Illinois.)*

Fig. 4–7. *Examples of light-protective amber prescription containers for, from left to right: small numbers of solid dosage forms, as tablets and capsules; liquid preparations administered by drops; liquid preparations; powders, or large numbers of solid dosage forms; and semisolid preparations, such as ointments and pastes. (Courtesy of Armstrong Cork Company.)*

plastic blister wells is another popular method of single-unit packaging. Oral liquids are generally single-unit dispensed in paper, plastic, or foil cups, or pre-packaged and dispensed in glass containers having threaded caps or crimped aluminum caps (Fig. 4–6). A number of hospital pharmacies package oral liquids for pediatric use in disposable plastic syringes with rubber tips on the orifice for closure. In these instances the nursing staff must be fully aware of the novel packaging and special labeling used to indicate "not for injection." Medications which *are* used for injection may also be pre-packaged in syringes for direct administration to the patient. However, great care must be exercised in the preparation and packaging of parenteral products and appropriate laboratory tests performed to insure their sterility and stability. Other dosage forms, as suppositories, powders, ointments, creams, and ophthalmic solutions, are also commonly found in single-unit packages provided by large manufacturers. However, the relatively infrequent use of these dosage forms in a given hospital, extended care facility, or community pharmacy does not generally justify the expense of purchasing the spe-

cialized packaging machinery necessary for the small-scale packaging of these forms.

Some pharmaceutical manufacturers are now placing some of their pharmaceutical products in *unit-of-use* packaging. This is packaging in which an amount of drug product to be used during the usual course of a patient's treatment, or an otherwise commonly prescribed amount of that drug, is packaged in a container and requires only labeling before dispensing. For example, the antibiotic tetracycline is frequently prescribed to be taken 4 times a day for 10 days. Unit-of-use packaging would contain 40 capsules, sufficient for the usual course of treatment. For long-term treatment, as in the case of treating hypertension with antihypertensive drugs, the dosage forms may be packaged in quantities to last the patient a given number of months.

Many pharmaceutical products require *light-resistant containers* to protect them from photochemical deterioration. In most instances a container made of a good quality of amber glass will reduce light transmission sufficiently to protect the light-sensitive pharmaceutical. The containers shown in Figure 4–7 are widely used for this purpose. In some instances opaque glass or glass rendered opaque by a special coat-

Table 4–7.   Constitution of Official Glass Types

Type	General Description
I	Highly resistant, borosilicate glass
II	Treated soda-lime glass
III	Soda-lime glass
NP	General purpose soda-lime glass

ing is employed. Opaque plastic containers are becoming increasingly popular in the packaging of pharmaceutical products. The use of outer wrapping or carton can also be used to protect light-sensitive pharmaceuticals.

It is generally good practice for the pharmacist to dispense medication to his patients in the same type and quality of container as that used by the manufacturer of the product. In some instances the original container may be used by the pharmacist in dispensing the medication.

The official compendia provide tests and standards for glass and plastic containers with respect to their ability to prevent the transmission of light. Containers intended to provide protection from light or those offered as "light-resistant" containers must meet prescribed compendia standards which define the acceptable limits of light transmission at any wavelength of light between 290 and 450 nm.

The glass used in packaging pharmaceuticals is classified into four categories, depending upon the chemical constitution of the glass and its ability to resist deterioration. Table 4–7 presents the chemical make-up of the various glasses; types I, II, and III are intended for parenteral products and type NP is intended for nonparenteral products and those intended for oral or topical use. Each type is tested according to its resistance to water attack. The degree of attack is determined by the amount of alkali released from the glass under the test conditions specified. Obviously the leaching of alkali from the glass into a pharmaceutical solution or preparation placed in the container could alter the pH and thus the stability of the product. Pharmaceutical manufacturers must select and utilize containers which do not adversely affect the composition or stability of their products. Type I is generally the most resistant glass of the four categories.

Plastic containers are tested for suitability as containers of parenteral preparations. The object of the tests is to determine the reaction of living animal tissue and of normal animals to the presence of portions of the plastic and of injection extracts of it. On the basis of the biological test procedures, plastics intended for packaging parenteral products are also divided into classes of quality.

The interest and widespread use of plastic containers in the pharmaceutical industry has been generated by a number of factors including: (1) the advantage of plastic over glass containers in lightness of weight and resistance to impact and thus lower transportation costs and losses due to container damage; (2) the versatility in container design and in consumer acceptance afforded by plastics; (3) the interest and convenience in utilizing low and medium density polyethylene in the formation of squeeze bottles which serve a dual function of both package and applicator for preparations as ophthalmics, nasal solutions, and lotions; and (4) the advent of newer techniques in drug distribution, dispensing, and inventory control particularly in hospitals which required the development of packaging as the strip package, blister package, and plastic disposable syringe for unit-dose delivery.

Today a wide variety of dosage forms may be found packaged in plastic. The modern compact-type container used for oral contraceptives, which contains sufficient tablets for a monthly cycle of administration and permits the scheduled removal of one tablet at a time, is a prime example of the imaginative packaging possible with plastics (Fig. 4–8). Plastic bags for intravenous fluids, plastic ointment tubes, plastic film protected suppositories and plastic tablet and capsule vials are other examples of the widespread use of plastics in pharmaceutical packaging.

The use of plastics in pharmaceutical packaging is a developing science and technology. Problems arise and indeed are resolved because of the nature and alterability of plastics. The term "plastic" does not apply to a single type of material but rather to a vast number of existing and possible materials. Under specified experimental conditions monomers are added to each other forming long polymers. The desired properties of a plastic material may be produced by the right choice of the monomers, by the regulation of the synthesis, or by the addition of certain functional groups. For example, the addition of methyl groups to every other carbon atom in the polymer chains of polyethylene will give polypropylene a material which can be effectively autoclaved, whereas

Fig. 4–8. *A and B. Examples of plastic packaging used for oral contraceptive products. (B) The "Wallette" dispenser allows an easy to follow format (Courtesy of Syntex Laboratories.)*

polyethylene cannot. If a chlorine atom is added to every other carbon in the polyethylene polymer, polyvinyl chloride is produced. This material is rigid and has good clarity making it a useful material in certain packaging situations. The placement of other functional groups on the main chain of polyethylene or added to other types of polymers can give a variety of alterations to the final plastic material. In addition, added agents may be employed to alter the properties of the plastic. These agents include plasticizers, stabilizers, antioxidants, fillers, antistatic agents, antimold agents, colorants, and others.

Among the problems associated with the use of plastics in packaging are (1) permeability of the containers to atmospheric gases and to moisture vapor; (2) leaching of the constituents of the container to the internal contents; (3) sorption of drugs from the contents to the container; (4) transmission of light through the container; and (5) alteration of the container upon storage.

True *permeability* is considered a process of solution and diffusion, with the penetrant initially dissolving in the plastic material on one side and diffusing through to the other side. Permeability should be contrasted with *porosity*, which is a condition in which minute holes or cracks are present in the plastic and through which gas or moisture vapor may move directly.

The permeability of a plastic is a function of several factors including the nature of the polymer itself, the amounts and types of plasticizers, fillers, lubricants, pigments and other additives used, the pressure conditions, and the temperature. Generally, increases in the temperature, pressure, and the use of additives to the polymer tend to increase the permeability of the plastic. In general, glass containers are less permeable than plastic containers. The closure plays as important a role in protecting pharmaceuticals as does the primary container. A tightly fitting closure can often be the difference between a protected or an unprotected drug product.

The movement of moisture vapor or gas, especially oxygen, through a pharmaceutical container can pose one of the greatest threats to the stability of a pharmaceutical product. For most pharmaceuticals which are dry powders or solid dosage forms, as tablets and capsules, moisture, and gaseous penetration may be anticipated to occur predominantly from the environment toward the content. In the presence of moisture, these products may tend to cake or liquefy or in the case of solid dosage forms lose their color or physical integrity. A host of pharmaceutical adjuncts, especially those used in tablet formulations, as diluents, binders, and disintegrating agents, are affected by moisture. The majority of these adjuncts are carbohydrates, starches, and natural or synthetic gums, and because of their hygroscopicity they hold moisture and may even serve as nutrient media for the growth of microorganisms. Many of the tablet disintegrating agents fulfill their pharmaceutical function by swelling in an aqueous media, and, if exposed to high moisture vapor upon storage, the disintegrants may prematurely swell, and cause the tablets to become deformed. Further, many medicinal agents, as aspirin, some barbiturates, and vitamins, are quite prone to hydrolytic decomposition and dosage forms of these agents must be especially guarded against moisture penetration. Nitroglycerin is especially prone to moisture and the sublingual tablets must be dispensed to the patient in its original glass container. Under proper storage conditions nitroglycerin sublingual tablets are stable for 2 years, however, once the original container is opened the patient must be advised to discard any unused tablets 6 months after the original bottle is opened.

Drug substances which exhibit oxidation propensity may undergo a greater degree of degradation when packaged in plastic as compared to glass. In glass, the void space is filled with air which is in a confined space and presents only a limited amount of oxygen to the drug contents. On the other hand, a drug packaged in a gas permeable plastic container may be constantly exposed to oxygen due to the replenished supply entering the container.

Liquid pharmaceutical products packaged in plastic which is permeable to the contents tend to lose molecules of solute (drug) or solvent (vehicle) outward toward the container. Such permeation can drastically alter the concentration of the drug in the pharmaceutical product thereby affecting its efficacy.

Leaching is a term used to describe the release or movement of components of a container into the contents. Compounds leached from plastic containers are generally the polymer additives as the plasticizers, stabilizers, or antioxidants. The leaching of these additives occurs predominantly when liquid or semi-solid dosage forms are packaged in plastic. Little leaching occurs when tablets or capsules are packaged in plastic.

Leaching may be influenced by temperature, excessive agitation of the filled container, and by the solubilizing effect of the contents on one or more of the polymer additives. The leaching of polymer additives from plastic containers of fluids intended for intravenous administration is an especially worrisome problem because the additive is injected along with the medication. The toxicologic effect of any leached additive is of prime concern and is presently an important area of investigation. Soft-walled plastic containers of polyvinyl chloride are frequently used to package various intravenous solutions as well as blood for transfusion. Leached material, whether dissolved in the contents or present as minute particles, poses a health hazard to the patient and sufficient studies should be performed on the leaching characteristics of each plastic material prior to its use in packaging a given pharmaceutical product.

Sorption is a term used to indicate the binding of molecules to polymer materials. Both *adsorption* and *absorption* may be considered within this term. Sorption occurs through chemical or physical means, or both, with the phenomena related to the chemical structure of the solute molecules and the physical and chemical properties of the polymer. Generally, the unionized species of a solute has a greater tendency to be bound than does the ionized species. Because the degree of ionization of a solute may be affected by the pH of the solution in which it is contained, the pH of a pharmaceutical solution may influence the sorption tendency of a particular solute. Further, the pH of a solution may affect the chemical nature of a plastic container in such a way to either increase or decrease the active bonding sites available to the solute molecules. Plastic materials with polar groups are particularly prone to the sorption process. Because the process of sorption is dependent upon the penetration or diffusion of a solute into the plastic, the pharmaceutical vehicle or solvent for the solute also plays a major role in the sorption process. Certain solvents may alter the plastic and increase its permeability to solute.

The process of sorption may be initiated by the adsorption of a solute to the inner surface of a plastic container. After the saturation of the surface, the solute may then diffuse into the plastic, perhaps with the assistance of the phar-maceutical solvent or vehicle, to be absorbed and bound to sites within the plastic. The sorption of a drug component from a pharmaceutical solution would naturally reduce the concentration of that agent in the solution and render the product unreliable as to potency and unacceptable for use. The sorption of antimicrobial preservatives or stabilizers from a pharmaceutical product would likewise render the product unsuitable for use. Even the sorption of colorants and flavorants which would alter a preparation's color stability and taste would be unacceptable to a pharmaceutical manufacturer. Thus, each formulative ingredient must be examined in the proposed plastic packaging to ascertain its tendency for sorption and to insure the continued stability and potency of a product during its anticipated shelf life. Active ingredients also can adsorb onto plastic. For example, insulin adsorption onto plastic intravenous infusion sets has been reported to be as high as 80% of a dose. However, it appears that between 20 to 30% of an insulin dose is actually adsorbed. Because of the wide variability of the adsorption phenomenon with insulin, it is prudent for the pharmacist to monitor patient progress while receiving an intravenous dose of insulin.

Insofar as the ability of plastic containers to protect pharmaceutical products from destructive light transmission, clear and uncolored plastic containers behave in much the same manner as clear and uncolored glass containers in allowing such transmissions. In fact, certain plastics allow permeability to short-wave rays that is even greater than for glass. Agents termed UV-absorbers may be added to the plastic to decrease the transmission of these short ultraviolet rays and thus may be used to protect drugs sensitive to these offending rays. As for glass, the official compendia set standards for the transmission of light through plastic containers intended to be "light resistant" for wavelengths of light between 290 and 450 nm. Many of the clear but colored plastic containers available to pharmacists meet these standards as do opaque containers.

Deformations, softening, hardening, and other physical changes in plastic containers have been observed. These changes may result from the permeation or sorption of the contents into the container changing its chemical or physical makeup. They may also result from the leaching of a component of the container into the contents, or from changes in temperature or physical stress placed upon the container in handling, shipping or storage.

The everchanging field of plastic technology will continue to yield innovative and effective materials for the packaging of pharmaceuticals in the future and eliminate the aforementioned problems. Today's so-called "superplastics" can be produced to withstand continuous temperatures of greater than 300°F, and possess a tensile strength of 10,000 pounds per square inch (compared to 32,000 psi for brass). Plastics are being produced that are stronger than steel, and employed in such products as bullet-proof vests. There are more than 4000 major polymers on the market today, with hundreds added each year with greater features and application. Plastics prepared by *coextrusion*, using barrier layers, and formed into sheets offer unique, strong, and flexible containers for the present and future. These plastic containers (exemplified by the potato chip bag) can be prepared to shield out light, oxygen, and moisture, a feature also particularly attractive to the packaging of pharmaceuticals.

In conclusion, each pharmaceutical preparation must be considered separately with respect to packaging and type of container selected. The container must be suited to the prolonged stability of the pharmaceutical preparation and must be conducive to the safe and effective utilization by the patient. A good guideline for the practicing pharmacist is to utilize the original or the same type of container in which the drug product was supplied originally by the manufacturer. For prescribed mixtures of drugs, especially liquid preparations and products containing volatile substances, a tightly closed, light-resistant glass container is usually the most protective container to use. Perhaps the best example which may be cited for the protective packaging of a volatile drug is that for nitroglycerin tablets, which must be dispensed in the original unopened (glass) container and must be maintained in this container by the patient to prevent the loss of potency due to the volatilization of nitroglycerin.

Safety Closures

To reduce the occurrence of accidental poisonings through the ingestion of drugs and other household chemicals, the Poison Prevention Packaging Act was passed into law in 1970. The responsibility for the administration and enforcement of the Act, originally with the Food and Drug Administration, was transferred to the Consumer Product Safety Commission in 1973 when this agency was created through the enactment of the Consumer Product Safety Act. The initial regulations called for the use of "child-proof" closures for aspirin products and certain household chemical products shown to have a significant potential for causing accidental poisoning in youngsters. As the technical capability in producing effective closures was developed, the regulations were extended to include the use of such safety closures in the packaging of both legend and over-the-counter medications. Presently, all legend drugs intended for oral use must be dispensed by the pharmacist to the patient in containers having safety closures unless the prescribing physician or the patient specifically requests otherwise or unless the product has been made specifically exempt from the requirement. Some manufacturers provide the safety closures with the smaller size packages of their prescription products which lend themselves directly to use as a dispensing quantity.

The manufacturer or packager of an over-the-counter drug product may provide a single-size noncomplying (not child-safe) package of the product provided it bears conspicuous labeling stating "This package for households without young children" or, if the package is small, stating, "Package not child-resistant," and provided the manufacturer also supplies the substance in complying packages.

Examples of commonly used safety closures in dispensing medication are presented in Figures 4–9 and 4–10.

Today, a child-safety container may be defined as one that is difficult for most children under 5 years of age to open or to obtain a harmful amount of the contents. It is not necessarily packaging that *all* children under 5 years of age cannot open. Further, the packaging should not be difficult for normal adults to open. A testing procedure has been designed by the Consumer Product Safety Commission to evaluate the effectiveness of such containers. The procedure is outlined in the USP.

The Consumer Product Safety Commission may propose the exemption of certain drugs and drug products from the safety closure regulation based on toxicologic data or on practical considerations. For instance, certain cardiac drugs, as sublingual tablets of nitroglycerin, are

Fig. 4–9. *Example of child-resistant safety closure on a prescription container. (Courtesy of Owens-Illinois.)*

exempt from the regulations because of the importance to the welfare of the patient for direct and immediate access to his medication. The few extra seconds required to open a safety container might be dangerously extended should the heart patient panic in his manipulative efforts with the closure. Exemptions are also permitted in the case of over-the-counter medications for one package size or specially marked package to be available to consumers for whom safety closures might be unnecessary or too difficult to manipulate. These consumers would include childless persons, arthritic patients, and the debilitated.

Drugs which are utilized or dispensed in inpatient institutions, as hospitals, nursing homes, and extended care facilities, need not be dispensed with safety closures unless they are intended for patients who are leaving the confines of the institution (outpatients).

Tamper-Resistant Packaging

On November 5, 1982, the Food and Drug Administration published regulations on tamper-resistant packaging in the *Federal Register.* These regulations were promulgated following the criminal tampering with over-the-counter drug products earlier in that year resulting in consumer illness and death. In the primary incident, cyanide surreptitiously had been placed in acetaminophen capsules in commercial packages for consumer purchase.

The regulations required tamper-resistant packaging for all over-the-counter drugs, with the exception of dermatologics, dentifrices, and insulin. A tamper-resistant package is defined as "one having an indicator or barrier to entry which, if breached or missing, can reasonably be expected to provide visible evidence to consumers that tampering has occurred." The regulations were to be fully in effect by February 6, 1984, the date after which no nonprescription drugs covered by the regulations could be sold without tamper-resistant packaging. Exempt from the regulations were products distributed to hospitals, nursing homes, and health care clinics "that are not distributed in a manner that affords the general public access to them while they are held for sale."

The fact that *tamper-resistant* packaging is not *tamper-proof* was demonstrated by a second episode of criminal tampering with over-the-counter products resulting in death in early 1986. Once again, the primary incident involved the placement of cyanide in acetaminophen capsules, except this time, the capsules were apparently triple sealed in containers with foil coverings over the bottle mouths, stretch seals over the bottle caps, and glued end-flaps of the outer packaging cartons. Immediately following this occurrence, the manufacturer recalled all of the product from the marketplace and replaced the encapsulated product with a tableted product considered much more difficult to adulterate. Subsequent FDA regulations required that after February 2, 1990, packaging for two-piece hard gelatin capsules sold over the counter must have at least two tamper-resistant features.

Pharmaceutical manufacturers have the option of determining the type of tamper-resistant packaging to utilize. Table 4–8 presents some examples of tamper-resistant packaging.

Labeling

The labeling of all drug products distributed in the United States must meet the specific labeling requirements as set forth in the federal regulations. These labeling requirements apply not only to proprietary products sold over-the-counter, but also to prescription drugs distributed to various health practitioners for ultimate dispensing to the patient. The labeling regulations are changed from time to time to meet the changing informational needs of the health professional and the patient. The federal labeling

Fig. 4–10. *Child-resistant prescription containers. (Courtesy of Kerr Glass Manufacturing Corporation.)*

Table 4–8.   Tamper-Resistant Packaging Examples

Package Type	Tamper Protection
Film Wrappers	Film wrapped and sealed around product and/or product containers; the film must be cut or torn to remove product.
Blister/Strip Packs	Individually sealed dosage units; removal requires tearing or breaking individual compartment.
Bubble Packs	Product and container sealed in plastic, usually mounted on/in display card; plastic must be cut or broken open to remove product.
Shrink Seals/Bands	Bands or wrappers which are shrunk by heat or drying to conform to cap and containers must be torn to open.
Foil, Paper, or Plastic Pouches	Sealed individual packets; must be torn to reach product.
Bottle Seals	Paper or foil sealed to mouth of a container under cap; must be torn or broken to reach product.
Tape Seals	Paper or foil sealed over carton flap or bottle cap; must be torn or broken to reach product.
Breakable Caps	Plastic or metal "tearaway" caps over container; must be broken to remove.
Sealed Tubes	Seal over mouth of tube; must be punctured to reach product.
Sealed Cartons	Carton flaps are sealed; carton cannot be opened without damage.
Aerosol Containers	Tamper-resistant by design.

requirements for drug products may be further enhanced by state and local drug laws. The contents of the label that the pharmacist affixes to dispensed medication is another topic, but it too is subject to specific requirements of the federal, state, and local regulations.

According to federal regulations, drug labeling includes not only the labels placed on the immediate container and packaging, but also the package inserts accompanying the product as well as all company literature and advertising or promotional material pertaining to the drug product. This includes such things as brochures, booklets, mailing pieces, file cards, bulletins, price lists, catalogs, sound recordings, film strips, motion-picture films, lantern slides, exhibits, displays, literature reprints and any other material containing product information provided by the manufacturer or distributor.

The essential information on a prescription-only drug is generally provided to the health professional through the product's *package insert*. This insert must provide *full disclosure;* that is, it must contain a full and balanced presentation of the positive as well as the negative aspects of the drug product to enable the prescriber to utilize the drug most safely and effectively.

Included in the prescription drug package insert is the following information:

1. Description of the product, including proprietary and non-proprietary names of the drugs present
2. Clinical pharmacology
3. Indications and usage
4. Contraindications
5. Warnings
6. Precautions
7. Adverse reactions
8. Drug abuse and dependence potential
9. Overdosage signs and treatment
10. Dosage and administration
11. Dosage forms, strengths and package sizes supplied

Included among the information usually appearing on the manufacturer's or distributor's label affixed to the container of Legend drugs are the following:

1. The nonproprietary name(s) of the drug(s) present and the proprietary trademark name of the product if one is used.
2. The name and address of the manufacturer or distributor of the product.

3. A quantitative statement of the amount of each drug present per unit of weight, volume, or dosage unit, whichever is most appropriate.
4. The pharmaceutical type of dosage form constituting the product.
5. The net amount of drug product contained in the package, in units of weight, volume or number of dosage units, as is appropriate.
6. The Federal Legend: "Caution—Federal law prohibits dispensing without prescription," or a similar statement.
7. The usual dose of the product including special dosage guidelines for children or for other patients under certain conditions, when appropriate.
8. A label reference to see the accompanying package insert or other product literature for additional information.
9. Special storage instructions, when applicable.
10. The National Drug Code identification number for the product.
11. The manufacturer's control number identifying the batch or lot of the drug.
12. An expiration date.
13. For controlled drug substances, the DEA symbol "C" together with the schedule assigned (e.g. III). The statement: "Warning—May be habit forming" may appear also.

When filling a prescription, the pharmacist is required by the federal Food, Drug and Cosmetic Act to include the following information on the label of the dispensed medication:

1. The name and address of the pharmacy
2. The serial number of the prescription
3. The date of the prescription or the date of its filling or refilling (state law often determines which date is to be used)
4. The name of the prescriber
5. The name of the patient
6. Directions for use, including precautions, if any, as indicated on the prescription

In addition to the above, state laws may require additional information as:

7. The address of the patient
8. The initials or name of the dispensing pharmacist
9. The telephone number of the pharmacy
10. The drug name, strength and manufacturer's lot or control number

11. The expiration date of the drug, if any
12. The name of the manufacturer or distributor

The label on the container of products sold over-the-counter without prescription usually contains much of the same type of product information as the prescription-only items with the exception of the Federal Legend and the DEA symbol. However, to advance the safe and proper use of over-the-counter medications, additional patient-oriented information is included in the labeling, including the following:

1. Product name and statement of identity, e.g., liquid antacid, listing of active ingredients and net quantity of contents.
2. Statements of all conditions, purposes, or uses for which the drug is intended or commonly used. Also included are conditions against which the drug is contraindicated or to be used only with professional supervision.
3. Directions for use—quantity of dose, including usual quantities for each of the uses for which it is intended and the usual quantities for persons of different ages and physical conditions, if pertinent.
4. Dosage instructions—frequency of administration, if used internally, or application, if used externally, and time of administration or application, with respect to meals, onset of symptoms or other time factors.
5. Warnings—maximum duration of administration or application prior to consulting a physician, and anticipated side effects of the drug's action which might be experienced by the user.
6. Cautionary statements—storage in a safe place out of the reach of children, appropriate instructions in the event of accidental overdosage, sodium content, etc.
7. Drug interaction precautions—heighten patient awareness of other medicines that could interfere with or enhance the effect of the OTC drug.
8. Route of administration or application.
9. Preparation for use—shaking, dilution, adjustment of temperature, or other manipulations or processes.
10. Declaration of presence of the dye Yellow No. 5 (to alert persons hypersensitive to this agent) and alcohol.
11. If the medication is to be taken internally, the label must contain the statement: "As

with any drug, if you are pregnant or nursing a baby, seek the advice of a health professional before using this product."

As noted above, over-the-counter package labeling must include appropriate warning statements whenever the medication is such that indiscriminate use may lead to serious medical complications or mask a condition more serious than that for which the medication was intended. For example, the use of laxatives is a dangerous practice when symptoms of appendicitis are present and can result in an intensification of the problem and even a rupturing of the appendix. For this reason the following statement is required by law to appear on laxative preparations:

"Warning: Do not use when abdominal pain, nausea, or vomiting is present. Frequent or prolonged use of this preparation may result in dependence on laxatives."

The seriousness of a cough may be underestimated by a patient if a proprietary cough syrup temporarily relieves the cough; however, coughing is a symptom of many serious conditions requiring specific treatment. Cough remedies sold over-the-counter must therefore bear the following warning statement:

"Warning: A persistent cough may indicate a serious condition. Persons with a high fever or persistent cough should not use this preparation unless directed by physician."

These are but two examples of the statements required on various types of proprietary products. The statements themselves and the types of preparations requiring them are written into the law and are available through the government literature. The labels of drugs sold directly to the layman should recommend their use against only those conditions that have been shown scientifically to be treated effectively by the drug. Serious conditions that cannot be diagnosed or successfully treated by the layman should not be mentioned in the labeling, nor should it contain any false or misleading statement. The label must be perfectly clear in meaning and this will become even more important in the future. Trends indicate that in future years more legend drugs will become available for over the counter purchase. Thus, the importance of labeling of these products for consumer use in understandable terms cannot be overemphasized.

As a part of the FDA's Current Good Manufacturing Practice (CGMP) Regulations of 1978, as revised in 1983, all over-the-counter drug products are required to bear expiration dates. However, enforcement of this requirement is currently waived for human O-T-C products if their labeling does not bear dosage limitations and they are stable for at least 3 years as supported by appropriate stability data.

Storage

To insure the stability of a pharmaceutical preparation for the period of its intended shelf life, the product must be stored under proper conditions. The labeling of each product generally includes the desired conditions of storage for that particular product. The terms generally employed in such labeling have definite meaning, as defined by the official compendia:

Cold—Any temperature not exceeding 8°C (46°F). A *refrigerator* is a cold place in which the temperature is maintained thermostatically between 2° and 8°C (36° and 46°F). A *freezer* is a cold place in which the temperature is maintained thermostatically between −10° and −20°C (14° and −4°F).
Cool—Any temperature between 8° and 15°C (46° and 59°F). An article for which storage in a cool place is directed may, alternatively be stored in a refrigerator unless otherwise specified in the individual monograph.
Room Temperature—The temperature prevailing in a working area. *Controlled room temperature* is a temperature maintained thermostatically between 15° and 30°C (59° and 86°F).
Warm—Any temperature between 30° and 40°C (86° and 104°F).
Excessive Heat—Any temperature above 40°C (104°F).
Protection from Freezing—Where in addition to the risk of breakage of the container, freezing subjects a product to loss of strength or potency, or to destructive alteration of the dosage form, the container label bears an appropriate instruction to protect the product from freezing.

When no specific storage or limitations are provided, it is understood that the storage conditions include protection from moisture, freezing, and excessive heat.

Standards for Current Good Manufacturing Practice

To insure high standards for drug product quality, the Food and Drug Administration enforces compliance with the requirements of its Current Good Manufacturing Practice (CGMP or GMP) regulations. The first GMP regulations were promulgated in 1963 under one of the provisions of the Kefauver-Harris Drug Amendments of 1962. Since that time they have been revised periodically, most recently in 1983. A topical outline of these regulations is presented in Table 4–9. As may be seen from this table, the CGMP regulations establish standards for all aspects of pharmaceutical manufacture in this country. A more detailed presentation may be found in the USP. Compliance with these standards is our best assurance that the products dispensed by the pharmacist to the patient are of appropriate and uniform high quality.

The FDA's CGMP regulations apply to a pharmacy only if it is engaged in the repackaging and relabeling of drugs and drug products beyond the usual conduct of dispensing and selling them at retail. Pharmacies which do engage in such activities must register with the FDA as a manufacturer and be subject to FDA inspection at regular intervals. These pharmacies would also be bound to the standards of Current Good Manufacturing Practices. Examples of pharmacies engaged in such activities include: hospital pharmacies that repackage drug products for their own use as well as the use of other hospitals; chain pharmacies that repackage and relabel bulk quantities of products from the manufacturer's original containers for distribution to individual pharmacies within the chain; and similar repackaging and relabeling activities conducted by individual pharmacists or pharmacies for distribution to other pharmacies or retailers.

Some Definitions[7]

Component—any material used in the manufacture of a drug product, including those which may not be present in the finished product.
Batch—a specific quantity of a drug of uniform specified quality produced according to a single manufacturing order durng the same cycle of manufacture.
Lot—a batch or any portion of a batch having uniform specified quality and a distinctive identifying "lot number."
Lot Number, Control Number, or Batch Number—any distinctive combination of letters, numbers or symbols from which the complete history of the manufacture,

Table 4–9. Topical Outline of Current Good Manufacturing Practice Regulations[1]

A. General Provisions
 1. Scope.
 2. Definitions.
B. Organization and Personnel
 1. Responsibilities of quality control unit.
 2. Personnel qualifications.
 3. Personnel responsibilities.
 4. Consultants.
C. Buildings and Facilities
 1. Design and construction features.
 2. Lighting.
 3. Ventilation, air filtration, air heating and cooling.
 4. Plumbing.
 5. Sewage and refuse.
 6. Washing and toilet facilities.
 7. Sanitation.
 8. Maintenance.
D. Equipment
 1. Equipment design, size, and location.
 2. Equipment construction.
 3. Equipment cleaning and maintenance.
 4. Automatic, mechanical, and electronic equipment.
 5. Filters.
E. Control of Components and Drug Product Containers and Closures
 1. General requirements.
 2. Receipt and storage of untested components, drug product containers, and closures.
 3. Testing and approval or rejection of components, drug product containers, and closures.
 4. Use of approved components, drug product containers, and closures.
 5. Retesting of approved components, drug product containers, and closures.
 6. Rejected components, drug product containers, and closures.
 7. Drug product containers and closures.
F. Production and Process Controls

 1. Written procedures; deviations.
 2. Charge-in of components.
 3. Calculation of yield.
 4. Equipment identification.
 5. Sampling and testing of in-process materials and drug products.
 6. Time limitations on production.
 7. Control of microbiological contamination.
 8. Reprocessing.
G. Packaging and Labeling Control
 1. Materials examination and usage criteria.
 2. Labeling issuance.
 3. Packaging and labeling operations.
 4. Tamper-resistant packaging requirements for over-the-counter human drug products.
 5. Drug product inspection.
 6. Expiration dating.
H. Holding and Distribution
 1. Warehousing procedures.
 2. Distribution procedures.
I. Laboratory Controls
 1. General requirements.
 2. Testing and release for distribution.
 3. Stability testing.
 4. Special testing requirements.
 5. Reserve samples.
 6. Laboratory animals.
 7. Penicillin contamination.
J. Records and Reports
 1. General requirements.
 2. Equipment cleaning and use log.
 3. Component, drug product container, closure, and labeling records.
 4. Master production and control records.
 5. Batch production and control records.
 6. Production record review.
 7. Laboratory records.
 8. Distribution records.
 9. Complaint files.
K. Returned and Salvaged Drug Products
 1. Returned drug products.
 2. Drug product salvaging.

[1]Code of Federal Regulations, *21*, part 211, revised April 1, 1983

Fig. 4–11. *Example of computer use in the pharmaceutical industry. In this instance, a CRT terminal is shown in the center on the operator's desk, with the programmer's console at the left, the floppy disk drive at the right, and the computer-controlled lyophilizer in the background. (Courtesy of D.J. Fraade, Burroughs Wellcome Co.)*

processing, packaging, holding, and distribution of a batch or lot of a drug product may be determined.

Active Ingredient—any component which is intended to furnish pharmacological activity or other direct effect in the diagnosis, cure, mitigation, treatment or prevention of disease or to affect the structure or function of the body of man or other animals.

Inactive Ingredient— any component other than the active ingredients in a drug product.

Drug Product—a finished dosage form that contains an active drug ingredient generally, but not necessarily, in association with inactive ingredients. The term may also include a dosage form that does not contain an active ingredient intended to be used as a placebo.

Master Record—records containing the formulation, specifications, manufacturing procedures, quality assurance requirements, and labeling of a finished product.

Verified—signed by a second individual or recorded by automated equipment.

Quarantined—an area that is marked, designated, or set aside for the holding of incoming components prior to acceptance examination.

Reprocessing—the activity whereby the finished product or any of its components is recycled through all or part of the manufacturing process.

Quality Control—the regulatory process through which industry measures actual quality performance, compares it with standards, and acts on the difference.

Batchwise Control—the use of validated in-process sampling and testing methods in such a way that results prove the process has done what it purports to do for the specific batch concerned, assuming control parameters have been appropriately respected.

Quality Assurance—the activity of providing, to all concerned, the evidence needed to establish confidence that the activities relating to quality are being performed adequately..

Quality Audit—a documented activity performed in accordance with established procedures on a planned and periodic basis to verify compliance with the procedures to assure quality.

Validation—establishing documented evidence that a system does what it purports to do (e.g., equipment, software, controls).

Process Validation—establishing documented evidence that a process does what it purports to do (e.g., sterilization).

Validation Protocol—a prospective experimental plan that, when executed, is intended to produce documented evidence that the system has been validated.

Validation Task Report—a scientific report of the results derived from executing a validation protocol.

Prospective Validation—establishing documented evidence that a system does what it purports to do based on a preplanned protocol.

Concurrent Processes Validation—establishing documented evidence that a process does what it purports to do based on information generated during actual implementation of the process.

Retrospective Validation—establishing documented evidence that a system does what it purports to do based on review and analysis of historic information.

Revalidation—repetition of the validation process or a specific portion of it.

Worst Case—the highest or lowest value of a given control parameter actually evaluated in a validation exercise.

Proven Acceptable Range (PAR)—all values of a given control parameter that fall between proven high and low worst-case conditions.

Compliance—determination through inspection of the extent to which a manufacturer is complying with prescribed regulations, standards, and practices.

Certification—documented testimony by qualified authorities that a system qualification, calibration, validation, or revalidation has been performed appropriately and that the results are acceptable.

Although not a part of the subject matter of this textbook, the reader should be aware that the FDA has developed Good Manufacturing Practice regulations for medical devices and has proposed CGMP regulations for large volume parenterals. Included in the list of critical medical devices are: airways, catheters, dialyzers, cardiac pacemakers, prosthetics, infusion pumps, respirators, valves, and ventilators.[8]

Computerization in the Pharmaceutical Industry

Computers are playing an increasing role in all areas within the pharmaceutical industry. Computers are used in many administrative procedures and record keeping, pharmaceutical process controls, production, packaging, and many other areas. Whereas the use of computers is commonplace in administrative procedures and in areas as inventory control, billing, record keeping, and so forth, it is relatively new in areas of process design and control and in production. The advantages of computer use in these areas may be summarized as follows:[9]

- increased productivity reducing labor
- improved process and product quality
- reduction in operator error and levels of product rejections
- increased process yields (as from chemical synthesis of drug compounds)
- enhanced repeatability of processes
- improved operator protection due to less "hands on" activity
- automated diagnostic and alarm actions alerting of possible mechanical malfunction, process decontrol or product defect
- assist in process and product validation efforts

- assist in bookkeeping efforts
- assist in scheduling efficacy
- reduced cost per product unit

There are a number of production areas that are computerized within the pharmaceutical industry. These include: sterile manufacturing areas, general packaging areas, pilot plant, solid dosage form manufacturing (e.g. tablet coating), chemical process control, and analytical testing. In addition to computers, robotic devices are being employed to replace certain human manual operations such as that on packaging lines. In these instances, robotic devices can be used to do routine tasks, as picking up and placing a filled bottle into the package carton.

Selected Reading

Chapman, K.G.: A Suggested Validation Lexicon. *Pharmaceutical Technology*, August, 1983, pp. 51–57.

Colorants for Drug Tablets and Capsules. *Drug and Cosmetic Industry*, 133(2):44, 1983.

Fink, J.L., Marquardt, K.W., and Simonsmeier, L.M.: *Pharmacy Law Digest*. St. Louis, Facts and Comparisons Division, J.B. Lippincott Co., 1987.

Fraade, D.J.: The Application of Digital Control Systems in the Pharmaceutical Industry. *Pharmaceutical Manufacturing*, 1(3):22, 1984.

Head, W.F., Jr.: *Pharmaceutical Quality Control*. Smithtown, NY, Exposition Press, 1983.

Madan, P.L., and Komotar, A.: Quality Control of Pharmaceuticals. *Drug and Cosmetic Industry*, 124 (4):66, 1979.

Mollica, J.A., Ahuja, S., and Cohen, J.: Stability of Pharmaceuticals. *J. Pharm. Sci.*, 67(4):443, 1978.

Murphy, D.H.: A Practical Compendium on Sweetening Agents. *Amer. Pharm.*, NS23:32–37, 1983.

Sacharow, S.: Developments in Barrier Plastic Bottles for Pharmaceutical Packaging. *Pharmaceutical Manufacturing*, 2(2):12–15, 1985.

Smith, D.L.: Compliance Packaging: A Patient Education Tool. *Amer. Pharm.*, NS29:42–53, 1989.

Notes

1. Adapted, in part, from Poole, J.W.: *Preformulation*, FMC Corporation (Publisher), 1982.
2. Paramethadione as Paradione (Abbott) and ethchlorvynol as Placidyl (Abbott).
3. *FDA Drug Bulletin*, 17, No. 1 (April) 1987 pp. 2–3; 16, No. 2 (November) 1986, pp. 17–18; *Federal Register*, 51(234):43900–43904, Dec. 5, 1986, 51(131):25012–25026, July 9, 1986.

   In a regulation that became final in August 1986, FDA banned the use of sulfites in fresh fruits and vegetables. In an accompanying regulation that went into effect on Jan. 1, 1987, the Agency required packaged foods containing sulfites to be labeled if sulfites are present at 10 parts per million or more. Most reported sulfite reactions have been to foods. About 28% of reported reactions occurred after eating at a restaurant salad bar, and about 13% occurred after eating other fruits and vegetables. About 14% of the reactions occurred after eating packaged foods prepared at home.

After analyzing reports of 22 deaths temporally associated with ingestion of sulfited products, FDA determined that 9 fatalities were probably, and 5 deaths possibly, due to sulfite ingestion. The remaining 8 deaths were probably not related to sulfites. All 14 deaths that were probably or possibly associated with sulfites occurred in severe asthmatics who developed severe respiratory distress and anaphylactoid reactions.

Under the regulations, sulfiting agents are no longer allowed on raw fruits and vegetables, and packaged sulfited foods are required to be labeled if sulfites are present in specified amounts. Wine and beer also may contain sulfites. They come under the jurisdiction of the Treasury Depart-ment's Bureau of Alcohol, Tobacco and Firearms, which requires a warning label on all alcoholic beverages containing sulfites.

4. Hornstein, I., and Teranishi, R.: The Chemistry of Flavor. *Chem. Eng. News, 45*:92–108, 1967.
5. Murphy, D.H.: A Practical Compendium on Sweetening Agents. *Amer. Pharm., NS23*:32–37, 1983; Sweetness Minus Calories = Controversy. *FDA Consumer, 19*, No. 1, 18–23, 1985.
6. Countdown on Color Additives, *FDA Consumer, 10*(1):5–7, 1976.
7. Obtained in part from Chapman, K.G.: A Suggested Validation Lexicon. *Pharmaceutical Technology*, August, 1983, pp. 51–57.
8. *Federal Register, 43*:52710, November 14, 1978.
9. Adapted from Fraade, D.J.: *An Overview and Case Histories of Computer Applications in a Pharmaceutical Industry.* Eighth International Good Manufacturing Practices Conference, The University of Georgia, 1984.

5 | Peroral Solids, Capsules, Tablets, and Controlled-Release Dosage Forms

WHEN MEDICATIONS are to be administered orally in dry form, capsules and tablets are most frequently used. They are effective and provide the patient with convenience of handling, identification, and administration. From a pharmaceutic standpoint, solid dosage forms are generally more stable than are their liquid counterparts and thus are preferred for poorly stable drugs. Dry powders are taken orally (usually after mixing in water) to a much lesser extent than are capsules and tablets, but are preferred by some patients who are unable to swallow the solid dosage forms. However, most medicated powders are utilized as external applications to the skin. While the use of powders *per se* in therapeutics is limited, the use of powders in dosage form preparation is extensive. Most of the medicinal substances in use today occur in crystalline or powdered form and are blended with other powdered materials, as inert fillers and disintegrants, prior to fabrication into solid dosage forms. Powdered drugs are also frequently added to ointments, pastes, suppositories, and other dosage forms during their preparation. Similarly, granules, which are agglomerates of powdered materials prepared into larger free flowing particles, are utilized chiefly in the preparation of tablets and in dry preparations intended to be reconstituted to liquid forms prior to use by the addition of the appropriate vehicle.

Powders

As a pharmaceutical preparation, a *powder* (Latin, *pulvis*) is a mixture of finely divided drugs and/or chemicals in dry form. This should be differentiated from the general use of the term "powder" or "powdered" which is commonly used to describe the physical state of a single chemical substance or a single drug.

A powder may be a finely subdivided preparation, a coarsely comminuted product, or a product of intermediate particle size. It may be prepared from a naturally occurring dried vegetable drug, or it may be a physical admixture of two or more powdered pure chemical agents present in definite proportions. Powders may contain small proportions of liquids dispersed thoroughly and uniformly over the solid components of the mixture, or the powder may be composed entirely of solid materials.

Some powders are intended to be used internally; others, externally. Certain powders are dispensed by the pharmacist to the patient in bulk quantities; others, in divided, individually packaged portions, depending primarily on the use, dose, or potency of the powder.

The disadvantages of powders as a dosage form include the potential for patient misunderstanding of the correct method of use, the undesirability of taking bitter or unpleasant tasting drugs in this manner, the difficulty of protecting from decomposition powders containing hygroscopic, deliquescent, or aromatic materials, and the manufacturing expense required in the preparation of uniform individually wrapped doses of powders. To be of high efficacy, the powder must be a homogeneous blend of all of the components and must be of the most advantageous particle size. As noted earlier (Chapter 3), the particle size of a drug not only contributes to its rate of solubility in a glass of water or within the stomach or intestine, but also may influence its biological activity or therapeutic performance.

Preparation of Powders

Particle Size

The particles of pharmaceutical powders may be very coarse, of the dimensions of about 10,000 microns or 10 mm, or they may be ex-

Table 5–1. Openings of Standard Sieves*

Sieve Number	Sieve Opening
2	9.5 mm
3.5	5.6 mm
4	4.75 mm
8	2.36 mm
10	2.00 mm
20	850 μm
30	600 μm
40	425 μm
50	300 μm
60	250 μm
70	212 μm
80	180 μm
100	150 μm
120	125 μm
200	75 μm
230	63 μm
270	53 μm
325	45 μm
400	38 μm

*Adapted from USPXXII-NF XVII

tremely fine, approaching colloidal dimensions of 1 micron or less. In order to standardize the particle size of a given powder, the USP employs descriptive terms such as "Very Coarse, Coarse, Moderately Coarse, Fine, and Very Fine," which are related to the proportion of powder that is capable of passing through the openings of standardized sieves of varying dimensions in a specified time period under shaking, generally in a *mechanical sieve shaker*. Table 5–1 presents the Standard Sieve Numbers and the sieve openings in each, expressed in millimeters and in micrometers. Sieves for such pharmaceutical testing and measurement are generally made of wire cloth woven from brass, bronze, or other suitable wire. They are not coated or plated.

Powders of vegetable and animal drugs are officially defined as follows:

Very Coarse (or a No. 8) powder—All particles pass through a No. 8 sieve and not more than 20% through a No. 60 sieve.

Coarse (or a No. 20) powder—All particles pass through a No. 20 sieve and not more than 40% through a No. 60 sieve.

Moderately Coarse (or a No. 40) powder—All particles pass through a No. 40 sieve and not more than 40% through a No. 80 sieve.

Fine (or a No. 60) powder—All particles pass

through a No. 60 sieve and not more than 40% through a No. 100 sieve.

Very Fine (or a No. 80) powder—All particles pass through a No. 80 sieve. There is no limit as to greater fineness.

The powder fineness for chemicals is defined as follows. It should be noted that there is no "Very Coarse" category.

Coarse (or a No. 20) powder—All particles pass through a No. 20 sieve and not more than 60% through a No. 40 sieve.

Moderately Coarse (or a No. 40) powder—All particles pass through a No. 40 sieve and not more than 60% through a No. 60 sieve.

Fine (or a No. 80) powder—All particles pass through a No. 80 sieve. There is no limit as to greater fineness.

Very Fine (or a No. 120) powder—All particles pass through a No. 120 sieve. There is no limit as to greater fineness.

Granules typically fall within the range of 4- to 12-sieve size, although granulations of powders prepared in the 12- to 20-sieve range are not uncommon when used in tablet making.

Particle size determination and distribution studies of powders may be performed by *sieving;* that is, by passing the powder by mechanical shaking through a series of sieves of known and successively smaller size, and determining the proportion of powder passing through or being withheld on each sieve. Other methods of particle size determinations include the measurement of the particles under the microscope through the use of a calibrated grid background or other measuring device, determination of sedimentation rates and the application of the Stokes' equation (p. 227), electrical conductivity methods, and others.[1-3] The study of particle size is referred to as *micromeritics*.

Comminution of Drugs

On a small scale, as in the community pharmacy, the pharmacist usually reduces the size of chemical substances by exposing them to the rigor of the mortar and pestle. A finer grinding action is accomplished in a mortar with a rough surface (as a porcelain mortar) than one with a smooth surface (as a glass mortar). The process of grinding a drug in a mortar to reduce its particle size is termed *trituration*.[4] On a large

Fig. 5–1. *Stokes Tornado Mill used to pulverize, granulate, and disperse materials presented to it in the dry or wet state. (Courtesy of Eli Lilly and Company.)*

scale, various types of mills and pulverizers may be used to reduce powder fineness. Figure 5–1 shows one such piece of equipment. The type shown is the Stokes Tornado Mill. This machine is employed to pulverize, granulate, and disperse materials presented to it in the dry or wet state.

A process termed *levigation* is commonly employed in the reduction of particle size particularly in the small-scale preparation of ointments. This is done to prevent the feeling of grittiness in the preparation due to the solid drug present. In the process, a mortar and pestle or ointment tile is generally used, and a paste formed of the solid material and a small amount of liquid (the *levigating agent*) in which the solid material is insoluble. The paste is then triturated, effecting a reduction in particle size. The levigated paste may then be added to the ointment base and the mixture made uniform and smooth, usually by rubbing them together with a spatula on the ointment tile. The entire levigation procedure may be performed with the spatula, usually employing a "figure 8" track to incorporate and levigate the materials. Mineral oil and glycerin are commonly used levigating agents.

The Mixing of Powders

When two or more substances are to be mixed together to form a uniform powder mixture, it is best to reduce the particle size of each indi-

vidually before weighing and blending. Depending upon the nature of the ingredients, the amount of powder to prepare, and the equipment available, powders may be prepared by *spatulation, trituration, sifting, tumbling* or by *mechanical mixers.*

Spatulation is a method by which small amounts of powders may be blended by the movement of a pharmaceutical spatula through the powders on a sheet of paper or an ointment tile. The method is not generally suitable for large quantities of powders or for powders containing one or more potent substances, because homogeneous blending is not as certain as with other methods. Very little compression or compacting of the powder results from this method, which is especially suited to the mixing of those solid substances that liquify or form *eutectic* mixtures when in close and prolonged contact with one another. These substances include phenol, camphor, menthol, thymol, aspirin, phenylsalicylate and other similar chemicals. To diminish contact, a powder prepared from such substances is commonly mixed in the presence of an inert diluent such as light magnesium oxide or magnesium carbonate to separate physically the troublesome agents.

Trituration may be employed both to comminute and to mix powders. If comminution is especially desired, a porcelain or a Wedgewood mortar having a rough inner surface is preferred over the generally smooth working surface of the glass mortar. However, for chemicals that may stain the porcelain or Wedgewood surface, a glass mortar may be preferred. Also, if simple admixture is desired without special need for comminution, the glass mortar is usually preferred, because it cleans more readily after use. The application of form or "heavy" trituration may have a compacting effect on a bulky fluffy powder and may be performed for this very purpose. When potent substances are to be mixed with a large amount of diluent (as in the preparation of a 10% trituration of a potent drug), the *geometric dilution method* is employed to ensure the uniform distribution of the potent drug. The use of this method is especially indicated in instances in which the potent and the nonpotent substances are of the same color and a visible sign of thorough mixing is lacking. By this method, the potent drug is placed upon an approximately equal volume of the diluent in a mortar and the mixture is thoroughly mixed by trituration. Then a second portion of diluent equal in volume to the powder mixture in the mortar is added, and the trituration is repeated. This process is continued by adding equal volumes of diluent to that powder present in the mortar and repeating the mixing until all of the diluent is incorporated.

Powders may also be mixed by passing them through sifters like the type used in the kitchen to sift flour. This process of *sifting* generally results in a light fluffy product. This process is not generally considered acceptable for the incorporation of potent drugs into a diluent base.

Another method of mixing powders is that of *tumbling* the powder enclosed in a large container which rotates generally by a motorized process. Special *powder blenders* have been devised and mix powders by a tumbling motion (Fig. 5–2). Mixing by this process is thorough, although time-consuming. Such blenders are widely employed in industry, as are large volume powder mixers which have motorized blades to blend the powder contained in a large mixing vessel (Fig. 5–3).

Use and Packaging of Powders

Depending upon their intended use, powders are packaged and dispensed by pharmacists in two main ways, as *bulk powders* or as *divided powders*. Nowadays, powders are generally supplied pre-packaged by the manufacturer to the community pharmacist for dispensing.

BULK POWDERS. Among the bulk powders commonly dispensed are (a) antacid and laxative powders, which the patient generally takes by mixing the directed amount of powder (usually a teaspoon or so) in a portion of water or other beverage and swallowing; (b) douche powders, generally dissolved in warm water by the patient for vaginal use; (c) medicated or nonmedicated powders for external application, usually dispensed in sifter cans for convenient application to the skin; (d) dentifrices or dental cleansing powders, used in dental hygiene; (e) denture powders, some used as dentifrices and others as adhesives to hold the dentures in place and, (f) Brewer's Yeast powder containing B-complex vitamins.

Depending upon the intended use of the powder, it may be supplied to the patient in a perforated or sifter-type can or container for external dusting, in an aerosol container for spraying onto the skin, or in a wide-mouthed glass or plastic jar which permits the entrance of a

Fig. 5–2. *Industrial size solid state processor or "twin shell" blender used to mix solid particles. (Courtesy of Abbott Laboratories.)*

Fig. 5–3. *The meticulous cleaning of a ribbon mixer used to blend powders preparative to granulation and tablet compression. (Courtesy of Eli Lilly and Company.)*

spoon and the easy removal of a spoonful of powder. All powders should be stored in tightly closed containers.

Dispensing powdered drugs in bulk amounts is generally limited to nonpotent substances. Powders containing potent substances or those that should be administered in controlled dosage are usually supplied to the patient in divided amounts. Powders supplied to the patient in either bulk or in divided portions that are intended for external use should bear an EXTERNAL USE ONLY or a similar label.

DIVIDED POWDERS. (Latin, *chartulae* (pl.); abbrev: *charts*.) After the powder has been properly mixed (using the geometric dilution method for potent substances), it may be di-

vided into individual units based upon the dose to be administered or the amount to be used at a single time. Each divided portion of powder may be placed on a small piece of paper, which is then folded so as to enclose the medication.

The reader is referred to Chapter 13 for a discussion of the preparation of divided powders.

Although divided powders have generally come into disuse because of more convenient and readily available unit doses of tablets and capsules, it is not unusual to find them being dispensed in a pharmacy as divided powders containing antacid medication or a premeasured amount of powder for use in preparing a vaginal douche solution. Further, a number of commercial preparations for the relief of pain, as Goody's Headache Powders and B. C. Powders, and laxatives, as Metamucil Powder, are packaged in unit-dose packets.

Official Powders

The following are examples of powders recently official in the USP/NF.

Compound Clioquinol Powder, USP—used by vaginal insufflation as an antitrichomonal.

Methylbenzethonium Chloride Powder, USP—local anti-infective used chiefly for diaper rash in infants and chafing.

Neomycin and Polymyxin B Sulfates and Bacitracin Zinc Topical Powders USP—an anti-infective combination for topical application as a powder and as an ointment.

Nystatin Topical Powder, USP—employed as topical dusting powder especially to moist areas in treatment of mycotic infections.

Microcrystalline Cellulose, NF—Pharmaceutic aid as tablet disintegrant, diluent, adsorbent, and suspending agent.

Tolnaftate Powder, USP and Tolnaftate Topical Aerosol Powder, USP—These are generally used with other dosage forms (e.g. cream, solution) in treatment of fungus infections when drying (with powder) may enhance the therapeutic response.

Granules

As indicated previously, granules are prepared agglomerates of smaller particles. They are generally irregularly shaped and behave as single larger particles. They are usually in the 4- to 12-sieve size range although granules of various mesh sizes may be prepared depending upon their application.

Generally, granules are prepared by moistening the desired powder or blended powder mixture (Fig. 5–4) and passing the moistened mass through a screen of the mesh size that will produce the desired size granules. The larger particles thus formed are then dried by air or under heat (as the nature of the drug will allow), while they are occasionally moved about on the drying trays to prevent the adhesion of the granules. Granules may also be prepared without the use of moisture by passing compressed masses of powdered material through a granulating machine.

Granules flow well compared to powders. For the purpose of comparison, consider the pouring characteristics of granulated sugar and powdered sugar. Because of their flow properties, granulations are usually made when powder mixtures are intended to be compressed into tablets. The flow characteristics allow the material to flow freely from the hopper or feeding container into the tableting presses. This will be discussed later in this chapter in greater detail.

Granules are generally more stable physically and chemically than are the corresponding powders from which they were prepared. Gran-

Fig. 5–4. *Moistened powder mass to be used in the preparation of granules.*

ules are less likely to cake or harden upon standing than are powders. Because their surface area is less than that of powders, granules are usually more stable to the effects of the atmosphere. Because granules are more easily "wetted" by a solvent than are certain powders which tend to float on the solvent's surface, granules are frequently preferred for the making of solutions.

A number of commercial products containing antibiotic drugs which are unstable in aqueous solution are prepared as granules for reconstitution by the pharmacist with purified water just prior to dispensing [e.g. Principen (ampicillin) for Oral Suspension (Squibb)]. The granules are so prepared to contain not only the medicinal agent, but the colorants, flavorants, and any other desired pharmaceutic ingredient. Upon reconstitution, the resultant liquid (solution or suspension) has all of the desired medicinal and pharmaceutic features of a liquid pharmaceutical.

Other types of granular products are prepared and sold commercially including a number which are packaged in bulk and utilized as laxatives. One example of this type of product is Senokot Granules (Purdue Frederick), which are cocoa-flavored granules containing standardized senna concentrate. The granules are measured by the teaspoon and usually mixed with water upon administration. Effervescent products as Bromo Seltzer (Warner Lambert) represent another popular type of granulated product. Granulations of effervescent products may be compressed into tablet form. K-Lyte (Mead Johnson) is an example of a product of this type. Effervescent granules and tablets are placed in a portion of water and taken as the effervescence subsides. Effervescent granulated salts are discussed more fully below.

Effervescent Granulated Salts

Effervescent salts are granules or coarse to very coarse powders containing a medicinal agent in a dry mixture usually composed of sodium bicarbonate, citric acid, and tartaric acid. When added to water, the acids and base react to liberate carbon dioxide, resulting in effervescence. The resulting carbonated solution masks the usually saline or otherwise undesirable taste of the medicinal agent present. By using granules or coarse particles of the mixed powders rather than the ordinary smaller sized

particles of these substances, the rate of solution of the substances is decreased upon addition to water, and the otherwise violent reaction and rapid, uncontrollable effervescence is eliminated. Such violent effervescence would likely overflow the glass of water to which it was added with subsequent loss of solution and little residual carbonation of the solution. The methods for the preparation of effervescent salts appear in Chapter 13.

An example of an effervescent salt is Effervescent Sodium Phosphate. It is used as a cathartic and has a usual dose of 10 g. About 2 teaspoonfuls of the granules are added to a glass of water, and the mixture is swallowed as the effervescence subsides. Each 10 g of the granules contain 2 g of exsiccated sodium phosphate, the usual dose of this agent, which is the active component of the effervescent salt.

Capsules

Capsules are solid dosage forms in which one or more medicinal and/or inert substances are enclosed within a small shell or container generally prepared from a suitable form of gelatin. Depending upon their formulation, the gelatin capsule shells may be hard or soft. The majority of capsules dispensed are intended to be swallowed whole by the patient for the benefit of the medication contained therein.[5] In certain instances the contents of a capsule may be removed from the gelatin shell and employed as a premeasured medicinal powder. For example, the product THEO-DUR SPRINKLE (Key Pharmaceuticals), is recommended for use in the latter manner, for children or other patients unable to swallow a tablet or capsule. It is recommended that the contents of the capsule, anhydrous theophylline in sustained release form, be sprinkled on a small amount of soft food immediately prior to ingestion.

It has become somewhat common practice in hospitals and extended care facilities to open capsules or crush tablets to mix with food or drink for ease of swallowing.[6] This should only be done with the concurrence *of the pharmacist* because the release characteristics of the drug from the dosage form could be dramatically altered. Subsequently, the amount of drug and the rate with which the drug is absorbed *could adversely* affect the patient's welfare. These products generally include: enteric coated dosage forms, designed to pass through the stom-

Fig. 5–5. *Pork skin gelatin used as raw material in the manufacture of gelatin capsules. (Courtesy of Smith, Kline & French Laboratories.)*

ach intact for absorption in the intestine; extended release dosage forms, designed to provide extended or prolonged release of the medication; and sublingual or buccal tablets, formulated to dissolve under the tongue or in the oral cavity. In many instances, if a patient is unable to swallow a solid dosage form, an alternative product, as an oral liquid, suppository or injection may be employed.

Hard Gelatin Capsules

Hard gelatin capsules are the type used by pharmaceutical manufacturers in the preparation of the majority of their capsule products and by the community pharmacist in the extemporaneous compounding of prescriptions. The basic empty capsule shells are made from a mixture of gelatin, sugar, and water and are clear, colorless, and essentially tasteless. Gelatin, USP, is a product obtained by the partial hydrolysis of collagen obtained from the skin, white connective tissue, and bones of animals. It is found in commerce in the form of a fine powder, a coarse powder, shreds, flakes, or sheets (Fig. 5–5).

Gelatin is stable in air when dry but is subject to microbic decomposition when it becomes moist or when it is maintained in aqueous solution. For this reason, soft gelatin capsules, which contain more moisture than the hard capsules, may be prepared with a preservative agent added to prevent the growth of fungi in the capsule shells. Normally, hard gelatin capsules contain between 13 and 16% of moisture. However, if stored in an environment of high humidity, additional moisture is absorbed by the capsules, and they may become distorted and lose their rigid shape. On the other hand, in an environment of extreme dryness, some of the moisture normally present in the gelatin capsules may be lost, and the capsules may become brittle and may crumble when handled.

Because moisture may be absorbed or released by gelatin capsules, depending upon the environmental conditions, it follows that little physical protection is afforded hygroscopic or deliquescent materials enclosed within a capsule when stored in an area of high humidity. It is not unusual to find capsules of such moisture-affected materials packaged in containers along with a packet of a desiccant material as a precaution against the capsules absorbing atmospheric moisture. With or without such desiccant materials, capsules should be generally stored in areas of low humidity.

Although gelatin is insoluble in cold water, it does soften through the absorption of up to ten times its weight of the water. Some patients prefer to swallow a capsule wetted with water or saliva, because the capsule softens and slides down the throat more readily than does a dry capsule. Gelatin is soluble in hot water, and in warm gastric fluid a gelatin capsule rapidly releases its contents. Gelatin, being a protein, is digested and absorbed.

Hard gelatin capsule shells are manufactured in two sections, the capsule body and a shorter cap. The two parts overlap when joined, with the cap fitting snugly over the open end of the capsule body. The shells are produced by the mechanical dipping of pins or pegs of the desired shape and diameter into a reservoir of the melted gelatin mixture, maintained at a constant temperature to achieve the desired degree of fluidity. The pegs, made of manganese bronze, are affixed to plates, each capable of holding up to about 500 pegs. Each plate is mechanically lowered to the gelatin bath, the pegs being submerged to the desired depth and for the desired period of time to achieve the proper length and thickness of coating. Then the plate and the pegs are slowly lifted from the gelatin bath, and the gelatin on the pegs is gently dried by a flow of temperature and humidity controlled air (see Figs. 5–6 and 5–7A). When dried, each capsule part is trimmed mechanically to the proper length and removed from the pegs, and the capsule bodies and caps are joined together. It is important that the thickness of the gelatin walls be strictly controlled so that the capsule body and cap fit snugly to prevent disengagement. Naturally, the pegs on which the caps are formed are slightly larger in diameter than the pegs on which the bodies are formed, since the caps overlap the bodies. In production, there is a continuous dipping, drying, removing, and joining of capsules as many peg-containing plates are rotated in and out of the gelatin bath.

Several methods of making capsules distinctive are available to the pharmaceutical manufacturer. One way is to color the gelatin used in the preparation of the capsules. Colorants may be used to prepare capsule bodies and caps having the same or different colors. By combining the various capsule parts, beautiful, transparent, and distinctive capsules may be prepared.

Opaque capsules may also be prepared to make a pharmaceutical product distinctive. These capsules are formed by adding an insoluble substance such as titanium dioxide to the gelatin mixture. Colored, opaque capsules may be prepared by using both a colorant and the opaque-producing substance.

A manufacturer may also alter the usually rounded shape of the capsule-making pegs to produce capsule shells of distinctive shapes. By tapering the end of the body-producing peg while leaving the cap-making peg rounded, one manufacturer prepares capsules easily differentiated from those of other manufacturers (Pulvules, Eli Lilly). Another firm produces capsules with the ends of both the bodies and caps highly tapered, but not pointed (Spansule Capsules, Smith, Kline & French). Still another manufacturer makes distinctive and tamper-proof and leakproof capsules by sealing the joint between the two capsule parts with a colored band of gelatin (Kapseals, Parke-Davis). Removal of the band through tampering is evident, as the bands cannot be returned to place without a great deal of trouble and resealing

Fig. 5–6. *Body of capsules and their caps are shown as they move through automated capsule-making machine. Each machine is capable of producing 30,000 capsules per hour. It takes a 40-minute cycle to produce a capsule. (Courtesy of Smith, Kline & French Laboratories.)*

CONI-SNAP ™

Fig. 5–8. *Line drawings of the CONI-SNAP™ capsule in open, pre-closed, and closed positions. The tapered rims (1) avoid telescoping, the indentations (2) prevent premature opening, and the grooves (3) lock the two capsule parts together after the capsule has been filled. (Courtesy of Capsugel Division, Warner-Lambert Co.)*

Fig. 5–7. *A, Capsules being dipped for coloring on automated capsule-making equipment. (Courtesy of Smith, Kline & French Laboratories.) B, Z-Weld's gelatin seal fuses the two capsule halves together to create a one-piece capsule that is tamper-evident. (Courtesy of Raymond Automation Co.)*

with gelatin. Figure 5–7B depicts a gelatin seal for capsules.

A recent innovation in capsule shell design has been the Snap-Fit™, Coni-Snap™, and Coni Snap Supro™ hard gelatin capsules, depicted in Figures 5–8 and 5–9. The original Snap-Fit construction enables the two halves of the capsule shells to be positively joined through locking grooves in the shell walls. The two grooves fit into each other and thus ensure reliable closing of the filled capsule. During the closing process, the capsule body is inserted into the cap. With the high-capacity filling rates of the modern capsule filling machines (over 180,000 capsules per hour), capsule splitting ("telescoping") and/ or denting of the capsule shell occurs with the slightest contact between the two capsule-part rims when they are joined. This problem, which exists primarily with straight-walled capsule shells, led to the development of the Coni-Snap capsule, in which the rim of the capsule body is not straight, but tapered slightly (see Fig. 5–9). This reduces the risk of the capsule-rims touching on joining, and essentially eliminates

CONI-SNAP ™

1) Tapered rim to avoid telescoping (Coni-Snap ™).

2) Grooves which lock the two halves together once the capsule has been filled (Snap-Fit ™ principle).

3) Indentations to prevent premature opening.

Fig. 5–9. *Line drawings of the CONI-SNAP™ and CONI-SNAP SUPRO™ (on right) capsules. The latter is designed to be smaller and to have the lower portion of the capsule shell concealed except for the rounded end. This makes separation of the two parts more difficult and contributes to capsule integrity. (Courtesy of Capsugel Division, Warner-Lambert Co.)*

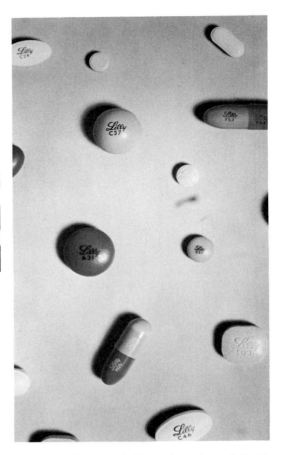

Fig. 5–10. *Examples of tablets and capsules marked with a letter-number code to facilitate identification. (Courtesy of Eli Lilly and Company.)*

the problem of splitting. In the Coni-Snap Supro capsules, the upper capsule part extends so far over the lower part that only the rounded edge of the latter is visible (Fig. 5–9). Opening of such a filled capsule is difficult because the lower surface offers less gripping surface to pull the two halves apart. This increases the security of the contents and the integrity of the capsule. As indicated previously in this text capsules may be imprinted with monograms of the manufacturer, the strength of the drug in the capsule, a code designation for product identification, or some other symbol making the product unique and distinguishable from other manufacturers' products (see Fig. 5–10).

Capsule Sizes

Empty gelatin capsules are manufactured in various sizes, varying in length, in diameter, and capacity. The size selected for use is determined by the amount of material to be encapsulated. Since the density and compressibility of a powder or a powder mixture will largely determine to what extent it may be packed into a capsule shell and because these are individual features of the materials themselves, there are no strict rules for predicting the proper capsule size for a given powder or formulation. However, comparison may be made with powders of well-known features (Table 5–2), and an initial judgment made as to the approximate capsule size to hold a specific amount of material, but the final decision is largely the result of trial. For human use, empty capsules ranging in size from 000, the largest, to 5, the smallest are commercially available, plain or colored (Fig. 5–11).[7] Larger capsules are available for veterinary use.

Table 5–2. Approximate Capacity of Empty Gelatin Capsules*

Drug Substance	Capsule Size								
	000	00	0	1	2	3	4	5	
Quinine Sulfate	650	390	325	227	195	130	97	65	mg
	10	6	5	3½	3	2	1½	1	grains
Sodium Bicarbonate	1430	975	715	510	390	325	260	130	mg
	22	15	11	8	6	5	4	2	grains
Aspirin	1040	650	520	325	260	195	162	97	mg
	16	10	8	5	4	3	2½	1½	grains

*Amount may vary according to the degree of pressure used in filling the capsules.

Hard gelatin capsules permit a wide prescribing latitude by the physician in that the pharmacist may extemporaneously prepare capsules containing a single chemical substance or a combination of drugs at the precise dosage level considered appropriate for the individual patient. This degree of flexibility is an advantage that capsules have as a dosage form over tablets, which are not prepared today in the community pharmacy.

Preparation of Filled Hard Gelatin Capsules

The preparation of filled hard gelatin capsules may be divided into the following steps:
1. Developing and preparing the formulation and selecting the size capsule.
2. Filling the capsule shells.
3. Cleaning and polishing the filled capsules.

Capsule Formulation and Selection of Capsule Size

In developing a capsule formulation, the goal is to prepare a formulation that results in ease of capsule filling during production and good drug release at accurate dosage when taken by the patient.

Generally, hard gelatin capsules are used to encapsulate between about 65 mg and 1 g of powdered material, including drug and any diluent required. As indicated in Table 5–2, the smallest capsule, a No. 5 capsule, is usually capable of holding at least 1 gr or 65 mg of powders of the type used in medicine. In order to fill completely a capsule of even the smallest size, a minimum of 65 mg of material is generally required. If the dose of the drug or the amount of drug to be placed in a single capsule is inadequate to fill the volume of the capsule, a diluent is necessary to add the proper degree of bulk to the drug to produce the proper fill. When the amount of drug to be administered in a single capsule is large enough to fill a capsule completely, a diluent may not be required. Lactose, microcrystalline cellulose, and pregelatinized starch are common diluents used in capsule filling.

In many instances the amount of drug placed in a single capsule falls within the usual dosage

Fig. 5–11. *Actual sizes of hard gelatin capsules. From left to right, sizes 000, 00, 0, 1, 2, 3, 4, and 5.*

range of that drug, a single capsule being taken as a dose of that particular medication. In other instances, especially when the amount of drug representing a usual dose is too large to place in a single capsule, two or more capsules may be required to provide the desired dose of that particular drug. For many medicinal agents, the initial or first dose may be larger than the subsequent doses, in which case more capsules may be required when drug therapy is initiated than when it is continued. In all instances, the amount of drug to be present in a single capsule is first determined, and the amount of diluent or inert materials, if any, is determined subsequently on the basis of its being needed to add bulk to the formulation, to separate chemically incompatible components of the formulation, or as a lubricant to facilitate the flow of the powder when an automatic capsule filling machine is utilized.

Magnesium stearate is a commonly used lubricant in capsule and tablet making to facilitate the flow of the drug-fill into the tableting or encapsulating machinery. Although small amounts of magnesium stearate are generally used (frequently less than 1%), the water-proofing characteristics of this insoluble material can pose a problem to the penetration of the solid dosage form by the gastrointestinal fluids intended to dissolve it. This obstacle to water and fluid penetration can delay the dissolution of the drug and its absorption. The practice of adding surfactants or wetting agents, as sodium lauryl sulfate, in capsule and tablet formulations to facilitate the wetting of the drug substance by the bathing of gastrointestinal fluids is a widely followed procedure in industry. The advantage of adding a wetting agent to capsule formulations of lithium carbonate to enhance dissolution has been demonstrated.[8] Even in instances in which magnesium stearate or some other water-insoluble lubricant is not used in capsule formulation, when the gelatin shell of a capsule dissolves, liquid must displace the air that surrounds the dry powder within the capsule and penetrate the drug before the capsule fill can be dispersed and dissolved. Powders of poorly soluble drugs have a tendency to float on the surface of the fluid and agglomerate to further minimize air-liquid contact and if wetting does not occur readily, dissolution is delayed.

Whether it be the presence of a lubricant, surfactant, or some other pharmaceutic excipient, formulation can influence the bioavailability of a drug substance and can account for differences in drug effects which may be encountered between two capsule products of the same medicinal substance.

Eutectic mixtures of drugs, or mixtures that tend to liquefy, may require a diluent or absorbant such as magnesium carbonate, kaolin, or light magnesium oxide to separate physically the interacting agents and to absorb any liquefied material. Generally, when such materials are used for this purpose, approximately 120 mg of diluent are used for each capsule. Drugs that are chemically incompatible with other drugs of the formulation may be physically separated by the same means. Another method for separating drugs within a capsule is to place one of the interfering substances in a small capsule that is then placed within a larger capsule containing the other formulative components. Instead of the smaller capsule, granules, pellets, or compressed tablets may be used for this purpose.

The use of tablets within capsules is also quite common in the extemporaneous filling of a small number of capsules, each to contain a very small quantity of a potent drug. In these instances, many pharmacists insert a small tablet of the desired strength of the potent drug in each capsule, filling the remaining capsule space with the specified amounts of other required less potent and more conveniently weighed drugs and/or with an inert diluent as is necessary.

Solid substances to be placed in a capsule must be thoroughly mixed before the capsules may be filled. Consideration must be given to the density and particle size of powders to be combined as the capsule fill. Powders may be more uniformly mixed if their particle size and density are approximately the same.

Capsules of gelatin are unsuitable for the encapsulation of aqueous liquids, because water softens the gelatin to produce distortion of the capsules. Naturally, this would prompt the loss of the liquid contents of the capsules. However, some liquids such as fixed or volatile oils that do not interfere with the stability of the gelatin shells may be placed in gelatin capsules which then may be sealed to ensure the retention of the liquid. In large scale production, liquids are placed in *soft gelatin* capsules which are sealed during their manufacture. Soft capsules are discussed later in this chapter.

Rather than placing a liquid in a capsule as such, it may be desirable in certain instances to absorb a small amount of liquid by mixing it with an absorbent, inert powder. The powder may then be placed in capsules in the usual manner. If the liquid is volatile, it may be necessary to seal the capsules.

AMOUNT OF FORMULA PREPARED. On a small or large industrial scale, the amount of formula prepared is that amount (drugs and diluents) necessary to fill the desired number of capsules. On an industrial scale this may mean many thousands of capsules. In the community pharmacy an individual prescription may call for the extemporaneous preparation of only six or a dozen capsules. Any slight loss in fill material during the preparation of the (powder) mixture or during the capsule-filling process will not materially affect the preparation of an industrial batch, but on a small scale, as in the filling of a prescription, a slight loss of fill material will likely result in an adequate amount of powder for the last capsule. To ensure enough fill for the last capsule in the extemporaneous compounding of small numbers of capsules, the community pharmacist generally calculates for the preparation of one more capsule than is required. This procedure may not be followed for capsules containing a controlled substance, because the amount of drug used and that called for in the prescription must strictly coincide.

SELECTION OF CAPSULE SIZE. The selection of the capsule size is best done during the development of the formulation, because the amount of any inert materials to be employed is dependent upon the size or capacity of the capsule to be selected. When the formulation of medicinal materials does not require diluent to increase the bulk, the capsule size may be selected after the development and preparation of the formulation. As indicated earlier, for drugs having large doses the amount of medication in a capsule may not necessarily correspond to a full dose of that medication. Smaller capsules may be required in instances in which the drug is to be taken by youngsters or by elderly patients, and more than a single capsule may be required to provide the dose of the drug. In instances in which there is a specific need for a small capsule, the capsule size may be selected first, and the formulation may be based on that capsule size. Depending upon the particular situation and requirements of the intended patient, the capsule size may be determined by the for-

mulation, or the formulation may be altered by the capsule size.

A properly filled capsule should have its body filled with the drug mixture and its cap fully extended down the body so as to enclose the powder in the body. The cap is not used to hold powder but to retain it, and a capsule size should be selected to meet this requirement.

Filling the Capsule Shells

When filling a small number of capsules in the pharmacy, the pharmacist generally uses the "punch" method. In this method the pharmacist takes the precise number of empty capsules to be filled from his stock container. By counting out the capsules as the initial step rather than taking a capsule from stock as each one is filled, the pharmacist guards against filling an erroneous number of capsules and avoids contaminating the stock container of empty capsules with drug particles that may cling to his fingertips. The powder to be encapsulated is placed on a sheet of clean paper or a glass or porcelain plate and with a spatula is formed into a cake having a depth of approximately one-fourth to one-third the length of the capsule body. Then the empty capsule body is held between the thumb and forefinger and "punched" vertically into the powder cake repeatedly until filled. Some pharmacists wear surgical gloves or rubber finger cots to avoid handling the capsules with bare fingers. Because the amount of powder packed into a capsule depends upon the degree of compression, the pharmacist should punch each capsule in the same manner and after capping weigh it to ensure equal and accurate filling. When nonpotent materials are being placed in capsules, the first filled capsule should be weighed (using an empty capsule of the same size on the opposite balance pan to counter the weight of the shell) to assist in the determination of the proper capsule size and degree of compression to be used in filling, and then other capsules should be weighed periodically to check the uniformity of this operation. When potent drugs are being used, each capsule should be weighed after filling to ensure accuracy. Such weighings protect against the uneven filling of capsules and the premature exhaustion or lack of total utilization of the powder mixture. After the body of a capsule has been filled and the cap has been placed on the body, the body is squeezed gently to distribute some powder to

Fig. 5–12. *Hand-operated capsule-filling machine. The model shown fills 96 capsules per operation and is made to obtain an hourly production of 1000 capsules. Shown with the basic machine are the tray used to hold the fill over the empty capsules, the spreader and roller used to distribute the fill material in the tray and permit it to enter the capsules uniformly, and the packer used to compact the fill in the capsules.*

the cap end of the capsule to give the product a full appearance. Some pharmacists place a small portion of powder in the cap before placing it on the body. Care must be exercised not to overfill a capsule. The cap should fit completely down on the body.

Granular material that does not lend itself well to the "punch" method of filling capsules may be poured into each capsule individually from the powder paper on which it was first weighed.

Pharmacists that prepare capsules on a regular or somewhat extensive basis may use hand-operated capsule machines. These machines are available in capacities of 24, 96, 100, and 144 capsules. When efficiently operated, they can produce from about 2000 capsules per working day for the smallest machine up to 2000 capsules per hour for the largest (Fig. 5–12).

Machines developed for industrial use can automatically remove the caps from empty capsules, fill the capsules, replace the caps, and clean the outside of the capsules at a rate of up to 165,000 capsules and greater per hour per

unit (Fig. 5–13). Most industrial capsule-filling machines are designed to fill the body of the empty capsule with powder and scrape off the excess at the level of fill before capping (Fig. 5–14). Therefore the formulation for each industrially produced capsule must be such that the filled body contains the amount of powder in which the right amount of drug and diluent are present. Periodic checks are made along the production line by taking capsules from production and weighing them for total powder and assaying them for active ingredient. Figure 5–15 depicts a process flow diagram for automated capsule filling in which a number of components are blended and placed in capsules.

The USP requires adherence to standards for *content uniformity* and *weight variation* to assure the uniformity of dosage units. These tests are described in the USPXXII-NFXVII.

Capsule Sealing

The capsule-tampering incidents of 1982 (refer to p. 125) rekindled industry interest in both tamper-resistant packaging and the protective sealing of capsules, particularly for over-the-counter products. The capsule-sealing process of *banding* (e.g., Kapseals, Parke-Davis; Qualicaps, Elanco) has been utilized for a number of years. In this process, the two capsule parts are sealed with a gelatin or polymer band at the seam of the cap and body. More recently, a tamper-resistant seal on hard gelatin capsules was developed in which the contact areas of the cap and body are wetted with a mixture of water and ethanol and then thermally bonded at 104° to 113°F.[9] Capsule-sealing equipment may be linked with capsule-filling equipment to maintain production levels of up to 180,000 capsules per hour per unit.

Cleaning and Polishing Capsules

Capsules prepared on a small scale or on a large scale may have small amounts of the powder formulation adhering to the outside of the capsules. This powder, which may be bitter or otherwise unpalatable, should be removed before packaging or dispensing to improve the appearance of the capsules and to preserve their quality of being tasteless on administration. On a small scale, capsules may be cleaned individually or in small numbers by rubbing them with a clean gauze or cloth. On a large scale, many capsule-filling machines are affixed with a cleaning vacuum that removes any extraneous

Fig. 5–13. *Osaka Automatic Capsule Filler (Model R-180), capable of filling up to 165,000 capsules per hour. (Courtesy of Sharples-Stokes Div., Stokes-Merrill, Pennwalt Corporation.)*

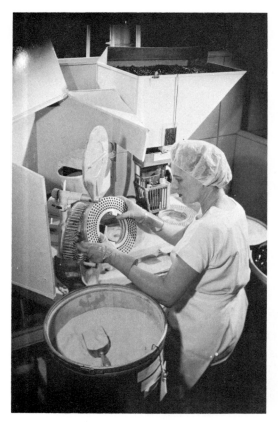

Fig. 5–14. *Filling of capsules is a semiautomatic operation. Capsules are automatically seated in holes in the metal form which is then separated to open the capsules. The form containing the bottom halves of the capsules is then filled with the dry therapeutic agent. The top section of the form is replaced, and the two halves of the capsules are automatically joined as they are ejected. (Courtesy of Parke, Davis & Company.)*

material from the capsules as they exit the equipment. Figure 5–16 shows an industrial method of cleaning and polishing hard filled capsules using the Accela-Cota apparatus.

Soft Gelatin Capsules

Soft gelatin capsules are prepared from shells of gelatin to which glycerin or a polyhydric alcohol such as sorbitol has been added to render the gelatin elastic or plastic-like. These capsules, which may be oblong, elliptical, or spherical in shape, may be employed to contain liquids, suspensions, pasty materials, or dry powders. Soft gelatin capsules are usually prepared, filled, and sealed in a continuous operation using spe-

cialized equipment. Empty soft gelatin capsules may be prepared and hermetically sealed (to prevent the walls from collapsing and adhering to one another) for filling at a later time, but this is not usually performed.

Soft gelatin capsules are useful when it is desirable to seal the medication within the capsule. The capsules are especially important to contain liquid drugs or drug solutions. Also, volatile drug substances or drug materials especially susceptible to deterioration in the presence of air may be better suited to a soft gelatin capsule than to the hard gelatin capsules.

Soft gelatin capsules are handsome and are easily swallowed by the patient. However, they are not easily prepared except on a large scale and then only with specialized equipment (Fig. 5–17).

Preparation of Soft Gelatin Capsules

Soft gelatin capsules may be prepared by the plate process, using a set of molds to form the capsules, or by the more efficient and productive die processes (rotary or reciprocating). By the plate process, a warm sheet of gelatin (plain or colored) is placed on the bottom plate of the mold, and the liquid medication is evenly poured on it. Then a second sheet of the prepared gelatin is carefully laid in place on top of the medication, and the top plate of the mold is put in place. The entire mold is then subjected to a press where pressure is applied to form, fill, and seal the capsules simultaneously. The capsules are then removed and washed with a solvent harmless to the capsules. Highly automated machines have been developed for the preparation of soft capsules by the plate process and are in use today in industry.

However, most industrially produced soft capsules are probably prepared by the rotary die process, a method developed in 1933 by Robert P. Scherer. By this method, liquid gelatin flowing from an overhead tank is formed into two continuous ribbons by the rotary die machine and brought together between twin rotating dies (Fig. 5–18). At the same time, metered fill material is injected between the ribbons precisely at the moment that the dies form pockets of the gelatin ribbons. These pockets of fill-containing gelatin are then sealed by pressure and heat, the capsules then being severed from the ribbon by the same process. The soft gelatin capsules may be manufactured in a number of shapes, including round, oval, ob-

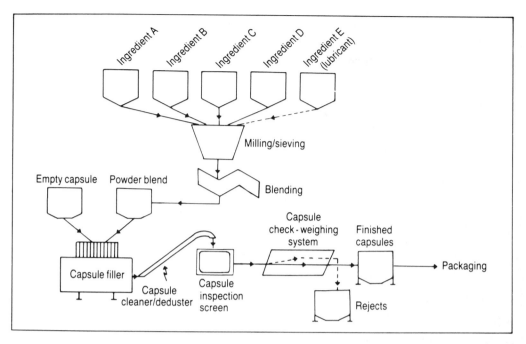

Fig. 5–15. *Process flow diagram for automated capsule filling. (From Yelvig, M.: Principles of process automation for liquid and solid dosage forms. Pharm. Technol., 8:47, 1984.)*

Fig. 5–16. *Cleaning and polishing hard filled capsules using the Accela-Cota apparatus. (Courtesy of Eli Lilly and Company.)*

long, tube-shape, and others. They may also be prepared of single or two-tone color, the latter resulting from the employment of two different colored ribbons of gelatin to form the sides of the capsule. A modern adaptation of this method, the Accogel Capsule Machine developed by Lederle Laboratories, permits the enclosure of dry powder or liquids in soft gelatin capsules. In addition, through the use of an adaptor, the machine is capable of enclosing preformed tablets in a gelatin film.

The reciprocating die process is similar to the rotary process in that ribbons of gelatin are formed and used to encapsulate the fill, but it differs in the actual encapsulating process. The gelatin ribbons are fed between a set of vertical dies that continually open and close to form rows of pockets in the gelatin ribbons. These pockets are filled with the medication and are sealed, shaped, and cut out of the film as they progress through the machinery. As the capsules are cut from the ribbons, they fall into refrigerated tanks which prevent the capsules from adhering to one another and from getting dull.

Application of Soft Gelatin Capsules

Soft gelatin capsules may be used to contain a variety of liquid and dry fills. Liquids which

Fig. 5–17.   *Rotary die process equipment. A, Gelatin tank; B, spreader box; C, gelatin ribbon casting drum; D, mineral oil lubricant bath; E, medicine tank; F, filling pump; G, encapsulating mechanism; H, capsule conveyor; I, capsule washer; J, infrared dryer; K, capsule drying tunnel; L, gelatin net receiver. (Courtesy of R.P. Scherer Corporation.)*

Fig. 5–18. *Schematic drawing of rotary die process. (Courtesy of R.P. Scherer Corporation.)*

Fig. 5–19. *Cleaning and inspection of hard filled capsules. (Courtesy of The Upjohn Company.)*

may be encapsulated into soft gelatin capsules include:[10]

1. Water immiscible, volatile and nonvolatile liquids such as vegetable and aromatic oils, aromatic and aliphatic hydrocarbons, chlorinated hydrocarbons, ethers, esters, alcohols, and organic acids.
2. Water miscible, nonvolatile liquids such as polyethylene glycols, and nonionic surface active agents as polysorbate 80.
3. Water miscible and relatively nonvolatile compounds, as propylene glycol and isopropyl alcohol, depending upon factors as concentration used and packaging conditions.

Liquids which can easily migrate through the capsule shell cannot be encapsulated into soft gelatin capsules. These materials include: water, above 5%, and low molecular weight water soluble and volatile organic compounds such as alcohols, ketones, acids, amines, and esters.

Solids may be encapsulated into soft gelatin capsules as solutions in one of the suitable liquid solvents, as suspensions, or as dry powders, granules, or pelletized materials.

Among the drugs commercially prepared in soft gelatin capsules are: ethchlorvynol (Placi-

dyl, Abbott), demeclocycline HCl (Declomycin, Lederle), chlorotrianisene (TACE, Merrell Dow), chloral hydrate (Noctec, Squibb), digoxin (Lanoxicaps, Burroughs Wellcome), vitamin A, and vitamin E, (Aquasol E, Armour) and docusate calcium (Surfak, Hoechst-Roussel).

Inspecting, Counting, Packaging, and Storing Capsules

Whether capsules are produced on a small or a large scale, they are required to pass not only tests of potency and uniformity but also a visual or electronic inspection to ensure that there are no flaws in the appearance of the capsules (Fig. 5–19). All capsules produced by the same method should be uniformly colored, uniformly filled, and uniformly shaped. As the pharmacist extemporaneously compounds a prescription for capsules in the community pharmacy, he must take care to prepare uniform capsules. On a large scale, however, the highly productive automatic capsule machines are capable of producing great numbers of capsules simultaneously, and these must be inspected visually or electronically as they are produced. Defective capsules are removed. If the number of capsules removed is excessively high, some production default in the capsule-producing mechanism of the machines is suspected and checked out by machinists.

In the pharmacy, capsules that have been extemporaneously compounded or those taken from a stock package of prefabricated capsules are usually counted by hand, using specially designed counting trays to facilitate the procedure and to ensure the hygienic transfer of the capsules into the final container. One of these trays, the Abbott counting tray, is depicted in Figure 5–20. In using this tray, the pharmacist pours a supply of capsules or tablets from the bulk source onto the clean tray, and using the spatula he counts the desired number of capsules or tablets, sweeping them into the trough as he counts. When the correct number is in the trough, the pharmacist closes the trough cover, picks up the tray, returns the uncounted dosage units to the bulk container by means of the lip

at the back of the tray, places the prescription contained at the opening of the trough, and carefully transfers the capsules or tablets into the container. By this method, the capsules or tablets remain untouched by the pharmacist. To prevent contamination of tablets and capsules, the tray must be wiped clean after each counting, as powder tends to get on the tray, especially when uncoated tablets are counted.

On a larger scale, as occurs in some community and hospital pharmacy settings, small automatic counting and container-filling apparatus is becoming increasing popular and useful. Some of these counting machines are shown in Figures 5–21 and 5–22.

On an industrial scale, solid dosage forms may be counted by means of large counting trays. The operator pours the dosage units on a tray containing the desired number of perforations, rotates the tray until each perforation is filled with a capsule or tablet, allows the excess to slide off the tray, and then transfers the

Fig. 5–20. *Steps in the counting of solid dosage units with the Abbott Sanitary Counting Tray: (1) placing units from stock package onto tray, (2) counting and transferring units to trough, (3) returning excess units to stock container, and (4) placing counted units into prescription container.*

Fig. 5–21. *Mini-Counter II, small automatic tablet and capsule counting and filling apparatus. (Courtesy of Production Equipment Co.)*

Fig. 5–22. *Versacount Model automatic tablet and capsule counting and filling apparatus. (Courtesy of Production Equipment Co.)*

counted number from the perforations into the container. This method has largely been replaced by highly automated counting devices that both count and transfer the desired number of dosage units into the containers. Machines have been developed to count and fill a dozen or more containers simultaneously, capping and moving the filled bottles along the production line where they can again be inspected, labeled, and finally packaged into cartons. One of these machines is shown in Figure 5–23.

Capsules are usually packaged in glass or in plastic containers, some containing packets of a desiccant to prevent the absorption of excessive moisture by the capsules. Soft capsules have a greater tendency than do hard capsules to soften and adhere to one another, and they must be maintained in a cool, dry place. In fact, all capsules remain stable longer if maintained tightly sealed in a cool place of low humidity.

The unit dose and strip packaging of solid dosage forms, particularly by pharmacies which service nursing homes and hospitals, provides sanitary handling of the medications, ease of identification, and security in accountability for medications. Typical small scale strip packaging equipment and commercial unit-dose packages of capsules and tablets are presented in Figures 5–24 and 5–25 respectively.

Official Capsules

There are over a hundred officially recognized medications in capsule form, representing a wide range of therapeutic categories. Examples of these are presented in Table 5–3.

Specialized Capsule Forms

There are some specialized capsule forms, as those containing drugs to be released in a controlled-release manner. These are discussed later in this chapter.

Tablets

Tablets are solid dosage forms of medicinal substances usually prepared with the aid of suitable pharmaceutical adjuncts. Tablets may vary in size, shape, weight, hardness, thickness, disintegration characteristics, and in other aspects, depending upon the intended use of the tablets and their method of manufacture. The majority of tablets are used in the oral ad-

Fig. 5–23. *Large Merrill filling machine that fills 16 bottles with 200 tablets each at one time. A flipper gate in the upper manifold directs the tablets into one row of bottles while the other filled row is evacuated and a new row of bottles moves into place. (Courtesy of The Upjohn Company.)*

ministration of drugs, and many of these tablets are prepared with colorants, flavorants, and coatings of various types. Other tablets such as those intended to be administered sublingually, buccally, or vaginally may not contain the same adjuncts or be prepared to possess the same types of features as tablets for oral administration. Many of the advantages of tablets for the oral administration of drugs have already been presented at the outset of this chapter and previously in Chapter 3.

Tablets are prepared primarily by compression. A limited number of tablets are prepared by molding. Compressed tablets are manufactured with tablet machines capable of exerting great pressure in compacting the powdered or granulated tableting material through the use of various shaped punches and dies (Fig. 5–26).

The tablet presses are heavy equipment of various capacities selected for use on the basis of the type of tablets to be manufactured and the production rate desired. Molded tablets are prepared by tablet machinery or manually by forcing dampened tablet material into a mold from which the formed tablet is then ejected and allowed to dry. Molded tablets are discussed in detail in Chapter 13.

Types of Tablets

The various types of tablets are described as follows, with the abbreviations for the tablet types in parentheses.

COMPRESSED TABLETS (C.T.). Compressed tablets, prepared by single compression, occur in various shapes and sizes and usually contain in addition to the medicinal substance(s), a num-

Fig. 5–24. *A strip packager for the unit dose dispensing of solid dosage forms. Drug information is imprinted on each individual packge unit. The model shown has a fully automatic cutoff from 1 to 24 dosage units and is especially suited to unit-dose packaging and dispensing in hospitals, dispensaries, nursing homes, and clinics. (Courtesy of Lakso Company, Inc.)*

ber of pharmaceutical adjuncts including (a) *diluents* or *fillers*, which add the necessary bulk to a formulation to prepare tablets of the desired size; (b) *binders* or *adhesives*, which promote the adhesion of the particles of the formulation, enabling a granulation to be prepared and the maintenance of the integrity of the final tablet; (c) *disintegrators* or *disintegrating agents*, which promote the breakup of the tablets after administration to smaller particles for more ready drug availability; (d) *antiadherents, glidants, lubricants* or *lubricating agents*, which enhance the flow of the tableting material into the tablet dies, prevent the sticking of this material to the punches and dies, and produce tablets having a sheen; and (e) *miscellaneous adjuncts* such as colorants and flavorants. After compression, some compressed tablets may be coated with various materials as described later. Most compressed tablets are employed for the oral administration of drugs, but some may be used for the sublingual, buccal, or vaginal administration of drugs.

MULTIPLE COMPRESSED TABLETS (M.C.T.). Multiple compressed tablets are prepared by subjection to more than a single compression. The result may be a multiple-layered tablet or a tablet-within-a-tablet, the inner tablet being the *core* and the outer portion being the *shell* (Fig. 5–27). Layered tablets are prepared by the initial compaction of a portion of fill material in a die and the addition of one or more portions of fill material to the same die, each additional fill being compressed to form a two- or three-layered tablet, depending upon the number of separate fills. Usually each portion of fill material contains a different medicinal agent separated from the others for reasons of incompatibility, for providing drug release in two or more stages, or simply for the unique appearance of a multiple-layered tablet. Generally each

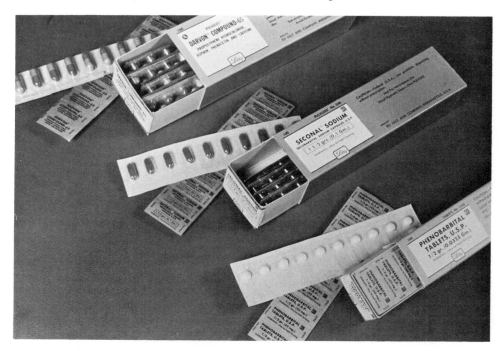

Fig. 5–25. *Example of unit-dose packaging of tablets and capsules. The drug name and other information are imprinted on the backing portion of each unit. (Courtesy of Eli Lilly and Company.)*

portion of fill is colored differently to prepare a multiple-colored as well as a multiple-layered tablet. In the preparation of tablets having another compressed tablet as the inner core, special machines are required to place the preformed tablet precisely within the die for the second compression and the new fill material around the core tablet.

SUGAR-COATED TABLETS (S.C.T.). Compressed tablets may be coated with a colored or an uncolored sugar. The coating is water-soluble and is quickly dissolved after swallowing. It serves the varied purposes of protecting the drug from the air and humidity and providing a taste or a smell barrier to objectional tasting or smelling drugs. Further, it enhances the appearance of many compressed tablets. Disadvantages to sugar-coating tablets are the time and expertise required by the process and the increase in the size and weight of the compressed tablets. Coated tablets may be 50% larger and heavier than the original uncoated tablets.

CHOCOLATE-COLORED TABLETS (C.C.T.). Chocolate-colored tablets are mainly of historic importance, because chocolate was once used to coat and color compressed tablets. Today chocolate has been replaced by other colorants such as iron oxides which are used to simulate the chocolate color.

FILM-COATED TABLETS (F.C.T.). Film-coated tablets are compressed tablets coated with a thin layer of a water-insoluble or water-soluble polymer capable of forming a film over the tablet. The film is generally colored and has the advantage over sugar-coatings in that it is more durable, less bulky, and less time-consuming to apply. The coating ruptures in the gastrointestinal tract.

ENTERIC-COATED TABLETS (E.C.T.). Enteric-coated tablets are tablets with a coating that resists dissolution or disruption in the stomach but not in the intestines, thereby allowing for tablet transit through the stomach in favor of tablet disintegration and drug dissolution and absorption from the intestines. This technique is employed in instances in which the drug substance is destroyed by gastric acid, is irritating to the gastric mucosa, or when by-pass of the stomach enhances drug absorption from the intestines to a significant extent.

BUCCAL OR SUBLINGUAL TABLETS. Buccal or sublingual tablets are generally flat, oval tablets intended to be dissolved in the buccal pouch

Table 5–3. Examples of Some Official Capsules

Official Capsule	Some Representative Commercial Capsules	Capsule Strengths Usually Available	Category
Acetaminophen	Tylenol (McNeil)	500 mg	Analgesic; antipyretic
Amoxicillin	Amoxil (Beecham)	250 and 500 mg	Antibacterial
Ampicillin	Amcill (Parke Davis); Polycillin (Bristol); Omnipen (Wyeth)	250 and 500 mg	Antibacterial
Aspirin	. . .	300 mg	Analgesic
Cephalexin	Keflex (Dista)	250 and 500 mg	Antibacterial
Chloral Hydrate	Noctec (Squibb)	250, 500, and 1000 mg	Hypnotic; sedative
Cloxacillin Sodium	Tegopen (Bristol)	250 and 500 mg	Antibacterial
Diphenhydramine HCl	Benadryl HCl (Parke Davis)	25 and 50 mg	Antihistaminic
Doxycycline Hyclate	Vibramycin (Pfizer)	50 and 100 mg	Antibacterial
Erythromycin Estolate	Ilosone (Dista)	125 and 250 mg	Antibacterial
Flurazepam HCl	Dalmane (Roche)	15 and 30 mg	Hypnotic
Gemfibrozil	Lopid (P-D)	300 mg	Antihyperlipidemic
Griseofulvin	Grisactin (Ayerst)	125 and 250 mg	Antifungal
Indomethacin	Indocin (Merck, Sharp & Dohme)	25 and 50 mg	Antiinflammatory; antipyretic; analgesic
Levodopa	Larodopa (Roche)	100, 250, and 500 mg	Antiparkinsonian
Loperamide HCl	Imodium (Janssen)	2 mg	Antidiarrheal
Nifedipine	Procardia (Pfizer)	10 and 20 mg	Calcium-channel blocker
Oxazepam	Serax (Wyeth)	10, 15 and 30 mg	Antianxiety
Propoxyphene HCl	Darvon (Lilly)	32 and 65 mg	Analgesic
Quinine Sulfate	Legatrin (Scholl)	130 mg	Antimyotonic
Rifampin	Rifadin (Merrell Dow)	150 mg	Antiinfective
Secobarbital Sodium	Seconal Sodium (Lilly)	30 mg	Hypnotic; sedative
Tetracycline HCl	Achromycin V (Lederle); Sumycin HCl (Squibb)	250 and 500 mg	Antibacterial; antiamebic; antirickettsial

Fig. 5–26. *Steps in the compression of a tablet on a single punch press. (Courtesy of Cherry-Burrell Corporation.)*

Fig. 5–27. *Diagram of multiple-compressed tablets. A, having a core of one drug and a shell of another, and B, a multiple-layered tablet of two drugs.*

(buccal tablets) or beneath the tongue *(sublingual tablets)* for absorption through the oral mucosa. They are useful in providing for the absorption of drugs that are destroyed by the gastric juice and/or poorly absorbed from the gastrointestinal tract. Although few drugs are absorbed from the oral cavity, some important ones to note are nitroglycerin and many steroid hormones. Tablets intended for buccal administration (as progesterone tablets) are prepared to erode or to dissolve slowly, while those for sublingual use (as nitroglycerin tablets) dissolve very promptly to give rapid drug effects.

CHEWABLE TABLETS. Chewable tablets, which have a smooth, rapid disintegration when chewed or allowed to dissolve in the mouth, yield a creamy base of a specially flavored and colored mannitol. The tablets are especially useful in tablet formulations for children and are commonly employed in the preparation of multiple vitamin tablets. They find other uses in the administration of antacids and antiflatulents. These tablets are prepared by compression.

EFFERVESCENT TABLETS. Effervescent tablets are prepared by compressing granular effervescent salts or other materials having the capacity to release gas when in contact with water. Commercially, alkalinizing-analgesic tablets are frequently made to effervesce to encourage fast disintegration and solution when added to water or an aqueous beverage.

TABLET TRITURATES (T.T.). Tablet triturates are small, usually cylindrical, molded (M.T.T.) or compressed tablets (C.T.T.) containing small amounts of usually potent drugs. Most tablet triturates are produced industrially by compression but they may also be prepared by molding for small-scale production, since the molds are more easily used and considerably less expensive than tablet presses. Tablet triturates must be readily and completely soluble in water; thus when these tablets are prepared by compression, a minimal amount of pressure is exerted. A combination of sucrose and lactose is usually the diluent, and any water-insoluble material is avoided in the formulation. Some tablet triturates are used for the oral administration of drugs and some for sublingual use (as nitroglycerin tablets). Pharmacists may employ tablet triturates in compounding procedures in the preparation of other solid or liquid dosage forms. For instance, the tablets may be easily inserted into capsules to provide accurate amounts of potent drug substances. They may

also be used by pharmacists to fortify liquid preparations, as prescribed, by dissolving the appropriate number of tablets in a small portion of water and then bringing the preparation to the required volume with the liquid medication being fortified.

HYPODERMIC TABLETS (H.T.). Hypodermic tablets are tablet triturates originally intended for use by the physician in his extemporaneous preparation of parenteral solutions. The physician dissolved the required number of tablets in a suitable vehicle, attained sterility of the preparation as best he could, and performed the injection. The tablets were intended as a convenience to the physician, since he could carry in his medicine bag a variety of lightweight hypodermic tablets and a suitable vehicle and prepare corresponding injections of the desired strength and volume according to the needs of the individual patients. However, the difficulty in achieving sterility and the current availability of a large number of drugs in injectable form, some in disposable syringes, have essentially eliminated the need for hypodermic tablets.

DISPENSING TABLETS (D.T.). Dispensing tablets are no longer in general use. In retrospect, they might better have been termed *compounding tablets*, because they were used by the pharmacist in compounding and not dispensed as such to the patient. The tablets containing relatively large amounts of highly potent drug substances were prepared as a convenience to the pharmacist, enabling him to obtain quickly accurately measured amounts of potent drugs in preparing other solid or liquid dosage forms. The diluent or base of the tablets was usually water-soluble to permit the preparation of clear aqueous solutions. Dispensing tablets were prepared by either molding or compression. Disintegrating agents, water-insoluble lubricants, colorants, flavorants, and coatings were not used in the preparation of dispensing tablets. Primarily because of the potential hazard in the inadvertent dispensing of these tablets to patients, dispensing tablets are not used today. Nowadays, the pharmacist more commonly employs commercially prepared compressed tablets or tablet triturates in the compounding of prescriptions calling for a drug substance unavailable in bulk, but available in these dosage forms.

CONTROLLED RELEASE TABLETS. Controlled release tablets and capsules will be discussed later in this chapter.

Fig. 5–28. *Packages of a drug product of two different tablet strengths, with one scored for ease of breaking in half. (Courtesy of Marion Laboratories.)*

Compressed Tablets

Characteristics and Quality

The physical features of compressed tablets are well known to even the layman. Some tablets are round, others oblong, and still others triangular. Some are thick; others are thin. Some tablets have larger diameters than others. Some tablets are flat; others have varying degrees of convexity. Some are *scored* or grooved in halves or in quadrants to permit the fairly accurate breaking of the tablet for the administration of a partial amount or for easier administration of smaller pieces of the tablet. Scored tablets are generally grooved on a single side (Fig. 5–28). Some tablets are engraved with a symbol of the manufacturer to denote the company, the product, or both. Tablets are produced in different colors to make them further distinctive.

Tablet diameters and shapes are determined by the die and punches used for the compres-

Fig. 5–29. *Contours of the punches determine the shape of the tablets. From left to right, flat face, shallow cup, standard cup, deep cup, and modified ball. (Courtesy of Cherry-Burrell Corporation.)*

sion of the tablet. The less concave the punches, the more flat the resulting tablets; conversely, the more concave the punches, the more convex the resulting tablets (Fig. 5–29). Punches having raised impressions will produce recessed impressions on the tablets; punches having recessed etchings will produce tablets having raised impression or monograms. Monograms may be placed on one or on both sides of a tablet, depending upon whether monogram-producing lower and/or upper punches are used (Fig. 5–30).

The thickness of a tablet is determined by the amount of fill permitted to enter the die and the amount of pressure applied during compression.

In addition to these apparent features of tablets, pharmacists are aware that tablets must meet other physical specifications that are generally unknown to the layman. These include tablet weight, tablet thickness, tablet hardness, tablet disintegration, content uniformity and for drug dissolution. These factors must be controlled within the production of a batch of tablets as well as from production batch to production batch in order to guarantee not only the outward appearance of the product but also its therapeutic efficacy (Fig. 5–31).

TABLET WEIGHT. The amount of fill placed in the die of a tablet press will determine the weight of the resulting tablet. The volume of fill (granulation or powder) permitted to enter the dies must be adjusted with the first few tablets produced to yield tablets of the desired weight and content. Adjustment is necessary, since tablet formulations are based on the weight of the tablets to be prepared. For example, if a tablet is to contain 20 mg of a drug substance and if 10,000 tablets are to be produced, 200 g of that drug are employed in the formula. After the addition of the pharmaceutical additives such as the diluent, disintegrant, lubricant, and binder, the formulation may weigh 2000 g, which means that each tablet must weigh 200 mg in order for 20 mg of drug to be present. Thus, the depth of fill in the tablet die must be adjusted to hold a volume of granulation weighing 200 mg.[11] Once the fill is properly set, production may start.

The USP contains a weight variation standard to which the official tablets must conform. A control of quality is necessary during production, and periodic checks are made of tablet weights, since a great expense would be in-

Fig. 5–30. *Various Stokes punches and dies for the production of distinctive tablets. (Courtesy of Stokes Equipment Division, Pennwalt Chemicals Corporation.)*

curred if the tablets were found *after* production not to meet the specifications (Fig. 5–32). During production, there is time to determine the cause of any problems and to make the necessary adjustments.

Naturally, the size of tablets produced depends not only on the volume and weight of the fill but also on the diameter of the die and upon the pressure applied to the fill on compaction.

TABLET THICKNESS. As indicated above, the thickness desired in a tablet must be coordinated with the volume of fill issued to the die, the diameter of the die, and the pressure applied to the fill by the punches. To produce tablets of uniform thickness during production and between productions for the same formulation, care must be exercised to employ the same volume of fill and the same pressure. Tablets of the same product which vary in size not only might alarm the patient but also might cause problems in packaging. Tablets are measured with a caliper during production to make certain of consistent thickness (Fig. 5–33). It should be pointed out that since pressure ap-

plied affects not only the thickness of the tablet but also its hardness and since the latter factor is probably the more important of the two, the thickness of a tablet is varied more by the size of the die and the fill permitted than by the pressure. Pressure adjustments are made primarily to control the softness or the hardness of the tablets.

TABLET HARDNESS. It is not unusual for a tablet press to exert as little as 3000 and as much as 40,000 pounds of force in the production of tablets. Generally, the greater the pressure applied, the harder the tablets, although the characteristics of the granulation also determine the hardness of the tablet. Certain tablets, such as lozenges and buccal tablets that are intended to dissolve slowly, are intentionally made hard; other tablets, such as compressed tablet triturates that are intended to dissolve rapidly, are made soft. In general, tablets should be sufficiently hard to resist breaking during packaging, shipment, and normal handling and yet soft enough to dissolve or disintegrate properly after administered or to be broken between the fingers when a part of a tablet is to be taken.

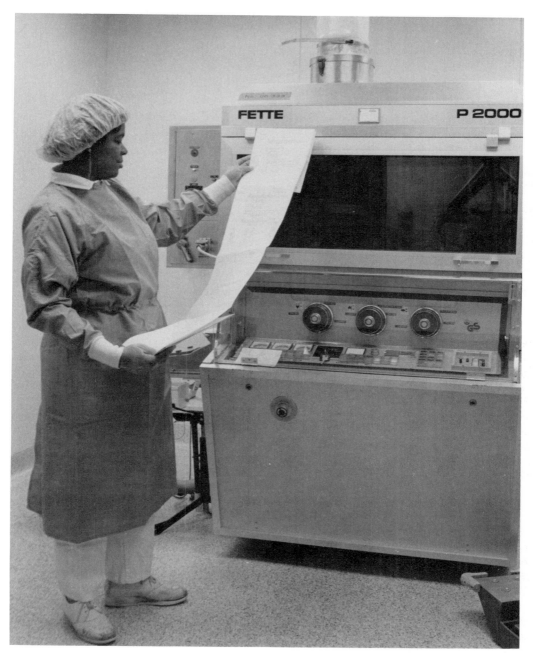

Fig. 5–31. *Quality control in the manufacturing of tablets. (Courtesy of Eli Lilly and Company.)*

Fig. 5–32.   *An automatic balance that weighs product and prints statistics to determine compliance with USP weight variation requirements for tablets. (Courtesy of Mocon Modern Controls, Inc.)*

Fig. 5–33.   *Tablet gauge used to measure the thickness of tablets. (Courtesy of Eli Lilly and Company.)*

A number of tablet hardness testers in use today measure the degree of force (in kilograms, pounds, or in arbitrary units) that is required to break a tablet (Figs. 5–34 and 5–35). In the industry, a force of about 4 kilograms is considered to be the minimum permitted for a satisfactory tablet. Hardness determinations are made during production to determine the need for pressure adjustments on the tablet presses.

Another means of determining the hardness of tablets is through the use of a *friabilator.* This apparatus determines the tablet's *friability* (that is, its tendency to crumble), by allowing the tablet to roll and fall within a rotating tumbling apparatus (Fig. 5–36). The tablets are weighed before and after a specified number of rotations, and the loss in weight is determined. Resistance to loss of weight indicates the tablet's ability to withstand abrasion in handling, packaging, and shipment.

TABLET DISINTEGRATION. For the medicinal component of a tablet to become fully available for absorption from the gastrointestinal tract, the tablet must first disintegrate and discharge the drug to the body fluids for dissolution. Tablet disintegration is also important for those tablets containing medicinal agents (such as antacids and antidiarrheals) that are not intended

Fig. 5–34. *Tablet hardness tester. (Courtesy of Eli Lilly and Company.)*

to be absorbed but rather to act locally within the gastrointestinal tract. In these instances, tablet disintegration provides drug particles with a greater surface area for localized activity within the body.

All USP tablets must pass the official test for disintegration, which is conducted *in vitro* with a special testing apparatus (Fig. 5–37). Briefly, the apparatus consists of a basket-rack assembly containing 6 open-ended glass tubes held vertically upon a 10-mesh stainless steel wire screen. During testing, a tablet is placed in each of the six tubes of the basket and through the use of a mechanical device, the basket is raised and lowered in the immersion fluid at a fre-

Fig. 5–36. *Erweka tablet testing apparatus for rolling and impact durability. Tablets are weighed and placed in the plexiglass drum in which a curved baffle is mounted. When the motor is activated by setting the timer, the tablets roll and drop. If the free fall within the drum results in the breakage or excessive abrasion of the tablets, they are considered not suited to withstand shipment without being damaged. The motor makes 20 rpm. After the tablets have been tested, they are removed and weighed again. The difference in weight within a given time indicates the rate of abrasion. (Courtesy of Chemical and Pharmaceutical Industry Co., Inc.)*

Fig. 5–35. *Automatic weight, hardness, thickness, and tablet diameter test instrument for quality control. Using a microprocessor and monitor for visualization, the instrument can test up to 20 samples at a time. (Courtesy of Scientific Instruments & Technology Corporation.)*

Fig. 5–37. *A, Tablet disintegration testing apparatus. B, Close-up view. (Courtesy of Eli Lilly and Company.)*

quency of between 29 and 32 cycles per minute, the wire screen always being maintained below the level of the fluid. For uncoated tablets, buccal tablets, and sublingual tablets, water maintained at about 37° C serves as the immersion fluid unless another fluid is specified in the individual monograph. For these tests, complete disintegration of tablets or capsules as "that state in which any residue of the unit, except fragments of insoluble coating or capsule shell, remaining on the screen of the test apparatus is a soft mass having no palpably firm core." Buccal tablets must disintegrate within 4 hours, and the sublingual and other uncoated tablets within the limits of the official monograph, usually 30 minutes but varying from about 2 minutes for Nitroglycerin Tablets, USP, to 30 minutes or longer for other tablets. For plain coated tablets, initial soaking in water at room temperature for 5 minutes is permitted to remove any water-soluble external coating. Then the tablets are immersed in simulated gastric fluid at 37° C for 30 minutes, and if they fail to disintegrate, they are subjected to the test using simulated intestinal fluid also at 37° C for the prescribed period according to the individual monograph. Enteric-coated tablets are similarly tested, except that the tablets are permitted to be tested in the simulated gastric fluid for one hour after which no sign of dissolution or disintegration must be seen. They are then actively immersed in the simulated intestinal fluid for 2 hours or for an individually designated length of time as stated in the monograph during which the tablets should have disintegrated. In each of the above cases, if 1 or 2 of the 6 tablets fails to disintegrate completely, tests are repeated on 12 additional tablets, and not less than 16 of the total of 18 tablets tested must disintegrate completely to meet the standard.[12]

Newly developed dissolution requirements in the USP have replaced the previous disintegration requirements for many official tablets.

TABLET DISSOLUTION. The USP contains a test for tablet and capsule dissolution for use when stated in the individual drug monographs. The test affords an objective means of determining the dissolution characteristics of a drug present in a solid dosage form. Because drug absorption and physiologic availability are largely dependent upon having the drug in the dissolved state, simple dissolution characteristics are an important property of a satisfactory drug product.

Briefly, an apparatus for testing the dissolution characteristics of a capsule or tablet dosage form consists of (1) a variable speed stirrer motor, (2) a paddle or a cylindrical stainless steel basket to be affixed to the end of the stirrer shaft, (3) a 1000-mL vessel of glass or other inert, transparent material, fitted with a cover having a center port for the shaft of the stirrer, and three additional ports, two for the removal of samples, and one for the placement of a thermometer, and (4) a suitable water bath to maintain the temperature of the dissolution medium in the vessel (Fig. 5–38). In each test, a volume of the dissolution medium (as stated in the individual monograph) is placed in the vessel and allowed to come to 37° C ±0.5° C. Then, the single tablet or capsule to be tested is immersed

Fig. 5–38. *Tablet dissolution apparatus. (Courtesy of Schering-Plough.)*

in the vessel or placed in the basket and the stirrer rotated at the speed specified in the monograph. At stated intervals, samples of the medium are withdrawn for chemical analysis of the proportion of drug dissolved. The tablet or capsule must meet the monographic requirement for rate of dissolution.

With the increased emphasis on dissolution testing and the determination of the bioavailability of drugs from solid dosage forms has come the introduction of sophisticated systems for the testing and analysis of tablet dissolution. One of these systems is shown in Figure 5–39. Figure 5–40 shows a modern quality control facility used to assure maintenance of standards in the production of tablets.

Methods of Preparation

The three most used methods for the preparation of compressed tablets are the *wet granulation method,* the *dry granulation method,* and *direct compression.* See Figure 5–41 for schematic drawings of each method. In addition to these three basic methods, recent technology has permitted the production of tablet granulations by the *fluid-bed process* (Fig. 5–42 and Fig. 5–43). The fluid-bed granulator performs the following three steps with a single piece of equipment: (1) preblending the formulation powder (including the active ingredients, diluents, disintegrants, etc.), (2) granulating by means of a suitable liquid binder (e.g., aqueous solutions of acacia, hydroxypropyl cellulose, povidone, etc.), and (3) drying the granulated product to the desired moisture content. In the process, the dry powder mixture is first preblended in the granulating bowl by the fluidizing air. Then, the binding solution is sprayed onto the fluidized powder

at a specified rate forming the agglomerates of powder, or granules, which are then dried.

Wet Granulation

Wet granulation is a widely employed method for the production of compressed tablets. The steps required in the preparation of tablets by this method may be separated as follows: (1) weighing and blending the ingredients, (2) preparing the wet granulation, (3) screening the damp mass into pellets or granules, (4) drying, (5) dry screening, (6) lubrication and blending, and (7) tableting by compression.

WEIGHING AND BLENDING. The active ingredient and any diluent and disintegrating agent required in the tablet formulation are weighed in amounts required for the preparation of the number of tablets to be produced and are mixed thoroughly, generally in a motor-driven powder blender or mixer. Among the diluents used are lactose, kaolin, mannitol, starch, powdered sugar, and calcium phosphate. The selection of the diluent is based partly on the experience of the manufacturer in the preparation of other tablets and also on its cost and compatibility with the other formulative ingredients. For example, calcium salts must not be employed as fillers in the preparation of tablets or capsules of tetracycline antibiotics, because the calcium interferes with the absorption of these drugs from the gastrointestinal tract.

Disintegrating agents include corn and potato starches, starch derivatives as sodium starch glycolate, cellulose derivatives as sodium carboxymethylcellulose, polyvinyl polypyrolidone (PVPP), crospovidone, cation-exchange resins, and other materials that swell or expand on exposure to moisture and effect the rupture or breakup of the tablet after it enters the gastrointestinal tract. Results of water-sorption studies show that the disintegrants with the highest water uptake are generally the most effective in most tablet systems.[13] Sodium starch glycolate and the cation exchange resins were shown to be particularly effective in the taking up of moisture. In studies of the mechanism of starch as a tablet disintegrant, it has been observed that the rupture of tablet surfaces occurs where agglomerates of starch grains were found and that tablet breakup probably results from the hydration of the hydroxy groups of the starch molecules causing them to move apart.[14] When starch is employed, 5% is usually suitable to

Fig. 5–39. *Beckman Model 25–7 dissolution system. A spectrophotometric system accommodating seven channels of analysis. Six dosage forms and a blank may be tested at one time. The constant temperature water bath is seen on the far left with six tablet basket assemblies in operation simultaneously. Using a multi-channel pump, solution from each of the six test vessels may be continuously sampled to a series of flow cells for UV or colorimetric analysis. (Courtesy of Beckman Instruments, Inc.)*

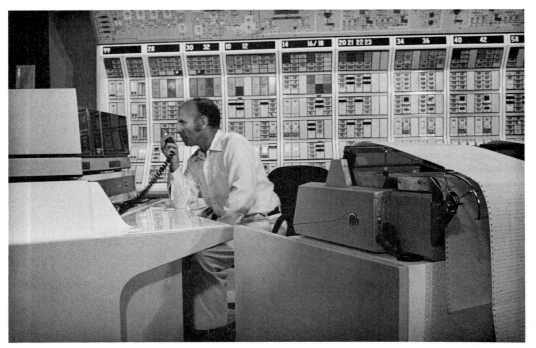

Fig. 5–40. *An ultramodern quality control facility for pharmaceutical manufacture. Central control bringing together advanced concepts of computer process technology, chemical engineering, and pharmaceutical manufacturing. The operator is controlling all aspects of tablet manufacture from weighing and mixing, to granulating and tableting meeting exacting specifications of tablet thickness, weight, hardness, and content uniformity. (Courtesy of Merck, Sharp & Dohme.)*

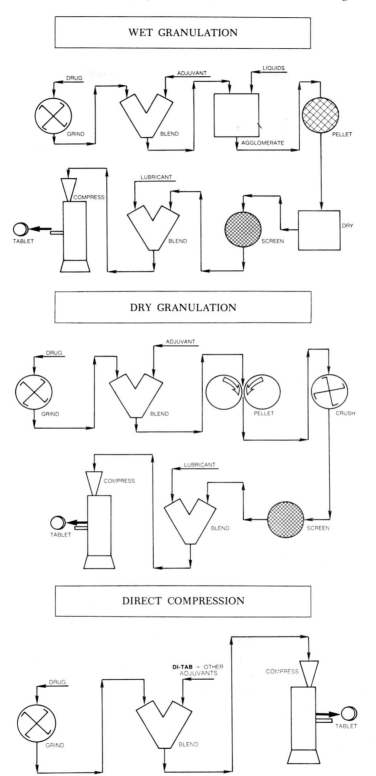

Fig. 5–41. *Schematic drawings of the three main methods for the preparation of tablets: wet granulation (top); dry granulation (center); direct compression (bottom). (Courtesy of Stauffer Chemical Co.)*

Fig. 5–42. *Cutaway view of a typical fluid bed granulator. (Courtesy of Ashok Y. Gore, Ph.D. Pharmaceutical Technology, Astor Publishing Co.).*

promote disintegration, but up to about 15% may be used to promote more rapid tablet disintegration. The total amount of disintegrant is not always added to the drug-diluent mixture, but a portion (sometimes half of that used) is reserved for later addition, with the lubricant, to the prepared granulation of the drug. This process results in a double disintegration of the tablet—the first from that portion of the disintegrant added last and effecting the breakup of the tablets into small pieces or chunks of tablet and the second disintegration from the initial addition of disintegrant and breaking up the pieces of tablet into fine particles.

Care must be exercised to achieve thorough

Fig. 5–43. *Example of fluid bed granulator. (Courtesy of Schering Laboratories.)*

mixing of the components to insure proper dosage administration as well as the uniform disintegration of all of the tablets produced. Sometimes the blended powders are passed through a sifter or a screen of appropriate fineness to eliminate clumps or compacts of powder.

PREPARING THE WET GRANULATION. For the powder mixture to flow evenly and freely from the hopper (the funnel-like container holding the drug and guiding its flow into the machine for tableting) into the dies, filling the latter evenly and fully at each occurrence, it is usually necesary to convert the powder mixture to free-flowing granules called the *granulation*. This is accomplished by adding a liquid binder or an adhesive to the powder mixture, passing the wetted mass through a screen of the desired mesh size, drying the granulation, and then passing through a second screen of smaller mesh to reduce further the size of the granules. The binding agent present in the tablets also contributes to the adhesion of the granules to one another, maintaining the integrity of the tablet after compression. Among the binding agents used are a 10 to 20% aqueous preparation of corn starch, a 25 to 50% solution of glucose, molasses, various natural gums (as acacia), cellulose derivatives (as methylcellulose, carboxymethylcellulose and microcrystalline cellulose), gelatins, and povidone. If the drug substance is adversely affected by an aqueous binder, the binding agents may be nonaqueous or may be added dry. In general, the binding action is more effective when the adhesive is mixed with the powders in liquid form. The amount of binding agent used is part of the operator's art and is dependent upon the other formulative ingredients. However, an amount that will render the drug mixture moist enough so that the powder is compactible by squeezing in the hand is usually sufficient. Care must be exercised not to overwet or underwet the powder. Overwetting usually results in granules that are too hard for proper tableting; underwetting usually results in the preparation of tablets that are too soft and tend to crumble. If desired, a suitable colorant or flavorant may be added to the binding agent to prepare a colored or flavored granulation.

SCREENING THE DAMP MASS INTO PELLETS OR GRANULES. Generally the wet granulation is pressed through a No. 6- or 8-mesh screen. This may be done by hand or by special granulation equipment, some of which prepares the granulation by extrusion through perforations in the apparatus. After all of the material has been converted into granules, the granulation is

Fig. 5–45. *Temperature-controlled oven for the drying of wet granulation preparative to tablet compression. (Courtesy of Stokes Equipment Division, Pennwalt Corporation.)*

Fig. 5–44. *Fitzpatrick malaxating machine, a continuous wet granulator that combines dry material and granulating excipient and discharges the wet granulation for spreading on a drying tray. Tray of wet granulation is then placed on truck for drying. (Courtesy of The Upjohn Company.)*

spread evenly on large pieces of paper in shallow trays and dried (Fig. 5–44).

DRYING THE GRANULATION. In most instances, the granules are dried in special drying cabinets that have circulating air systems and are thermostatically controlled (Fig. 5–45). Among the newer methods of drying in use today is *fluidization* conducted in *fluid bed driers* (Fig. 5–46). In this method the granules are dried by being suspended and agitated by a stream of warm air. If the effectiveness of the binder is dependent upon the presence of minute amounts of moisture, the granulation is not completely dried. However, an excessive amount of moisture remaining in a granulation is frequently the cause of ruptures occurring to coatings later placed on the compressed tablets.

DRY SCREENING. After drying, the granules are passed through a screen of a smaller mesh than that used to prepare the original granulation.

The degree to which the granules are reduced depends upon the size of the punches to be used and the tablets to be produced. The proper selection is based on experience; however, in general, the smaller the tablet to be produced, the smaller are the granules used to produce it. Screens from 12- to 20-mesh size are generally used for this purpose. Sizing of the granules is necessary so that the small die cavity for the production of small tablets may be completely filled by the flowing granulation. The voids or air spaces left by a large granulation in a small die cavity would likely result in the production of tablets of varying evenness.

LUBRICATION. After dry screening, a dry lubricant is generally added to the granulation. So that each granule is covered with lubricant, it may be dusted over the spread-out granulation through a fine mesh screen or blended in a powder mixer. Among the more commonly used lubricants are talc, magnesium stearate, and calcium stearate, but many other agents are occasionally employed. The quantity of lubricant used varies from one tableting operation to another and may range from a low of about 0.1% of the weight of the granulation to as much as 5%. Lubricants contribute to the preparation of compressed tablets in several ways; they improve the flow of the granulation in the hopper to the die cavity, they prevent the adhesion of the tablet formulation to the punches and dies

Fig. 5–46. *Stokes fluid bed dryer in which heated air is passed at controlled high velocity through the material to be dried, converting it into a fluidized bed and surrounding each individual particle with a stream of drying air. Because of the efficient mass heat transfer involved, materials previously requiring a 16-hour or longer drying cycle may be dried in less than 45 minutes, depending upon air-stream velocity, drying temperature and the physical properties of the material being processed. (Courtesy of Pennwalt Corporation.)*

Fig. 5–47. *Punch and die set: (A) upper punch, (B) die cavity, (C) die, and (D) lower punch. (Courtesy of Cherry-Burrell Corporation.)*

during compression, they reduce friction between the tablet and the die wall during the tablet's ejection from the tablet machine, and they give a sheen to the finished tablet.

TABLETING. There are a number of types of tablet presses or tableting machines, each varying in its productivity but similar in its basic operation. That operation is the compression of the tablet granulation within a steel die cavity by the pressure exerted by the movement of two steel punches, a lower punch and an upper punch.

There are single-punch tablet machines, some hand operated and some motor driven, which are capable of producing a single tablet upon completion of each up and down movement of the set of punches. As the lower punch drops, the feed shoe filled with granulation (from the hopper) is positioned over the die cavity which then fills. The feed shoe then retracts, scraping

the excessive granulation from the stage and leveling the layer of granulation in the die cavity. The upper punch lowers and compresses the material in the die cavity to form the tablet. The upper punch then retracts, and the lower punch rises to the precise level of the stage, lifting the tablet to be ejected from the stage by the feed shoe which moves over the die cavity once again to repeat the process (see Fig. 5–26). The tablet is ejected into a barrel or other suitable container. The first few tablets collected, as well as some tablets prepared during the course of production, are examined for weight variation, hardness, thickness, and disintegration, and the necessary adjustments are made in the volume of fill or the pressure of compression to prepare tablets of the desired quality.

Ordinary rotary tablet machines and high speed rotary tablet machines equipped with multiple punches and dies can greatly outproduce the single punch machines through the continuous rotating movement of the punches and continuous tablet compression (Figs. 5–47 and 5–48). In contrast to the single punch tablet machines generally having a capacity of about 100 tablets per minute, a single rotary press with 16 stations (16 sets of punches and dies) may produce up to 1150 tablets per minute. Double rotary tablet presses with 27, 33, 37, 41, or 49 sets of punches and dies are capable of producing 2 tablets for each die for each complete revolution of the die head because of having two tableting mechanisms. Some of these machines can produce 10,000 and more tablets per minute of operation (Fig. 5–49). For such high speed production, induced die feeders are required (Fig. 5–50). These induced feeders force

Fig. 5–48. *Manesty Rotapress rotary compression machine making compressed tablets. Tablets leaving the machine run over a tablet duster to screen where they are inspected. Material to be compressed is being fed from overhead hopper through yoke to each of the two compressing machine hoppers. Hardness of tablet is monitored electronically by oscilloscope at the right. (Courtesy of The Upjohn Company.)*

Fig. 5–49. *New Stokes Ultra Press, a double-sided rotary press capable of producing over 10,000 tablets per minute. (Courtesy of Stokes Equipment Division, Pennwalt Corporation.)*

granulation into the dies by the rotary action of an agitator. This feeding is much more rapid than standard gravity feeding and is necessary for the fast production rates achieved with these tableting machines.

As indicated earlier, tablet machines have been developed to form multiple-layered tablets by the multiple feed and multiple compression of fill material within a single die. Also, a layer of material can be compressed onto a tablet core placed strategically and automatically in the die by a special feed apparatus using a special tableting machine.

Dry Granulation

In the dry granulation method the granulation is formed not by moistening or adding a binding agent to the powdered drug mixture but by compacting large masses of the mixture and subsequently crushing and sizing these pieces into smaller granules (see Fig. 5–41). By this method, either the active ingredient or the

Fig. 5–50. *Induced die feeder. The standard gravity-fed open feed frame can be replaced with an induced die feeder. Using this accessory, granulation is forced into the die by the rotary action of the agitator. (Courtesy of Cherry-Burrell Corporation.)*

diluent must have cohesive properties in order for the large masses to be formed. This method is especially applicable to materials that cannot be prepared by the wet granulation method due to their sensitivity to moisture or to the elevated temperatures required for drying.

After weighing and mixing the ingredients in the same manner as in the wet granulation method, the powder is "slugged" or compressed into large flat tablets or pellets of about 1 inch in diameter. It is possible to do this because the flow of the powder into the slugging machine is facilitated by the large cavity and the tablets need not be of exact size or weight. The slugs must be hard enough to be broken up without producing an excessive amount of powder. The slugs are broken up by hand or by a mill (Fig. 5–51) and passed through a screen of desired mesh for sizing. Lubricant is added in the usual manner, and tablets are prepared by compression. Aspirin, which is hydrolyzed on exposure to moisture, is commonly prepared into tablets after slugging. Instead of the slugging method, compaction mills may be used to increase the density of a powder by pressing it between high-pressure rollers. The densified material is then broken up, sized, and lubricated, and tablets are prepared by compression in the usual manner.

Direct Compression

Some granular chemicals like potassium chloride and methenamine possess free flowing as well as cohesive properties that enable them to be compressed directly in a tablet machine without need of either wet or dry granulation. In past years the number of medicinal substances that could be tableted without prior granulation was quite small. Today the use of special pharmaceutical excipients imparts to certain tablet formulations the required qualities for tablet production by direct compression, and many additional products may now be produced in this manner. In the direct-compression of tablets, the tableting excipients used must be materials with properties of fluidity and compressibility. Tableting excipients having the desired characteristics include: *fillers*—spray-dried lactose, microcrystals of alpha-monohydrate lactose, sucrose-invert sugar-corn starch mixtures (NuTab, Ingredient Technology Corp.), microcrystalline cellulose, and dicalcium phosphate (Di-Tab, Stauffer Chemical Co.); *disintegrating agents*—direct-compression starch (Starch 1500,

Colorcon, Inc.), sodium carboxymethyl starch, cross-linked carboxymethylcellulose fibers (Ac-Di-Sol, FMC Corp.), and cross-linked polyvinylpyrrolidone; *lubricants*—magnesium stearate and talc; and *glidants*—fumed silicon dioxide (Cab-O-Sil, Cabot Corp.).[15]

In addition to the use of special excipients, forced or induced feeders which have been developed permit the preparation of certain additional tablets by direct compression because the deaerating action of the feeder on light, bulky powders makes them more dense and permits them to flow evenly and completely into the die cavities under moderate pressure. This deaeration also eliminates air entrapment within the die as the tablets are compressed, thereby reducing a major cause of *capping*, (loose at the top like a "cap") or splitting of tablets upon compression.

The capping or splitting of tablets may be caused by a number of factors and is not limited to tablets prepared by direct compression. For instance punches that are not immaculately clean and perfectly smooth may result in capped tablets, as may dies that are old or imperfect. Too much pressure on compression can cause capping, as can a granulation which is too soft. Generally there is a portion of "fines" or a fine powder which results when the dry granulation is sized and generally amounts to 10 to 20% of the weight of the granulation and are necessary to properly fill the die cavity. However, an excess of these fines can also lead to capping. When a large quantity of air is trapped in the tablet, a condition called *laminating* results. The tablets appear split and cracked around the sides caused by expansion when the pressure of tableting is released. Figure 5–52 shows tablets which have split. Tablets which have aged (usually beyond the expiration date) may also exhibit splitting or other physical deformation.

Tablet Dedusting

To remove traces of loose powder adhering to tablets following compression, the tablets are conveyed directly from the tableting machine to a tablet deduster. Examples of this type of apparatus are shown in Figures 5–53 and 5–54.

Tablet Coating

Since the reasons for coating tablets and the different types of coatings (i.e., enteric, sugar,

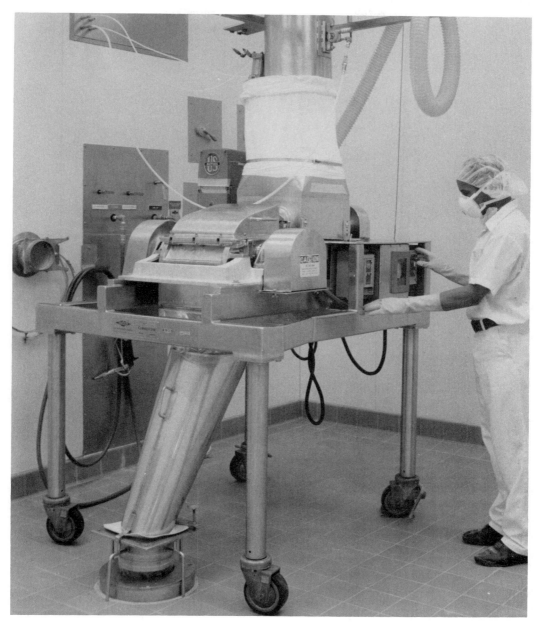

Fig. 5–51. *Frewitt Oscillator or Fitz Mill utilized in the pulverization or granulation process. (Courtesy of Eli Lilly and Company.)*

Fig. 5–52. *Tablets which have split on aging, due to conditions of manufacture or storage.*

film) have already been mentioned, this section will be limited to the general methods involved in the application of these coatings.

Sugarcoating Tablets

The sugarcoating of tablets may be divided into the following steps: (1) waterproofing and sealing (if needed), (2) subcoating, (3) smoothing and final rounding, (4) finishing and coloring (if desired), and (5) polishing. Generally the entire coating process is conducted in a series of mechanically operated coating pans, which are acorn-shaped vessels of galvanized iron, stainless steel, or copper partially open in the front and with diameters ranging from about 1 to 4 feet and therefore of various capacities (Figs. 5–55 and 5–56). The smaller pans are used for experimental, developmental, and pilot plant operations; the larger pans, for industrial production. The pans are fixed and operate at about a 40° angle, which permits the tablets to remain inside the pan during its revolutions yet also permits the operator to observe and handle the tablets from the open end of the pan. During each of the operations involved in the coating of tablets, the pan is rotated by a motor at moderate speeds, allowing the tablets to tumble and roll about in the pan

Fig. 5–53. *Tablets leaving tableting machine run over a tablet duster to screen where they are inspected. (Courtesy of The Upjohn Company.)*

and make contact with each other and with the coating solutions. As they rotate, the coating solution is gently poured or sprayed on the tablets in portions, and warm air is introduced into the pan to hasten the drying of each coat so that the tablets do not stick to one another and so that the entire process may be hastened, since the tablets require many coats of material and each subsequent coat may be applied only after the previous coat has dried. Tablets intended to be coated are generally compressed tablets that have been prepared to be highly convex and have as thin an edge as possible to permit the coatings to form rounded rather than angular edges.

WATERPROOFING AND SEALING COATS. For tablets containing components that may absorb

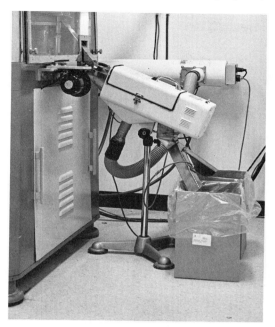

Fig. 5–54. *Model 25 Manesty Tablet Deduster. Tablets leaving tableting machine are dedusted and passed into collection containers. (Courtesy of Eli Lilly and Company.)*

moisture or be adversely affected on contact with moisture, a waterproofing layer or coating of a material such as shellac is placed on the compressed tablets before the subcoating application. The shellac or other waterproofing agent is applied in solution (usually alcoholic) form and is gently poured on the compressed tablets rotating in the coating pans or is sprayed on as a fine spray. Warm air is blown into the pan during the coating to hasten the drying and to prevent tablets from sticking together. A second coat of the waterproofing substance may be added to the tablets after the first coat has dried to ensure against moisture penetration into the compressed tablets.

SUBCOATING. After the waterproofing or sealing coats (if they are necessary) have been applied, the tablets are given about 3 to 5 subcoats of a sugar-based syrup for the purpose of rounding the tablets and bonding the sugar coating to the compressed tablet. In applying the subcoating, a heavy syrup generally containing gelatin and sometimes acacia is added to the tablets as they roll in the coating pan. When the tablets are partially dry they are sprinkled with a dusting powder, which is usually a mixture of powdered sugar and starch but may

also contain talc, acacia, or precipitated chalk. Warm air is applied to the rolling tablets, and when they are dry, the subcoating process is repeated and repeated again until the tablets are of the desired shape and size (Fig. 5–57). At this point, the tablets are usually removed from the coating pan, the excess powder is shaken off the tablets by gently jostling them on a cloth screen, and the coating pan is then washed to remove extraneous coating material.

SMOOTHING AND FINAL ROUNDING. After the tablets have been subcoated to the desired shape (roundness), 5 to 10 additional coatings of a very thick syrup are applied to the rolling tablets for the purpose of completing the rounding of the tablets and smoothing the coatings. This syrup may be composed of a sucrose-based simple syrup, or it may have additional components like starch and calcium carbonate. As the syrup is applied, the operator moves his hand through the rolling tablets to distribute the syrup and to prevent the sticking of the tablets to one another. A dusting powder may or may not be used between syrup applications, but warm air is generally applied to hasten the drying time of each coat. If the coating is to be colored, the suitable dye may be added to the syrup during this step of the coating process as well as during the next step.

FINISHING AND COLORING. To attain final smoothness and the appropriate color to the tablets, several coats of a thin syrup containing the desired colorant (if any) are applied. This step is usually performed in a clean pan, free from previous coating materials.

An innovation in tablet coating equipment is the Accela-Cota coating pan shown in Figure 5–58. This system provides for the automated spraying of coating material into the pan with a simultaneous flow of air being drawn across the revolving bed of tablets. The result is a more uniform tablet coating and a decrease in the time of the coating operation. The tablets may be coated with this procedure using film coatings, a cellulose acetate phthalate, or sugar-based coatings.

Tablets, coated by any of the methods, may then be passed through special imprinting machines to impart any distinctive symbol or identification code on the tablets (Fig. 5–59).

POLISHING. Coated tablets may be polished in special drum-shaped pans made by stretching a cloth fabric over a metal frame or in ordinary coating pans lined with canvas. The fabric or

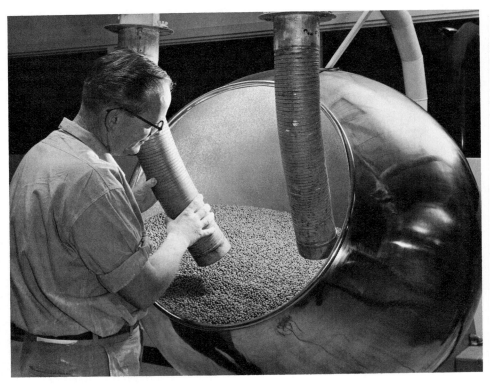

Fig. 5–55. *Tablet coating, showing the warm air supply and the exhaust. (Courtesy of Wyeth Laboratories.)*

Fig. 5–56. *Modern tablet coating facility. Air and exhaust ducts to assist drying are automatically operated from central board. (Courtesy of Eli Lilly and Company.)*

Fig. 5–57. *Tablet gauge used to measure the size of coated tablets. (Courtesy of Eli Lilly and Company.)*

the canvas may be impregnated with a wax such as carnauba wax with or without the addition of beeswax and the tablets polished as they roll about in the pan. Or, the wax may be dissolved in a nonaqueous solvent such as acetone or petroleum benzin and sprayed on the rolling tablets in small amounts. After each coat has dried, the addition of a small amount of talc to the tumbling tablets contributes to their high luster (Fig. 5–60). Two or three coats of wax may be applied depending upon the desired gloss. Another method of polishing tablets simply in-

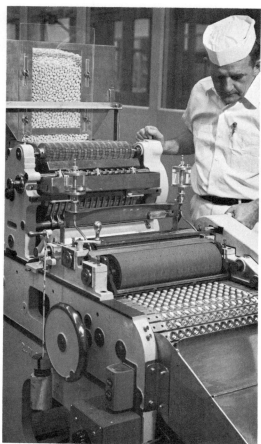

Fig. 5–59. *Branding of coated compression tablets on a Hartnett branding machine. (Courtesy of The Upjohn Company.)*

volves placing pieces of wax in the polishing pan along with the tablets and permitting the tablets to tumble over the wax until the desired sheen is attained.

Film-Coating Tablets

As one can ascertain from the previous discussion of sugarcoating, the process is not only tedious and time-consuming, requiring the expertise of a highly skilled technician, but it also results in the preparation of coated tablets that may be twice the size and weight of the original uncoated compressed tablets. These factors are important to a manufacturer in his consideration of the expense of both packaging materials and shipping. From a patient's point of view, large tablets are not as convenient to swallow

Fig. 5–58. *Tablet coating by spray technique using the Accela-Cota equipment. (Courtesy of Eli Lilly and Company.)*

Fig. 5–60. *Example of coated, polished, and monogrammed tablets. (Courtesy of Wyeth-Ayerst Laboratories.)*

availability of the drug. Example: polyethylene glycol.

3. A *plasticizer* to produce flexibility and elasticity of the coating and thus provide durability. Example: castor oil.

4. A *surfactant* to enhance spreadability of the film during application. Example: polyoxyethylene sorbitan derivatives.

5. *Opaquants* and *colorants* to make the appearance of the coated tablets handsome and distinctive. Examples: Opaquant, titanium dioxide; colorant, F.D.&C. or D.&C. dyes.

6. *Sweeteners, flavors,* and *aromas* to enhance the acceptability of the tablet to the patient. Examples: sweeteners, saccharin; flavors and aromas, vanillin.

7. A *glossant* to provide luster to the tablets without a separate polishing operation. Example: beeswax.

8. A *volatile solvent* to allow the spread of the other components over the tablets while allowing rapid evaporation to permit an effective yet speedy operation. Example: alcohol-acetone mixture.

as are small tablets. Also, the coating of tablets by the application of the sugarcoating may vary slightly from batch to batch and within the batch. The film-coating process, which places a thin, skin-tight coating of a plastic-like material over the compressed tablet, was developed to produce coated tablets having essentially the same weight, shape, and size as the originally compressed tablet. The coating is thin enough to reveal any depressed or raised monograms punched into the tablet by the tablet punches. In addition, film-coated tablets are far more resistant to destruction by abrasion than are sugar-coated tablets, and like sugar-coated tablets, the coating may be colored to make the tablets attractive and distinctive.

Film-coating solutions may be nonaqueous or aqueous. The nonaqueous solutions generally contain the following types of materials to provide the desired coating to the tablets:

1. A *film former* capable of producing smooth, thin films reproducible under conventional coating conditions and applicable to a variety of tablet shapes. Example: cellulose acetate phthalate.

2. An *alloying substance* providing water solubility or permeability to the film to ensure penetration by body fluids and therapeutic

Tablets are film coated by the application or spraying of the film-coating solution upon the tablets in ordinary coating pans. The volatility of the solvent enables the film to adhere quickly to the surface of the tablets.

Due to both the expense of the volatile solvents used in the film-coating process and the problem of the release of these potentially toxic agents into the atmosphere, the high cost of solvent recovery systems, and their explosiveness, pharmaceutical manufacturers are favoring the use of aqueous-based film-coating solutions. One of the problems attendant to these, however, is the slow evaporation of the water-base compared to the volatile organic solvent-based film-coating solutions. The first commercially available (to the pharmaceutical industry) water-based, colloidal coating dispersion, is called AQUACOAT (FMC Corporation) and contains a 30% ethyl cellulose pseudolatex. Pseudolatex dispersions have the advantage of high solids content (for greater coating ability) and relatively low viscosity. The low viscosity allows less water to be used in the coating dispersion, resulting in a lesser requirement for water-evaporation and a reduced likelihood of water interference with the tablet formulation. In addition, the low viscosity permits greater coating penetration into the crevices of monogrammed or scored tablets. In using the pseudolatex coating dispersion, a plasticizer is incorporated to assist in the production of a denser, less-permeable film, with higher gloss and greater mechanical strength. Other aqueous systems utilized to film-coat tablets include the use of cellulosic materials as methylcellulose, hydroxypropyl cellulose, and hydroxypropyl methylcellulose.

A typical aqueous film-coating formulation contains the following:[16]

1. *Film-forming polymer* (7–18%). Examples: cellulose ether polymers as hydroxypropyl methylcellulose, hydroxypropyl cellulose, and methylcellulose.
2. *Plasticizer* (0.5–2.0%). Examples: glycerin, propylene glycol, polyethylene glycol, and dibutyl subacetate.
3. *Colorant and opacifier* (2.5–8%). Examples: FD&C or D&C Lakes and iron oxide pigments.
4. *Vehicle* (water, to make 100%)

There are some problems attendant to aqueous film-coating. Some relate to the formulations employed, the techniques and equipment used, and the processes involved. These problems may result in the appearance of small amounts (*picking*) or larger amounts (*peeling*) of film fragments flaking from the tablet surface; roughness of the tablet surface due to failure of spray droplets to coalesce (*orange peel effect*); an uneven distribution of color on the tablet surface (*mottling*); filling-in of the score-line or indented logo on the tablet by the film (*bridging*); and, the disfiguration of the core tablet when subjected for too long a period of time to the coating solution (tablet *erosion*). The cause of each of these problems can be determined and rectified through appropriate changes in formulation, equipment, technique or process.[16]

Enteric Coating

The purpose of enteric coating for solid dosage forms has been previously discussed. Since the pH within the various depths of the gastrointestinal tract may vary between patients and within a given patient at different times, it is generally considered preferable to base the design of an enteric coating upon the length of time required for disintegration or drug release rather than on specific environmental conditions of the intestine. However, enteric preparations may be based on one factor or the other,

or on both. If the tablet is coated to various thicknesses with certain coating materials that are not immediately dissolved by the gastric fluid, the tablet may be prevented from disintegrating until it has time to reach the intestinal tract. Among the materials used in enteric coatings are phenyl salicylate (salol), a combination of 45 parts of n-butyl stearate, 30 parts of carnauba wax, and 25 parts of stearic acid, shellac, hydroxypropyl methylcellulose phthalate, cellulose acetate trimellitate, and cellulose acetate phthalate. These materials are applied on a large industrial scale by the usual coating methods.

Air Suspension Coating

This process, also known as the Wurster process after its developer, may be employed for the rapid coating of granules, powders, or tablets. The items to be coated are fed into a vertical cylinder and are supported by a column of air that enters from the bottom of the cylinder. Within the air stream, the solids rotate both vertically and horizontally. As the coating solution enters the system, it is rapidly placed on the suspended, rotating solids, with rounding coats being applied in less than an hour with the assistance of warm air blasts released in the chamber.

Compression Coating

In a manner similar to the preparation of multiple compressed tablets having an inner core and an outer shell of drug material, core tablets may be sugarcoated by compression. The coating material in the form of a granulation or a powder is compressed onto a tablet core of drug with a special tablet press. This method eliminates the time-consuming and tedious operation previously described in this section. Compression coating is an anhydrous operation and thus may be safely employed in the coating of tablets having a drug that is sensitive to moisture. The resulting coat is more uniform than the usual sugarcoating applied using pans, and less of a coating is required. Resulting tablets are lighter and smaller and are therefore easier to swallow and less expensive to package and ship.

Irrespective of the method used in coating, all tablets are visually inspected for physical imperfections (Fig. 5–61).

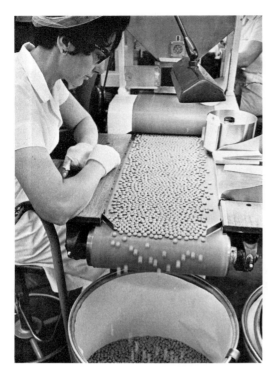

Fig. 5–61. *Checking for physical imperfections in coated tablets. (Courtesy of Smith, Kline & French.)*

Fig. 5–62. *Cut-away view of "Gelcaps" dosage form. A gelatin-coated capsule-shaped tablet. Dosage form is more easily swallowed than a comparable tablet, smaller than an equivalent capsule, and tamper-evident. (Courtesy of McNeil Consumer Products Co.)*

Gelatin Coated Tablets

A recent innovation in tablet coating is the gelatin coated tablet. Termed GELCAPS, the innovator product is a gelatin-coated capsule-shaped tablet (Fig. 5–62). The use of a tablet makes the size of the product about one-third smaller than a capsule filled with an equivalent amount of powder. The gelatin coating facilitates ease of swallowing. Compared to dry-filled, unsealed capsules, GELCAPS are more tamper-resistant and tamper-evident.

Chewable Tablets

Chewable tablets are tablets which are intended to disintegrate smoothly in the mouth at a moderate rate, either with or without actual chewing. Characteristically, chewable tablets have a smooth texture upon disintegration, are pleasant tasting, and leave no bitter or unpleasant aftertaste. Mannitol, a white crystalline hexahydric alcohol, which possesses many of the characteristics desired for the excipient in chewable tablets, is widely employed for this pur-

pose. Mannitol is about 70% as sweet as sucrose with a cool taste and mouth-feel, the latter resulting from its negative heat of solution and a moderate solubility in water. Mannitol's nonhygroscopicity also makes it an ideal excipient for the preparation of chewable tablets containing moisture-sensitive drugs. Chewable tablets are prepared by wet granulation and compression, using minimum degrees of tablet hardness. In many chewable tablet formulations, mannitol may account for 50% or more of the weight of the formulation. Sometimes, other sweetening agents, as sorbitol, lactose, dextrose and glucose, may be substituted for part or all of the mannitol. Lubricants and binders which do not detract from the texture or desired hardness of the tablet are used in formulating chewable tablets. To enhance the appeal of the tablets, colorants and tart or fruity flavorants are commonly employed. Among the types of products prepared into chewable tablets are antacids and vitamins, analgesic and cold tablets intended for children.

The following is a formula for a typical chewable antacid tablet:[17]

	Per Tablet
Aluminum hydroxide	325.0 mg
Mannitol	812.0 mg
Sodium saccharin	0.4 mg
Sorbitol (10% w/v solution)	32.5 mg
Magnesium stearate	35.0 mg
Mint flavor concentrate	4.0 mg

Preparation: Blend the aluminum hydroxide, mannitol, and sodium saccharin. Prepare a wet granulation with the sorbitol solution. Dry at 120° F and screen through a 12-mesh screen. Add the flavor and magnesium stearate, blend, and compress into tablets.

Molded Tablets

The commercial preparation of tablets by molding has been replaced by the tablet compression process. The student who may be using the molding process in the laboratory, may refer to Chapter 13 for a description of this method.

Official Tablets

Examples of official tablets are presented in Table 5–4.

Rate-Controlled Dosage Forms and Drug Delivery Systems

Some solid dosage forms are designed to release their medication to the body for absorption rapidly and completely, whereas other products are designed to release the drug slowly for more prolonged drug release and sustained drug action. The latter types of dosage forms are commonly referred to as *controlled-release, sustained-release, prolonged-release, timed-release, slow-release, sustained-action, prolonged-action,* or *extended-action* tablets or capsules.

Table 5–4. Examples of Some Official Tablets

Official Tablet	Some Representative Commercial Products	Tablet Strengths Usually Available	Category and Comments
Acetaminophen	Tylenol (McNeil)	325 mg	Analgesic and antipyretic
Allopurinol	Zyloprim (Burroughs Wellcome)	100 and 300 mg	Antigout; antiurolithic
Amitriptyline HCl	Elavil HCl (Merck, Sharp & Dohme)	10, 25, 50, 100, and 150 mg	Antidepressant
Betamethasone	Celestone (Schering)	0.6 mg	Adrenocorticoid
Bisacodyl	Dulcolax (Boehringer Ingelheim)	5 mg	Cathartic; enteric coated tablets
Carbamazepine	Tegretol (Geigy)	200 mg	Anticonvulsant
Chlorambucil	Leukeran (Burroughs Wellcome)	2 mg	Antineoplastic
Chlorpheniramine Maleate	Chlor-Trimeton Maleate (Schering)	4, 8, and 12 mg	Antihistaminic; some tablets (8 and 12 mg) controlled-release
Chlorpropamide	Diabinese (Pfizer)	100 and 250 mg	Antidiabetic
Cimetidine	Tagamet (Smith, Kline & French)	200 and 300 mg	Histamine H_2 receptor antagonist
Diazepam	Valium (Roche)	2, 5, and 10 mg	Sedative; skeletal muscle relaxant
Digoxin	Lanoxin (Burroughs Wellcome)	0.125, 0.25 and 0.5 mg	Cardiotonic
Dimenhydrinate	Dramamine (Searle)	50 mg	Antinauseant
	—	25 and 30 mg	Bronchodilator; vasoconstrictor
Furosemide	Lasix (Hoechst-Roussel)	20, 40, and 80 mg	Diuretic; antihypercalcemic; antihypertensive
Griseofulvin	Fulvicin U/F (Schering)	250 and 500 mg	Antifungal
Haloperidol	Haldol (McNeil)	0.5, 1, 2, 5, 10 and 20 mg	Tranquilizer
Hydrochlorothiazide	Hydro-Diuril (Merck, Sharp & Dohme)	25, 50 and 100 mg	Diuretic; antihypertensive
Ibuprofen	Motrin (Upjohn)	300, 400, 600 and 800 mg	Analgesic; antipyretic
Levodopa	Larodopa (Roche)	100, 250, and 500 mg	Antidyskinetic
Levothyroxine sodium	Synthroid (Flint)	0.025, 0.05, 0.075, 0.1, 0.125, 0.15, 0.2 and 0.3 mg	Thyroid hormone
Meclizine HCl	Antivert (Roerig)	12.5, 25 and 50 mg	Antivertigo

Table 5–4.   Continued

Official Tablet	Some Representative Commercial Products	Tablet Strengths Usually Available	Category and Comments
Meperidine Hydrochloride	Demerol (Winthrop-Breon)	50 and 100 mg	Narcotic analgesic
Meprobamate	Equanil (Wyeth)	200 and 400 mg	Sedative; hypnotic
Methyldopa	Aldomet (Merck, Sharp & Dohme)	125, 250, and 500 mg	Antihypertensive
Metronidazole	Flagyl (Searle)	250 and 500 mg	Antiamebic; antitrichomonal
Nitroglycerin	Nitrostat (Parke-Davis)	0.150, 0.3, 0.4 and 0.6 mg	Anti-anginal sublingual tablets
Penicillin V Potassium	Pen Vee K (Wyeth)	250, and 500 mg	Antibacterial
Prednisone	Meticorten (Schering)	1 mg	Adrenocorticoid
Prochlorperazine maleate	Compazine (Smith, Kline & French)	5, 10 and 25 mg	Antiemetic
Propanolol HCl	Inderal (Ayerst)	10, 20, 40, 60, 80, and 90 mg	Antianginal; antiarrhythmic; antihypertensive
Sulindac	Clinoril (Merck, Sharp & Dohme)	150 and 200 mg	Antirheumatic, anti-inflammatory
Terbutaline sulfate	Brethine (Geigy)	2.5 and 5 mg	Antiasthmatic
Tolbutamide	Orinase (Upjohn)	250 and 500 mg	Antidiabetic
Warfarin Sodium	Coumadin Sodium (DuPont)	2, 2.5, 5, 7.5, and 10 mg	Anticoagulant

Although these terms have been frequently used interchangeably, the meaning of "sustained-release" and "controlled-release" are different. Sustained release describes the release of a drug substance from a dosage form or delivery system over an extended period of time. Controlled-release describes a system in which the *rate* of the drug's release is more precisely controlled compared to the sustained release product.

The term "drug delivery systems" refers to the technology utilized to present the drug to the desired body site for drug release and absorption. The modern transdermal patch, discussed in Chapter 9, is an example of a drug delivery system. The first drug delivery system developed was the *syringe,* invented in 1855, used to deliver medication by injection.

The goal of rate-controlled technology is to produce a convenient, generally self-administered dosage form that yields a constant infusion of the drug. The advantages of rate-controlled drug delivery are presented in Table 5–5.

Controlled-release dosage forms that provide sustained drug release require less frequent drug administration than ordinary dosage forms (Fig. 5–63A). This is considered an advantage in assuring patient compliance in the taking of medication. Patients required to take 1 or 2 dosage units a day are thought to be less likely to forget a dose than if they were required to take their medication 3 or 4 times a day. Further, controlled-release dosage forms allow whole day coverage and help to reduce the need for the patient to be awakened for an early morning dosing. Also, depending upon the medication and the dosage form, the daily cost to the patient may be less with less frequent dosage administration.

Rather than providing *sustained-release,* some solid dosage forms are designed to sequentially release two full doses of a drug. Such dosage forms also enable the patient to be maintained on the drug for longer than usual periods following the administration of a single dosage unit. These types of products are usually termed *repeat-action* tablets or capsules (Fig. 5–63B).

Many of these specialized types of dosage forms are protected by patents and have been given trademark names that help to identify both the manufacturer and the type of pharmaceutical product.

Sustained-Release Forms

Most sustained-release forms are designed so that the administration of a single dosage unit provides the immediate release of an amount

Table 5–5.   Advantages of Rate-Controlled Drug-Delivery Systems Over Conventional Dosage Forms

Advantage	Explanation
Reduction in drug blood level fluctuations	By controlling the rate of drug release, "peaks and valleys" of drug-blood or -serum levels are eliminated.
Reduction in dosing frequency	Rate-controlled products deliver more than a single dose of medication and thus are taken less often than conventional forms.
Enhanced patient convenience and compliance	With less frequency of dose administration, the patient is less apt to neglect taking a dose. There is also greater patient convenience with daytime and nighttime medication, and control of chronic illness.
Reduction in adverse side effects	Because there are seldom drug blood level peaks above the drug's therapeutic range, and into the toxic range, adverse side effects are less frequently encountered.
Reduction in health care costs i.e., economy	Although the initial cost of rate-controlled drug delivery systems is usually greater than conventional dosage forms, the average cost of treatment over an extended time period may be less. With less frequency of dosing, enhanced therapeutic benefit, and reduced side-effects, the time required of health care personnel to dispense, administer and monitor patients is reduced.

of drug that promptly produces the desired therapeutic effect and gradual and continual release of additional amounts of drug to maintain this level of effect over an extended period, usually 8 to 12 hours.

In this type of dosage form, the design is based on the particular qualities of each individual drug. What may be an effective type of dosage form design for one drug may be ineffective in promoting the sustained release of another drug because of peculiar physical, chemical, and biological qualities. To maintain the constant level of drug in the system, the drug must be released from the dosage form at a rate that will replace the amount of drug being metabolized and excreted from the body. For each drug, this is a highly individualized quality. In general, the drugs best suited for incorporation into a sustained release product have the following characteristics.

1. *They exhibit neither very slow nor very fast rates of absorption and excretion.* Drugs with slow rates of absorption and excretion are usu-

ally inherently long-acting and their preparation into sustained-action type dosage forms is not necessary. Similarly, a drug with a short half life, i.e., < 2 hours, should not be formulated into a sustained release product because such a delivery system would require unacceptably large release rates and doses.

2. *They are uniformly absorbed from the gastrointestinal tract.* Drugs absorbed poorly or at varying and unpredictable rates are not good candidates for sustained-release products, because their drug release and therefore drug absorption will fluctuate, depending upon the position of the drug in the gastrointestinal tract and the dosage form's rate of movement within the tract.

3. *They are administered in relatively small doses.* Drugs with large single doses frequently are not suitable for the preparation of the sustained-action product because the individual dosage unit needed to maintain the extended therapeutic blood level of the

Fig. 5–63A. *Hypothetical drug blood level-time curves for a conventional solid dosage form and a controlled release product.*

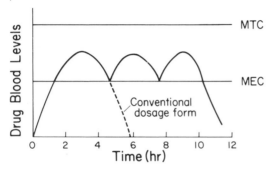

Fig. 5–63B. *Hypothetical drug blood level-time curves for a conventional solid dosage form and a multiple-action product.*

drug would have to be too large for the patient to easily swallow.

4. *They possess a good margin of safety.* The most widely used measure of the margin of safety is its therapeutic index [Chapter 2], i.e., median toxic dose, TD50/median effective dose, ED50. This index can range from one (where the effective dose produces toxic effects) to several thousand. For very "potent" drugs whose therapeutic concentration is narrow, the value of the therapeutic index is very small. The larger the therapeutic index the safer the drug. Thus, those drugs which are potent in very small doses or possess very narrow or small therapeutic indices are poor candidates for formulation into controlled-release formulations because of technologic limitations of precise control over release rates.

5. *They are used in the treatment of chronic rather than acute conditions.* Drugs for acute conditions generally require more physician control of the dosage than that provided by sustained-release products.

The most common mechanisms utilized in rate-controlled pharmaceutical products are: solvent action of biologic fluids on coated drug particles, osmotic systems controlled by the diffusion of biologic fluids through a polymer, erodible systems controlled by the erosion of a polymeric matrix, diffusion systems controlled by the diffusion of the drug through a polymeric membrane or monolithic matrix, and chemical reaction or interaction between the drug substance or its pharmaceutical barrier and site-specific biologic fluids. These mechanisms are utilized in the development of dosage forms and drug delivery systems for oral and other routes of administration.

Examples of the pharmaceutical technology utilized to achieve rate-controlled and sustained release solid dosage forms are described below.

COATED BEADS OR GRANULES OR MICROENCAP-SULATED DRUG. In this method a solution of the drug substance in a non-aqueous solvent such as a mixture of acetone and alcohol is coated onto small inert non-pareil seeds or beads made of a combination of sugar and starch. In instances in which the dose of the drug is large, the starting granules of material may be composed of the drug itself. Then with some of the beads or granules remaining uncoated and intended to provide the immediately released dose of drug when taken, coats of a lipid material like beeswax or a cellulosic material like ethylcellulose are applied to the remainder (about two-thirds to three-fourths) of the granules, with some granules receiving a few coats and others many coats. Then the beads or granules of different thicknesses of coatings are blended in the desired proportions to achieve the proper blend. The coating material may be colored with a dye material so that the beads of different coating thicknesses will be darker in color and distinguishable from those having fewer coats and being lighter in color. When properly blended, the granules may be placed in capsules or tableted. The variation in the thickness of the coats and in the type of material used in the coating is reflected in the rate at which the body fluids are capable of penetrating the coating and in dissolving the drug. Naturally, the thicker the coat, the more resistant to penetration and the more delayed will be the drug release. The presence of drug granules of various coating thicknesses therefore produces the sustained drug release. The time-blood level profile is similar to that obtained with multiple dosing. An example of this type of dosage form is the *Spansule* capsule, shown in Figure 5–64.

Microencapsulation is a process by which solids, liquids, or even gases may be encapsulated into microscopic size particles through the formation of thin coatings of "wall" material around the substance being encapsulated. The process had its early origin in the late 1930s as a "clean" substitute for carbon paper and carbon ribbons as sought by the business machines industry. The ultimate development in the 1950s of reproduction paper and ribbons which contained dyes in tiny gelatin capsules released upon impact by a typewriter key or the pressure of a pen or pencil was the stimulus for the development of a host of microencapsulated materials, including drugs. Gelatin is a common wall-forming material but synthetic polymers as polyvinyl alcohol, ethylcellulose, or polyvinyl chloride have been used. The typical encapsulation process usually begins with the dissolving of the prospective wall material, say gelatin, in water. The material to be encapsulated is added and the two-phase mixture thoroughly stirred. With the material to be encapsulated broken up to the desired particle size, a solution of a second material is added, usually acacia. This additive material is chosen to have the ability to concentrate the gelatin (polymer) into tiny liquid droplets. These droplets (coacervate) then form a film or coat around the particles of the substance to be encapsulated as a consequence of the extremely low interfacial tension of the residual water or solvent in the wall material so that a continuous, tight, film coating remains on the particle (Fig. 5–65). The final dry microcapsules are free-flowing, discrete particles of coated material. Of the total particle weight, the wall material usually represents between 2 and 20%. By varying the wall thickness of microencapsulated drug particles, their dissolution rates may be altered and sustained release obtained. An example of a drug commercially available in microencapsulated dosage form is potassium chloride as Micro-K (Robins Laboratories).

EMBEDDING DRUG IN SLOWLY ERODING MATRIX. By this process, the portion of the drug intended to have sustained action is combined with lipid or cellulosic material processed into granules that can be placed into capsules or tableted. When these granules are combined with granules of drug prepared without the special lipid or cellulosic excipient, the untreated portion provides the immediate drug effect, and the treated portion the prolonged effect. The treated granules slowly erode in the body fluids. The types of materials used in the preparation of the granules may be varied to achieve different rates of erosion. The product SLOW-K (CIBA) is a sugar-coated tablet containing 8 mEq of potassium chloride in a wax matrix. The formulation is intended to provide a controlled release of potassium from the matrix to minimize the likelihood of producing high (and irritating) localized concentrations of potassium within the gastrointestinal tract.

Two-layered tablets may be prepared from the granules, with one layer containing the untreated drug for immediate release and the other layer having the drug for sustained release. Three-layered tablets may be similarly prepared, with both outer layers containing the drug for immediate release. Some commercial tablets are prepared with an inner core containing the sustained release portion of drug and

Fig. 5–64. *The* Spansule *capsule showing the hard gelatin capsule containing hundreds of tiny pellets for sustained drug release and the rupturing of one of the pellets as occurs in the gastric fluid. (Courtesy of Smith, Kline & French Laboratories.)*

Fig. 5–65. *Microscapsules of mineral oil in a gelatin-acacia coacervate. (Photo courtesy of James C. Price, Ph.D., College of Pharmacy, The University of Georgia.)*

an outer shell completely enclosing the core and containing the drug portion for immediate release. Tablets prepared from the type of material described in the next method may be similarly constructed.

EMBEDDING DRUG IN INERT PLASTIC MATRIX. By this method, the drug is granulated with an inert plastic material such as polyethylene, polyvinyl acetate, or polymethacrylate, and the granulation is compressed into tablets. The drug is slowly released from the inert plastic matrix by leaching by the body fluids. The compression of the tablet creates the matrix or plastic form that retains its shape during the leaching of the drug and through its elimination from the alimentary tract. The initially released drug is present on the surfaces of the tablet or is only superficially embedded. The primary example of a dosage form of this type is the *Gradumet* (Abbott).

COMPLEX FORMATION. Certain drug substances when chemically combined with certain other chemical agents form chemical complexes that may be only slowly soluble in body fluids, depending upon the pH of the environment. This slow dissolution rate is effective to provide the sustained action of the drug.

It should be remembered that certain drug substances that are only slowly soluble in body fluids without special complexation or other treatment are inherently long acting.

ION-EXCHANGE RESINS. A solution of the cationic drug is passed through a column containing the ion-exchange resin, to which it complexes by the replacement of hydrogen atoms. The resin-drug complex is then washed and may be tableted, encapsulated, or suspended in an aqueous vehicle. The release of the drug is dependent upon the pH and the electrolyte concentration in the gastrointestinal tract. Generally, release is greater in the acidity of the stomach than the less acidic small intestine. Examples of drug products of this type include *Biphetamine* capsules (resin complexes of amphetamine and dextroamphetamine) and *Ionamin* capsules (phentermine resin) both by Pennwalt.

The mechanism of action of drug release from ion exchange resins may be depicted as follows.

In the stomach:
(1) Drug resinate + HCl⇌acidic resin + drug hydrochloride
(2) Resin salt + HCl⇌resin chloride + acidic drug

In the intestine:
(1) Drug resinate + NaCl⇌sodium resinate + drug hydrochloride
(2) Resin salt + NaCl⇌resin chloride + sodium salt of drug.

Pennwalt's "Pennkinetic" system incorporates a polymer barrier coating and bead technology in addition to the ion-exchange mechanism. The initial dose comes from an uncoated portion, and the remainder from the coated beads. The coating does not dissolve, and release is controlled over a 12-hour period by ionic exchange. The drug-containing polymer particles are minute, and may be suspended to produce a liquid with controlled-release characteristics [e.g., Delsym (McNeil)] as well as solid dosage forms.

HYDROCOLLOID SYSTEM. Hydrocolloids can play a significant role in the design of a controlled-release product. An example is the product Valrelease, a 15-mg slow-release dosage form of Valium (diazepam/Roche). Valrelease has been formulated using a unique Hydrodynamically Balanced drug-delivery System (HBS). This dosage form was designed to achieve, in one administration, plasma concentrations of diazepam equivalent to those ob-

Fig. 5–66. *Depiction of the OROS osmotic pump drug delivery system. (Courtesy of Alza Corporation.)*

tained with conventional Valium 5 mg tablets taken 3 times daily. The Hydrodynamically Balanced drug-delivery System consists of a matrix so designed that upon contact with gastric fluid, the dosage form demonstrates a bulk density of less than one and, thus, remains buoyant. When the Valrelease capsule shell dissolves, the outermost hydrocolloids come in contact with gastric fluid. They swell to form a boundary layer, which prevents immediate penetration of fluid into the formulation. The outer hydrocolloid boundary layer gradually erodes, with the subsequent formation of another "outer" boundary layer. This is a continuous process causing the gelatinous mass to constantly erode, while diazepam is gradually released through each layer as the fluid slowly penetrates the matrix. Valrelease remains in the stomach for a variable period of time, depending on individual physiologic characteristics. However, when Valrelease passes into the intestine, gradual release of the active drug and absorption continue.

OSMOTIC PUMP. The Oros system, developed by Alza, is an oral osmotic pump composed of a core tablet and a semi-permeable coating with a 0.4 mm diameter hole for drug exit. The hole is produced by a laser beam and the product operates on the principle of osmotic pressure (Fig. 5–66). The semi-permeable membrane permits water to enter from the patient's stomach into the core, dissolving the drug. The pressure that is built up forces or pumps the drug solution out of the delivery orifice (Fig. 5–67). A currently marketed product of this type is Acutrim (CIBA-Geigy).

Oros is a sophisticated oral controlled release drug delivery system in which the release rate may be controlled by changing the *surface area, the thickness* or *the nature* of the membrane and/or by changing the diameter of the drug release

Fig. 5–67. *The OROS (Oral Osmotic) drug delivery system. A tablet core of drug is surrounded by a semipermeable membrane that is pierced by a small laser-drilled hole. After ingestion, water is drawn into the tablet from the digestive tract by osmosis. As water enters the tablet core, the drug gradually goes into solution. The solution is pushed out through the small hole at a controlled rate of about 1 to 2 drops per hour. (Courtesy of ALZA Corporation.)*

orifice. Other pharmaceutical companies have developed similar systems. For example, Elan Pharmaceutical has developed a system called Modas–*Multidirectional Osmotic Drug Absorption System*. Modas is an osmotic device with solubilized drug delivered through a fixed permeable membrane designed to admit moisture and excrete the soluble drug back through the same membrane at constant pressure. The drug comes out of the entire surface area of the tablet at a constant rate.

Repeat Action Forms

Some specialized tablets are prepared so that an initial dose of the drug is released from the tablet shell and a second dose from an inner core of the tablet, which is separated from the outer shell by a slowly permeable barrier coating. Generally the barrier coating is penetrated and drug from the inner core is exposed to the body fluids some 4 to 6 hours after the swallowing of the tablet. Such a tablet permits the release of two doses of drug from a single tablet, eliminating the need for more frequent drug administration. An example of this type of dosage form is *Repetabs* (Schering). As for the sustained-action type of dosage forms, the repeat-action forms are best suited for those drugs having low dosage and employed in chronic conditions and for drugs having regular absorption patterns with fairly rapid rates of absorption and excretion.

Delayed Action Forms

The release of a drug from a dosage form may be intentionally delayed until it reaches the intestinal environment for any of several reasons. Among these may be the fact that the drug is destroyed by the gastric juices, or it may be excessively irritating to the lining of the stomach or a nauseating drug, or it may be better absorbed from the intestines than from the stomach. Capsules and tablets coated so as to remain intact in the stomach but yield their ingredients in the intestines are said to be *enteric coated*. The coating may be composed of a material that is pH dependent and breaks down in the less acidic environment of the intestine, or the coating may erode due to moisture and on a time basis coinciding with the time required for the tablet or capsule to reach the intestines. Other coatings may deteriorate due to the hydrolysis-catalyzing action of certain intestinal enzymes. Among the many agents used to enteric coat tablets and capsules are fats, fatty acids, waxes and mixtures of these, shellac, and cellulose acetate phthalate. An example of a commercially prepared brand of enteric coated tablets is *Enseals* (Lilly). A popular enteric-coated aspirin tablet is Ecotrin (Smith Kline Consumer Products).

Liposomes

In the early 1960s, research scientists noted that various phospholipids formed multilayered vesicles (sacs) when dispersed in water. These cell-like structures become known as *liposomes*. Like a biologic cell, a liposome is composed of a thin but durable membrane that surrounds an aqueous compartment, protecting it from the outside environment. Both cellular and liposome membranes are capable of regulating the transport of molecules in and out of the enclosed compartment. Thus liposomes may be used to control the passage of drugs, entrapped in the aqueous phase, through the membrane and to the intended body site for absorption or action. In recent years, drug-containing liposome systems have been developed for the delivery of drugs by various routes of administration including inhalation, ocular, injectable, dermal, and oral.

Liposomes may be constructed to have a single aqueous compartment surrounded by a lipid layer (*unilamellar*) or they may consist of concentric lipid and aqueous layers (*multilamellar*). The structure of liposomes permits the incorporation of fat-soluble drugs in the lipid layer and water-soluble drugs in the interior aqueous compartment. Drugs encapsulated in the aqueous phase are released by slowly diffusing through the lipid membrane. Lipid-soluble drugs embedded in the lipid membrane or bound to the membrane surface are slowly released as the membrane is broken down by body fluids. Because lipids from natural sources are used to form the liposome membrane, liposomes are considered biocompatible and biodegradable.

Liposomes are produced by dispersing the lipid (usually phospholipids) phase in the drug solution. Simple mixing to vigorous agitation is applied to the system. Upon dispersion, the lipid molecules align to form the biomolecular membrane. The lipophilic ends of the lipid molecules intercalate to form the inside of the membrane and the hydrophilic ends line up on the two outer surfaces. The membrane then wraps around, encapsulating the drug solution as the liposome is formed.

Generally, simple hand mixing of the phospholipid and aqueous phase produces a dispersion of multilamellar vesicles of large and widely mixed size. Various homogenizers and pressure flow-through devices have been utilized to achieve a more narrowly defined liposome size distribution. For use as drug carriers, liposomes should be homogeneous and reproducible in batch-to-batch production, stability, and drug release characteristics. Recently, microfluidization techniques have been used to produce liposomes of well-defined size distribution. This process involves the ultra high velocity interaction of two fluid streams in closely defined interaction. The pressures of the system, as high as 8000 psi, result in the jet interaction of the phases and liposome formation rates of as high as 75%, in contrast to other mixing systems which may result in a capture of the aqueous phase between 8 to 25%.

Because of the variation in the method of preparation, the size of liposomes varies from about 0.3 to 10 microns. The size of liposomes influences both their distribution in the body and their deposition. For instance, following injection, large size liposomes can have the tendency to deposit in the lungs whereas smaller particles may concentrate in other body sites, such as the liver. Alterations in the membrane composition, the phospholipid configuration, or in the electrical charge on liposomes can also greatly influence their distribution in the body. Agents as cholesterol and cetylphosphate have been incorporated into the phospholipid bilayers to alter the liposome's properties, changing not only the diffusion characteristics of the membrane but also the distribution of the liposome within the body following administration.

Several liposome products are under commercial development for inhalation, ocular, dermal and parenteral routes of administration. For example, liposome-based bronchodilators, delivered as nebulized and aerosolized solutions, are being designed to treat bronchospasm. Ocular delivery products containing "bioadhesive" liposomes that adhere to the eye's surface are being developed to provide lubricating eye drops and sustained effects for glaucoma medication. Liposome products for application of therapeutic agents to the skin and scalp to provide extended drug release and perhaps greater percutaneous absorption are being investigated. Liposome-based products are also being developed to target drugs to specific body organs following intravenous administration. The objective is to concentrate the drug's action at the desired body site to maximize therapeutic action and minimize toxicity. Drugs being studied include anticancer agents, antibiotics, and peptide hormones.

Other technologies for rate-controlled targeted delivery include the use of transdermal drug delivery systems, implantable (subcutaneous) drug delivery systems, ocular drug delivery systems, intravenous infusion pumps, and monoclonal antibodies which are utilized as specific carriers for drugs, enzymes, and radiopharmaceuticals in the diagnosis and treatment of disease. These technologies are discussed elsewhere in this text.

Pharmacist Monitoring of Patients Using Controlled-Release Drugs

When a patient is prescribed a controlled-release drug the attainment of the peak and therapeutic concentration of the drug might be somewhat delayed. If an immediate effect is desirable, either an intravenous dose or immediate-release dosage form of the drug would be preferable. Thus, a pharmacist when consulted about a dosing recommendation should keep this in mind as it relates to patient needs.

As mentioned earlier in this chapter variations in the bioavailability from a controlled-release product are possible so the pharmacist must be cognizant of patient complaints of unusual adverse effects or possible ineffectiveness. Therapeutic levels of the certain drugs, e.g., theophylline, must be maintained for the desired therapeutic outcome to occur and once a patient is stabilized on a controlled-release product it should not be substituted. A different product, even with an identical amount of active ingredient, could cause a marked shift in the patient's drug blood/serum level due to different release characteristics of the dosage form. Unless two controlled-release products of the same drug have demonstrated similar bioavailability and therapeutic effect they should not be used interchangeably or substituted for one another.

Packaging and Storing Tablets

Tablets are best stored in tight containers and in places of low humidity protected from extremes in temperature. Products that are especially prone to decomposition by moisture may be copackaged with a desiccant. Drugs that are adversely affected by light are packaged in light-resistant containers. With a few exceptions, solid dosage forms that are properly stored will be stable for several years or more.

In most instances of dispensing, the pharmacist is well advised to use a similar type of container as provided by the manufacturer of the product and the patient advised to maintain the drug in the container dispensed. Proper storage conditions as recommended for the particular drug should be maintained by the pharmacist and patient and expiration dates observed.

The pharmacist should be aware also that the hardness of certain tablets may change upon aging usually resulting in a decrease in the disintegration and dissolution rates of the product. The increase in tablet hardness can frequently be attributed to the increased adhesion of the binding agent and other formulative components within the tablet. Examples of increased tablet hardening with age have been reported for a number of drugs including aluminum hydroxide, sodium salicylate and phenylbutazone.[18]

Certain tablets containing volatile drugs, as nitroglycerin, may experience the migration of the drug between tablets in the container thereby resulting in a lack of uniformity among the tablets.[19] Further, packing materials, as cotton and rayon, in contact with nitroglycerin tablets may absorb varying amounts of nitroglycerin rendering the tablets sub-potent.[20]

In 1972, the Food and Drug Administration issued a number of regulations covering the packaging, labeling, and dispensing of nitroglycerin products. These regulations include:

1. All nitroglycerin tablets must be packaged in glass containers with tightly-fitting metal screw caps.
2. No more than 100 tablets may be packaged in each container.
3. Nitroglycerin tablets must be dispensed in their original containers and bear the label–"Warning: To prevent loss of potency, keep these tablets in the original container. Close tightly immediately after use."
4. All nitroglycerin tablets should be stored at controlled room temperatures of between 59° and 86° F.

Implementation of these regulations contributed to the maintenance of better content uniformity standards for nitroglycerin tablets than had been previously achieved. However, since nitroglycerin is a volatile liquid at room temperature, some nitroglycerin is lost to the atmosphere when the containers are opened and particularly if they are not tightly closed. In a further effort to reduce the loss of nitroglycerin from tablets and to prevent the migration of the substance from tablet to tablet, pharmaceutical manufacturers of these tablets have recently been developing "stabilized" nitroglycerin tablets. The main method used is to include a small amount of a nonvolatile substance in the formulation which has the effect of reducing the vapor pressure of the nitroglcyerin and thus its tendency to escape from the tablet. One such

marketed product is *Nitrostat* by Parke-Davis which contains polyethylene glycol as the stabilizer.

Other Solid Dosage Forms for Oral Administration

Pills

Pills are small, round, solid dosage forms containing a medicinal agent and intended to be administered orally. Although the manufacture and administration of pills was at one time quite prevalent, today pills have largely been replaced by compressed tablets and capsules. A procedure for the extemporaneous preparation of pills on a small-scale may be found in the first edition of this text.

Lozenges

Lozenges are disc-shaped, solid dosage forms containing a medicinal agent and generally a flavoring substance and intended to be slowly dissolved in the oral cavity for localized effects. Lozenges are frequently called *troches* and less frequently referred to as *pastilles*. Many of the commercially available lozenges have a hard candy as the base or a base of sugar and an adhesive substance such as mucilage or gum.

Commercially, lozenges may be made by compression, using a tablet machine and large, flat punches. The machine is operated at a high degree of compression to produce lozenges that are harder than ordinary tablets so that they slowly dissolve or disintegrate in the mouth. Medicinal substances that are heat stable may be prepared into a hard, sugar candy lozenge by candy-making machines that process a warm, highly concentrated, flavored syrup as the base and form the lozenges by molding and drying.

Lozenges are gaining renewed acceptance as a means to deliver a multitude of different drugs. As an example, for the treatment of oropharyngeal candidiasis a lozenge dosage form is available with either nystatin or clotrimazole as its active ingredient. The patient allows the lozenge (or troche) to slowly dissolve in the mouth, and the dosage form is much more convenient to the patient when compared to the necessity of swishing an oral suspension in the mouth. Further, these lozenges maintain adequate salivary levels of the antifungal drug for about 3 hours and help to promote effectiveness of therapy. Lozenge dosage forms are also available for self-care drugs, e.g., benzocaine, dextromethorphan, phenylpropanolamine, to treat acute, self-limiting conditions ranging from minor sore throat to cough and congestion. These forms are particularly advantageous for those persons who find it difficult to swallow solid dosage forms and for young children.

Solid Dosage Forms for Other than the Oral Route of Administration

There are a few solid dosage forms which are used by routes of administration other than oral. For instance, dosage forms called *pellets* or *inserts* are implanted under the skin by special injectors or by surgical incision for the purpose of providing for the continuous release of medication. Such implants provide the patient with an economical means of obtaining long-lasting effects (up to several months following implantation) and obviate the need for frequent injections or oral dosage administration. Hormonal substances are most frequently administered in this manner. Other solid dosage forms, *vaginal tablets* or *inserts*, are specially formulated and shaped tablets intended to be placed in the vagina by special applicators, where the medication is released, generally for localized effects. Another example of a solid dosage form intended for use by means other than swallowing is a specially prepared capsule containing a micronized powder [Intal (Fisons)] intended to be released from the capsule and inhaled deep into the lungs through the use of a special inhaler-device (Spinhaler turbo-inhaler). These dosage forms and drug delivery systems will be discussed in subsequent chapters.

Proper Administration of Peroral Dosage Forms

The dosage forms discussed in this chapter are all to be administered by mouth. The easiest way is to place the dosage form upon the tongue and swallow it with a glassful of water. Most patients will understand this method of administration and do so with water. However, some persons do not realize that these dosage forms should be taken with water and may proceed to merely swallow the tablet or the capsule. This can be dangerous because it is possible for the tablet or capsule to lodge within the esophagus.

Several documented cases of esophageal ulceration in young women, for example, have occurred with the ingestion of tetracycline and tetracycline derivatives, particularly when taken just before bedtime. Thus, it is important to counsel the patient to take all oral dosage forms with at least some water. This is particularly so with those dosage forms that contain aspirin, ferrous sulfate, any NSAID, potassium chloride and any tetracycline drug, to ensure passage of the medicine into the stomach. It is equally important to also instruct patients to take these medications no later than at least 1 hour before retiring for the evening.

Senior citizens are at an increased risk because the process of swallowing medications like those mentioned takes longer, and if they have esophageal strictures, there is the potential for these to lodge in the esophagus. Further, patients who suffer from gastroesophageal reflux disease must also be cautioned to take medicines with water and at least 1 hour before retiring. Otherwise, there is a possibility that some of the medicine may be refluxed back into the esophagus from the stomach once the patient retires for the evening.

As mentioned earlier in this chapter, certain oral dosage forms have protective coatings, e.g., enteric-coated, or may be formulated to provide delayed or continuous release of the active ingredient. The patient must be advised not to chew or crush these tablets as the amount and the rate of release of the drug may be dramatically altered. The patient should also be forewarned that they may notice remnants of these types of dosage forms in the stool. They should be told not to be concerned as the drug portion of the preparation has already been absorbed.

When a tablet can be crushed or a capsule opened to facilitate oral administration the pharmacist must keep in mind that medicines usually have an unpleasant taste. The bitter taste of the drug could be masked partially by recommending to the patient to mix the drug with applesauce, fruit juice, or carbonated beverages. However, the patient must be advised to consume the entire mixture. Otherwise the patient will not receive the total dose.

For those who experience gagging or choking when taking a solid dosage form, there is an innovative product called the Drink-A-Pill Drinking Glass. This contains a specially-designed shelf on which a tablet or capsule is placed after the glass is filled with water. When the patient drinks the content of the glass, the dosage form flows with the water into the mouth and goes right down without the gag reflex. Alternatively, if the patient simply cannot swallow the solid dosage form, the pharmacist can suggest to the prescribing physician a liquid form of the drug. If such a preparation is not available, is may be possible to extemporaneously compound the drug into a liquid vehicle. Several liquid formulations from solid dosage forms are listed in the *Handbook on Extemporaneous Formulations*. If this is not possible, the pharmacist could recommend the use of an available liquid dosage form of a different chemical compound with similar therapeutic effect.

Selected Reading

Banakar, U.V.: Drug Delivery Systems. *Amer. Pharm.*, NS27(2):39, 1987.

Bindschaldler, C., Gurny, R., and Doelker, E.: Mechanically strong films produced from cellulose acetate-latexes. *J. Pharm. Pharmacol.*, 39:335–338, 1986.

Chow, M.S.S.: Monitoring of Oral Controlled-Release Drugs. *U.S. Pharmacist*, 12(2):58, 1987.

Conine, J.W., and Hadley, H.R.: Preparation of Small Solid Pharmaceutical Spheres. *Drug and Cosmetic Ind.*, 106:38, 1970.

Davis, S.S.: Colloids as Drug-delivery Systems. *Pharm. Tech.* 11:110, 1987.

Davis, S.S., Norring-Christensen, F., Khosla, R., and Feely, L.C.: Gastric emptying of large single unit dosage forms. *J. Pharm. Pharmacol.*, 40:205–207, 1988.

Drug Delivery Systems. Eugene, OR, Aster Publishing Corp., 1987.

Flynn, G.L.: Considerations in Controlled-Release Drug Delivery Systems. *Pharm. Tech.*, 6:33–39, 1982.

Foley, V.L., and Belcastro, P.F.: From Bullets to Pills: The Mechanization of Tablet Manufacturing. *Pharm. Tech.*, 11:110, 1987.

Gore, A.Y., McFarland, D.W., and Batuyios: Fluid-bed Granulation: Factors Affecting the Process in Laboratory Development and Production Scale-up. *Pharm. Tech.*, 9:114, 1985.

Heller, J.: Chemically self-regulated drug delivery systems. *J. Controlled Release*, 8:111–125, 1988.

Industrial wet granulation, N.O. Lindberg (ed.). *Acta Pharm. Suecica*, 25:185–280, 1988.

Jones B.E.: Hard Gelatin Capsules and the Pharmaceutical Formulator. *Pharm. Tech.*, 9:106–112, 1985.

Jones, T.M.: The Influence of Excipients on the Design and Manufacture of Tablets and Capsules. *Drug and Cosmetic Ind.*, 124:40, 1979.

Krowczynski, L.: Extended Release Dosage Forms. Boca Raton, FL, CRC Press, Inc., 1987, pp. 97–150.

Luzzi, L.: Microencapsulation. *J. Pharm. Sci.*, 59:1367–1375, 1970.

Madan, P.L.: Sustained-Release Drug Delivery Systems: Part I. An Overview. *Pharm. Manufacturing*, 2:23–27, 1985.

Mathur, L.K., Forbes, S.J., and Yelvigi, M.: Characterization Techniques for the Aqueous Film Coating Process. *Pharm. Tech.* 8:42, 1984.

Mayhew, E., Nikolopoulos, G.T., King, J.J., and Siciliano, A.A.: A Practical Method for the Large-Scale Manufacture of Liposomes. *Pharm. Manufacturing*, 2:18–22, 1985.

Mehta, A.M.: Factors in the Development of Oral Controlled-Release Dosage Forms. *Pharm. Manufacturing*, 3:23, 1986.

Mitchell, J.F., and Pawlicki, K.S.: Oral Dosage Forms that Should not be Crushed. *Hosp. Pharm.*, 22:987–988, 1987.

Mufson, D.: The Application of Liposome Technology to Targeted Delivery Systems. In *Drug Delivery Systems*. Palo Alto, Aster Publishing Corp., 1985, pp. 16–21.

Page, D.P., et al.: Stability Study of Nitroglycerin Sublingual Tablets. *J. Pharm Sci.*, 64:140–147, 1975.

Park, K., Wood, R., and Robinson, J.: Oral controlled systems. In *Medical Applications of Controlled Release*. R.S. Langer and D.L. Wise (eds.), Boca Raton, FL, CRC Press, Inc., 1984, pp. 159–201.

Schwartz, J.B.: Granulation. *Drug Devel. Ind. Pharm.*, 14:2071–2090, 1988.

Urquhart, J. (ed.): *Controlled-Release Pharmaceuticals*: Washington, D.C., Amer. Pharm. Assoc., 1981.

Yeung, V.W., and Nixon, J.R.: Preparation of Microencapsulated Liposomes. *J. Microencapsulation*, 5:331–337, 1988.

Notes

1. Orr, C., and Dallavalle, J.M.: *Fine Particles Measurement*. New York, The Macmillan Co., 1959.

2. Irani, R.R., and Callis, C.F.: *Particle Size Measurement, Interpretation and Application*. New York, John Wiley & Sons, Inc., 1963.

3. Parrott, E.L.: Milling. In *The Theory and Practice of Industrial Pharmacy*, 3rd Ed., L. Lachman, H.A. Lieberman, and J.L. Kanig. (eds.). Philadelphia, Lea & Febiger, 1986, pp. 21–46.

4. It should be noted that a type of pharmaceutical preparation termed a *trituration* is a powder mixture, usually containing 10% of a potent medicinal substance in a vehicle of lactose. Triturations provide a convenient means whereby pharmacists can accurately obtain small amounts of potent drugs. For example, 50 mg of a potent drug may be obtained by weighing 500 mg of a 10% trituration of that drug.

5. Dosage units, such as tablets and capsules, containing therapeutically inert materials or drug substances unrelated to the disease or condition being treated are termed *placebos*. A placebo is deliberately prescribed by a physician for its nonspecific psychologic or psychophysiologic effect without the patient's knowledge. Actually, a placebo may include not only oral dosage forms, but parenteral medication, topical preparations, inhalants, and other types of pharmaceutical preparations as well as mechanical, surgical, or other

therapeutic techniques. A pharmacist may issue a placebo for a specific drug by replacing the contents of a capsule with an inert or inappropriate (to the symptom or illness) substance. The reader may wish to refer to the following paper which deals with the usefulness of placebo treatment: Vogel, A.V., Goodwin, J.S., and Goodwin, J.M.: The Therapeutics of Placebo. *American Family Physician*, July, 1980, pp. 105–109.

6. Mitchell, J.F., and Pawlicki, K.S.: Oral Dosage Forms that Should not be Crushed: 1987 revision. *Hosp. Pharmacy*, 22:987, 1987.

7. It is possible for pharmacists to color extemporaneously small numbers of plain empty gelatin capsules by placing the separated capsules in a small volume of 70% alcohol containing the desired dye (food colorings used in baking may be used), allowing the capsules to be submerged in the solution for a minute or so, decanting the solution, and drying the capsules on a paper towel. Excessive water in the dye solution or excessive exposure to the solution may result in the distortion of the capsules.

8. Caldwell, H.C.: Dissolution of Lithium and Magnesium from Lithium Carbonate Capsules Containing Magnesium Stearate. *J. Pharm. Sci.*, 63:770–773, 1974.

9. Capsule Sealing with the Licaps® Sealing Process. Capsugel, Greenwood, S.C., 1986.

10. Stanley, J.P.: Soft Gelatin Capsules. In *The Theory and Practice of Industrial Pharmacy*. 3rd Ed. L. Lachman, H.A. Lieberman, and J.L. Kanig (eds.), Philadelphia, Lea & Febiger, 1986, pp. 398–429.

11. It should be apparent that when reference is made to a "20-mg tablet," the reference is to the amount of drug contained in the tablet and not to the actual weight of the tablet. Tablets such as aspirin tablets, which generally have small amounts of pharmaceutical adjuncts present, may actually weigh only slightly more than the amount of active ingredient present. Generally tablets made from drugs with large doses have proportionately less diluent present than do tablets made from drugs with small doses, and there is a closer relationship between drug present and tablet weight for the former type of drug than for the latter.

12. The USP XXII-NFXVII should be consulted for the full details of the apparatus and the testing procedure.

13. Khan, K.A., and Rhodes, C.T.: Water-Sorption Properties of Tablet Disintegrants. *J. Pharm. Sci.*, 64:447, 1975.

14. Lowenthal, W., and Wood, J.H.: Mechanism of Action of Starch as a Tablet Disintegrant VI: Location and Structure of Starch in Tablets. *J. Pharm. Sci.*, 62:287, 1973.

15. Shangraw, R.F., Wallace, J.W., and Bowers, F.M.: Morphology and Functionality in Tablet Excipients for Direct Compression. *Pharm. Tech.*, 11:136, 1987.

16. Mathur, L.K., Forbes, S.J., and Yelvigi, M.: Characterization Techniques for the Aqueous Film Coating Process. *Pharm. Tech.*, 8:42, 1984.

17. "Atlas Mannitol, USP Tablet Excipient," ICI Americas Inc., Wilmington, Delaware, 1973.

18. Barrett, D. and Fell, J.T.: Effect of Aging on Physical Properties of Phenylbutazone Tablets. *J. Pharm. Sci.*, 64:335, 1975.

19. Page, D.P., *et al.*: Stability Study of Nitroglycerin Sublingual Tablets. *J. Pharm. Sci.*, 64:140, 1975.

20. Fusari, S.A.: Nitroglycerin Sublingual Tablets I: Stability of Conventional Tablets. *J. Pharm. Sci.*, 62:122, 1973.

6 | *Oral Solutions, Syrups, and Elixirs*

IN PHYSICOCHEMICAL terms, solutions may be prepared from any combination of solid, liquid, and gas, the three states of matter. For example, a solid solute may be dissolved in either another solid, a liquid, or a gas, and with the same being true for a liquid solute and for a gas, nine types of homogeneous mixtures are possible. In pharmacy, however, interest in solutions is for the most part limited to preparations of a solid, a liquid, and less frequently a gas solute dissolved in a liquid solvent.

In pharmaceutical terms, *solutions* are defined as "liquid preparations that contain one or more soluble chemical substances usually dissolved in water and that do not, by reasons of their ingredients; method of preparation or use, fall into another group of products." Indeed, many pharmaceutical products, which from a physicochemical standpoint are solutions in that they are homogeneous mixtures of solute dissolved in solvent, are, from a pharmaceutical standpoint, classified as other product types. For example, aqueous pharmaceutical solutions containing a sugar are classified as *syrups;* sweetened hydroalcoholic (combinations of water and ethanol) solutions are termed *elixirs;* solutions of aromatic materials are termed *spirits* if the solvent is alcoholic or *aromatic waters* if the solvent is aqueous. Solutions prepared by extracting active constituents from crude drugs are termed *tinctures* or *fluid extracts,* depending upon their method of preparation and their concentration. *Tinctures* may also be solutions of chemical substances dissolved in alcohol or in a hydroalcoholic solvent. Certain solutions prepared to be sterile and pyrogen-free and intended for parenteral administration are classified as *injections.* Although other examples could be cited, it is apparent that a solution, as a distinct type of pharmaceutical preparation, is much more limited in its meaning than is the physicochemical definition of the term *solution.*

This chapter deals with the general area of solution preparation and concentrates on the oral solution and the two other dosage forms most frequently utilized in the administration of oral medication in solution, the syrup and elixir. Solutions employed topically, by injection, ophthalmically, and by other means are covered in subsequent chapters.

Oral solutions, syrups, and elixirs are prepared and utilized for the specific effects of the medicinal agents present. In these preparations the medicinal agents are intended to provide systemic effects. The fact that they are administered in solution form usually means that their absorption from the gastrointestinal tract into the systemic circulation may be expected to occur more rapidly than from suspension or solid dosage forms of the same medicinal agent.

Solutes other than the medicinal agent are usually present in orally administered solutions. These additional agents usually are included to provide color, flavor, sweetness, or stability to the solution. In formulating or compounding a pharmaceutical solution, the pharmacist must utilize information on the solubility and stability of each of the solutes present with regard to the solvent or solvent system employed. He must guard against using combinations of medicinal or pharmaceutic agents which will result in chemical or physical interactions affecting the therapeutic quality or pharmaceutic stability of the product.

For single-solute solutions and especially for multiple-solute solutions, the pharmacist must be aware of the solubility characteristics of the solutes and the features of the common pharmaceutical solvents. Each chemical agent has its own solubility in a given solvent. For many medicinal agents, their exact solubilities in the usual solvents are stated in the USP as well as in other reference books.

Solubility

Attractive forces between atoms lead to the formation of molecules and ions. The intermolecular forces, which are developed between like molecules, are responsible for the physical state (i.e., solid, liquid, or gas) of the substance under given conditions, as temperature and pressure. Under ordinary conditions, most organic compounds, and thus most drug substances, form molecular solids.

When molecules interact, attractive forces and repulsive forces are in effect. The attractive forces cause the molecules to cohere, whereas the repulsive forces prevent molecular interpenetration and destruction. When the attractive and repulsive forces are equal, the potential energy between two molecules is minimum and the system is most stable.

Dipolar molecules frequently tend to align themselves with other dipolar molecules such that the negative pole of one molecule points toward the positive pole of the other. Large groups of molecules may be associated through these weak attractions known as *dipole-dipole* or van der Waals forces. In addition to the dipolar interactions, other attractions occur between polar and nonpolar molecules and ions. These include ion-dipole forces and hydrogen bonding. The latter is of particular interest. Because of small size and large electrostatic field, the hydrogen atom can move in close to an electronegative atom, forming an electrostatic type of association referred to as a *hydrogen bond* or *hydrogen bridge*. Hydrogen bonding involves strongly electronegative atoms as oxygen, nitrogen, and fluorine. Such a bond exists in water, represented by the dotted lines:

Water

Hydrogen bonds also exist between some alcohol molecules, esters, carboxylic acids, aldehydes, and polypeptides.

When a solute dissolves, the substance's intermolecular forces of attraction must be overcome by forces of attraction between the solute and solvent molecules. This involves breaking the solute-solute forces and the solvent-solvent forces to achieve the solute-solvent attraction.

The *solubility* of an agent in a particular solvent indicates the *maximum* concentration to which a solution may be prepared with that agent and that solvent. When a solvent, at a given temperature, has dissolved all of the solute it can, it is said to be *saturated*. In order to emphasize the possible variation in solubility between two chemical agents and therefore in the amounts of each required to prepare a saturated solution, two official aqueous saturated solutions are cited as examples, Calcium Hydroxide Topical Solution, USP, and Potassium Iodide Oral Solution, USP. The first solution, prepared by agitating an excess amount of calcium hydroxide with purified water, contains only about 140 mg of dissolved solute per 100 mL of solution at 25°C, whereas the latter solution contains about 100 g of solute per 100 mL of solution, over 700 times as much solute as present in the calcium hydroxide topical solution. It is apparent from this comparison that the maximum possible concentration to which a pharmacist may prepare a solution varies greatly and is dependent, in part, on the chemical constitution of the solute. Through selection of a different solubilizing agent or a different chemical salt form of the medicinal agent, alteration of the pH of a solution, or substitution, in part or in whole, of the solvent, a pharmacist can in certain instances dissolve greater quantities of a solute than would otherwise be possible. For example, iodine granules are soluble in water only to the extent of 1 g in about 3000 mL of water. Using only these two agents, the maximum concentration possible would be approximately 0.03% of iodine in aqueous solution. However, through the use of an aqueous solution of potassium or sodium iodide as the solvent, much larger amounts of iodine may be dissolved as the result of the formation of a water-soluble complex with the iodide salt. This reaction is taken advantage of, for example, in Iodine Topical Solution USP, prepared to contain about 2% of iodine and 2.4% of sodium iodide.

Temperature is an important factor in determining the solubility of a drug and in preparing its solution. Most chemicals absorb heat when they are dissolved and are said to have a *negative heat of solution*, resulting in increased solubility with a rise in temperature. A few chemicals have a *positive heat of solution* and exhibit a decrease in solubility with a rise in temperature. Other factors, in addition to temperature, affect solubility. These include the various chemical

Table 6–1. Terms of Solubility

Descriptive Term	Parts of Solvent Required for 1 Part of Solute
Very soluble	Less than 1
Freely soluble	From 1 to 10
Soluble	From 10 to 30
Sparingly soluble	From 30 to 100
Slightly soluble	From 100 to 1000
Very slightly soluble	From 1000 to 10,000
Practically insoluble, or Insoluble	More than 10,000

Table 6–2. Water and Alcohol Solubilities of Some Selected Weak Acids, Weak Bases, and Their Salts

	Number of mL of Solvent Required to Dissolve 1 g of Drug	
Drug	Water	Alcohol
Atropine	455	2
Atropine sulfate	0.5	5
Codeine	120	2
Codeine sulfate	30	1,280
Codeine phosphate	2.5	325
Morphine	5,000	210
Morphine sulfate	16	565
Phenobarbital	1,000	8
Phenobarbital sodium	1	10
Procaine	200	soluble
Procaine hydrochloride	1	15
Sulfadiazine	13,000	sparingly soluble
Sodium sulfadiazine	2	slightly soluble

and other physical properties of both the solute and the solvent, factors of pressure, the acidity or basicity of the solution, the state of subdivision of the solute, and the physical agitation applied to the solution during the dissolving process. The solubility of a pure chemical substance at a given temperature and pressure is constant; however, its *rate of solution,* that is, the speed at which it dissolves, depends upon the particle size of the substance and the extent of agitation. The finer the powder, the greater the surface area that comes in contact with the solvent, and the more rapid the dissolving process. Also, the greater the agitation, the more unsaturated solvent passes over the drug, and the faster the formation of the solution.

The solubility of a substance in a given solvent may be determined by preparing a saturated solution of it at a specific temperature and determining by chemical analysis the amount of chemical dissolved in a given weight of solution. By simple calculation, the amount of solvent required to dissolve the amount of solute can be determined. The solubility may then be expressed as grams of solute dissolving in milliliters of solvent—for example, "1 g of sodium chloride dissolves in 2.8 mL of water." When the exact solubility has not been determined, general expressions of relative solubility may be used. These terms are defined in the USP as presented in Table 6–1.

A great many of the important organic medicinal agents are either weak acids or weak bases, and their solubility is dependent to a large measure upon the pH of the solvent. These drugs react either with strong acids or strong bases to form water-soluble salts. For instance, the weak bases, including many of the alkaloids (atropine, codeine, and morphine), antihistamines (diphenhydramine and tripelen-

amine), local anesthetics (cocaine, procaine, and tetracaine), and other important drugs are not very water-soluble,[1] but they are soluble in dilute solutions of acids. Pharmaceutical manufacturers have prepared many acid salts of these organic bases to enable the preparation of aqueous solutions. It must be recognized, however, that if the pH of the aqueous solutions of these salts is changed by the addition of alkali, the free base may separate from solution unless it has adequate solubility in water. Organic medicinals that are weak acids include the barbiturate drugs (as phenobarbital and pentobarbital) and the sulfonamides (as sulfadiazine and sulfacetamide). These and other weak acids form water-soluble salts in basic solution and may separate from solution by a lowering of the pH. Table 6–2 presents the comparative solubilities of some typical examples of weak acids and weak bases and their salts.

Although there are no exact rules for predicting unerringly the solubility of a chemical agent in a particular liquid, experienced pharmaceutical chemists utilize the type of information presented in Table 6–2 in estimating the solubility features of a similar chemical compound. The information gathered on a great number of individual chemical compounds has led to the characterization of the solubilities of groups of compounds, and though there may

Table 6–3. Solubilities of Selected Organic Compounds in Water as a Demonstration of Chemical Structure-Solubility Relationship

Compound	Formula	Number of mL of Water Required to Dissolve 1 g of Compound
Benzene	C_6H_6	1430
Benzoic acid	C_6H_5COOH	275
Benzyl alcohol	$C_6H_5CH_2OH$	25
Phenol	C_6H_5OH	15
Pyrocatechol	$C_6H_4(OH)_2$	2.3
Pyrogallol	$C_6H_3(OH)_3$	1.7
Carbon Tetra-chloride	CCl_4	2000
Chloroform	$CHCl_3$	200
Methylene Chloride	CH_2Cl_2	50

be an occasional inaccuracy with respect to an individual member of a group of compounds, the generalizations nonetheless serve a useful function. As demonstrated by the data in Table 6–2 and other similar data, salts of organic compounds are generally more soluble in water than are the corresponding organic bases. Conversely, the organic bases are generally more soluble in organic solvents, including alcohol, than are the corresponding salt forms. Perhaps the most written guideline for the prediction of solubility is that "like dissolves like," meaning that a solvent having a chemical structure most similar to that of the intended solute will be most likely to dissolve it. Thus, organic compounds are more soluble in organic solvents than in water. Organic compounds may, however, be somewhat water-soluble if they contain polar groups capable of forming hydrogen bonds with water.[2] In fact, the greater the number of polar groups present, the greater will likely be the organic compound's solubility in water. Further, the introduction of halogen atoms into a molecule tends to decrease water-solubility because of an increase in the molecular weight of the compound without a proportionate increase in polarity. An increase in the molecular weight of an organic compound without a change in polarity generally results in decreased solubility in water. Table 6–3 demonstrates some of these generalities through the use of specific chemical examples.

As with organic compounds, the pharmacist is aware of some general patterns of solubility

that apply to inorganic compounds. For instance, most salts of monovalent cations such as sodium, potassium, and ammonium are water soluble, whereas the divalent cations like calcium, magnesium, and barium usually form water-soluble compounds with nitrate, acetate, and chloride anions but not with carbonate, phosphate, or hydroxide anions.[3] To be sure, there are certain combinations of anion and cation which would seem to be quite similar in make-up but which do not have similar solubility characteristics. For instance, magnesium sulfate (Epsom salt) is soluble, but calcium sulfate is only slightly soluble; barium sulfate is very insoluble (1 g dissolves in about 400,000 mL of water) and is used as an opaque media for x-ray observation of the intestinal tract, but barium sulfide and barium sulfite are not as insoluble, and their oral use can result in poisoning; mercurous chloride (HgCl) is insoluble and was formerly used as a cathartic, but mercuric chloride ($HgCl_2$) is soluble in water and is a deadly poison if taken internally. There are many instances in which solubilities of certain drugs and their differentiation from other drugs are critical to the pharmacist in order that he might avoid compounding failures or therapeutic disasters.

For organic as well as for inorganic solutes, the ability of a solvent to dissolve them depends upon its effectiveness in overcoming the electronic forces that hold the atoms of the solute together and the corresponding lack of resolute on the part of the atoms themselves to resist the solvent action. During the dissolution process, the molecules of the solvent and the solute become uniformly mixed and cohesive forces of the atoms are replaced by new forces due to the attraction of the solute and solvent molecules for one another.

The student may find the following general rules of solubility useful.

A. For Inorganic Molecules

1. If *both* the cation and anion of an ionic compound are *monovalent*, the solute-solute attractive forces are usually easily overcome, and therefore, these compounds are generally water soluble. (Examples, NaCl, LiBr, KI, NH_4NO_3, $NaNO_2$)
2. If only *one* of the two ions in an ionic compound is *monovalent*, the solute-solute interactions are also usually easily overcome and the compounds are generally water

soluble. (Examples: $BaCl_2$, MgI_2, Na_2SO_4, Na_3PO_4)

3. If *both* the cation and anion are *multivalent* the solute-solute interaction may be too great to be overcome by the solute-solvent interaction and the compound may have poor water solubility. (Examples: $CaSO_4$, $BaSO_4$, $BiPO_4$; Exceptions: $ZnSO_4$, $FeSO_4$)
4. Common salts of alkali metals (Na, K, Li, Cs, Rb) are usually water soluble. (Exception: Li_2CO_3)
5. Ammonium and quaternary ammonium salts are water soluble.
6. Nitrates, nitrites, acetates, chlorates, and lactates are generally water soluble. (Exceptions: silver and mercurous acetate)
7. Sulfates, sulfites, and thiosulfates are generally water soluble. (Exceptions: calcium and barium salts)
8. Chlorides, bromides, and iodides are generally water soluble. (Exceptions: salts of silver and mercurous ions)
9. Acid salts corresponding to an insoluble salt will be more water soluble than the original salt.
10. Hydroxides and oxides of compounds other than alkali metal cations and the ammonium ion are generally water insoluble.
11. Sulfides are water insoluble except for their alkali metal salts.
12. Phosphates, carbonates, silicates, borates, and hypochlorites are water insoluble except for their alkali metal salts and ammonium salts.

B. For Organic Molecules

1. Molecules having one polar functional group are usually soluble to total chain lengths of five carbons.
2. Molecules having branched chains are more soluble than the corresponding straight-chain compound.
3. Water solubility decreases with an increase in molecular weight.
4. Increased structural similarity between solute and solvent is accompanied by increased solubility.

It is the pharmacist's knowledge of the chemical characteristics of drugs that permits the selection of the proper solvent for a particular solute. However, in addition to the factors of solubility, the selection is based on such additional solvent characteristics as clarity, low toxicity, viscosity, compatibility with other formulative ingredients, chemical inertness, palatability, odor, color, and economy. In most instances, and especially for solutions to be taken orally, used ophthalmically, or injected, water is the preferred solvent, because it comes closer to meeting the majority of the above criteria than the other available solvents. In many instances, when water is used as the primary solvent, an auxiliary solvent is also employed to augment the solvent action of water or to counter any of its deficiencies. Alcohol, glycerin, and propylene glycol, perhaps the most used auxiliary solvents, have been quite effective in contributing to the desired characteristics of pharmaceutical solutions and in maintaining their stability.

Other solvents, as acetone, ethyl oxide, and isopropyl alcohol, are too toxic to be permitted in pharmaceutical preparations to be taken internally, but they are useful as reagent solvents in organic chemistry and in the preparatory stages of drug development, as in the extraction or removal of active constituents from medicinal plants. For purposes such as this, certain solvents are officially recognized in the compendia. A number of fixed oils, as corn oil, cottonseed oil, peanut oil, and sesame oil, serve useful solvent functions particularly in the preparation of oleaginous injections and are recognized in the official compendia for this purpose.

Some Solvents For Oral Preparations

The following official agents find use as solvents in the preparation of oral solutions, syrups, and elixirs.

Alcohol, USP (Ethyl Alcohol, Ethanol, Spiritus Vini Rectificatus, S.V.R.), C_2H_5OH

Next to water, alcohol is the most useful solvent in pharmacy. It is used as a primary solvent for many organic compounds. Together with water it forms a hydroalcoholic mixture that dissolves both alcohol-soluble and water-soluble substances, a feature especially useful in the extraction of active constituents from crude drugs. By varying the proportion of the two agents, the active constituents may be selectively dissolved and extracted or allowed to remain behind according to their particular solubility characteristics in the menstruum. Alcohol, USP, is 94.9 to 96.0% C_2H_5OH by volume (i.e., v/v) when determined at 15.56° C, the U.S. Government's standard temperature for alcohol determinations. *Dehydrated Alcohol*, USP, contains not less than 99.5% C_2H_5OH by volume and is utilized in instances in which an essentially water-free alcohol is desired.

Diluted Alcohol, NF

Diluted Alcohol, NF, is prepared by mixing equal volumes of Alcohol, USP, and Purified Water, USP. The final volume of such mixtures is not the sum of the individual volumes of the two components, but due to contraction of the liquids upon mixing, the final volume is generally about 3% less than what would normally be expected. Thus when 50 mL of each component is combined, the resulting product measures approximately 97 mL. It is for this reason that the strength of Diluted Alcohol, NF, is not exactly half that of the more concentrated alcohol, but slightly greater, approximately 49%. Diluted alcohol is a useful hydroalcoholic solvent in various pharmaceutical processes and preparations.

Glycerin, USP (Glycerol), $CH_2OH \cdot CHOH \cdot CH_2OH$

Glycerin is a clear syrupy liquid with a sweet taste. It is miscible both with water and alcohol. As a solvent, it is comparable with alcohol, but because of its viscosity, solutes are slowly soluble in it unless it is rendered less viscous by heating. Glycerin has preservative qualities and is often used as a stabilizer and as an auxiliary solvent in conjunction with water or alcohol. It is used in many internal preparations.

Propylene Glycol, USP, $CH_3CH(OH)CH_2OH$

Propylene glycol, a viscous liquid, is miscible with water and alcohol. It is a useful solvent with a wide range of application and is frequently substituted for glycerin in modern pharmaceutical formulations.

Purified Water, USP, H_2O

Naturally occurring water exerts its solvent effect on most substances it contacts and thus is impure and contains varying amounts of dissolved inorganic salts, usually sodium, potassium, calcium, magnesium, and iron, chlorides, sulfates, and bicarbonates, as well as dissolved and undissolved organic matter and microorganisms. Water found in most cities and towns where water is purified for drinking purposes usually contains less than 0.1% of total solids, determined by evaporating a 100 mL sample of water to dryness and weighing the residue (which would weigh less than 100 mg). Drinking water must meet the United States Public Health Service regulations with respect to bacteriological purity. Acceptable drinking water should be clear, colorless, odorless, and neutral or only slightly acid or alkaline, the deviation from neutral being due to the nature of the dissolved solids and gases (carbon dioxide contributing to the acidity and ammonia to the alkalinity of water).

Ordinary drinking water obtained from the tap is not generally acceptable for the manufacture of most aqueous pharmaceutical preparations or for the extemporaneous compounding of prescriptions because of the chemical incompatibilities that may result from the combination of dissolved solids present and the medicinal agents being added. Signs of such incompatibilities are precipitation, discoloration, and occasionally effervescence. Its use is permitted in the washing and in the extraction of crude vegetable drugs, in the preparation of certain products for external use, and in other instances in which the difference between the use of water and purified water is of no consequence. Naturally, when large volumes of water are required to clean pharmaceutical machinery and equipment, tap water may be economically employed so long as a residue of solids is prevented by using purified water as the final rinse or by wiping the water dry with a meticulously clean cloth.

Purified Water, USP is obtained by distillation, ion-exchange treatment, reverse osmosis, or other suitable process. It is prepared from water complying with the federal Environmental Protection Agency with respect to drinking water. Compared to ordinary drinking water, Purified Water, USP is more free of solid impurities. When evaporated to dryness, it must not yield greater than 0.001% of residue (1 mg of total solids per 100 mL of sample evaporated). Thus purified water is 100 times more free of dissolved solids than is water. Purified Water, USP is intended for use in the preparation of aqueous dosage forms, *except* those intended for parenteral administration (injections). For the latter purpose, Water for Injection, Bacteriostatic Water for Injection, or Sterile Water for Injection, are utilized. These are discussed in Chapter 8.

The main methods used in the preparation of purified water are distillation and ion-exchange; these methods are described briefly as follows.

DISTILLATION METHOD. To prepare purified water, there are many commercially available stills in various sizes and styles with various capacities of from about one-half to 100 gallons of distillate per hour. Generally the first portion of aqueous distillate (about the first 10 to 20%) must be discarded, since it contains many foreign volatile substances usually found in urban drinking water, the usual starting material in the preparation of purified water. Also, the last portion of water (about 10% of the original volume of water) remaining in the distillation apparatus must be discarded and not subjected to further distillation because distillation to dryness would undoubtedly result in the decomposition of the remaining solid impurities to volatile substances that would distill and contaminate the previously collected portion of distillate.

ION-EXCHANGE METHOD. On a large or small scale, the ion-exchange method for the preparation of purified water offers a number of advantages over the distillation method. For one thing, the requirement of heat is eliminated and with it costly and troublesome maintenance frequently encountered in the operation of the more complex distillation apparatus. Because of the simpler equipment and the nature of the method, the ion-exchange process permits ease of operation, minimal maintenance, and a more mobile facility. Many pharmacies and small laboratories which purchase large volumes of distilled water from commercial suppliers for use in their work would no doubt benefit financially and in convenience through the installation of an ion-exchange demineralizer in the work area.

The ion-exchange equipment in use today generally involves the passage of water through a column of cation and anion exchangers, consisting of water-insoluble, synthetic, polymerized phenolic, carboxylic, amino, or sulfonated resins of high molecular weight. These resins are mainly of two types: (a) the cation, or acid exchangers, which permit the exchange of the cations in solution (in the tap water) with hydrogen ion from the resin; (b) the anion, or base exchange resins, which permit the removal of anions. These two processes are successively or simultaneously employed to remove both cations and anions from water. The processes are indicated as follows, with M^+ indicating the metal or cation (as Na^+) and the X^- indicating the anion (as Cl^-).

(a) *Cation Exchange:*
$$H\text{-}Resin + M^+ + X^- + H_2O \rightarrow M\text{-}Resin + H^+ + X^- + H_2O$$

(b) *Anion Exchange:*
$$Resin\text{-}NH_2 + H^+ + X^- + H_2O \rightarrow Resin\text{-}NH_2 \cdot HX + H_2O \text{ (pure)}$$

Water purified in this manner is referred to as *demineralized* or *de-ionized water*, and may be used in any pharmaceutical preparation or prescription calling for distilled water.

Preparation of Solutions

Most pharmaceutical solutions are unsaturated with solute. Thus the amounts of solute to be dissolved are usually well below the capacity of the volume of solvent employed. The strengths of pharmaceutical preparations are usually expressed in terms of *% strength*, although for very dilute preparations, expressions of *ratio strength* or *mg%* may be used. These expressions and examples are shown in Table 6–4.

The term %, when used without qualification (as with w/v, v/v, or w/w) means % weight-in-volume for solutions or suspensions of solids in liquids; % weight-in-volume for solutions of gases in liquids; % volume-in-volume for solutions of liquids in liquids; and, weight-in-weight for mixtures of solids and semisolids.

Some chemical agents that may be soluble in a given solvent are only slowly soluble and require an extended time for dissolving. To hasten the dissolution process, a pharmacist may employ one or several techniques. He may apply heat, reduce the particle size of the solute, utilize a solubilizing agent, or subject the ingredients to rigorous agitation during the preparation of the solution. Normally, most chemical agents are more soluble in solvents at elevated temperatures than at room temperature or below because an endothermic reaction between the solute and solvent utilizes the energy of the heat to enhance the dissolution process. However, elevated temperatures cannot be maintained for pharmaceuticals, and the net effect of heat is simply an increase in the *rate* of solution rather than an increase in solubility. An

Table 6–4. Common Methods of Expressing the Strengths of Pharmaceutical Preparations

Expression	Abbreviated Expression	Meaning and Example
Percent weight-in-volume	% w/v	number of grams of a constituent in 100 mL of preparation (e.g., 1% w/v = 1 g of constituent in 100 mL of preparation).
Percent volume-in-volume	% v/v	number of mL of a constituent in 100 mL of preparation (e.g., 1% v/v = 1 mL of constituent in 100 mL of preparation).
Percent weight-in-weight	% w/w	number of grams of a constituent in 100 g of preparation (e.g., 1% w/w = 1 g of constituent in 100 g of preparation).
Ratio strength, weight-in-volume	—:—— w/v	number of grams of constituent in stated number of mL of preparation (e.g., 1:1000 w/v = 1 g of constituent in 1000 mL of preparation).
Ratio strength, volume-in-volume	—:—— v/v	number of mL of constituent in stated number of mL of preparation (e.g., 1:1000 v/v = 1 mL of constituent in 1000 mL of preparation).
Ratio strength, weight-in-weight	—:—— w/w	number of grams of constituent in stated number of grams of preparation (e.g., 1:1000 w/w = 1 g of constituent in 1000 g of preparation).
Milligram percent	mg%	number of mg of constituent in 100 mL of preparation (e.g., 5 mg% = 5 mg of constituent in 100 mL of preparation).

increased rate is satisfactory to the pharmacist, because most of his solutions are unsaturated anyhow and do not require the presence of solute above the normal capacity of the solvent at room temperature. Pharmacists are generally reluctant to employ heat to facilitate solution, and when they do, they are careful not to exceed the minimally-required temperature, for many medicinal agents are destroyed at elevated temperatures, and the advantage of rapid solution may be completely offset by drug deterioration. If volatile solutes are to be dissolved or if the solvent is volatile (as alcohol), the heat would encourage the loss of these agents to the atmosphere and must therefore be avoided. Pharmacists are aware that certain chemical agents, particularly calcium salts, undergo exothermic reactions as they dissolve and give off heat. For such materials the use of heat would actually discourage the formation of a solution. The best pharmaceutical example of this type of chemical is calcium hydroxide, which is used in the preparation of Calcium Hydroxide Topical Solution, USP. This solute is soluble in water to the extent of 140 mg per 100 mL of solution at 25° C (about 77° F) and 170 mg per 100 mL of solution at 15° C (about 59° F). Obviously the temperature at which the solution is prepared or stored can affect the concentration of the resultant solution.

In addition to, or instead of, raising the temperature of the solvent to increase the rate of solution, a pharmacist may choose to decrease the particle size of the solute. This may be accomplished by the *comminution* (grinding a solid to a fine state of subdivision) of the solute with a mortar and pestle on a small scale or industrial micronizer on a large scale. The reduced particle size causes an increase in the surface area of the substance exposed to the solvent. If the powder is placed in a suitable vessel (as a beaker, graduate cylinder, or bottle) with a portion of the solvent and is stirred or shaken, as suited to the container, the rate of solution may be increased due to the continued circulation of fresh solvent to the drug's surface and the constant removal of newly-formed solution from the drug's surface.

Most solutions prepared for oral administration are prepared by simple solution of the solutes in the solvent or solvent mixture. A few, as Magnesium Citrate Oral Solution, are prepared by chemical reaction of the formulative components.

Oral Solutions and Preparations for Oral Solution

Solutions intended for oral administration usually contain flavorants and colorants to make the medication more attractive and palatable for the patient. When needed, they may also contain stabilizers to maintain the chemical and physical stability of the medicinal agents and preservatives to prevent the growth of microorganisms in the solution. The formulation pharmacist must be wary of chemical interactions which may occur between the various components of a solution which may result in an alteration in the preparation's stability and/or potency. For instance, it has been demonstrated that esters of p-hydroxybenzoic acid (methyl-, ethyl-, propyl-, and butylparabens), the most frequently used preservatives in oral preparations, have a tendency to partition into certain flavoring oils.[4] This partitioning effect could reduce the effective concentration of the preservatives in the aqueous medium of a pharmaceutical product below the level needed for preservative action.

Liquid pharmaceuticals for oral administration are usually formulated such that the patient receives the usual dose of the medication in a conveniently administered volume, as 5 mL (one teaspoonful), 10 mL or 15 mL (one tablespoonful). A few solutions have unusually large doses, as Magnesium Citrate Oral Solution with a usual adult dose of 200 mL. On the other hand many solutions used in pediatric patients are given by drop, utilizing a calibrated dropper usually furnished by the manufacturer in the product package.

Dry Mixtures for Solution

A number of medicinal agents, particularly certain antibiotics, have insufficient stability in aqueous solution to meet extended shelf-life periods. Thus, commercial manufacturers of these products provide them to the pharmacist in dry powder or granule form for reconstitution with a prescribed amount of purified water immediately before dispensing to the patient. The dry powder mixture contains all of the formulative components including drug, flavorant, colorant, buffers, and others, except for the solvent. Once reconstituted by the pharmacist the resultant solutions remain stable when stored in the refrigerator for periods of from 7 to 14 days depending upon the preparation. This is generally a sufficient period of time for the patient to complete the volume of medication usually prescribed. However, if medication remains after the patient completes his course of therapy, he should be instructed to discard the remaining portion which would be unfit for use at a later date.

Among the official dry powder mixtures intended for reconstitution to oral solutions are the following:

Acetaminophen for Effervescent Solution, USP [Bromo Seltzer (Warner-Lambert)]; an analgesic/antipyretic agent

Cloxacillin Sodium for Oral Solution, USP [Tegopen (Bristol)]; an antiinfective antibiotic

Nafcillin Sodium for Oral Solution, USP [Unipen (Wyeth)]; a bactericidal semisynthetic penicillin

Oxacillin Sodium for Oral Solution, USP [Prostaphlin (Bristol)]; an antiinfective antibiotic

Penicillin G Potassium for Oral Solution, USP [Pentids (Squibb)]; an antiinfective antibiotic

Penicillin V Potassium for Oral Solution, USP [Pen-Vee K (Wyeth); V-Cillin K (Lilly); various others]; an antiinfective antibiotic

Potassium Chloride for Oral Solution, USP [K-LOR (Abbott)]; a potassium supplement

Oral Solutions

Most of the official oral solutions are prepared commercially by pharmaceutical manufacturers (Fig. 6–1) and made available to pharmacists for dispensing to their patients. Thus the concern of the pharmacist with these products is generally not in the area of their specific manufacture, but rather in their therapeutic and pharmaceutic characteristics so that he can advise the patient of the proper use, dosage, method of administration, and storage of the product. Knowledge of the solubility and stability characteristics of the medicinal agents and the solvents employed in the commercial products is useful to the pharmacist in informing the patient of the advisability of mixing the solution with juice, milk, or other beverages upon administration. Information regarding the solvents used in each commercial product appears on the product label and in the accompanying package insert. Table 6–5 presents examples of some oral solutions. A few of special pharmaceutical interest are described below.

Table 6–5.   Examples of Oral Solutions by Category

Oral Solution	Some Representative Commercial Products	Concentration of Commercial Product	Comments
Anticonvulsants			
Paramethadione Oral Solution	Paradione Oral Solution (Abbott)	300 mg paramethadione/mL	The solution is administered in the treatment of petit mal epilepsy.
Trimethadione Oral Solution	Tridone Oral Solution (Abbott)	200 mg trimethadione/5 mL	This is an aqueous solution used for the same purpose as paramethadione solution.
Antidepressant *(tricyclic)*			
Nortriptyline HCl Oral Solution	Aventyl HCl Liquid (Lilly)	10 mg nortriptyline HCl/5 mL	Indicated for relief of symptoms of depression.
Antihistamine/Decongestant Combination			
Pseudoephedrine HCl and Chlorpheniramine Maleate Liquid	Dorcol Children's Liquid Cold Formula (Dorsey)	15 mg of pseudoephedrine HCl and 1 mg of chlorpheniramine maleate per 5 mL	This solution is used in children for the temporary relief of nasal congestion, running nose and sneezing due to the common cold, hay fever and other upper respiratory allergies.
Antiperistaltic			
Diphenoxylate HCl and Atropine Sulfate Oral Solution	Lomotil Liquid (Searle)	2.5 mg of diphenoxylate HCl and 0.025 mg of atropine sulfate/5 mL	This preparation is indicated in the management of diarrhea. Diphenoxylate is related structurally and pharmacologically to the narcotic meperidine. Atropine sulfate is added to the solution in subtherapeutic amounts to discourage (by virtue of side effects) deliberate overdosage.
Loperamide HCl Oral Solution	Imodium A-D liquid (McNeil)	1 mg of loperamide HCl per 5 mL	This preparation is indicated for the treatment of diarrhea for both adults and children 6 years of age and older. Loperamide is structurally related to haloperidol.
Antipsychotics			
Haloperidol Oral Solution	Haldol Concentrate (McNeil)	2 mg haloperidol/mL	These solutions are used primarily in severe neuropsychiatric conditions when oral medication is preferred and other oral dosage forms (as tablets and
Perphenazine Oral Solution	Trilafon Concentrate (Schering)	16 mg perphenazine/5 mL	
Thioridazine HCl Oral Solution	Mellaril Concentrate (Sandoz)	30 and 100 mg thioridazine HCl/mL	

Table 6–5.   Continued

Oral Solution	Some Representative Commercial Products	Concentration of Commercial Product	Comments
Antipsychotics (continued)			
Thiothixene HCl Oral Solution	Navane Concentrate (Roerig)	equivalent of 5 mg thiothixene/mL	capsules) are considered impractical. The concentrated solutions are employed by adding the desired amount of the concentrate by calibrated dropper to soup or a beverage as tomato or fruit juices, milk, coffee, tea, or carbonated beverages.
Bronchodilator			
Aminophylline Oral Liquid	Somophylline Liquid (Fisons)	105 mg (equivalent to 90 mg theophylline) per 5 mL	This preparation is indicated for the symptomatic treatment of bronchial asthma and reversible bronchospasm associated with chronic bronchitis and emphysema. The alcohol-free formulation is very advantageous for its use in children.
Theophylline Oral Solution	Theophylline Oral Solution (Roxane)	80 mg of theophylline per 15 mL	This alcohol-free solution is used for the same purpose as the Somophylline Liquid. However, the amount needed for each dose is greater, i.e., 15 mL *vs* 5 mL
Cathartics			
Magnesium Citrate Oral Solution, USP	—	amount of magnesium citrate equivalent to between 1.55 g and 1.9 g/100 mL of magnesium oxide	Discussed in text.
Sodium Phosphate Oral Solution	Phospho-Soda (Fleet)	18 g sodium phosphate and 48 g sodium biphosphate/100 mL	Works as laxative within 1 hour when taken before meals or overnight when taken at bedtime. Usual dose is 10 to 20 mL of solution, best taken diluted with one-half glass of water and followed with a full glass of water.
Corticosteroid			
Prednisone Sodium Phosphate Liquid	Pediapred Oral Liquid (Fisons)	5 mg prednisolone (as sodium phosphate) per 5 mL	This solution is used in children for the treatment of acute exacerbations of multiple sclerosis.
Dental Caries Protectant			
Sodium Fluoride Oral Solution	Pediaflor Drops (Ross)	0.5 mg/mL	Prophylaxis of dental caries; intended for use when community water supplies are inadequately fluoridated.

Table 6–5.   Continued

Oral Solution	Some Representative Commercial Products	Concentration of Commercial Product	Comments
Sodium Fluoride Oral Rinse/Supplement	Phos-Flur Rinse/Supplement (Hoyt)	0.2 mg of fluoride (from 0.44 mg sodium fluoride) per mL	This preparation is used after brushing or flossing the teeth and just prior to sleep for the prevention of dental caries. When used as a dental rinse it is not to be swallowed after it is vigorously rinsed around and between the teeth for one minute.
Diuretic Furosemide Oral Solution	Lasix Oral Solution (Hoeschst-Roussel)	10 mg of furosemide per mL	This preparation is indicated to treat edema and hypertension in adults and in children.
Electrolyte Replenisher Potassium Chloride Oral Solution	Kaochlor Liquid (Adria)	5% KCl (20 mEq of K/30 mL); 10% KCl (40 mEq of K/30 mL); 20% KCl (80 mEq of K/30 mL)	Used in conditions of hypopotassemia (low level of potassium in the blood). Condition may be prompted by severe or chronic diarrhea, a low level of potassium intake in the diet, increased renal excretion of potassium, and other causes. The solution is diluted with water or fruit juice before taking.
Expectorant Potassium Iodide Oral Solution	SSKI (Upsher-Smith)	300 mg KI/0.3 mL	Discussed in text.
Fecal Softener Docusate Sodium Solution	Colace Liquid (Mead Johnson)	10 mg docusate sodium/mL	Usually 50 to 200 mg of the drug is measured by calibrated dropper and mixed with milk, fruit juice, or other liquid (to mask the taste) before administration. The drug softens the fecal mass by lowering the surface tension, thus permitting normal bowel habits, particularly in geriatric, pediatric, cardiac, obstetric, and surgical patients. Dosage is taken for several days or until bowel movements are normal.

Table 6–5.   Continued

Oral Solution	Some Representative Commercial Products	Concentration of Commercial Product	Comments
Hematinic Ferrous Sulfate Oral Solution	Fer-In-Sol Drops (Mead Johnson Nutritional)	75 mg ferrous sulfate/ 0.6 mL	Used for prevention and treatment of iron deficiency anemias. Usual prophylactic dose of 0.3 or 0.6 mL measured by calibrated dropper and mixed with water, fruit juice, or vegetable juice before administration. Dosage form intended primarily for infants and children.
Histamine H$_2$ Antagonist Cimetidine HCl Liquid	Tagamet HCl Liquid (SKF)	300 mg of cimetidine HCl per 5 mL	This preparation is indicated to treat peptic ulcer disease and pathological hypersecretory conditions, e.g., Zollinger-Ellison syndrome.
Narcotic Agonist Analgesic Methadone HCl Oral Solution	Methadone HCL (Roxane)	1 or 2 mg/mL	For relief of severe pain; detoxification and maintenance treatment of narcotic addiction.
Psychotherapeutic Agent Ergoloid Mesylate Oral Solution	Hydergine Liquid (Sandoz)	1 mg/mL	Utilized in symptomatic treatment of idiopathic decline in mental capacity.
Vitamin D Source Ergocalciferol Solution	Calciferol Drops (Kremers-Urban)	8,000 units/mL	A solution of water-insoluble ergocalciferol (vitamin D$_2$) in propylene glycol. The usual prophylactic dose of ergocalciferol is about 400 units and the therapeutic dose may be as high as 200,000 to 500,000 units daily in treating rickets.

Oral Rehydration Solutions

Rapid fluid loss associated with diarrhea can lead to dehydration and ultimately death in some patients, particularly infants. It has been estimated that over five million children under 4 years of age die due to diarrheal illnesses each year worldwide.[5] Diarrhea is characterized by an increased frequency of loose, watery stools, and because there is an intensive fluid loss, dehydration can be an outcome. During diarrhea, the small intestine secretes far above the normal amount of fluid and electrolytes, and this simply exceeds the ability of the large intestine to reabsorb it. This fluid loss occurs mostly from the body's extracellular fluid compartment and can lead to a progressive loss of blood volume culminating in hypovolemic shock.

Diarrhea is a normal physiologic body response to rid itself of a noxious or toxic substance, e.g., *Rotavirus, Escherichia coli*. Thus, the treatment approach is to allow the diarrhea to proceed and not to terminate it too quickly, but promptly replace the fluid and electrolytes that are lost to prevent dehydration. The loss of fluid during diarrhea is accompanied by a depletion

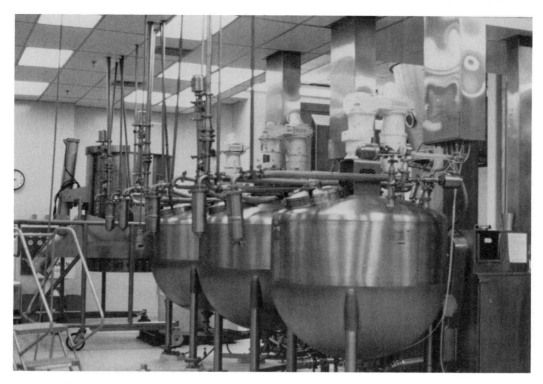

Fig. 6–1. *Large scale pharmaceutical mixing vessels. (Courtesy of Schering Laboratories.)*

of sodium, potassium and bicarbonate ions, which if severe can result, as mentioned, in hypovolemic shock, as well as acidosis, hyperpnea and vomiting. If continuous, bouts of vomiting and diarrhea can cause malnutrition as well. Consequently, the goal is to replace lost fecal water with an oral rehydration solution and utilize nutritional foods such as soybean formula and bran.

Oral rehydration solutions are usually effective in treatment of patients with mild volume depletion of 5 to 10% of body weight. These are available over-the-counter, are relatively inexpensive and their use has diminished the incidence of complications associated with parenterally-administered electrolyte solutions. Therapy with these solutions is based on the observation that glucose is actively absorbed from the small intestine, even during bouts of diarrhea. This active transport of glucose is advantageous because it is coupled with sodium absorption. Almost like in domino fashion, sodium absorption promotes anion absorption which in turn promotes water absorption to

short circuit dehydration. To produce maximal absorption of sodium and water studies have demonstrated that the optimal concentrations of glucose and sodium in an isotonic solution are 110 mM (2%) glucose and 60 mEq/L of sodium ion, respectively. Bicarbonate and/or citrate ions are also included in these solutions to help correct the subsequent metabolic acidosis which is caused by diarrhea and dehydration.

A typical oral rehydration solution contains 45 mEq Na^+, 20 mEq K^+, 35 mEq Cl^-, 30 mEq citrate, and 25 g of dextrose per liter. These formulations are available in liquid or powder/packet form for reconstitution. It is important that the user add the specific amount of water needed to prepare the powder forms. Further, these products should not be mixed with or given with other electrolyte-containing liquids, such as milk or fruit juices. Otherwise, there is no method to calculate how much electrolyte the patient actually received. The pharmacist must also discourage the production of homemade versions of these solutions. The success of these solutions is dependent upon the accuracy of the formulation. If prepared incorrectly, homemade preparations could cause hypernatremia or cause the diarrhea to worsen.

Oral Colonic Lavage Solution

Traditionally, the preparation of the bowel for procedures such as a colonoscopy have consisted of the administration of clear liquid diets for 24 to 48 hours preceding the procedure, the administration of oral laxatives, e.g., magnesium citrate or bisacodyl, the night before, and cleansing enemas administered 2 to 4 hours prior to procedure commencement. Typically, to circumvent the cost of having to hospitalize the patient the night prior to the procedure, patients were allowed to perform this regimen at home. However, while the results have been generally satisfactory, that is, the bowel is cleared for the procedure, poor patient compliance with and acceptance of this regimen can cause problems during the procedure. Further, additive effects of malnutrition and poor oral intake prior to the procedure can cause more patient problems.

Consequently, an alternative method to prepare the gastrointestinal tract has been devised. This procedure requires less time and dietary restriction and obviates the need for cleansing enemas. This method involves the oral administration of a balanced solution of electrolytes with polyethylene glycol (PEG-3350). Prior to its dispensing to the patient, the pharmacist reconstitutes this powder with water creating an iso-osmotic solution having a mildly salty taste. The polyethylene glycol acts as an osmotic agent within the gastrointestinal tract and the balanced electrolyte concentration results in virtually no net absorption or secretion of ions. Thus, a large volume of this solution can be administered without a significant change in water or electrolyte balance.

The formulation of this oral colonic lavage solution is as follows:

Polyethylene Glycol 3350	236.00 g
Sodium Sulfate	22.74 g
Sodium Bicarbonate	6.74 g
Sodium Chloride	5.86 g
Potassium Chloride	2.97 g

In 4800 mL disposable container

The recommended adult dosage of this product is 4 L of solution prior to the gastrointestinal procedure. The patient is instructed to drink 240 mL of solution every 10 minutes until about 4

L are consumed. The patient is advised to drink each portion quickly rather than sipping it continuously. Usually, the first bowel movement will occur within 1 hour. Several regimens are utilized, and one method is to schedule patients for a midmorning procedure, allowing the patient 3 hours for drinking and a 1-hour waiting period to complete bowel evacuation.

To date this approach to bowel evacuation has been associated with a low incidence of side effects, primarily nausea, transient abdominal fullness, bloating, and occasionally, cramps and vomiting. Ideally, the patient should not have taken any food 3 to 4 hours before beginning the administration of the solution. In no case should solid foods be taken by the patient for at least 2 hours before the solution is administered. No foods, except clear liquids, are permitted after this product is administered and prior to the examination. The product must be stored in the refrigerator after reconstitution, and this aids somewhat in decreasing the salty taste of the product.

Magnesium Citrate Oral Solution

Magnesium citrate oral solution is a colorless to slightly yellow, clear, effervescent liquid having a sweet, acidulous taste and a lemon flavor. It is commonly referred to as "Citrate" or as "Citrate of Magnesia." It is required to contain an amount of magnesium citrate equivalent to between 1.55 and 1.9 g of magnesium oxide in each 100 mL.

The solution is prepared by reacting official magnesium carbonate with an excess of citric acid (equation 1), flavoring and sweetening the solution with lemon oil and syrup, filtering with talc, and then carbonating it by the addition of either potassium or sodium bicarbonate (equation 2). The solution may be further carbonated by the use of carbon dioxide under pressure.

(1) $(MgCO_3)_4 \cdot Mg(OH)_2 + 5H_3C_6H_5O_7$
$\rightarrow 5\ MgHC_6H_5O_7 + 4CO_2 + 6H_2O$

(2) $3KHCO_3 + H_3C_6H_5O_7 \rightarrow K_3C_6H_5O_7$
$+ 3CO_2 + 3H_2O$

The solution provides an excellent medium for the growth of molds, and any mold spores present during the manufacture of the solution must be killed if the preparation is to remain stable. For this reason, during the preparation of the solution the liquid is heated to boiling (prior to carbonation), boiled water is employed to bring the solution to its proper volume, and boiling water is used to rinse the final container. The final solution may be sterilized.

Magnesium citrate solution has always been troublesome, since it has a tendency to deposit a crystalline solid upon standing. Apparently this is due to the formation of some almost insoluble, normal magnesium citrate (rather than the exclusively dibasic form as in equation 1). The cause of the problem has largely been attributed to the indefinite composition of the official magnesium carbonate, which by definition is "a basic hydrated magnesium carbonate or a normal hydrated magnesium carbonate" (see equation 1). It contains the equivalent of 40 to 43.5% of magnesium oxide. Apparently solutions prepared from magnesium carbonates with differing equivalents of magnesium oxide vary in stability, with the most stable ones being prepared from samples of magnesium carbonate having the lower equivalent of magnesium oxide. The formula for the preparation of 350 mL of magnesium citrate solution calls for the use of 15 g of official magnesium carbonate, which corresponds to approximately 6.0 to 6.47 g of magnesium oxide.

In carbonating the solution, the bicarbonate may be added in tablet form rather than as a powder in order to delay the effervescence resulting from its contact with the citric acid. If the powder were used, the reaction would be immediate and violent, and it would be virtually impossible to close the bottle in time to prevent the loss of carbon dioxide or solution. The solution may be further carbonated by the use of CO_2 under pressure. Most of the magnesium citrate solutions prepared commercially today are packaged in the same type of bottles as "soft drink" carbonated beverages. The solution is generally packaged in bottles of 300 mL. Since the solution is carbonated, it loses some of its character if allowed to stand for a period of time after the container has been opened. Magnesium citrate solution is generally stored in a cold place, preferably in a refrigerator, keeping the bottle on its side so the cork or rubber liners of the caps are kept moist and swollen, thereby maintaining the airtight seal between the cap and the bottle.

The solution is employed as a saline cathartic, with the citric acid, lemon oil, syrup, carbonation, and the low temperature of the refrigerated solution all contributing to the patient's acceptance of the large volume of medication. For many patients it represents a pleasant way of taking an otherwise bitter saline cathartic.

Sodium Citrate and Citric Acid Oral Solution

This official solution contains 100 mg of sodium citrate and 67 mg of citric acid in each mL of aqueous solution. The solution is administered orally in doses of 10 to 30 mL as frequently as four times daily as a systemic alkalinizer. Systemic alkalinization is useful in patients having conditions in which long term maintenance of an alkaline urine is desirable, such as patients with uric acid and cystine calculi of the urinary tract. The solution is also a useful adjuvant when administered with uricosuric agents in gout therapy since urates tend to crystallize out of an acid urine.

Syrups

Syrups are concentrated, aqueous preparations of a sugar or sugar-substitute with or without added flavoring agents and medicinal substances. Syrups containing flavoring agents but not medicinal substances are called *nonmedicated* or *flavored vehicles* (syrups). Some official and previously official nonmedicated syrups are presented in Table 6–6. These syrups are intended to serve as pleasant-tasting vehicles for medicinal substances to be added later, either in the extemporaneous compounding of prescriptions or in the preparation of a standard formula for a *medicated syrup*, which is a syrup containing a therapeutic or medicinal agent. Nowadays these syrups are used to extemporaneously prepare liquid dosage forms of medicines that are only available in solid dosage forms, e.g., tablets, capsules. These prescriptions, while not frequent, are necessary for the oral administration of drugs to patients who cannot swallow solid dosage forms, e.g., elderly, infants.[6] Medicated syrups are commercially prepared from the starting materials; that is, by combining each of the individual components of the syrup, as sucrose, purified water, flavoring agents, coloring agents, the therapeutic agent, and other necessary and desirable ingredients. Naturally, medicated syrups are employed in therapeutics for the value of the medicinal agent present in the syrup.

Table 6–6. Examples of Nonmedicated Syrups (Vehicles)

Nonmedicated Syrup	Comments
Cherry Syrup	A sucrose-based syrup containing about 47% by volume of cherry juice. The syrup's tart and fruit flavor is attractive to most patients and the acidic pH of the syrup makes it useful as a vehicle for drugs requiring an acid medium.
Cocoa Syrup	This syrup is a suspension of cocoa powder in an aqueous vehicle sweetened and thickened with sucrose, liquid glucose, and glycerin, and flavored with vanillin and sodium chloride. The syrup is particularly effective in administering bitter tasting drugs to children.
Orange Syrup	This sucrose-based syrup utilizes sweet orange peel tincture, and citric acid as the source of flavor and tartness. The syrup resembles orange juice in taste and is a good vehicle for drugs stable in an acidic medium.
Raspberry Syrup	A sucrose-based syrup containing about 48% by volume of raspberry juice. It is a pleasantly flavored vehicle used to disguise the salty or sour taste of saline medicaments.
Syrup	This is an 85% solution of sucrose in purified water. This "simple syrup" may be used as the basis for the preparation of flavored or medicated syrups.

Syrups provide a pleasant means of administering a liquid form of a disagreeable tasting drug. They are particularly effective in the administration of drugs to youngsters, since their pleasant taste usually dissipates any reluctance on the part of the child to take the medicine. The fact that syrups contain little or no alcohol adds to their favor among parents.

Any water-soluble drug that is stable in aqueous solution may be added to a flavored syrup. However care must be exercised to insure the compatibility between the medicinal drug substance and the other formulative components of the syrup. Also, certain flavored syrups have an acidic medium, whereas others may be neutral or slightly basic and the proper selection must be made to insure the stability of any added medicinal agent. Perhaps the most frequently found types of medications administered as medicated syrups are antitussive agents and antihistamines. This is not to imply that other types of drugs are not formulated into syrups; indeed, a wide variety of medicinal substances can be found in syrup form and among the many commercial products. Examples of medicated syrups are presented in Table 6–7.

Components of Syrups

Most syrups contain the following components in addition to the purified water and any medicinal agents present: (1) the sugar, usually sucrose, or sugar-substitutes used to provide sweetness and viscosity, (2) antimicrobial preservatives, (3) flavorants, and (4) colorants. Also, many syrups, especially those prepared commercially, contain special solvents, solubilizing agents, thickeners, or stabilizers.

Sucrose and Non-Sucrose Based Syrups

Sucrose is the sugar most frequently employed in syrups, although in special circumstances it may be replaced in whole or in part by other sugars, as dextrose, or non-sugars as sorbitol, glycerin and propylene glycol. In some instances, all glycogenetic substances (materials converted to glucose in the body), including those agents mentioned above, are replaced by nonglycogenetic substances such as methylcellulose or hydroxyethylcellulose. These two materials are not hydrolyzed and absorbed into the blood stream, and their use results in an excellent syrup-like vehicle for medications intended for use by diabetic patients and others whose diets must be controlled and restricted to nonglycogenetic substances. The viscosity generally resulting from the use of these cellulose derivatives is much like that of a sucrose syrup. The addition of one or more artificial sweeteners usually produces an excellent facsimile of a true syrup.

Table 6–7. Examples of Medicated Syrups by Category

Syrup	Some Representative Commercial Products	Concentration of Commercial Product*	Comments
Analgesic			
Meperidine HCl Syrup	Demerol Syrup (Winthrop)	50 mg meperidine HCl/5 mL	Narcotic analgesic indicated for relief of moderate to severe pain and as an adjunct to general anesthesia.
Antibacterials			
Isoniazid Syrup	Laniazid Syrup (Lannett)	50 mg isoniazid/5 mL	Used in treatment of tuberculosis. Usual dose is 5 mg/kg of body weight once a day, up to 300 mg
Anticholinergic			
Dicyclomine HCl Syrup	Bentyl Syrup (Lakeside)	10 mg dicyclomine HCl/5 mL	Used as adjunctive therapy in treatment of peptic ulcer.
Oxybutynin Chloride Syrup	Ditropan Syrup (Marion)	5 mg of oxybutynin chloride per 5 mL	Used for the relief of symptoms associated with voiding in patients with uninhibited neurogenic and reflex neurogenic bladder.
Antiemetics			
Chlorpromazine HCl Syrup	Thorazine Syrup (Smith Kline and French)	10 mg chlorpromazine HCl/5 mL	Used to control nausea and vomiting.
Dimenhydrinate Syrup	Dramamine Liquid (Searle)	15 mg dimenhydrinate/5 mL	Used to control nausea, vomiting, and motion sickness.
Prochlorperazine Edisylate Syrup	Compazine Syrup (Smith Kline and French)	5 mg prochlorperazine edisylate/5 mL	Used to control nausea and vomiting.
Promethazine HCl Syrup	Phenergan Syrup (Wyeth)	6.25 mg, 12.5 mg, and 25 mg promethazine HCl/5 mL	Used to control nausea, vomiting, motion sickness, and allergic reactions.
Anticonvulsant			
Sodium Valproate Syrup	Depakene Syrup (Abbott)	250 mg of valproic acid (as sodium salt) per 5 mL	Used as the sole or adjunctive therapy in simple (petit mal) and complex absence seizure disorders.
Antihistamines			
Chlorpheniramine Maleate Syrup	Chlor-Trimeton Allergy Syrup (Schering)	2 mg chlorpheniramine maleate/5 mL	
Cyproheptadine HCl Syrup	Periactin Syrup (Merck Sharp & Dohme)	2 mg cyproheptadine HCl/5 mL	
Dexchlorpheniramine Maleate Syrup	Polaramine Syrup (Schering)	2 mg dexchlorpheniramine maleate/5 mL	All of the antihistamines listed are used for prevention and treatment of allergic reactions.
Hydroxyzine HCl Syrup	Atarax Syrup (Roerig)	10 mg hydroxyzine HCl/5 mL	
Triprolidine HCl Syrup	Actidil Syrup (Burroughs Wellcome)	1.25 mg triprolidine HCl/5 mL	
Antipruritics			
Methdilazine HCl Syrup	Tacaryl Syrup (Westwood)	4 mg methdilazine HCl/5 mL	These antipruritics are used for relief of itching in urticaria.
Trimeprazine Tartrate Syrup	Temaril Syrup (Herbert)	2.5 mg trimeprazine tartrate/5 mL	
Antipsychotics			
Lithium Citrate Syrup	Cibalith-S (CIBA)	8 mEq lithium/5 mL	Used in the management of psychotic disorders.

Table 6–7.   Continued

Syrup	Some Representative Commercial Products	Concentration of Commercial Product*	Comments
Antitussive			
Dextromethorphan Syrup	Delsym (McNeil)	30 mg dextromethrophan/5 mL	For relief of cough.
Diphenhydramine Syrup	Benylin Cough Syrup (Parke-Davis Consumer)	12.5 mg of diphenhydramine HCl per 5 mL	Used for the control or coughs due to colds or allergy.
Antiviral			
Amantadine HCl Syrup	Symmetrel Syrup (DuPont)	50 mg amantadine HCl/5 mL	Prevention of respiratory infections caused by A_2 (Asian) viral strains. Treatment of idiopathic Parkinson's disease.
Bronchodilators			
Albuterol Sulfate Syrup	Proventil Syrup (Schering) Ventolin Syrup (Glaxo)	2 mg of albuterol sulfate per 5 mL	Used for the relief of bronchospasm in patients with obstructive airway disease, and for the prevention of exercise-induced bronchospasm.
Metaproterenol Sulfate Syrup	Alupent Syrup (Boehringer-Ingelheim)	10 mg of metaproterenol sulfate per 5 mL	
Cathartic			
Lactulose Syrup	Chronulac Syrup (Merrell Dow)	10 g of lactulose per 15 mL	Dose is 15 to 30 mL daily as a laxative.
Cholinergic			
Pyridostigmine Bromide Syrup	Mestinon Syrup (Roche)	60 mg pyridostigmine bromide/5 mL	Used in treatment of myasthenia gravis.
Decongestant			
Pseudoephedrine Sulfate Syrup	Sudafed Syrup (Burroughs-Wellcome)	30 mg of pseudoephedrine sulfate per 5 mL	Used for the temporary relief of nasal congestion due to the common cold, hay fever or other upper respiratory allergies, and nasal congestion associated with sinusitis.
Emetic			
Ipecac Syrup	—	21 mg ether-soluble alkaloids of ipecac/15 mL	Used to induce vomiting in poisoning. The dose of 15 mL may be repeated in 20 minutes if vomiting does not occur. If after the second dose, vomiting does not occur, the stomach should be emptied by gastric lavage.
Expectorant			
Guaifenesin Syrup	Robitussin Syrup (Robins)	100 mg guaifenesin/5 mL	For symptomatic relief of respiratory conditions associated with cough and bronchial congestion.
Fecal Softener			
Docusate Sodium Syrup	Colace Syrup (Mead Johnson)	20 mg docusate sodium/5 mL	Stool softener by surface-action.
Gastrointestinal Stimulant			
Metoclopramide HCl Monohydrate Syrup	Reglan Syrup (Robins)	5 mg of metoclopramide HCl per 5 mL	Used to provide relief of symptoms associated with diabetic gastroparesis (gastric stasis) and gastroesophageal reflux.

Table 6–7.   Continued

Syrup	Some Representative Commercial Products	Concentration of Commercial Product*	Comments
Glucocorticoids			
Betamethasone Syrup	Celestone Syrup (Schering)	600 μg betamethasone/5 mL	These are adrenocortical steroids useful in treating inflammatory conditions and those resulting from adrenocortical insufficiency.
Triamcinolone Diacetate Syrup	Aristocort Syrup (Lederle)	2 and 5 mg triamcinolone diacetate/5 mL	
Hemostatic			
Aminocaproic Acid Syrup	Amicar Syrup (Lederle)	1.25 g aminocaproic acid/5 mL	Used in treatment of excessive bleeding resulting from systemic hyperfibrinolysis and urinary fibrinolysis.
Hypnotic/Sedative			
Chloral Hydrate Syrup	Noctec Syrup (Squibb)	500 mg chloral hydrate/10 mL	Sedative in doses of 250 mg and hypnotic to induce sleep at doses of 500 mg. Alcoholic beverages should be avoided when taking this syrup. The syrup is usually diluted with water or other beverage before taking.

*The amount per stated volume of syrup constitutes a usual single dose of the medication unless otherwise stated.

The characteristic "body" that the sucrose and the substitutive agents seek to impart to the syrup is essentially the result of attaining the proper viscosity. This quality, together with the sweetness and the flavorants generally added, results in a type of pharmaceutical preparation that is quite effective in masking the taste of added medicinal agents. When the syrup is swallowed, only a portion of dissolved drug actually makes contact with the taste buds, the remainder of the drug being carried past them and down the throat in the containment of the viscous syrup. This type of physical concealment of the taste is not possible for a solution of a drug in an unthickened, mobile, aqueous preparation. In the case of antitussive syrups, the thick sweet syrup has a soothing effect on the irritated tissues of the throat as it passes over them.

Most syrups contain a high proportion of sucrose, usually 60 to 80%, not only because of the desirable sweetness and viscosity of such solutions but also because of their inherent stability in contrast to the unstable character of dilute sucrose solutions. The aqueous sugar medium of dilute sucrose solutions is an efficient nutrient medium for the growth of microorganisms, particularly yeasts and molds. On the other hand, concentrated sugar solutions are quite resistant to microbial growth, due to the unavailability of the water required for the growth of microorganisms. This aspect of syrups is best demonstrated by the simplest of all syrups, Syrup, NF which has the synonym of "simple syrup" and is prepared by dissolving 85 g of sucrose in enough purified water to make 100 mL of syrup. The resulting preparation requires no additional preservation; in fact, preservatives may not be added to this official syrup. When properly prepared and maintained, the syrup is inherently stable and resistant to the growth of microorganisms. An examination of this syrup reveals its concentrated nature and the relative absence of available water for microbial growth. Syrup has a specific gravity of about 1.313, which means that each 100 mL of syrup weighs 131.3 g. Because 85 g of sucrose are present, the difference between 85 g and 131.3 g or 46.3 g, represents the weight of the purified water present. Thus, 46.3 g, or mL, of purified water are used to dissolve the 85 g of sucrose. The solubility of sucrose in water is 1 g in 0.5 mL of water; therefore, to dissolve 85 g of sucrose, about 42.5 mL of water would be required. Thus, only a very slight excess of water (about 3.8 mL per 100 mL of syrup) is employed in the preparation of syrup. Although not enough to be particularly amenable to the growth of microorganisms, the slight excess of water permits the syrup to remain physically stable under conditions of varying temperatures. If the syrup were completely saturated with sucrose, under cool storage conditions some sucrose might crystallize from solution and, by acting as nuclei, initiate a type of chain reaction that would result in the separation of an amount of sucrose disproportionate to its solubility at the storage temperature. The syrup would then be very much unsaturated and probably suitable for microbial growth. As formulated, the official syrup is both stable and resistant to crystallization as well as to microbial growth. However, many of the other official syrups and a host of commercial syrups are not intended to be as nearly saturated as Syrup, NF, and therefore must employ added preservative agents to prevent microbial growth and to ensure their stability during their period of use and storage.

As noted earlier, sucrose-based syrup may be substituted in whole or in part by other agents in the preparation of medicated syrups. A solution of a polyol, as sorbitol, or a mixture of polyols, as sorbitol and glycerin, are commonly used. Sorbitol Solution, USP, which contains 64% by weight of the polyhydric alcohol sorbitol is employed as shown in the following example formulations for medicated syrups:[7]

Antihistamine Syrup

Chlorpheniramine Maleate, USP	0.4 g
Glycerin, USP	25.0 mL
Syrup, NF	83.0 mL
Sorbitol Solution, USP	282.0 mL
Sodium Benzoate, NF	1.0 g
Alcohol, USP	60.0 mL
Color and flavor	q.s.
Purified Water, USP, to make	1000.0 mL

Ferrous Sulfate Syrup

Ferrous Sulfate, USP	135.0 g
Citric Acid, USP	12.0 g
Sorbitol Solution, USP	350.0 mL
Glycerin, USP	50.0 mL
Sodium Benzoate, NF	1.0 g
Flavor	q.s.
Purified Water, USP, to make	1000.0 mL

Antimicrobial Preservative

The amount of a preservative required to protect a syrup against microbial growth varies with the proportion of water available for growth, the nature and inherent preservative activity of some formulative materials (as many flavoring oils that are inherently sterile and possess antimicrobial activity), and the capability of the preservative itself. Among the preservatives commonly used in the preservation of syrups with the usually effective concentrations are benzoic acid (0.1 to 0.2%), sodium benzoate (0.1 to 0.2%), and various combinations of methyl-, propyl-, and butylparabens (totaling about 0.1%). Frequently alcohol is used in the preparation of syrups to assist in the dissolving of alcohol-soluble ingredients, but normally it is not present in the final product in amounts that would be considered to be adequate for preservation (15 to 20%).

Flavorant

Most syrups are flavored with synthetic flavorants or with naturally occurring materials as volatile oils (e.g. orange oil), vanillin, and others, to render the syrup pleasant tasting. Because syrups are aqueous preparations, these flavorants must possess sufficient water-solubility. However, sometimes a small amount of alcohol is added to a syrup to ensure the continued solution of a poorly (water) soluble flavorant.

Colorant

To enhance the appeal of the syrup, a coloring agent is generally used which correlates with the flavorant employed (i.e. green with mint, brown with chocolate, etc.). The colorant used is generally water soluble, nonreactive with the other syrup components, and color-stable at the pH range and under the intensity of light that the syrup is likely to enounter during its shelf-life.

Preparation of Syrups

Syrups are most frequently prepared by one of four general methods, depending upon the physical and chemical characteristics of the ingredients. Broadly stated, these methods are (1) solution of the ingredients with the aid of heat, (2) solution of the ingredients by agitation without the use of heat, or the simple admixture of liquid components, (3) addition of sucrose to a prepared medicated liquid or to a flavored liquid, and (4) by percolation of either the source of the medicating substance or of the sucrose.

In certain instances a syrup may be successfully prepared by more than one of the above methods, and the selection may simply be a matter of preference on the part of the pharmacist.

For many of the official syrups there is no officially designated method for their preparation. This is due to the fact that most of the official syrups are available on a commercial basis and are not prepared extemporaneously by the pharmacist.

Solution with the Aid of Heat

Syrups are prepared by this method when it is desired to prepare the syrup as quickly as possible and when the syrup's components are not damaged or volatilized by heat. In this method the sugar is generally added to the purified water, and heat is applied until solution is effected. Then, other required heat-stable components are added to the hot syrup, the mixture is allowed to cool, and its volume is adjusted to the proper level by the addition of purified water. In instances in which heat-labile agents or volatile substances, as volatile flavoring oils and alcohol, are to be added, they are generally added to the syrup after the solution of the sugar is effected by heat, and the solution is rapidly cooled to room temperature.

The use of heat facilitates the rapid solution of the sugar as well as certain other components of syrups; however, caution must be exercised against becoming impatient and using excessive heat. Sucrose, a disaccharide, may be hydrolyzed into monosaccharides, dextrose (glucose), and fructose (levulose). This hydrolytic reaction is referred to as *inversion*, and the combination of the two monosaccharide products is *invert sugar*. When heat is applied in the preparation of a sucrose syrup, some inversion of the sucrose is almost certain. The speed of inversion is greatly increased by the presence of acids, the hydrogen ion acting as a catalyst to the reaction. Should inversion occur, the sweetness of the syrup is altered, because invert sugar is sweeter than sucrose; and the normally colorless syrup darkens due to the effect of heat on the levulose portion of the invert sugar. When the syrup is greatly overheated, it becomes amber colored due to the caramelization of the sucrose. Syrups so decomposed are more susceptible to fermentation and to microbial growth than the stable, nondecomposed syrups. Because of the prospect of decomposition by heat, syrups cannot be sterilized by autoclaving. The use of boiled purified water in the preparation of a syrup can enhance its permanency, and the addition of preservative agents, when permitted, can protect it during its shelf life. Storage in tight containers is a requirement for all syrups.

Solution by Agitation without the Aid of Heat

To avoid heat-induced inversion of sucrose, a syrup may be prepared without heat by agitation. On a small scale, sucrose and other formulative agents may be dissolved in purified water by placing the ingredients in a vessel of greater capacity than the volume of syrup to be prepared, thus permitting the thorough agitation of the mixture. This process is more time-consuming than that utilizing heat to facilitate the solution of sucrose, but the product has maximum stability. Huge glass-lined or stainless steel tanks affixed with mechanical stirrers or agitators are employed in the large-scale preparation of syrups.

Sometimes simple syrup or some other non-medicated syrup, rather than sucrose, is employed as the sweetening agent and vehicle. In instances such as this, other liquids that are soluble in the syrup or miscible with it may be added and thoroughly mixed to form a uniform product. When solid agents are to be added to a syrup, it is best to dissolve them in a minimal amount of purified water and then incorporate the resulting solution into the syrup. When solid substances are added directly to a syrup, they generally dissolve slowly because the viscous nature of the syrup does not permit the solid substance to distribute readily throughout the syrup to the available solvent and also because a limited amount of available water is present in concentrated syrups.

Addition of Sucrose to a Medicated Liquid or to a Flavored Liquid

Occasionally a medicated liquid, as a tincture or fluidextract, is employed as the source of medication in the preparation of a syrup. Many such tinctures and fluidextracts contain alcohol-soluble constituents and are prepared with alcoholic or hydroalcoholic vehicles. If the alcohol-soluble components are desired medicinal agents to be present in the corresponding syrup, some means of rendering them water-soluble is generally employed. However, if the alcohol-soluble components are undesirable or unnecessary components of the corresponding syrup, they are generally removed by mixing the tincture or fluidextract with water, allowing the mixture to stand until separation of the water-insoluble agents is complete, and filtering them from the mixture. The filtrate then represents the medicated liquid to which the sucrose is added in the preparation of the syrup. In other instances when the tincture or fluidextract is miscible with aqueous preparations, it may be added directly to simple syrup or to a flavored syrup to medicate it.

Percolation

In the percolation method,[8] either sucrose may be percolated to prepare the syrup, or the source of the medicinal component may be percolated to form an extractive to which sucrose or syrup may be added. This latter method really involves two separate procedures: first the preparation of the extractive of the drug and then the preparation of the syrup.

An example of a syrup prepared by percolation is Ipecac syrup. Ipecac syrup is prepared by adding glycerin and syrup to an extractive of powdered ipecac obtained by percolation. The drug ipecac consists of the dried rhizome and roots of *Cephaëlis ipecacuanha* and contains the medicinally active alkaloids, emetine, cephaeline, and psychotrine. These alkaloids are extracted from the powdered ipecac by percolation with a hydroalcoholic solvent.

The syrup is categorized as an emetic with a usual dose of 15 mL. This amount of syrup is commonly used in the management of poisoning in children when the evacuation of the stomach contents is desirable. About 80% of children given this dose will vomit within a half hour. For a household emetic in event of poisoning, 1-oz. bottles of the syrup may be sold without the requirement of a prescription. Ipecac syrup also has some application as a nauseant expectorant, in doses smaller than the emetic dose.

Recent evidence indicates that many bulimics—most commonly young woman in their late teens to early 30s—use syrup of ipecac to bring on attacks of vomiting in an attempt to lose more weight.[9] Pharmacists must be aware of this misuse of syrup of ipecac and warn these individuals because one of the active ingredients besides ipecac in the syrup is emetine. With continual use of the syrup, emetine builds up toxic levels within body tissues and in 3 to 4 months can do irreversible damage to heart muscles resulting in symptoms mimicking a heart attack. Shortness of breath is the most common symptom in patients who misuse syrup of ipecac, but some persons may describe low blood pressure-related symptoms and irregularities of heart beat.

Elixirs

Elixirs are clear, sweetened, hydroalcoholic solutions intended for oral use, and are usually flavored to enhance their palatability. *Nonmedicated* elixirs are employed as vehicles and *medicated* elixirs for the therapeutic effect of the medicinal substances they contain. Compared to syrups, elixirs are usually less sweet and less viscous because they contain a lower proportion of sugar and consequently less effective than syrups in masking the taste of medicinal substances. However, because of their hydroalcoholic character, elixirs are better able than aqueous syrups to maintain both water-soluble and alcohol-soluble components in solution. Also because of their stable characteristics and the ease which which they are prepared (by simple solution), from a manufacturing standpoint, elixirs are preferred over syrups.

The proportion of alcohol present in elixirs varies widely since the individual components of the elixirs have different water and alcohol solubility characteristics. Each elixir requires a specific blend of alcohol and water to maintain all of the components in solution. Naturally, for those elixirs containing agents which have poor water-solubility the proportion of alcohol required is greater than for elixirs prepared from components having good water solubility. In addition to alcohol and water, other solvents, as glycerin and propylene glycol, are frequently employed in elixirs as adjunct solvents.

Although many elixirs are sweetened with sucrose or with a sucrose-syrup, some utilize sorbitol, glycerin and/or artificial sweeteners. Elixirs having a high alcoholic content usually utilize an artificial sweetener as saccharin, which is required only in small amounts, rather than sucrose which is only slightly soluble in alcohol and requires greater quantities for equivalent sweetness.

All elixirs contain flavoring materials to increase their palatability and most elixirs have coloring agents to enhance their appearance. Elixirs containing over 10 to 12% of alcohol are usually self-preserving and do not require the addition of an antimicrobial agent for their preservation.

Although the USP monographs for medicated elixirs provide standards, they do not generally provide official formulas. Formulations are left up to the individual manufacturers. Example formulations for some medicated elixirs are as follows:[10]

Phenobarbital Elixir

Phenobarbital, USP	4.00 g
Orange Oil, NF	0.25 mL
Propylene Glycol, NF	100.00 mL
Alcohol, USP	200.00 mL
Sorbitol Solution, USP	600.00 mL
Color	q.s.
Purified Water, USP, to make	1000.00 mL

Theophylline Elixir

Theophylline, USP	5.3 g
Citric Acid, USP	10.0 g
Liquid Glucose, NF	44.0 g
Syrup, NF	132.0 mL
Glycerin, USP	50.0 mL
Sorbitol Solution, USP	324.0 mL
Alcohol, USP	200.00 mL
Sodium Saccharin, USP	5.0 g
Lemon Oil, NF	0.5 g
FDC Yellow No. 5	0.1 g
Purified Water, USP, to make	1000.0 mL

Medicated elixirs are formulated such that a patient receives the usual adult dose of the drug in a convenient measure of elixir. For most elixirs, one or two teaspoonfuls (5 or 10 mL) provide the usual adult dose of the drug. One advantage of elixirs over their counterpart drugs in solid dosage forms is the flexibility and ease of dosage administration, particularly to children. A parent can administer a half-teaspoonful of medication, for instance, to a child with much greater ease than would be required by the breaking of a corresponding tablet or by separating and dividing a capsule of medication. In instances in which elixir medication is intended for children, commercial packages often contain a calibrated measuring device, as a dropper or spoon, to enable the parent to measure the medication accurately according to the amounts recommended for the child's age, weight, or condition.

The disadvantage associated with the use of elixirs is that they can, if used in too great a dose, cause patient inebriation. So an important consideration in the selection of medicine that is available as an elixir would be the amount of alcohol a patient would receive per dose. Further, because elixirs contain alcohol and usually some volatile oils that deteriorate in the presence of air and light, they are best stored in tight, light-resistant containers protected against extremes of temperature.

Preparation of Elixirs

Elixirs are usually prepared by simple solution with agitation and/or by the admixture of two or more liquid ingredients. Alcohol-soluble and water-soluble components are generally dissolved separately in alcohol and in purified water, respectively. Then the aqueous solution is added to the alcoholic solution, rather than the reverse, in order to maintain the highest possible alcoholic strength at all times so that minimal separation of the alcohol-soluble components occurs. When the two solutions are completely mixed the mixture is made to volume with the specified solvent or vehicle. Frequently the final mixture will not be clear, but cloudy, due principally to the separation of some of the flavoring oils by the reduced alcoholic concentration. If this occurs, the elixir is usually permitted to stand for a prescribed number of hours, to ensure the saturation of the hydroalcoholic solvent and to permit the oil globules to coalesce so that they may be more easily removed by filtration. Talc, a frequent filter aid in the preparation of elixirs, has the ability to absorb the excessive amounts of oils and therefore assist in their removal from the solution. The presence of glycerin, syrup, sorbitol, and propylene glycol in elixirs generally contributes to the solvent effect of the hydroalcoholic vehicle, assists in the dissolution of the solute, and enhances the stability of the preparation. However, the presence of these materials adds to the viscosity of the elixir and slows the rate of their filtration.

Nonmedicated Elixirs

Nonmedicated elixirs may be useful to the pharmacist in the extemporaneous filling of prescriptions involving: (1) the addition of a therapeutic agent to a pleasant tasting vehicle, and (2) the dilution of an existing medicated elixir. In selecting a liquid vehicle for a drug substance, the pharmacist should concern himself with the solubility and stability of the drug substance in water and alcohol. If a hydroalcoholic vehicle is selected, the proportion of alcohol present should be only slightly above that amount which is needed to effect and maintain the drug's solution. When a pharmacist is called upon to dilute an existing medicated elixir, the nonmedicated elixir he selects as the diluent should have the approximate alcoholic concentration as the elixir being diluted. Also, the flavor and color characteristics of the diluent should not be in conflict with the medicated elixir and all components should be chemically and physically compatible.

In years past, when pharmacists were called upon more frequently than today to compound prescriptions, the three most commonly used nonmedicated elixirs were: Aromatic Elixir, Compound Benzaldehyde Elixir, and Iso-Alcoholic Elixir. The student may wish to refer to the previous edition of this text for information on these preparations.

Medicated Elixirs

As noted previously, medicated elixirs are employed for the therapeutic benefit of the medicinal agent present. In most instances, the official and commercial elixirs contain a single therapeutic agent. The main advantage of having only a single therapeutic agent present is that the dosage taken of that single drug may be increased or decreased by simply taking more or less of the elixir, whereas when two or more therapeutic agents are present in the same preparation, it is impossible to increase or decrease the amount taken of one without an automatic and corresponding adjustment in the dose taken of the other; a change which may not be desired. Thus, for patients required to take more than a single medication, many physicians prefer them to take separate preparations of each drug so that if an adjustment in the dosage of one is desired, it may be accomplished without the concomitant adjustment of the other.

Table 6–8 presents some examples of medicated elixirs. Some of these are briefly discussed below.

Antihistamine Elixirs

As indicated in Table 6–8, antihistamines are useful primarily in the symptomatic relief of certain allergic disorders. In their action, they suppress symptoms caused by histamine, one of the chemical agents released during the antigen-antibody reaction of the allergic response. Although only minor differences exist in the properties of most antihistamines, one or another may be preferred by a prescriber through his experience in managing a specific type of allergic reaction. A prescriber's preference may also be based on the incidence of adverse effects which may be expected to occur. The incidence and severity of these effects do vary somewhat with the drug and the dose of each drug. The most common untoward effect is sedation, and patients taking antihistamines should be warned against engaging in activities requiring mental alertness, as driving an automobile or tractor or operating machinery. Other common adverse effects include dryness of the nose, throat, and mouth, dizziness and disturbed concentration. Included among the most sedating antihistamines are diphenhydramine, doxylamine, and methapyrilene. In fact, diphenhydramine is used as a sleep aid in numerous over-the-counter products for its ability to cause drowsiness. Conversely, chlorpheniramine maleate does not produce as much sedation as the aforementioned antihistamines and it is for this reason that it is a popular choice for daytime antihistamine activity.

Most antihistaminic agents are basic amines. By forming salts through interaction with acid, the compounds are rendered water soluble. These salt forms are generally used in elixirs and thus the elixirs of the antihistamines are not required to contain a large proportion of alcohol. Because the acid salts of the antihistamines are used, the pH of these elixirs is on the acid side and must remain so if the drugs are to remain freely soluble in water. A pharmacist should keep this in mind when utilizing

Table 6–8. Examples of Medicated Elixirs by Category

Elixir	Some Representative Commercial Products	Usual Adult Dose of Drug/Volume of Commercial Elixir	Comments
Adrenocortical Steroid			
Dexamethasone Elixir	Decadron Elixir (Merck Sharp & Dohme)	500 µg/5 mL	Dexamethasone is a synthetic analogue of hydrocortisone that is considered to be about 30 times more potent than the latter drug. The commercial dexamethasone elixir is packaged with a calibrated dropper for the accurate measurement of small doses and is intended primarily for children, but also has utility for adults who may have trouble swallowing tablets. The elixir is used for many indications, including the treatment of rheumatoid arthritis, skin diseases, allergies and inflammatory conditions.
Analgesic/Antipyretic			
Acetaminophen Elixir	Children's Tylenol Elixir (McNeil)	160 mg/5 mL	Use for reduction of pain and lowering of fever particularly in patients sensitive to or unable to take aspirin. Elixir especially useful for pediatric patients.
Antihistamines			
Diphenhydramine HCl Elixir	Benadryl Elixir (Parke-Davis)	25 mg/10 mL	Antihistamine elixirs are employed for a variety of allergic reactions including: perennial and seasonal allergic rhinitis, vasomotor rhinitis, allergic skin manifestations of urticaria, reactions to insect bites, and others.
Antipsychotic			
Fluphenazine HCl Elixir	Prolixin Elixir (Princeton)	2.5 mg/5 mL	Used in the management of psychotic disorders.
Bronchodilator			
Oxtriphylline Elixir	Choledyl Elixir (Parke-Davis)	100 mg/5 mL	Used in treatment of bronchial asthma and in other conditions requiring bronchodilation.
Cardiotonic			
Digoxin Elixir	Lanoxin Pediatric Elixir (Burroughs Wellcome)	50 µg/mL	Among other effects, digoxin increases the force of myocardial contraction. Used in congestive heart failure, atrial fibrillation and other cardiac conditions. See text for additional discussion.

Table 6–8.   Continued

Elixir	Some Representative Commercial Products	Usual Adult Dose of Drug/Volume of Commercial Elixir	Comments
Central Stimulant			
Dextroamphetamine Sulfate, Elixir	Dexedrine Elixir (Smith Kline & French)	5 mg/5 mL	Used in instances of narcolepsy, hyperkinesia, and exogenous obesity.
Electrolyte Replenisher			
Potassium Gluconate Elixir	Kaon Elixir (Adria)	20 mEq K/15 mL	Used for the prevention and treatment of hypokalemia which may occur secondary to diuretic or corticosteroid administration. Elixir is mixed with water prior to taking.
Expectorants			
Terpin Hydrate Elixir	—	170 mg/10 mL	
Terpin Hydrate and Codeine Elixir	—	170 mg terpin hydrate and 20 mg codeine/ 10 mL	Terpin hydrate has expectorant action. The addition of codeine and dextromethorphan provides antitussive action as well.
Terpin Hydrate and Dextromethorphan HBr Elixir	—	170 mg terpin hydrate and 20 mg dextromethorphan HBr/10 mL	
Sedative/Hypnotics			
Butabarbital Sodium Elixir	Butisol Sodium Elixir (Wallace)	30 mg/5 mL	The barbiturate elixirs are utilized in low dosage as sedatives and in higher dosage as hypnotics. See text for additional discussion.
Phenobarbital Elixir	—	20 mg/5 mL	
Smooth Muscle Relaxant			
Theophylline Sodium Glycinate Elixir	Asbron G Elixir (Sandoz)	300 mg/15 mL	Used in bronchial asthma and other conditions requiring smooth muscle relaxation; said to be less irritating to gastric mucosa than other forms of theophylline.

one of these elixirs in the compounding of a prescription involving adding or mixing other components.

Barbiturate Sedative/Hypnotic Elixirs

The barbiturates are sedative/hypnotic agents which are used to produce various degrees of central nervous system depression. As the dose of these drugs is increased, the effects go from sedation to hypnosis to respiratory depression, the latter being the cause of death in fatal barbiturate overdosage.

Barbiturates are administered in small doses in the daytime hours as sedatives to reduce restlessness and emotional tension. The appropriate dose for this purpose is that amount which alleviates anxiety or tension but does not produce drowsiness or lethargy. Greater doses of the barbiturates may be given before bedtime as hypnotics to relieve insomnia.

Barbiturates have been classified according to the duration of their (hypnotic) effects; that is, *long-acting, intermediate-acting, short-acting,* or *ultrashort-acting* agents. The long-acting barbiturates including phenobarbital are considered most useful in maintaining daytime sedation and in treating some convulsive states and least useful in acting as hypnotics. The intermediate-acting barbiturates include amobarbital and are used primarily for short-term daytime sedation and are effective in treating insomnia. The barbiturates classified as short-acting include pentobarbital and secobarbital and are used similarly to the intermediate-acting barbiturates.

The ultrashort-acting barbiturates, as thiopental, are given intravenously to induce anesthesia.

The most common untoward effect noticed in patients taking barbiturates is drowsiness and lethargy. Large doses may produce residual sedation resembling the hangover following alcohol intoxication. Prolonged use of barbiturates may lead to psychic or physical dependence. This dependence, in susceptible individuals, leads to compulsive abuse of the drug with severe withdrawal symptoms following abstinence. In heavy chronic users, abrupt withdrawal may lead to convulsions, delirium, and occasionally to coma and death.

Some pharmaceutic aspects of Phenobarbital Elixir are presented below.

Phenobarbital Elixir

Phenobarbital elixir is formulated to contain 0.4% of phenobarbital, which provides about 20 mg of drug per teaspoonful (5 mL) of elixir. The elixir is commonly flavored with orange oil, colored red with an FDA-approved colorant, and sweetened with syrup. The official elixir contains about 14% of alcohol, which is used to dissolve the phenobarbital. However, this amount represents almost the very minimum required to keep the phenobarbital in solution. Thus glycerin is often added to enhance the solubility of phenobarbital.

Phenobarbital is a long-acting barbiturate with a duration of action of about 4 to 6 hours and a usual adult dose as a sedative of about 30 mg and a hypnotic dose of about 100 mg. The strength of the elixir permits the convenient adjustment of dosage to achieve the proper degree of sedation in the treatment of infants, children, and certain adult patients.

The elixir is commercially available from a variety of manufacturers under its nonproprietary name.

Digoxin Elixir

No official method of preparation is indicated for Digoxin Elixir; however, it is required to contain about 5 mg of digoxin per 100 mL of elixir or about 0.25 mg per teaspoonful. The usual oral adult dose of digoxin as a cardiotonic agent is about 1.5 mg on initial therapy and about 0.5 mg for maintenance therapy.

Digoxin is a cardiotonic glycoside obtained from the leaves of *Digitalis lanata*. It is a white crystalline powder that is insoluble in water, but

Fig. 6–2. *Serum digoxin concentrations following administration of 0.5 mg of digoxin by oral tablet and elixir-like oral solution. (Adapted from D.H. Huffman and D.L. Azarnoff: Absorption of Orally Given Digoxin Preparations, J.A.M.A., 222:957, 1972.)*

soluble in dilute alcohol solutions. The official elixir contains about 10% of alcohol. Digoxin is a poisonous drug, and its dose must be carefully determined and administered to each individual patient. Adults generally take digoxin tablets rather than the elixir, which must be measured by the highly variable household teaspoon. The elixir is generally employed in pediatric practice, and the commercial product available for this purpose is packaged with a calibrated dropper to facilitate accurate dosage measurements.

Digoxin is one of many drugs which is available to the prescriber in more than a single type of dosage form. The prescriber frequently has the choice of selecting a solid dosage form, as a tablet or capsule, or a liquid form of the medication for his patient. The advantages of each have been noted previously but it is important here to point out again that drugs administered in different dosage forms may exhibit different bioavailability characteristics with varying patterns of drug release and rates and extents of drug absorption. Such differences have been noted for digoxin, between tablets from different manufacturers, as well as between tablets and oral liquid dosage forms.[11-13] Figure 6–2 shows the differences noted in one study of the serum digoxin levels following administration of 0.5 mg of digoxin by oral tablet and oral solution having an elixir-like vehicle. It can be readily seen that the serum digoxin levels following administration of the oral solution were considerably greater than from the oral tablet.

A patient taking a drug known to exhibit bioavailability problems, and whose therapeutic dosage regimen has been successfully established with a particular drug product, should not be changed to another product.

Proper Administration and Use of Liquid Peroral Dosage Forms

The dosage forms discussed in this chapter are all to be administered by mouth. Conveniently, these can be measured in a spoon, i.e., teaspoon, tablespoon, depending upon the desired dosage and swallowed. Preferably, however, these medicines should be measured out in calibrated devices for administration. These devices assure the patient that the correct dose will be received because teaspoons, for example, can vary dramatically in the volume they deliver. Even though these are liquids, it is recommended that the patient follow the administration of the liquid dosage form with a glassful of water.

The pharmacist must be careful in the selection of liquid products given the patient's history and other concurrent medicines. For example, some syrups contain sucrose or another sugar as an ingredient, and the pharmacist must recall that such syrups would not be optimal for use in an oral prescription intended for a diabetic patient. Similarly, a product that is formulated as an elixir would not be advantageous to use in a patient who receives concurrent medicines that possess an antabuse-like activity, i.e., the patient may get violently ill from the concurrent ingestion of alcohol. Metronidazole and chlorpropramide are two drugs that have been implicated to cause this reaction when mixed with alcohol. Further, if the patient is receiving another drug that causes drowsiness the pharmacist must make a decision to intervene and contact the prescribing physician to determine whether the prescribed elixir could be harmful to the patient.

Notes

1. However, they are usually more soluble in the less polar solvents as alcohol and the various organic solvents.
2. Polar groups include OH, CHO, COH, CHOH, CH_2OH, COOH, NO_2, CO, NH_2 and SO_3H.
3. An excellent chart depicting the solubility characteristics of inorganic salts may be found in *Husa's Pharmaceutical Dispensing*, 6th ed. E. W. Martin, (ed.) Easton, PA, Mack Publishing Company, 1966, p. 549.
4. Chemburkar, P.B. and Joslin, R.S.: Effect of Flavoring Oils on Preservative Concentrations in Oral Liquid Dosage Forms. *J. Pharm. Sci.*, 64:414–41, 1975.
5. Gossel, T.A.: Oral Rehydration Solutions. *US Pharmacist*, 12(2):90–98, 1987.
6. *Handbook on Extemporaneous Formulations*. Bethesda, MD, American Society of Hospital Pharmacists, Inc., 1987.
7. *Oral Liquid Pharmaceuticals*. Wilmington, DE, ICI Americas, Inc., 1975.
8. The process of percolation of drugs is discussed at greater length in Chapter 13.
9. Murphy, D.: Ipecac Misuse by Bulimics: APhA Launches Educational Campaign. *Amer. Pharm.*, NS25:264–265, 1985.
10. *Oral Liquid Pharmaceuticals*. Wilmington, DE, ICI Americas, Inc., 1975.
11. Huffman, D.H., and Azarnoff, D.L.: Absorption of Orally Given Digoxin Preparations. *JAMA*, 222:957–960, 1972.
12. Lindenbaum, J., et al.: Variation in Biologic Availability of Digoxin from Four Preparations. *N. Engl. J. Med.*, 285:1344–1347, 1971.
13. Wagner, J., et al.: Equivalence Lack in Digoxin Plasma Levels. *JAMA*, 224:199–204, 1973.

7 | *Oral Suspensions, Emulsions, Magmas, and Gels*

THIS CHAPTER includes the main types of liquid preparations containing undissolved drug distributed throughout a vehicle and intended for oral administration. In these preparations, the substance distributed is referred to as the *disperse* or *dispersed phase* and the vehicle is termed the *dispersing phase* or *dispersion medium*. For most oral preparations of this type, the dispersion medium is aqueous.

The particles of the disperse phase are usually solid materials which are insoluble in the dispersion medium. In the case of emulsions, the disperse phase is a liquid substance which is neither soluble nor miscible with the liquid of the dispersing phase. The emulsification process results in the dispersion of liquid drug as fine droplets throughout the dispersing phase.

The particles of the disperse phase vary widely in size, from large particles visible to the naked eye down to particles of colloidal dimension, falling between 1 millimicron (mμ) and about 500 millimicrons or 0.5 micron (μ) in size. Dispersions containing coarse particles, usually 1 to 100 microns in size, are referred to as *coarse dispersions* and include the *suspensions* and *emulsions*. Dispersions containing particles of smaller size are termed *fine dispersions*, and, if the particles are in the colloidal range, *colloidal dispersions*. *Magmas* and *gels* represent such fine dispersions.

Largely because of their greater size, dispersed particles in a coarse dispersion have a greater tendency to separate from the dispersion medium than do the particles of a fine dispersion. Most solids in dispersion tend to settle to the bottom of the container because of their greater density than the dispersing medium, whereas most emulsified liquids for oral use are oils and generally have a lesser density than the aqueous medium in which they are dispersed and tend to rise toward the top of the preparation. Complete and uniform redistribution of the disperse phase is essential to the accurate administration of uniform doses. For a properly

Fig. 7–1. *Examples of some commercial oral suspensions.*

prepared dispersion, this should be accomplished by the moderate agitation of the container.

While the focus of this chapter is on dispersions of drugs administered orally, the same basic pharmaceutical characteristics apply to those disperse systems administered by other routes and discussed later in this text. Included among these are lotions for topical application to the skin, ophthalmic suspensions, and sterile suspensions for injection.

Oral Suspensions

Suspensions may be defined as preparations containing finely divided drug particles (referred to as the *suspensoid*) distributed somewhat uniformly throughout a vehicle in which the drug exhibits a minimum degree of solubility. Some suspensions are available in ready-to-use form—that is, already distributed through a liquid vehicle with or without stabilizers and other pharmaceutical additives (Fig. 7-1). Other preparations are available as dry powders intended for suspensions in liquid vehicles. This type of product generally is a powder mixture containing the drug and suitable

Fig. 7–2. *Commercial antibiotic preparation for oral suspension following reconstitution with purified water. On the left is the dry powder mixture, and on the right the suspension after reconstitution with the specified amount of purified water.*

suspending and dispersing agents, which upon dilution and agitation with a specified quantity of vehicle (generally purified water) results in the formation of a suspension suitable for administration. Figure 7–2 demonstrates the preparation of this type of product. Drugs that are unstable if maintained for extended periods of time in the presence of an aqueous vehicle (for example, many antibiotic drugs) are most frequently supplied as dry powder mixtures for reconstitution at the time of dispensing. This type of preparation is designated in the USP by a title of the form ". . . for Oral Suspension." Prepared suspensions not requiring reconstitution at the time of dispensing are simply designated as ". . . Oral Suspension."

Reasons for Oral Suspension

The reasons for preparing the oral suspension are several. For one thing, certain drugs are chemically unstable when in solution but stable when suspended. In instances such as this, the oral suspension insures chemical stability while permitting liquid therapy. For many patients, the liquid form is preferred over the solid form

of the same drug because of the ease of swallowing liquids and the flexibility in the administration of a range of doses. This is particularly advantageous for infants, children and the elderly. The disadvantage of the disagreeable taste of certain drugs when given in solution form is overcome when the drug is administered as undissolved particles of a suspension. In fact, chemical forms of certain poor-tasting drugs have been specifically developed for their insolubility in a desired vehicle for the sole purpose of preparing a palatable liquid dosage form. For example, the water-insoluble ester form of chloramphenicol, chloramphenicol palmitate, was developed to prepare a palatable liquid dosage form of the chloramphenicol, the result being the development of Chloramphenicol Palmitate Oral Suspension, USP. By the creation of insoluble forms of drugs for use in suspensions, the difficult taste-masking problems of developmental pharmacists are greatly reduced, and the selection of the flavorants to be used in a given suspension may be based on taste preference rather than on a particular flavorant's ability to act as a masking agent for an unpleasant tasting drug. For the most part, oral suspensions are aqueous preparations with the vehicle flavored and sweetened to suit the anticipated taste preferences of the intended patient.

Features Desired in a Pharmaceutical Suspension

There are many considerations in the development and preparation of a pharmaceutically elegant suspension. In addition to therapeutic efficacy, chemical stability of the components of the formulation, permanency of the preparation, and esthetic appeal of the preparation—desirable qualities in all pharmaceutical preparations—a few other features apply more specifically to the pharmaceutical suspension:

1. A properly prepared pharmaceutical suspension should settle slowly and should be readily redispersed upon the gentle shaking of the container.
2. The characteristics of the suspension should be such that the particle size of the suspensoid remains fairly constant throughout long periods of undisturbed standing.

3. The suspension should pour readily and evenly from its container.

These main features of a suspension, which depend upon the nature of the dispersed phase, the dispersion medium, and pharmaceutical adjuncts, will be discussed briefly.

Sedimentation Rate of the Particles of a Suspension

The various factors involved in the rate of velocity of settling of the particles of a suspension are embodied in the equation of Stokes' law:

$$V = \frac{d^2(\rho_1 - \rho_2)g}{18\eta}$$

where V = the velocity of the fall of a spherical particle,
g = the gravitational constant,
d = the diameter of the sphere,
ρ_1 = the density of the sphere,
ρ_2 = the density of the liquid, and
η = the viscosity of the dispersion medium.

Stokes' equation was derived for an ideal situation in which uniform, perfectly spherical particles in a very dilute suspension settle without effecting turbulence in their downward course, without collision of the particles of the suspensoid, and without chemical or physical attraction or affinity for the dispersion medium. Obviously, Stokes' equation does not apply precisely to the usual pharmaceutical suspension in which the suspensoid is irregularly shaped, of various particle diameters, and not spherical, in which the fall of the particles *does* result in both turbulence and collision, and also in which there may be a reasonable amount of affinity of the particles for the suspension medium. However, the basic concepts of the equation do give a valid indication of the factors that are important to the suspension of the particles and a clue to the possible adjustments that can be made to a formulation to decrease the rate of particle sedimentation.

From the equation it is apparent that the velocity of fall of a suspended particle is greater for larger particles than it is for smaller particles, all other factors remaining constant. By reducing the particle size of the dispersed phase, one can expect a slower *rate* of descent of the par-

ticles. Also, the greater the density of the particles, the greater the rate of descent, provided the density of the vehicle is not altered. Because aqueous vehicles are generally used in pharmaceutical oral suspensions, the density of the particles is generally greater than that of the vehicle, a desirable feature, for if the particles were less dense than the vehicle, they would tend to float, and floating particles would be quite difficult to distribute uniformly in the vehicle. The rate of sedimentation may be appreciably reduced by increasing the viscosity of the dispersion medium, and within limits of practicality this may be done. However, a product having a high viscosity is not generally desirable, because it pours with difficulty and it is equally difficult to redisperse the suspensoid. Therefore, if the viscosity of a suspension is increased, it is done so only to a modest extent to avoid these difficulties.

The viscosity characteristics of a suspension may be altered not only by the vehicle used, but also by the solids content. As the proportion of solid particles is increased in a suspension, so is the viscosity. The viscosity of a pharmaceutical preparation may be determined through the use of a Brookfield Viscometer, which measures viscosity by the force required to rotate a spindle in the fluid being tested (Fig. 7–3).

For the most part, the physical stability of a pharmaceutical suspension appears to be most appropriately adjusted by an alteration in the dispersed phase rather than through great changes in the dispersion medium. In most instances, the dispersion medium is supportive to the adjusted dispersed phase. These adjustments mainly are concerned with particle size, uniformity of particle size, and separation of the particles so that they are not likely to become greatly larger or to form a solid cake on standing.

Physical Features of the Dispersed Phase of a Suspension

Probably the most important single consideration in a discussion of suspensions is the size of the drug particles.[1] In most good pharmaceutical suspensions, the particle diameter is between 1 and 50 microns.[2]

Particle size reduction is generally accomplished by dry-milling prior to the incorporation of the dispersed phase into the dispersion medium. One of the most rapid, convenient, and

SYNCHRONOUS MOTOR
SPEED SELECTOR KNOB
ON-OFF TOGGLE SWITCH
CLUTCH LEVER
KNURLED NUT
HANDLE
POINTER
JEWEL BEARING SUPPORT
SPINDLE COUPLING NUT
IMMERSION MARK
SPINDLE BODY

GEAR TRAIN
CIRCULAR BUBBLE LEVEL
DIAL
CALIBRATED SPIRAL SPRING
UPPER SHAFT
PIVOT POINT
REMOVABLE SPINDLE GUARD
SAMPLE CONTAINER

Fig. 7–3. *Schematic drawing of the Brookfield Viscometer. (Courtesy of Brookfield Engineering Laboratories.)*

inexpensive methods of producing fine drug powders of about 10 to 50 micron size is *micropulverization.* Micropulverizers are high-speed, attrition or impact mills which are efficient in reducing powders to the size acceptable for most oral and topical suspensions. For still finer particles, under 10 microns, the process of *fluid energy* grinding, sometimes referred to as *jet-milling* or *micronizing*, is quite effective. By this process, the shearing action of high velocity compressed air streams on the particles in a confined space produces the desired ultrafine or micronized particles. The particles to be micronized are swept into violent turbulence by the sonic and supersonic velocity of the air streams. The particles are accelerated into high velocities and collide with one another, resulting in fragmentation and a decrease in the size of the particles. This method may be employed in instances in which the particles are intended for parenteral or ophthalmic suspensions. Particles of extremely small dimensions may also be produced by *spray-drying* techniques. A

spray dryer is a cone-shaped piece of apparatus into which a solution of a drug is sprayed and rapidly dried by a current of warmed, dry air circulating in the cone. The resulting dry powder is then collected. It is not possible for a community pharmacist to achieve the same degree of particle-size reduction with such simple comminuting equipment as the mortar and pestle. However, many micronized drugs are commercially available and when needed may be purchased by the pharmacist in bulk quantities.

As shown by Stokes' equation, the reduction in the particle size of a suspensoid is beneficial to the stability of the suspension in that the rate of sedimentation of the solid particles is reduced as the particles are decreased in size. The reduction in particle size produces slow, more uniform rates of settling. However, one should avoid reducing the particle size to too great a degree of fineness, since fine particles have a tendency to form a compact cake upon settling to the bottom of the container. The result may be that the cake resists breakup upon shaking, and forms rigid aggregates of particles which are of larger dimension and less suspendable than the original suspensoid. The particle shape of the suspensoid can also affect caking and product stability. It has been shown that symmetrical barrel-shaped particles of calcium carbonate produced more stable suspensions than did asymmetrical needle-shaped particles of the same agent. The needle-shaped particles formed a tenacious sediment-cake on standing which could not be redistributed whereas the barrel-shaped particles did not cake on standing.[3]

To avoid the formation of a cake, measures must be taken to prevent the agglomeration of the particles into larger crystals or into masses. One common method of preventing the rigid cohesion of small articles of a suspension is through the intentional formation of a less rigid or loose aggregation of the particles held together by comparatively weak particle-to-particle bonding forces. Such an aggregation of particles is termed a *floc* or a *floccule,* with flocculated particles forming a type of lattice structure that resists complete settling (although flocs settle more rapidly than fine, individual particles) and thus are less prone to compaction than unflocculated particles. The flocs settle to form a higher sediment volume than unflocculated particles, the loose structure of which permits the aggregates to break up easily and distribute readily with a small amount of agitation.

There are several methods of preparing flocculated suspensions, the choice depending on the type of drug involved and the type of product desired. For instance, in the preparation of an oral suspension of a drug, clays such as diluted bentonite magma are commonly employed as the flocculating agent. The structure of the bentonite magma and of other clays used for this purpose also assists the suspension by helping to support the floc once formed. When clays are unsuitable as agents, as in a parenteral suspension, frequently a floc of the dispersed phase can be produced by an alteration in the pH of the preparation (generally to the region of minimum drug solubility). Electrolytes can also act as flocculating agents, apparently by reducing the electrical barrier between the particles of the suspensoid and forming a bridge so as to link them together. The carefully determined concentration of nonionic and ionic surface-active agents (surfactants) can also induce the flocculation of particles in suspension and increase the sedimentation volume.

Dispersion Medium

Oftentimes, as with highly flocculated suspensions, the particles of a suspension settle too rapidly to be consistent with what might be termed a pharmaceutically elegant preparation. The rapid settling hinders the accurate measurement of dosage and from an esthetic point of view produces too unsightly a supernatant layer. In many of the commercial suspensions, suspending agents are added to the dispersion medium to lend it a structure to assist in the suspension of the dispersed phase. Carboxymethylcellulose, methylcellulose, xanthan gum, and bentonite are a few of the agents employed to thicken the dispersion medium and help suspend the suspensoid. When polymeric substances and hydrophilic colloids are used as suspending agents, appropriate tests must be performed to show that the agent does not interfere with the availability for therapeutic effects of the suspension's medicinal substance. These materials have been found to bind certain medicinal agents, rendering them unavailable or more slowly available for their therapeutic function. Also, the amount of the suspending agent must not be such to render the suspension too viscous to agitate (to distribute the *suspensoid*) or to pour. The study of the flow characteristics is termed *rheology.*

Support of the suspensoid by the dispersion medium may depend upon several factors: the density of the suspensoid, whether it is flocculated, and the amount of material requiring support.

The solid content of a suspension intended for oral administration may vary considerably, depending on the dose of the drug to be administered, the volume of product desired to be administered, and also on the ability of the dispersion medium to support the concentration of drug while maintaining desirable features of viscosity and flow. The usual adult oral suspension is frequently designed to supply the dose of the particular drug in a convenient measure of 5 mL or one teaspoonful. Pediatric suspensions are formulated to deliver the appropriate dose of drug by administering a dose-calibrated number of drops. Figure 7–4 shows commonly packaged oral suspensions administered as pediatric drops. Some are accompanied by a calibrated dropper, whereas other

Fig. 7–4. *Examples of oral pediatric suspensions showing package designs of a built-in dropper device and a calibrated dropper accompanying the medication container.*

packages have the drop capability built into the container. On administration the drops may be placed directly into the infant's mouth or mixed with a small portion of food. Because many of the suspensions of antibiotic drugs intended for pediatric use are prepared in a highly flavored, sweetened, colored base, they are frequently referred to by their manufacturers and also popularly as "syrups," even though in fact they are suspensions.

The Preparation of the Suspension

In the preparation of a suspension, the pharmacist must be acquainted with the characteristics of both the intended dispersed phase and the dispersion medium. In some instances the dispersed phase has an affinity for the vehicle to be employed and is readily "wetted" by it upon its addition. Other drugs are not penetrated easily by the vehicle and have a tendency to clump together or to float on top of the vehicle. In the latter case, the powder must first be wetted by a so-called "wetting agent" to make the powder more penetrable by the dispersion medium. Alcohol, glycerin, and other hygroscopic liquids are employed as wetting agents when an aqueous vehicle is to be used as the dispersion phase. They function by displacing the air in the crevices of the particles, dispersing the particles, and subsequently allowing the penetration of dispersion medium into the powder. In the large-scale preparation of suspensions the wetting agents are mixed with the particles by an apparatus such as a colloid mill; on a small scale in the pharmacy, they are mixed with a mortar and pestle. Once the powder is wetted, the dispersion medium (to which have been added all of the formula-

tion's soluble components such as colorants, flavorants, and preservatives) is added in portions to the powder, and the mixture is thoroughly blended before subsequent additions of vehicle. A portion of the vehicle is used to wash the mixing equipment free of suspensoid, and this portion is used to bring the suspension to final volume and insure that the suspension contains the desired concentration of solid matter. The final product is then passed through a colloid mill or other blender or mixing device to insure uniformity.

Whenever appropriate, suitable preservatives should be included in the formulation of suspensions to preserve against bacterial and mold contamination.

An example formula for an oral suspension follows.[4] In the example, the suspensoid is the antacid aluminum hydroxide, the preservatives are methylparaben and propylparaben, with syrup and sorbitol solution providing the viscosity as well as the sweetness.

Aluminum hydroxide compressed gel	362.8 g
Sorbitol Solution, USP	282.0 mL
Syrup, NF	93.0 mL
Glycerin, USP	25.0 mL
Methylparaben, NF	0.9 g
Propylparaben, NF	0.3 g
Flavor	q.s.
Purified Water, USP, to make	1000.0 mL

In preparing a formula such as this, the parabens are dissolved in a heated mixture of the sorbitol solution, glycerin, syrup, and a portion of the water. The mixture is then cooled and the aluminum hydroxide added with stirring. The flavor is added and sufficient purified water to volume. The suspension is then homogenized, using a hand homogenizer, homomixer, or colloid mill.

Unfortunately, not all medicines are available in a convenient, easy to take liquid dosage form. Consequently, patients who are not able to swallow solid medicines, e.g., infants, elderly, may present a special need. Thus, the pharmacist may have to use a solid dosage form, e.g., tablet, capsule, of the drug and extemporaneously compound a liquid product. A difficulty that confronts the pharmacist is a lack of ready information of stability of a drug when it is incorporated into a liquid vehicle. It is known that drugs in liquid form have faster decomposition rates than when in solid form, and

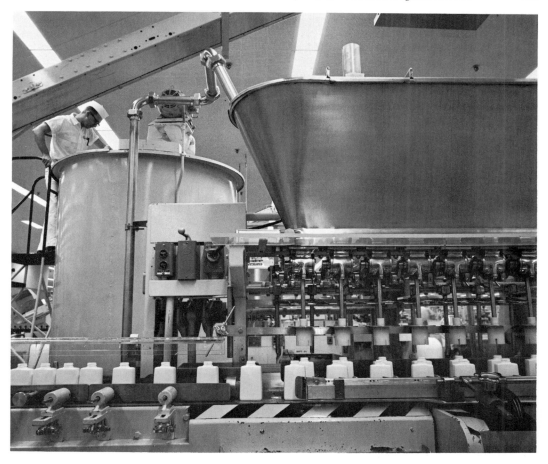

Fig. 7–5. *Liquid filling. The 1000-gallon portable storage tank holding the bulk product is shown in the background. The fluid preparation is pumped from the bottom of the tank through sanitary piping to the large stainless steel hopper located in the foreground. Immediatley below the hopper are eight piston-type filling cylinders. Extending from the filling heads are eight filling tubes, each with a bottle-centering bell. On the left, bottles are shown being conveyed after cleaning. As they pass through an indexing worm, the bottles are then spaced accurately for transfer by a pusher bar to the filling position. After filling, incoming bottles push those filled onto the conveyor to the bottle-capping operation. (Courtesy of The Upjohn Company.)*

some are affected by the pH of the medium. Leucovorin calcium when compounded from crushed tablets or the injectable form is most stable in milk or antacid and is unstable in acidic solutions, e.g., Aromatic Elixir USP.

To overcome this information gap, the pharmacist can attempt to contact the pharmaceutical manufacturer of the solid dosage form to attain stability information. Depending upon the situation, a manufacturer may be unwilling to provide this information on the basis of legal implication. Fortunately, however, a number of extemporaneous formulations have appeared in the professional literature (e.g., for prednisone oral suspension[5]) and some manufacturers may

provide within the package insert a formula for the preparation of an oral liquid form, e.g., Rifadin [Merrell-Dow]. Further, the Committee on Extemporaneous Formulations, an American Society of Hospital Pharmacy special interest group has compiled and published a listing of extemporaneous formulations in a text titled, *Handbook of Extemporaneous Formulations*. It is a compilation of formulations based upon documented stability data and unpublished data compiled by pharmaceutical manufacturers and practitioners.

Typically, when formulating an extemporaneous suspension, the contents of a capsule are emptied into a mortar or the tablets of the drug

Table 7–1. Examples of Oral Suspensions by Category

Oral Suspension	Some Representative Commercial Products	Concentration of Respective Drug in Commercial Oral Suspension	Comments
Analgesic			
Propoxyphene Napsylate Oral Suspension	Darvon N Suspension (Lilly)	50 mg/5 mL	Propoxyphene napsylate is a water-insoluble agent that differs from propoxyphene HCl (Darvon) in solubility (the HCl salt is water-soluble) and allows more stable liquid dosage forms and tablet formulations. The drug is employed as an analgesic in the relief of mild to moderate pain. It is related structurally to the narcotic methadone.
Acetaminophen Oral Suspension	Tempra (Mead Johnson); Tylenol (McNeil)	100 mg/mL	Analgesic/antipyretic. Provided to patient in a dropper-bottle for pediatric use.
Antacids			
Alumina and Magnesia Oral Suspension	Delcid Oral Suspension (Lakeside)	Aluminum hydroxide, 600 mg, and magnesium hydroxide, 655 mg/5 mL	
Alumina, Magnesia, and Simethicone Oral Suspension	Mylanta (Stuart)	Aluminum hydroxide, 200 mg; magnesium hydroxide, 200 mg; and simethicone, 20 mg/5 mL	
Alumina and Magnesium Trisilicate Oral Suspension	Alma-Mag Liquid (Rugby)	250 mg of aluminum hydroxide and 500 mg of magnesium trisilicate/5 mL	
Alumina Magnesia and Calcium Carbonate Oral Suspension	Camalox (Rorer)	225 mg of aluminum hydroxide, 200 mg of magnesium hydroxide, and 250 mg of calcium carbonate/5 mL	These preparations are used to counteract gastric hyperacidity and to relieve distress in the upper gastrointestinal tract. See text for additional discussion.
Magaldrate Oral Suspension	Riopan Oral Suspension (Ayerst)	540 mg of hydroxymagnesium aluminate, a chemical entity of aluminum and magnesium hydroxides.	
Magnesia and Alumina Oral Suspension	Maalox Suspension (Rorer)	225 mg of aluminum hydroxide and 200 mg of magnesium hydroxide/5 mL.	
Aluminum Hydroxide and Magnesium Carbonate Oral Suspension	Gaviscon Liquid Antacid (Marion)	Aluminum hydroxide, 95 mg, magnesium carbonate, 412 mg/15 mL, and sodium alginate	
Anthelmintics			
Pyrantel Pamoate Oral Suspension	Antiminth Oral Suspension (Pfizer)	250 mg/5 mL	These anthelmintics are employed to rid the body of worm infections. See text for additional discussion.
Thiabenzadole Oral Suspension	Mintezol Oral Suspension (Merck Sharp & Dohme)	500 mg/5 mL	

Table 7–1.   Continued

Oral Suspension	Some Representative Commercial Products	Concentration of Respective Drug in Commercial Oral Suspension	Comments
Antibacterials (Antibiotics)			
Chloramphenicol Palmitate Oral Suspension	Chloromycetin Palmitate Oral Suspension (Parke-Davis)	150 mg/5 mL	A broad-spectrum antibiotic reserved for serious infections by susceptible organisms when less potentially hazardous agents are ineffective or contraindicated. The tasteless palmitate ester of chloramphenicol is hydrolyzed in the gut to chloramphenicol before absorption.
Erythromycin Estolate Oral Suspension	Ilosone (Dista)	125 mg/5mL	Broad-spectrum macrolide antibiotic having bacteriostatic and bacteriocidal activity.
Tetracycline HCl Oral Suspension	Achromycin V Oral Suspension (Lederle)	125 mg/5 mL	Tetracycline antibiotics act by inhibiting microorganisms' protein synthesis. They are effective against a wide range of gram-positive and gram-negative microorganisms.
Antibacterials (Non-antibiotic Anti-infectives)			
Methenamine Mandelate Oral Suspension	Mandelamine Suspension and Mandelamine Suspension Forte (Parke-Davis)	250 and 500 mg (Forte)/5 mL	Methenamine mandelate oral suspension is prepared with an oleaginous vehicle. Methenamine mandelate is a chemical combination of approximately equal parts of methenamine and mandelic acid which is effective in destroying most of the pathogens commonly found to infect the urinary tract. An acid urine is essential for the activity of the drug, with maximum efficacy occurring at pH 5.5. The methenamine component of the drug in an acid urine is hydrolyzed to ammonia and the bactericidal agent, formaldehyde. The mandelic acid component meantime exerts its antibacterial action and contributes to the acidification of the urine. The usual dose of the drug is 1 g, up to four times a day.

Table 7–1.   Continued

Oral Suspension	Some Representative Commercial Products	Concentration of Respective Drug in Commercial Oral Suspension	Comments
Antibacterials (Non-antibiotic Anti-infectives) *Cont.*			
			The suspension form of the drug is especially useful in treating pediatric patients as well as those adults who cannot or will not swallow a tablet (also official and commercially available).
Nitrofurantoin Oral Suspension	Furadantin Oral Suspension (Norwich Eaton)	25 mg/5 mL	The aqueous suspension of nitrofurantoin is a urinary tract antibacterial agent. Because nitrofurantoin is discolored by alkalies and by exposure to light and is decomposed upon contact with metals other than stainless steel and aluminum, the pharmacist should make certain that these offending environments are avoided in preparing and packaging of the drug. Amber glass containers are normally used in the packaging of the suspension. The usual adult dose of the drug is 50 to 100 mg (four times a day) corresponding to about 4 teaspoonfuls (20 mL) of the suspension. The nausea sometimes associated with nitrofurantoin therapy can usually be minimized by administering the drug during meals or with milk or other food snacks before retiring. The suspension is particularly useful in treating children in which case the dose of nitrofurantoin is based on body weight, between 5 to 7 mg of drug being given per day (in divided doses) per kg of body weight. Infants less than 1 month of age should not be given the drug because of their inability, due to immature enzyme systems, to detoxify the drug.

Table 7–1.   Continued

Oral Suspension	Some Representative Commercial Products	Concentration of Respective Drug in Commercial Oral Suspension	Comments
Sulfamethoxazole and Trimethoprim Suspension	Bactrim (Roche) Spectra (Burroughs-Wellcome)	40 mg of trimethoprim and 200 mg of sulfamethoxazole per 5 mL	This suspension is used to treat acute middle ear infection (otitis media) in children and urinary tract infections due to susceptible microorganisms.
Sulfamethoxazole Oral Suspension	Gantanol Suspension (Roche)	500 mg/5 mL	These sulfa-drug suspensions are bacteriostatic agents particularly useful in the treatment of urinary tract infections. Sulfonamides competitively inhibit bacterial synthesis of folic acid and para-aminobenzoic acid.
Sulfisoxazole Acetyl Oral Suspension	Gantrisin Syrup and Gantrisin Pediatric Suspension (Roche)	500 mg/5 mL	
Anticonvulsants Primidone Oral Suspension	Mysoline Suspension (Ayerst)	250 mg/5 mL	This drug is useful in the management of grand mal epilepsy and psychomotor attacks.
Antidiarrheal Bismuth Subsalicylate Suspension	Pepto-Bismol (Procter & Gamble)	262 mg/5 mL	For indigestion without causing constipation, nausea, and control of diarrhea. An unlabeled use has been for the prevention and treatment of traveler's (enterotoxigenic *Escherichia coli*) diarrhea, but in neither case is it the first line of therapy.
Antiflatulent Simethicone Oral Suspension	Mylicon Drops (Stuart)	40 mg/0.6 mL	Used for the symptomatic treatment of gastrointestinal distress due to entrapment of gas. The drug acts by reducing the surface tension of gas bubbles, enabling them to coalesce and to be released through belching or passing flatus.
Antifungals Nystatin Oral Suspension	Mycostatin Oral Suspension (Squibb)	100,000 units/mL	Mycostatin is an antibiotic with antifungal activity. The suspension is held in the mouth as long as possible before swallowing in the treatment of infections of the oral cavity caused by *Candida* (Monilia) *albicans* and other Candida species.

Table 7–1. Continued

Oral Suspension	Some Representative Commercial Products	Concentration of Respective Drug in Commercial Oral Suspension	Comments
Antifungals *Cont.*			
Griseofulvin Oral Suspension	Grifulvin V Suspension (Ortho)	125 mg/mL	Microsize griseofulvin acts systemically as an antifungal (fungistatic).
Antihypertensive			
Methyldopa Oral Solution	Aldomet Oral Suspension (Merck, Sharp & Dohme)	250 mg/5 mL	Antihypertensive agent useful in lowering high blood pressure.
Antipsychotics, Sedatives, Antiemetics			
Chlorprothixene Oral Suspension, USP	Taractan Concentrate (Roche)	100 mg/5 mL	Used in the control of moderate to severe agitation, anxiety, and tension, when such symptoms are manifestations of schizophrenia.
Hydroxyzine Pamoate Oral Suspension, USP	Vistaril Oral Suspension (Pfizer)	25 mg/5 mL	Used in the management of anxiety, tension, and psychomotor agitation.
Thioridazine Oral Suspension	Mellaril (Sandoz)	25 mg/5 mL	For the management of manifestations of psychotic disorders and short-term treatments of moderate to marked depression with variable degrees of anxiety in adults.
Bronchodilator			
Theophylline Oral Suspension	Elixicon (Berlex)	100 mg/5 mL	This suspension is used for the symptomatic relief or prevention of bronchial asthma and reversible bronchospasm associated with chronic bronchitis and emphysema.
Diuretic			
Chlorothiazide Oral Suspension	Diuril Oral Suspension (Merck Sharp & Dohme)	250 mg/5 mL	Acts as a diuretic by interfering with the renal tubular mechanism of electrolyte reabsorption (increases excretion of sodium and chloride).
Nonsteroidal Anti-inflammatory			
Indomethacin Oral Suspension	Indocin (MSD)	25 mg/5 mL	For the active treatment of moderate to severe rheumatoid arthritis (including acute flares of chronic illness), moderate to severe osteoarthritis, acute painful shoulder (bursitis or tendinitis), and acute gouty arthritis.

crushed in a mortar with a pestle. The selected vehicle is then slowly added to and mixed with the powder to create a paste and then diluted to the desired volume. The selected vehicle can be commercially available for this purpose, e.g., Roxane's Diluent (Flavored) for Oral Use (Roxane), or be a combination of a liquid that affords suspending qualities, e.g., Cologel (Eli Lilly and Co.), and a liquid that affords a pleasant taste to the preparation, e.g., Cherry Syrup. Because there are usually water-insoluble excipients from the tablet or the capsule the final product is a suspension. If the active ingredient is water-soluble and if a solution is desired, distilled water is added to dissolve the drug and then the mixture is filtered to remove the insoluble excipients.

The extent of the formulation depends upon the patient for whom the product is intended. For example, a liquid suspension for a neonate does not necessitate the inclusion of preservatives, colorings, flavorings and alcohol because of the potential for each of these to cause either acute or long-term adverse effects. Because this liquid product will probably be administered through a tube feeding threaded through the mouth into the stomach, and because taste sensation is usually underdeveloped in the neonate a flavoring agent is not required.

In the neonate, alcohol can alter liver function, cause gastric irritation and effect neurologic depression. So unless it is absolutely necessary it should be omitted from an extemporaneous formulation. Pharmacists must be cautious because some vehicles such as Aromatic Elixir USP contain a significant amount of alcohol, i.e., 21 to 23%, and would not be preferable for use in this patient type. The same problem would hold for liquid formulations for the elderly or any patient who may be receiving another medication that depresses the central nervous system.

Preservatives have been implicated for deleterious adverse effects in preterm infants. Benzyl alcohol should be omitted from neonate formulations because this agent can cause a gasping syndrome characterized by a deterioration of multiple organ systems and eventually death. Propylene glycol has also been implicated to cause problems, i.e., seizures, stupor, in some preterm infants. Thus, formulations for neonates should be purposely kept simple, and not compounded to supply more than just a few days of medicine.

To minimize stability problems of the extemporaneously prepared product, it should be placed in air-tight, light-resistant containers by the pharmacist and subsequently stored in the refrigerator by the patient. Because it is a suspension, the patient should be instructed to shake it well prior to use and on a daily basis watch for any color change or consistency change that might indicate a stability problem with the formulation.

Packaging and Storage of Suspensions

All suspensions should be packaged in wide mouth containers having adequate airspace above the liquid to permit adequate shaking and ease of pouring (Fig. 7–5).

Most suspensions should be stored in tight containers protected from freezing, excessive heat, and light. It is important that suspensions be shaken before each use to ensure a uniform distribution of solid in the vehicle and thereby uniform and proper dosage.

Examples of Oral Suspensions

Examples of official and commercial oral suspensions are presented in Table 7–1. Antacid and antibacterial suspensions are briefly discussed below as examples of this dosage form.

Antacid Oral Suspensions

Antacids are intended to counteract the effects of gastric hyperacidity and as such are employed by persons, as peptic ulcer patients, who must reduce the level of acidity in the stomach. They are also widely employed and sold over-the-counter to patients suffering from conditions popularly referred to as "acid indigestion," "heartburn," and "sour stomach." Many patients belch or otherwise reflux acid from the stomach to the esophagus and take antacids to counter the acid brought to the esophagus and throat.

Most antacid preparations are composed of water-insoluble materials that act within the confines of the gastrointestinal tract to counteract the acid and/or soothe the irritated or inflamed linings of the gastrointestinal tract. There are a few water-soluble agents employed, as sodium bicarbonate, but for the most part, water-insoluble salts of aluminum, calcium, and magnesium are employed, as aluminum hydroxide, aluminum phosphate, dihydroxyaluminum aminoacetate, calcium carbonate, calcium phosphate, magaldrate, magnesium carbonate, magnesium oxide and magnesium hydroxide. The ability of each of these to neutralize gastric acid varies with the chemical agent. For instance, sodium bicarbonate, calcium carbonate, and magnesium hydroxide neutralize acid effectively, whereas magnesium trisilicate and aluminum hydroxide do so less effectively and much more slowly. In selecting an antacid, it is also important to consider the possible adverse effects of each agent in relation to the individual patient being treated. Each agent has its own peculiar potential for adverse effects. For instance, sodium bicarbonate possesses the capability for sodium overload and systemic alkalosis which is of potential hazard to patients on sodium-restricted diets. Magnesium preparations may lead to diarrhea and are dangerous to patients with diminished renal function due to the patients' inability to excrete all of the magnesium which may be absorbed (the gastric acid converts insoluble magnesium hydroxide to magnesium chloride which is water-soluble and is partially absorbed). Calcium carbonate carries the potential for inducing hypercalcemia and stimulation of gastric secretion and acid production, the latter effect known as "acid rebound." Excessive use of aluminum hydroxide may lead to constipation and phosphate depletion with consequent muscle weakness, bone resorption, and hypercalciuria.

The use to which an antacid is to be put is a major consideration in its selection. For instance, in the occasional treatment of heartburn, or other infrequent episodes of gastric distress, a single dose of sodium bicarbonate or a magnesium hydroxide preparation may be desired, but for the treatment of acute peptic ulcer or duodenal ulcer in which the therapeutic regimen includes the frequent administration of antacids, sodium bicarbonate would provide too great an amount of sodium and the magnesium hydroxide would induce diarrhea. Thus, in the treatment of ulcerative conditions, a combination of magnesium hydroxide and aluminum hydroxide is frequently used because the latter agent possesses some constipating effects which counter the diarrhea effects of the magnesium hydroxide.

In instances in which frequent dosage administration is required, and in cases in which gastroesophageal reflux is being treated, liquid antacids generally are preferred over tablet forms. For one thing, the liquid suspensions assert more immediate action—they do not require the time needed for tablets to disintegrate. It is important that an antacid preparation have a reasonably fast onset of action because its presence in the stomach may not last long due to gastric emptying into the intestines. It has been shown by endoscopic studies that on a fasting stomach very little antacid remains in the stomach 1 hour following administration. It is for this reason that the FDA has set the requirement that antacid tablets that are not intended to be chewed upon administration must disintegrate within 10 minutes in simulated gastric conditions. Frequent food snacks generally prolong the time an antacid remains in the stomach and can prolong its action.

Because many antacid materials, especially aluminum and calcium-containing products, interfere with the absorption of other drugs, especially the tetracycline group of antibiotics, pharmacists must caution their patients against taking such drugs concomitantly.

In addition to the suspension forms of antacids, a number of liquid antacid preparations of the magma and gel type are official and commercially available and will be mentioned later in this chapter. All of these liquid forms are usually pleasantly flavored (generally with peppermint) to enhance their palatability and patient appeal. Because liquid antacid preparations characteristically contain a large amount of solid material, they must be shaken vigorously to redistribute the antacid prior to administration. Also, a large dose of antacids is frequently required. Thus, many patients would prefer to swallow one or two tablespoonfuls of a liquid antacid preparation than to swallow whole or chew the corresponding number of tablets (commonly 3 to 6) for the equivalent dose of drug.

Antibacterial Oral Suspensions

The antibacterial oral suspensions include preparations of antibiotic substances (e.g., chloramphenicol palmitate, erythromycin derivatives, and tetracycline and its derivatives), sulfonamides (e.g., sulfamethoxazole, sulfisoxazole acetyl), other chemotherapeutic agents (e.g., methenamine mandelate and nitrofurantoin), or combinations of these (e.g., sulfamethoxazole-trimethoprim).

Many antibiotic materials are unstable when maintained in solution for an appreciable length of time and therefore, from a stability standpoint, insoluble forms of the drug substances in aqueous suspension or as dry powders for reconstitution (discussed next) are attractive to pharmaceutical manufacturers. The antibiotic oral suspensions, including those prepared by reconstitution, provide a convenient way to administer dosages to infants and children as well as to adult patients who may prefer liquid preparations to solid dosage forms. Many of the oral suspensions that are intended primarily for infants are packaged with a calibrated dropper to assist in the delivery of the prescribed dose. Examples of some commercial pediatric antibiotic oral suspensions are pictured in Figure 7–4, and examples of calibrated droppers in Figure 7–6.

The dispersing phase of antibiotic suspensions is aqueous, and usually colored, sweetened and flavored to render the liquid more appealing and palatable. As noted previously, the palmitate form of chloramphenicol was selected for the suspension dosage form not only because of its water-insolubility, but also because of its quality of being flavorless, thereby eliminating the formulating problem of trying to mask the otherwise bitter taste of the chloramphenicol base.

Dry Powders for Oral Suspension

A number of official and commercial preparations consist of dry powder mixtures or granules, which are intended to be suspended in water or some other vehicle prior to oral administration. As indicated previously, these official preparations have "for Oral Suspension" in their official title to distinguish them from already prepared suspensions.

The majority of drugs prepared as a dry mix for oral suspension are antibiotics. The dry products are prepared commercially to contain the antibiotic drug, colorants (FD&C dyes), flavorants, sweeteners (as sucrose or sodium saccharin), stabilizing agents (as citric acid, sodium citrate), suspending agents (as guar gum, xanthan gum, methylcellulose), and preserving agents (as methylparaben, sodium benzoate) that may be needed to enhance the stability of either the dry powder or granule mixture or the ultimate liquid suspension. When called upon to "reconstitute" and dispense one of these products, the pharmacist loosens the powder at the bottom of the container by lightly tapping it against a hard surface, and then adds the label-designated amount of purified water, usually in portions, and shakes until all of the dry powder has been suspended (Fig. 7–2). It is important for the pharmacist to add precisely the prescribed amount of purified water to the dry mixture if the proper drug concentration per dosage unit is to be achieved. Also, the use of purified water rather than tap water is needed to avoid the addition of possible offending impurities which could adversely affect the stability of the resulting preparation. Generally, manufacturers provide the dry powder or granule mixture in a slightly oversized container to permit the adequate shaking of the contents after the entire amount of purified water has been added. Pharmacists must realize that an oversized bottle is provided with each of these products and they must carefully measure out the required amount of purified water. They should not "eyeball" the amount of water to be added or mistakenly fill up the bottle with purified water. Among the official antibiotic drugs for oral suspension are the following:

Fig. 7–6. *Examples of calibrated droppers utilized in the administration of pediatric medications.*

Amoxicillin for Oral Suspension, USP
[Amoxil for Oral Suspension (Beecham)]
Ampicillin for Oral Suspension, USP
[Omnipen for Oral Suspension (Wyeth)]
Bacampicillin for Oral Suspension, USP
[Spectrobid for Oral Suspension (Roerig)]
Cefaclor for Oral Suspension, USP
[Ceclor for Oral Suspension (Lilly)]
Cefadroxil for Oral Suspension, USP
[Ultracef (Bristol)]
Cephadrine for Oral Suspension, USP
[Anspor for Oral Suspension (Smith, Kline
& French)]
Cephalexin for Oral Suspension, USP
[Keflex for Oral Suspension (Dista)]
Cyclacillin for Oral Suspension, USP
[Cyclapen-W for Oral Suspension (Wyeth)]
Dicloxacillin Sodium for Oral Suspension,
USP
[Dynapen for Oral Suspension (Bristol)]
Doxycycline for Oral Suspension, USP
[Vibramycin Monohydrate for Oral Sus-
pension (Pfizer)]
Erythromycin Ethylsuccinate for Oral Sus-
pension, USP
[E.E.S. Granules for Oral Suspension (Ab-
bott)]
Hetacillin for Oral Suspension, USP
[Versapen for Oral Suspension (Bristol)]
Penicillin V for Oral Suspension, USP
[V-Cillin for Oral Suspension (Lilly)]

There are also several official combinations of antibiotics for oral suspension combined with other drugs. For example, the combination of erythromycin ethyl succinate and acetylsulfisoxazole granules for oral suspension is indicated for the treatment of acute middle ear infection caused by susceptible strains of *Hemophilus influenzae*. Probenecid is combined with ampicillin for reconstitution and ultimate use for the treatment of uncomplicated infections (urethral, endocervical or rectal) caused by *Neisseria gonorrhoeae* in adults.

Among the official drugs other than antibiotics prepared as dry powder mixtures for reconstitution to oral suspension are the following: ipodate calcium [Oragrafin Calcium (Squibb)], a diagnostic aid used in cholecystography; cholestyramine [Questran (Bristol)], a drug used in the management of high cholesterol levels; and barium sulfate [Barosperse (Mallinckrodt)], used orally or rectally as a ra-diopaque contrast medium to visualize the gastrointestinal tract as an aid to diagnosis.

The most frequently used of these agents is barium sulfate. Barium sulfate was introduced into medicine about 1910 as a contrast medium in the roentgen-ray examination of the gastrointestinal tract. It is practically insoluble in water and thus its administration, even in the large doses required, is safe because it is not absorbed from the gastrointestinal tract. The pharmacist must be careful not to confuse "barium sulfate," with other forms of barium as the *sulfide* and *sulfite* which are soluble salts and *are* poisonous. Barium sulfate is a fine, non-gritty, white, odorless and tasteless powder. When prepared into a suspension and administered orally, it is used to diagnose conditions of the hypopharynx, esophagus, stomach, small intestine and colon. The barium sulfate renders the gastrointestinal tract opaque to the x ray so that it may be photographed, revealing any abnormality in the anatomic features of the tract. When administered rectally, the barium sulfate allows visualization of the features of the rectum and colon.

Commercially, barium sulfate for diagnostic use is available as a bulk powder containing the required suspending agents for effective reconstitution to an oral suspension or enema prior to administration. Enema units, which contain prepared suspension in a ready-to-use and disposable bag, are also available [Barosperse Disposable Barium Enema Unit (Mallinckrodt)].

Emulsions

An emulsion is a dispersion in which the dispersed phase is composed of small globules of a liquid distributed throughout a vehicle in which it is immiscible (Fig. 7–7). In emulsion terminology, the dispersed phase is referred to as the *internal phase*, and the dispersion medium as the *external* or *continuous phase*. Emulsions having an oleaginous internal phase and an aqueous external phase are referred to as *oil-in-water* emulsions, and are commonly designated as "o/w" emulsions. Conversely, emulsions having an aqueous internal phase and an oleaginous external phase are termed *water-in-oil* emulsions and are referred to as "w/o" emulsions. Because the external phase of an emulsion is continuous, an oil-in-water emulsion may be diluted or extended with water or an aqueous preparation, and a water-in-oil emulsion with an oleaginous or oil-miscible liquid.

Fig. 7–7. *Mineral oil in water emulsion. The largest oil globule in the photograph measures approximately 0.04 mm. (Courtesy of James C. Price, Ph.D., College of Pharmacy, The University of Georgia.)*

Generally, to prepare a stable emulsion, a third phase is necessary, that being an *emulsifying agent*. Depending upon their constituents, the viscosity of emulsions can vary greatly, and pharmaceutical emulsions may be prepared as liquids or semisolids. Based on the constituents and the intended application, liquid emulsions may be employed orally, topically, or parenterally; semisolid emulsions, topically. Many pharmaceutical preparations that may actually be emulsions may not be classified as such because they seem to fit some other pharmaceutical category more appropriately. For instance, certain lotions, liniments, creams, ointments, and commercial vitamin drops may be emulsions but may be referred to in the terms indicated and will be discussed in this book under these various designations.

Purpose of Emulsions and of Emulsification

Pharmaceutically, the process of emulsification enables the pharmacist to prepare relatively stable and homogeneous mixtures of two immiscible liquids. It permits the administration of a liquid drug in the form of minute globules rather than in bulk. For orally administered emulsions, the oil-in-water type of emulsion permits the palatable administration of an otherwise distasteful oil by dispersing it in a sweetened, flavored aqueous vehicle in which it may be carried past the taste buds and into the stomach. The reduced particle size of the oil globules may render the oil more digestible and more readily absorbed, or if that is not the intent, more effective in its task, as for example the increased efficacy of mineral oil as a cathartic when in the emulsified form.

Emulsions to be applied externally to the skin may be prepared as o/w or w/o emulsions, depending upon such factors as the nature of the therapeutic agents to be incorporated into the emulsions, the desirability for an emollient or tissue softening effect of the preparation, and the condition of the skin surface. Medicinal agents that are irritating to the skin generally are less irritating if present in the internal phase of an emulsified topical preparation than in the external phase from which direct contact with the skin is more prevalent. Naturally, the miscibility or the solubility in oil and in water of a medicinal agent to be used in an emulsified preparation would dictate to a great extent the vehicle in which it must be present, and its nature would in turn suggest the phase of the emulsion that the resulting solution should become. On the unbroken skin, a water-in-oil emulsion can usually be applied more evenly because the skin is covered with a thin film of sebum, and this surface is more readily wetted by oil than by water. A water-in-oil emulsion is also more softening to the skin, because it resists drying out and is resistant to removal by contact with water. On the other hand, if it is desirable to have a preparation that is more easily removed from the skin with water, an oil-in-water emulsion would be preferred. As for absorption, absorption through the skin (percutaneous absorption) may be enhanced by the diminished particle size of the internal phase. Other aspects of topical preparations will be discussed in Chapter 9.

Theories of Emulsification

Many theories have been advanced in an attempt to explain how emulsifying agents act in promoting emulsification and in maintaining the stability of the resulting emulsion. Although certain of these theories apply rather specifically to certain types of emulsifying agents and to certain conditions (as the pH of the phases of the system and the nature and relative proportions of the internal and external phases), they may be viewed in a general way to describe the possible manner in which emulsions may be produced and stabilized. Among the most prevalent theories are the *surface-tension theory*, the *oriented-wedge theory*, and the *plastic* or *interfacial film theory*.

All liquids have a tendency to assume a shape having the least amount of surface area exposed. For a drop of a liquid, that shape is spherical. In a spherical drop of liquid there are internal forces that tend to promote the association of the molecules of the substance to resist the distortion of the drop into a less spherical form. If two or more drops of the same liquid come into contact with one another, the tendency is for them to join or to *coalesce*, making one larger drop having a lesser surface area than the total surface area of the individual drops. This tendency of liquids may be measured quantitatively, and when the surrounding of the liquid is air, it is referred to as the liquid's *surface tension. When the liquid is in contact with a second liquid in which it is insoluble and immiscible, the force causing each liquid to resist breaking up into smaller particles is called interfacial tension.* Substances that can promote the lowering of this resistance to breakup can encourage a liquid to be reduced to smaller drops or particles. These tension-lowering substances are referred to as *surface-active* (surfactants) or *wetting agents.* According to the *surface-tension theory* of emulsification, the use of these substances as emulsifiers and stabilizers results in the lowering of the interfacial tension of the two immiscible liquids, reducing the repellent force between the liquids and diminishing each liquid's attraction for its own molecules. Thus the surface-active agents facilitate the breaking up of large globules into smaller ones, which then have a lesser than usual tendency to reunite or coalesce.

The *oriented-wedge* theory assumes monomolecular layers of emulsifying agent curved around a droplet of the internal phase of the emulsion. The theory is based on the presumption that certain emulsifying agents orient themselves about and within a liquid in a manner reflective of their solubility in that particular liquid. In a system containing two immiscible liquids, presumably the emulsifying agent would be preferentially soluble in one of the phases and would be embedded more deeply and tenaciously into that phase than the other. Since many molecules of substances upon which this theory is based (for example, soaps) have a hydrophilic or water-loving portion and a hydrophobic or water-hating portion (but usually lipophilic or oil-loving), the molecules will position or orient themselves into each phase. Depending upon the shape and size of the molecules, their solubility characteristics, and thus their orientation, the wedge-shape arrangement envisioned for the molecules will cause the surrounding of either oil globules or water globules. Generally an emulsifying agent having a greater hydrophilic character than hydrophobic character will promote an oil-in-water emulsion, and a water-in-oil emulsion results through the use of an emulsifying agent that is more hydrophobic than hydrophilic. Putting it another way, the phase in which the emulsifying agent is more soluble will generally become the continuous or external phase of the emulsion. Although this theory may not represent a totally accurate depiction of the molecular arrangement of the emulsifier molecules, the concept that water-soluble emulsifiers generally do form oil-in-water emulsions is important and is generally found in practice.

The *plastic-* or *interfacial-film theory* places the emulsifying agent at the interface between the oil and water, surrounding the droplets of the internal phase as a thin layer of film adsorbed on the surface of the drops. The film prevents the contact and coalescing of the dispersed phase; the tougher and more pliable the film, the greater the stability of the emulsion. Naturally, enough of the film-forming material must be available to coat the entire surface of each drop of internal phase. Here again, the formation of an oil-in-water or a water-in-oil emulsion is dependent upon the degree of solubility of the agent in the two phases, with water-soluble agents encouraging oil-in-water emulsions and oil-soluble emulsifiers the reverse.

In actuality, it is unlikely that a single theory of emulsification may be used to explain the means by which the many and varied emulsifiers promote emulsion formation and stability. It is more than likely that even within a given emulsion system, more than one of the aforementioned theories of emulsification is applicable and plays a part. For instance, lowering of the interfacial tension is important in the initial formation of an emulsion, but the formation of a protective wedge of molecules or film of emulsifier is important for continued emulsion stability. No doubt certain emulsifiers are capable of both tasks.

Preparation of Emulsions

Emulsifying Agents

The initial step in preparation of an emulsion is the selection of the emulsifier. To be useful in a pharmaceutical preparation, the emulsifying agent must possess certain qualities. For one thing, it must be compatible with the other formulative ingredients and must not interfere with the stability or efficacy of the therapeutic agent. It should be stable and not deteriorate in the preparation. The emulsifier should be nontoxic with respect to its intended use and the amount to be consumed by the patient. Also, it should possess little odor, taste, or color. Of prime importance is the capability of the emulsifying agent to promote emulsification and to maintain the stability of the emulsion for the intended shelf life of the product.

Various types of materials have been used in pharmacy as emulsifying agents, with hundreds, if not thousands, of individual agents tested for their emulsification capabilities. Although no attempt will be made here to try to discuss the merits of each of these agents in pharmaceutical emulsion, it would be well to point out the types of materials that are commonly used and their general application. Among the emulsifiers and stabilizers for pharmaceutical systems are the following:

1. Carbohydrate materials such as the naturally occurring agents acacia, tragacanth, agar, chondrus, and pectin. These materials form hydrophilic colloids when added to water and generally produce o/w emulsions. Acacia is perhaps the most frequently used emulsifier in the preparation of extemporaneous emulsions by the community pharmacist. Tragacanth and agar are commonly employed as thickening agents in acacia-emulsified products.
2. Protein substances such as gelatin, egg yolk, and casein. These substances produce o/w emulsions. The disadvantage of gelatin as an emulsifier is that the emulsions prepared from it frequently are too fluid and become more fluid upon standing.
3. High molecular weight alcohols such as stearyl alcohol, cetyl alcohol, and glyceryl monostearate. These are employed primarily as thickening agents and stabilizers for o/w emulsions of certain lotions and ointments used externally. Cholesterol and cholesterol derivatives may also be employed in externally used emulsions and promote w/o emulsions.
4. Wetting agents, which may be anionic, cationic, or nonionic. These agents contain both hydrophilic and lipophilic groups, with the lipophilic portion of the molecule generally accounting for the surface-activity of the molecule. In anionic agents, this lipophilic portion is negatively charged, but in the cationic agent it is positively charged. Owing to their opposing ionic charges, anionic and cationic agents tend to neutralize each other if present in the same system and are thus considered incompatible with one another. Nonionic emulsifiers show no inclination to ionize. Depending upon their individual nature, certain of the members of these groups form o/w emulsions and others w/o emulsions. Anionic emulsifiers include various monovalent, polyvalent, and organic soaps such as triethanolamine oleate and sulfonates such as sodium lauryl sulfate. Benzalkonium chloride, known primarily for its bactericidal properties, may be employed as a cationic-type of emulsifier. Agents of the nonionic type include the sorbitan esters and the polyoxyethylene derivatives, some of which appear in Table 7–2.

   The ionic nature of a surfactant is of prime consideration in the selection of a surfactant to utilize in forming an emulsion. Nonionic surfactants are effective over pH range 3 to 10; cationic surfactants are effective over pH range 3 to 7; and, anionic surfactants require a pH of greater than 8.[6]
5. Finely divided solids such as colloidal clays including bentonite, magnesium hydroxide, and aluminum hydroxide. These generally form o/w emulsions when the insoluble material is added to the aqueous phase if there is a greater volume of the aqueous phase than of the oleaginous phase. However, if the powdered solid is added to the oil and the oleaginous phase volume predominates, a substance like bentonite is capable of forming w/o emulsion.

The relative volume of internal and external phases of an emulsion is important, regardless of the type of emulsifier used. As the internal concentration of an emulsion is increased, there

Table. 7–2.   Examples of HLB Values for Selected Emulsifiers

Agent	HLB
Ethylene glycol distearate	1.5
Sorbitan tristearate (Span 65*)	2.1
Propylene glycol monostearate	3.4
Triton X-15†	3.6
Sorbitan monooleate (Span 80*)	4.3
Sorbitan monostearate (Span 60*)	4.7
Diethylene glycol monolaurate	6.1
Sorbitan monopalmitate (Span 40*)	6.7
Sucrose dioleate	7.1
Acacia	8.0
Amercol L-101‡	8.0
Polyoxyethylene lauryl ether (Brij 30*)	9.7
Gelatin	9.8
Triton X-45†	10.4
Methylcellulose	10.5
Polyoxyethylene monostearate (Myrj 45*)	11.1
Triethanolamine oleate	12.0
Tragacanth	13.2
Triton X-100†	13.5
Polyoxyethylene sorbitan monostearate (Tween 60*)	14.9
Polyoxyethylene sorbitan monooleate (Tween 80*)	15.0
Polyoxyethylene sorbitan monolaurate (Tween 20*)	16.7
Pluronic F 68§	17.0
Sodium oleate	18.0
Potassium oleate	20.0
Sodium lauryl sulfate	40.0

*ICI Americas, Inc., Wilmington, DE
†Rohm and Haas, Philadelphia, PA
‡Amerchol Corporation, Edison, NJ
§BASF-Wyandotte Chemical Corporation, Parsippany, NJ

is an increase in the viscosity of the emulsion to a certain point, after which the viscosity decreases sharply. At this point the emulsion has undergone *inversion;* that is, it has changed from an o/w emulsion to a w/o, or vice versa. In practice, emulsions may be prepared without inversion with as much as about 75% of the volume of the product being internal phase.

The HLB System

Generally, each emulsifying agent has a hydrophilic portion and a lipophilic portion with one or the other being more or less predominant and influencing in the manner already described the type of emulsion. A method has been devised[7] whereby emulsifying or surface-active agents may be categorized on the basis of their chemical make-up as to their hydro-

Table 7–3.   Activity and HLB Value of Surfactants

Activity	Assigned HLB
Antifoaming	1 to 3
Emulsifiers (w/o)	3 to 6
Wetting agents	7 to 9
Emulsifiers (o/w)	8 to 18
Solubilizers	15 to 20
Detergents	13 to 15

phile-lipophile balance or "HLB." By this method, each agent is assigned an HLB value or number which is indicative of the substance's polarity. Although the numbers have been assigned up to about 40, the usual range is between 1 and 20. Materials that are highly polar or hydrophilic have been assigned higher numbers than materials that are less polar and more lipophilic. Generally, those surface-active agents having an assigned HLB value of from 3 to 6 are greatly lipophilic and produce water-in-oil emulsions, and those agents having HLB values of from about 8 to 18 produce oil-in-water emulsions. Examples of some assigned HLB values for some selected surfactants are shown in Table 7–2. The type of activity to be expected from surfactants of assigned HLB numbers is presented in Table 7–3.

In the HLB system, in addition to assigning values to the emulsifying agents, values are also assigned to oils and oil-like substances. In using the HLB concept in the preparation of an emulsion, one selects emulsifying agents having the same or nearly the same HLB value as the oleaginous phase of the intended emulsion. For example, mineral oil has an assigned HLB value of 4 if a w/o emulsion is desired and a value of 10.5 if an o/w emulsion is to be prepared. To prepare a stable emulsion, the emulsifying agent selected should have an HLB value similar to the one for mineral oil, depending on the type of emulsion desired. When needed, two or more emulsifiers may be combined to achieve the proper HLB value.

Methods of Emulsion Preparation

Emulsions may be prepared by several methods, depending upon the nature of the emulsion components and the equipment available for use. On a small scale, as in the laboratory or pharmacy, emulsions may be prepared using a dry Wedgewood or porcelain mortar and pestle, a mechanical blender or mixer such as a Waring blender or a milk-shake mixer, a hand

Fig. 7–8. *The laboratory preparation of an emulsion, using a hand homogenizer.*

homogenizer (Fig. 7–8), or sometimes a simple prescription bottle. On a large scale, large volume mixing tanks may be used to form the coarse emulsion through the action of a high speed impeller, and the coarse product may be rendered fine by passage through a colloid mill, in which the particles are sheared between the small gap separating a high speed rotor and the stator, or by passage through a large homogenizer, in which the liquid is forced under great pressure through a small valve opening.

In the small-scale extemporaneous preparation of emulsions, three methods may be used. They are the *continental* or *dry gum method*, the *English* or *wet gum method*, and the *bottle* or the *Forbes bottle method*. In the first method, the emulsifying agent (usually acacia) is mixed with the oil before the addition of water. In the second method, the emulsifying agent is added to the water (in which it is soluble) to form a mucilage, and then the oil is slowly incorporated to form the emulsion. The bottle method is reserved for volatile oils or less viscous oils and is a variation of the dry gum method.

CONTINENTAL OR DRY GUM METHOD. The method is also referred to as the "4:2:1" method because for every 4 parts (volumes) of oil, 2 parts of water and 1 part of gum are added in preparing the initial or *primary emulsion*. For instance, if 40 mL of oil are to be emulsified, 20 mL of water and 10 g of gum would be employed, with any additional water or other formulation ingredients being added afterward to the primary emulsion. In this method the acacia or other o/w emulsifier is triturated with the oil in a perfectly dry Wedgewood or porcelain mortar until thoroughly mixed. A mortar with a rough rather than smooth inner surface must be used to ensure proper grinding action and the reduction of the globule size during the preparation of the emulsion. A glass mortar has too smooth a surface to produce the proper size reduction of the internal phase. After the oil and gum have been mixed, the two parts of water are then added all at once, and the mixture is triturated immediately, rapidly, and continuously until the primary emulsion that forms is creamy white and produces a crackling sound to the movement of the pestle. Generally, about 3 minutes of mixing are required to produce such a primary emulsion. Other liquid formulative ingredients that are soluble in or miscible with the external phase may then be added to the primary emulsion with mixing. Solid substances such as preservatives, stabilizers, colorants, and any flavoring material are usually dissolved in a suitable volume of water (assuming water is the external phase) and added as a solution to the primary emulsion. Any substances that might interfere with the stability of the emulsion or the emulsifying agent are added as near last as is practically possible. For instance, since alcohol has a precipitating action on gums such as acacia, alcohol or any solution containing alcohol should not be added directly to the primary emulsion, since the total alcoholic concentration of the mixture would be greater at that point than it would be after other diluents had been previously added. When all necessary agents have been added, the emulsion is transferred to a graduate and made to volume with water previously swirled about in the mortar to remove the last portion of emulsion.

Provided the dispersion of the acacia in the oil is adequate, the dry gum method can almost be guaranteed to produce an acceptable emulsion. Sometimes, however, the amount of acacia needs to be adjusted upward to ensure an emulsion can be produced. For example, volatile oils, liquid petrolatum (mineral oil) and linseed oil usually require a "3:2:1 or 2:2:1" ratio for adequate preparation.

Rather than use a mortar and pestle, the pharmacist can generally prepare an excellent emulsion using the dry gum method and an electric mixer or blender.

ENGLISH OR WET GUM METHOD. By this method, the same proportions of oil, water, and gum are used as in the continental or dry gum method, but the order of mixing is different, and the proportion of ingredients may be varied during the preparation of the primary emulsion

as is deemed necessary by the operator. Generally a mucilage of the gum is prepared by triturating granular acacia with twice its weight of water in a mortar. The oil is then added slowly in portions, and the mixture is triturated to emulsify the oil. Should the mixture become too thick during the process, additional water may be blended into the mixture before another successive portion of oil is added. After all of the oil has been added, the mixture is thoroughly mixed for several minutes to insure uniformity. Then, as with the continental or dry

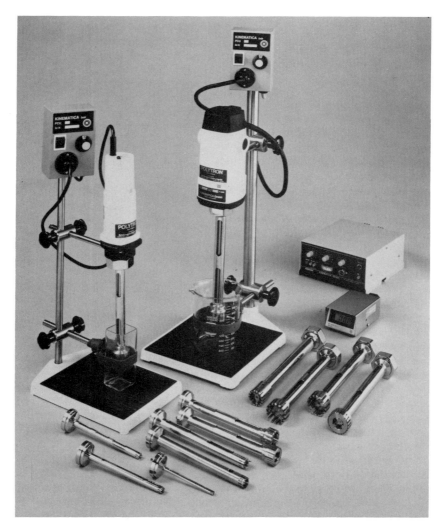

Fig. 7–9. *Brinkmann Homogenizer Models PT 10/35 and PT 45/80 with accessories. The equipment is used for the homogenization, dispersion and emulsification of solids or liquids. Volumes can be processed ranging from 0.5 mL to 25 liters. (Courtesy of Brinkmann Instruments Co., Division of Sybron Corporation.)*

gum method, the other formulative materials are added, and the emulsion is transferred to a graduate and made to volume with water.

BOTTLE OR FORBES BOTTLE METHOD. For the extemporaneous preparation of emulsions from volatile oils or oleaginous substances of low viscosities, the bottle method is useful. In this method, powdered acacia is placed in a dry bottle, two parts of oil are then added, and the mixture is thoroughly shaken in the capped container. A volume of water approximately equal to the oil is then added in portions, the mixture being thoroughly shaken after each addition. When all of the water has been added, the primary emulsion thus formed may be diluted to the proper volume with water or an aqueous solution of other formulative agents.

This method is not suited for viscous oils, because they cannot be thoroughly agitated in the bottle when mixed with the emulsifying agent. In instances in which the intended dispersed phase is a mixture of part fixed oil and part volatile oil, the dry gum method is generally employed for emulsification.

AUXILIARY METHODS. An emulsion prepared by either the wet gum or the dry gum methods can generally be increased in quality by passing it through a hand homogenizer. In this apparatus, the pumping action of the handle forces the emulsion through a very small orifice which reduces the globules of the internal phase to about 5 microns and sometimes less. The hand homogenizer is less efficient in reducing the particle size of very thick emulsions, and it should not be employed for emulsions containing a high proportion of solid matter because of possible damage to the valve.

IN SITU SOAP METHOD. The two types of soaps developed by this method are calcium soaps and soft soaps. Calcium soaps are water-in-oil emulsions which contain certain vegetable oils, e.g., oleic acid, in combination with lime water (syn Calcium Hydroxide Solution USP), and are prepared simply by mixing equal volumes of the oil and lime water. The emulsifying agent in this instance is the calcium salt of the free fatty acid which is formed from the combination of the two entities. In the case of olive oil, the free fatty acid is oleic acid, and the resultant emulsifying agent formed is calcium oleate. A difficulty which sometimes arises when preparing this self-emulsifying product is that the amount of free fatty acids in the oil may be insufficient on a 1:1 basis with calcium hydrox-

ide and typically to make up for this deficiency a little excess of the oil is needed to ensure a nice, homogeneous emulsion results. Otherwise, tiny droplets of water form on the surface of the preparation. Because the oil phase is the external phase, this formulation is ideal where occlusion and skin softening are desired, e.g., itchy, dry skin or sunburned skin. A typical example of this emulsion is calamine liniment:

Calamine
Zinc Oxide   aa   80.0 g
Olive Oil
Calcium Hydroxide Sol'n aa qs ad 1000.0 mL

Microemulsions

Microemulsions are thermodynamically stable, optically transparent, isotropic mixtures of a biphasic oil-water system stabilized with surfactants. The diameter of droplets in a *micro*emulsion may be in the range of 100 Å (10 millimicrons) to 1000 Å whereas in a *macro*emulsion the droplets may be 5000 Å in diameter. Both o/w and w/o microemulsions may be formed spontaneously by agitating the oil and water phases with carefully selected surfactants. The type of emulsion produced depends upon the properties of the oil and surfactants utilized.

Hydrophilic surfactants may be used to produce "transparent" o/w emulsions of many oils, including flavor oils and vitamin oils such as A, D, and E. Surfactants in the HLB range of 15 to 18 have been used most extensively in the preparation of such emulsions. These emulsions are dispersions of oil, not true solutions; however, because of the appearance of the product, the surfactant is commonly said to "solubilize" the oil. Surfactants commonly used in the preparation of such oral liquid formulations are polysorbate 60 and polysorbate 80.

A recent article reviewed the use of microemulsions in drug delivery.[6] Among the advantages cited were more rapid and efficient absorption of drugs administered orally through microemulsions than through solid dosage forms; enhanced transdermal drug delivery through increased drug diffusion into the skin; and the unique potential application of microemulsions in the development of artificial red blood cells and in the targeting of cytotoxic drugs to cancer cells.

Stability of Emulsions

Generally speaking, an emulsion is considered to be physically unstable if: (a) the internal or dispersed phase upon standing tends to form aggregates of globules, (b) large globules or aggregates of globules rise to the top or fall to the bottom of the emulsion to form a concentrated layer of the internal phase, and (c) if all or part of the liquid of the internal phase becomes "unemulsified" and forms a distinct layer on the top or bottom of the emulsion as a result of the coalescing of the globules of the internal phase. In addition, an emulsion may be adversely affected by microbial contamination and growth and by other chemical and physical alterations.

AGGREGATION AND COALESCENCE. Aggregates of globules of the internal phase have a greater tendency than do individual particles to rise to the top of the emulsion or fall to the bottom. Such a preparation of the globules is termed the "creaming" of the emulsion, and provided coalescence is absent, it is a reversible process. The term is taken from the dairy industry and is analogous to the creaming or the rising to the top of cream in milk that is allowed to stand. The creamed portion of an emulsion may be redistributed rather homogeneously upon shaking, but if the aggregates are difficult to disassemble or if insufficient shaking is employed before each dose, improper dosage of the internal phase substance may result. Further, the creaming of pharmaceutical emulsion is not esthetically acceptable to the pharmacist nor appealing to the consumer. More importantly, it increases the risk of the coalescing of the globules.

According to the Stokes' equation (p. 227), the rate of separation of the dispersed phase of an emulsion may be related to such factors as the particle size of the dispersed phase, the difference in the density between the phases, and the viscosity of the external phase. It is important to recall that the rate of separation is increased by increased particle size of the internal phase, a larger density difference between the two phases, and a decreased viscosity of the external phase. Therefore, to increase the stability of an emulsion, the globule or particle size should be reduced as fine as is practically possible, the density difference between the internal and external phases should be minimal, and the viscosity of the external phase should be reasonably high. Thickeners such as tragacanth and agar are frequently added to emulsions to increase the viscosity of the external phase. Upward creaming takes place in unstable emulsions of the o/w or w/o type in which the in-

ternal phase has a lesser density than the external phase. Downward creaming takes place in unstable emulsions in which the opposite is true.

Of greater destruction to an emulsion than creaming is the coalescence of the globules of the internal phase and the separation of that phase into a layer. The separation of the internal phase from the emulsion is called the "breaking" of the emulsion, and the emulsion is described as being "cracked" or "broken." This is irreversible, because the protective sheath about the globules of the internal phase no longer exists. Attempts to reestablish the emulsion by agitation of the two separate layers are generally unsuccessful. Additional emulsifying agent and reprocessing through appropriate machinery are usually necessary to reproduce an emulsion.

Generally, care must be taken to protect emulsions against the extremes of cold and heat. Freezing and thawing result in the coarsening of an emulsion and sometimes in its breaking. Excessive heat has the same effect. Because emulsion products may be transported to and used in various geographic locations having varying climates and conditions of extremely high and low temperature, pharmaceutical manufacturers must have predetermined knowledge of their emulsion stability before they may be shipped. For most emulsions, the industry performs tests of evaluation under experimental conditions of 5° C, 40° C, and 50° C to determine the product's stability. Stability at both 5° C and 40° C for 3 months is considered the minimal stability that an emulsion should possess. Shorter exposure periods at 50° C may be used as an alternate test.

Because other environmental conditions such as the presence of light, air, and contaminating microorganisms can adversely affect the stability of an emulsion, appropriate formulative and packaging steps are usually taken to minimize such possible hazards to product stability. For light-sensitive emulsions, light-resistant containers are used. For emulsions susceptible to oxidative decomposition, antioxidants may be included in the formulation and adequate label warning provided to ensure that the container is tightly closed to air after each use. Many molds, yeasts, and bacteria can bring about the decomposition of the emulsifying agent of an emulsion, thereby causing the disruption of the system. In cases in which the emulsifier is not affected by the microbes, the product can be rendered unsightly by their presence and growth and will of course not be efficacious from a pharmaceutical or therapeutic standpoint. Fungistatic preservatives are generally included in the aqueous phase of an o/w emulsion, since fungi (molds and yeasts) are more likely to contaminate emulsions than are bacteria. Combinations of methylparaben and propylparaben are frequently employed to serve this function. Alcohol in the amount of 12 to 15% based on the external phase volume is frequently added to orally used o/w emulsions for preservation.

Examples of Oral Emulsions

Mineral Oil Emulsion

This emulsion, also referred to as liquid petrolatum emulsion, is an oil-in-water emulsion prepared from the following formula:

Mineral Oil......................	500 mL
Acacia (finely powdered).........	125 g
Syrup	100 mL
Vanillin	40 mg
Alcohol	60 mL
Purified Water, a sufficient quantity, to make..............	1000 mL

The emulsion is prepared by the dry gum method (4:2:1), mixing the oil with the acacia and adding 250 mL of purified water all at once to effect the primary emulsion. To this is slowly added with trituration the remainder of the ingredients, with the vanillin dissolved in the alcohol. A substitute flavorant for the vanillin, a substitute preservative for the alcohol, and a substitute emulsifying agent for the acacia and an alternative method of emulsification may be used as desired.

The emulsion is employed as a lubricating cathartic wtih an usual dose of 30 mL. The usual dose of the plain (unemulsified) mineral oil for the same purpose is 15 mL. The emulsion is much more palatable than is the unemulsified oil. Both are best taken at bedtime. There are a number of commercial preparations of emulsified oil, with many containing additional cathartic agents as phenolphthalein, milk of magnesia, agar, and others.

Castor Oil Emulsion

This emulsion is utilized as a laxative, for isolated bouts of constipation, and in preparation of the colon for x-ray and endoscopic examination. The castor oil present in the emulsion works directly on the small intestine to promote bowel movement. This, and other laxatives, should not be used regularly or excessively as they can lead to dependence for bowel movement. Castor oil may cause excessive loss of water and body electrolytes if used excessively which can have a debilitating effect. Laxatives should not be used when nausea, vomiting, or abdominal pain is present since these symptoms may indicate appendicitis, and use of a laxative in this instance could promote rupturing of the appendix.

The amount of castor oil in commercial castor oil emulsions varies from about 35 to 67%. The amount of oil present influences the dose of the emulsion required. Generally, for an emulsion containing about two-thirds oil, the adult dose would be 45 mL, about 3 tablespoonfuls. For children 2 to 6 years of age, 15 mL is usually sufficient and for children less than 2 years of age, 5 mL may be given. Castor oil is best taken on an empty stomach, followed with one full glass of water.

Simethicone Emulsion

Simethicone emulsion is a water-dispersible form of simethicone used as a defoaming agent for the relief of painful symptoms of excess gas in the gastrointestinal tract. Simethicone emulsion works in the stomach and intestines by changing the surface tension of gas bubbles enabling them to coalesce; thus, freeing the gas for easier elimination. The emulsion, in drop form, is useful for the relief of gas in infants due to colic, air swallowing, or lactose intolerance. The commercial product [Mylicon Drops (Stuart)] contains 40 mg of simethicone per 0.6 mL. Simethicone is also present in a number of antacid formulations [e.g., Mylanta (Stuart)] as a therapeutic adjunct to relieve the discomfort of gas.

Gels and Magmas

Gels are defined as semisolid systems consisting of dispersions made up of either small inorganic particles or large organic molecules enclosing and interpenetrated by a liquid. Gels in which the macromolecules are distributed throughout the liquid in such a manner that no apparent boundaries exist between them and the liquid are called *single-phase gels*. In instances in which the gel mass consists of floccules of small distinct particles, the gel is classified as a two-phase system and frequently called a *magma* or a *milk*. Gels and magmas are considered colloidal dispersions since they each contain particles of colloidal dimension.

Colloidal Dispersions

Many of the various types of colloidal dispersions have been given appropriate names. For instance, *sol* is a general term to designate a dispersion of a solid substance in either a liquid, a solid, or a gaseous dispersion medium. However, more often than not it is used to describe the solid-liquid dispersion system. To be more descriptive, a prefix such as *hydro-* for water *(hydrosol)* or *alco-* for alcohol *(alcosol)* may be employed to indicate the dispersion medium. The term *aerosol* has similarly been developed to indicate a dispersion of a solid or a liquid in a gaseous phase.

Although there is no precise point at which the size of a particle in a dispersion can be considered to be "colloidal," there is a generally accepted size range. A substance is said to be colloidal when its particles fall between 1 millimicron (mµ) and about 500 millimicrons or 0.5 micron (µ).[8] Colloidal particles are usually larger than atoms, ions, or molecules and generally consist of aggregates of many molecules, although in certain proteins and organic polymers single, large molecules may be of colloidal dimension and form colloidal dispersions. One difference between colloidal dispersions and true solutions is the larger particle size of the disperse phase of the former type of preparation. Another difference is the optical properties of the two systems. True solutions do not scatter light and therefore appear clear, but colloidal dispersions contain opaque particles that do scatter light and thus appear turbid. This turbidity is easily seen, even with dilute preparations, when the dispersion is observed at right angles to a beam of light passed through the dispersion (Tyndall effect). Although reference is made here to dilute colloidal dispersions, most pharmaceutical preparations contain high concentrations of particles within the colloidal size range, and in these instances there is no difficulty in observing turbidity. In fact, certain preparations may be quite opaque, depending upon the concentration of the disperse phase. Also, the particle size of the disperse phase in

some pharmaceutical preparations may not be uniform, and a preparation may contain particles within and outside of the colloidal range, giving the preparation more of an opaque appearance than if all particles were uniformly colloidal.

Particle size is not the only important criterion for establishing the colloidal state. The nature of the dispersing phase with respect to the disperse phase is also of great importance. The attraction or lack of attraction between the disperse phase and the dispersion medium affects the ease of preparation of a colloidal dispersion as well as the character of the dispersion. Certain terminology has been developed to characterize the various degrees of attraction between the phases of a colloidal dispersion. If the disperse phase interacts appreciably with the dispersion medium, it is referred to as being *lyophilic,* meaning "solvent-loving." If the degree of attraction is small, the colloid is termed *lyophobic,* or "solvent-hating." These terms are more suitably used when reference is made to the specific dispersion medium, for a single substance may be lyophobic with respect to one dispersion medium and lyophilic with respect to another. For instance, starch is lyophilic in water but lyophobic in alcohol. Terms such as *hydrophilic* and *hydrophobic,* which are more descriptive of the nature of the colloidal property, have therefore been developed to refer to the attraction or lack of attraction of the substance specifically to water. Generally speaking, because of the attraction to the solvent of lyophilic substances in contrast to the lack of attraction of lyophobic substances, lyophilic colloidal systems are usually easier to prepare and have the greater stability. A third type of colloidal sol, termed as *association* or *amphiphilic colloid,* is formed by the grouping or association of molecules that exhibit both lyophilic and lyophobic properties.

Lyophilic colloids are generally large organic molecules capable of being solvated or associated with the molecules of the dispersing phase. These substances disperse readily upon addition to the dispersion medium to form colloidal dispersions. As more molecules of the substance are added to the sol, the viscosity is characteristically increased and when the concentration of molecules is sufficiently high, the liquid sol may become a semisolid or solid dispersion, termed a *gel.* Gels owe their rigidity to an intertwining network of the disperse phase which entraps and holds the dispersion medium. A change in the temperature can cause certain gels to resume the sol or liquid state. Also, some gels may become fluid after agitation only to resume their solid or semisolid state after remaining undisturbed for a period of time, a phenomenon known as *thixotropy*.[9]

Lyophobic colloids are generally composed of inorganic particles. When these are added to the dispersing phase, there is little if any interaction between the two phases. Unlike lyophilic colloids, lyophobic materials do not spontaneously disperse but must be encouraged to do so by special, individualized procedures. Their addition to the dispersion medium does not greatly affect the viscosity of the vehicle. Amphiphilic colloids form dispersions in both aqueous and nonaqueous media. Depending upon their individual character and the nature of the dispersion medium, they may or may not become greatly solvated. However, they generally cause an increase in the viscosity of the dispersion medium with an increase in concentration.

For the most part, the colloidal sols and gels used in pharmacy are aqueous preparations. The various preparations composed of colloidal dispersions are prepared, not according to any general method but according to the means best suited to the individual preparation. Some substances such as acacia are termed *natural colloids* because they are self-dispersing upon addition to the dispersing medium. Other materials that require special means for prompt dispersion are termed *artificial colloids*. They may require fine pulverization of coarse particles to colloidal size by a colloid mill or a micropulverizer, or colloidal size particles may be formed by chemical reaction under highly controlled conditions.

Preparation of Magmas and Gels

Many magmas and gels are prepared by freshly precipitating the disperse phase in order to achieve a fine degree of subdivision of the particles and a gelatinous character to those particles. The desired gelatinous precipitate results when solutions of inorganic agents react to form an insoluble chemical having a high attraction for water. As the microcrystalline particles of the precipitate develop, they strongly attract water to yield gelatinous particles, which combine to form the desired gelatinous precipitate. Other magmas and gels may be prepared by the

direct hydration in water of the inorganic chemical, the hydrated form constituting the disperse phase of the dispersion. In addition to the water vehicle, other agents as propylene glycol, propylgallate and hydroxypropylcellulose may be used to enhance gel formation.

Because of the high degree of attraction between the disperse phase and the aqueous medium in both magmas and gels, these preparations remain fairly uniform on standing with little settling of the disperse phase. However, on long standing a supernatant layer of the dispersion medium develops, but the uniformity of the preparation is easily reestablished by moderate shaking. To ensure uniform dosage, magmas and gels should be shaken before use, and a statement to that effect must be included on the label of such preparations. The medicinal magmas and gels are used orally for the value of the disperse phase.

Examples of Magmas and Gels

One official magma, Bentonite Magma, NF, is used as a suspending agent and finds application in the extemporaneous compounding of prescriptions calling for the suspension of medicinal agents. Sodium Fluoride and Phosphoric Acid Gel, USP, is applied topically to the teeth as a dental care prophylactic. Other official gels applied topically include Fluocinonide Gel, USP, an antiinflammatory corticosteroid, and Tretinoin Gel, USP, an irritant which stimulates epidermal cell turnover and causes peeling and is effective in the treatment of acne. Other official magmas and gels are employed as antacids, namely: Aluminum Phosphate Gel, USP, Aluminum Hydroxide Gel, USP; Dihydroxyaluminum Aminoacetate Magma, USP, and Milk of Magnesia (Magnesia Magma), USP. Some of these preparations are discussed briefly below.

Bentonite Magma, NF

Bentonite magma is a preparation of 5% bentonite, a native, colloidal hydrated aluminum silicate, in purified water. It may be prepared mechanically in a blender with the bentonite added directly to the purified water while the machine is running, or it may be prepared by sprinkling the bentonite, in portions, upon hot purified water, allowing each portion to become thoroughly wetted without stirring before another portion is added. By the latter method, the mixture must be allowed to stand for 24 hours before it may be stirred. The standing period ensures the complete hydration and swelling of the bentonite. Bentonite, which is insoluble in water, swells to approximately twelve times its volume upon addition to water. The NF monograph for bentonite contains a test for "swelling power," in which 2 g of a bentonite sample is added in portions to 100 mL of water contained in a 100-mL glass-stoppered cylinder. At the end of a 2-hour period, the mass at the bottom of the cylinder is required to occupy an apparent volume of not less than 24 mL. Other required tests are for gel formation, fineness of powder, and pH, the latter being between 9.5 and 10.5. After bentonite magma has been allowed to stand undisturbed for some period of time, it sets to a gel. Upon agitation the sol form returns. The process may be repeated indefinitely. As mentioned earlier, this phenomenon is termed *thixotropy*, and bentonite magma is termed a *thixotropic gel*. The thixotropy occurs only when the bentonite concentration is somewhat above 4%.

Bentonite magma is employed as a suspending agent. Its alkaline pH must be considered, because this might be undesirable for certain drugs. Further, because the suspending capacity of the magma is drastically reduced if the pH is lowered to about pH 7, another suspending agent should be selected for drugs requiring a less alkaline medium rather than make bentonite magma more acidic.

Aluminum Hydroxide Gel, USP

Aluminum Hydroxide Gel, USP, is an aqueous suspension of a gelatinous precipitate composed of insoluble aluminum hydroxide and the hydrated aluminum oxide, equivalent to about 4% of aluminum oxide. The disperse phase of the gel is generally prepared by chemical reaction, using various reactants. Usually the aluminum source of the reaction is aluminum chloride or aluminum alum, which yields the insoluble aluminum oxide and aluminum hydroxide precipitate. To the gel, the USP permits the addition of peppermint oil, glycerin, sorbitol, sucrose, saccharin, or other flavorants and sweeteners as well as suitable antimicrobial agents.

This antacid preparation is a white, viscous suspension. It is effective in neutralizing a portion of the gastric hydrochloric acid and by virtue of its gelatinous, viscous, and insoluble character, coats the inflamed and perhaps ulcerated gastric surface and is useful in the treatment of hyperacidity and peptic ulcers. The main disadvantage to its use is its constipating effects. The usual dose is 10 mL, four or more times a day. Ten mL of the analogous commercial product (Amphojel, Wyeth) has the capacity to neutralize about 13 mEq of acid. The preparation should be stored in tight containers, and freezing should be avoided.

Because it possesses a trivalent cation, aluminum hydroxide has the capability to interfere with the bioavailability of tetracycline by chelating with the antibiotic in the gastrointestinal tract. Thus, when these two medicines are indicated for patient use, the doses of each should be staggered to ensure the patient receives the benefit of both drugs. Aluminum hydroxide gel has also been implicated at decreasing the bioavailability of other drugs as well by adsorption onto the gel. This is usually illustrated by a decrease in the area under the concentration time curve (AUC) for the concomitantly administered drug. Suffice to say that the clinical significance of the interaction might not be that great, but observation of the patient to insure the proper therapeutic outcome from the other drug is important. Thus, for example, if aluminum hydroxide gel is suspected of causing incomplete absorption of the second drug, then an upward alteration in the dose of the drug might be necessary provided the aluminum hydroxide gel administration remains the same.

Aluminum Phosphate Gel, USP

Aluminum Phosphate Gel, USP, is an aqueous suspension of between 4 and 5% of aluminum phosphate. It may also contain flavorants, sweeteners, and preservatives as indicated for the aluminum hydroxide gel. Although the latter gel interferes with phosphate absorption from the intestines, aluminum phosphate gel does not and is preferred for use by patients with peptic ulcer who also suffer from chronic diarrhea and other conditions that may lead to potassium deficiency.

The usual dose of the preparation is 15 mL, which is capable of neutralizing about 10 mEq of acid. The commercial counterpart is Phosphaljel (Wyeth).

Milk of Magnesia, USP

Milk of Magnesia, USP, is a preparation containing between 7 and 8.5% of magnesium hydroxide. Although there is no method of preparation indicated in the USP for this preparation, it may be prepared by a reaction between sodium hydroxide and magnesium sulfate (1), diluted solutions being used to ensure a fine, flocculent, gelatinous precipitate of magnesium hydroxide. The precipitate so produced is washed with purified water to remove the sodium sulfate prior to its incorporation with additional purified water to prepare the required volume of product. Commercially, the product is more economically produced by the direct hydration of magnesium oxide (2).

(1) $2NaOH + MgSO_4 \rightarrow Mg(OH)_2 + Na_2SO_4$

(2) $MgO + H_2O \rightarrow Mg(OH)_2$

Irrespective of its method of preparation, milk of magnesia is a white, opaque, viscous preparation from which varying proportions of water separate on standing. For this reason it should be shaken before use. The preparation has a pH of about 10, which may bring about a reaction between the magma and the glass container imparting a bitter taste to the preparation. To minimize such an occurrence, the USP permits the addition of 0.1% citric acid to the preparation. Also, flavoring oils at a concentration not exceeding 0.05% may be added to enhance the palatability of the preparation.

Milk of Magnesia possesses reasonable acid-neutralizing ability and a dose of 5 mL will neutralize about 10 mEq of stomach acid. However, to neutralize more acid a higher dose, e.g., 15 mL is usually necessary, and this may predispose the patient to the development of diarrhea, a common side effect of this drug. Thus, to circumvent the problem of diarrhea from magnesium hydroxide and the constipating effects of aluminum hydroxide, frequently these two drugs are combined in an antacid preparation. The combination results in a more palatable product with optimum buffering of stomach contents between a pH of 4 to 5, and less of a chance for either diarrhea or constipation to occur. If a patient takes the combination, sometimes diarrhea may still occur, and for this reason several recent formulations, e.g., TC Suspension [Rorer], have been formulated with a greater amount of aluminum hydroxide added per dose. When a laxative effect is desired a bedtime dose of 30 to 60 mL of milk of magnesia will suffice very nicely by the next morning.

The preparation is best stored in tight con-tainers preferably at a temperature above freezing and below 35°C. Freezing results in a coarsening of the disperse phase, and temperatures above 35°C decrease the gel structure.

Proper Administration and Use of Peroral Disperse Systems

The variety of dosage forms discussed in this chapter are for oral consumption, and like those liquid dosage forms from the previous chapter, these can be measured in a spoon, i.e., teaspoon, tablespoon, depending upon the desired dosage. With these dosage forms it is very important that the patient understand how much of the product to use. For example, differences in dosage can occur between product category, e.g., OTC antidiarrheal suspensions [tablespoonfuls] *vs* OTC antacid suspensions [teaspoonfuls]. Differences in dosage can also occur within a category, most notably antacid suspensions. Some are recommended in teaspoon doses because of higher concentration whereas others are suggested in tablespoon quantities. It is important, therefore, that the pharmacist ensure that the patient knows how much to use, and then use a calibrated device to make sure the right amount is taken.

Reconstituted products, as mentioned earlier in the chapter typically are suspensions. Several potential problems can emerge if the pharmacist is not careful to counsel the patient about them. Usually the patient or the guardian of the patient receives the product in an oversized bottle that allows for the proper shaking of the product prior to its use. To allay fears that all of the medicine may not be in the bottle, the pharmacist must make the patient or the guardian aware of this, and indicate this feature enhances the shakability before its administration. Further, some patients do not make the connection that the medicine should be administered by mouth. Oral antibiotic suspensions intended to treat a middle ear infection have been mistakenly administered directly into the ear by some patients or guardians. Thus, the pharmacist should review with the patient the proper administration. Lastly, because these are reconstituted with purified water stability problems with the drug usually dictate it be stored in the refrigerator until it is consumed. The patient has to be informed of this. Tiny labels on the container directing one to store the product in the refrigerator are sometimes overlooked by the consumer. Alternatively, not all suspensions need to be stored in the refrigerator but because of prior experience with other liquid suspensions that necessitated refrigeration a patient or guardian may assume this is necessary.

Certain suspensions by virtue of their active ingredients, e.g., aluminum hydroxide gel, cholestyramine, kaolin, have the ability to interfere with the absorption of other drugs that might be concurrently administered. For example, cholestyramine has been shown to interfere with and decrease the bioavailability of such drugs as warfarin, digitoxin and thyroid hormones. The pharmacist should be aware of this and make recommendations to help avoid this drug interaction whenever possible. The typical suggestion would be to stagger the administration of the liquid cholestyramine away from other drug administration by several hours, and in the case of warfarin, giving warfarin at least 6 hours after the cholestyramine reportedly avoids the impaired warfarin bioavailability.[10] However, warfarin is a drug that undergoes enterohepatic recycling in the body, and if cholestyramine were present in the intestine because of earlier administration it could bind it and decrease warfarin's subsequent reabsorption. In this instance, concomitant use of one of the two drugs should be discontinued by the physician. However, if concurrent use is necessary, the pharmacist should monitor the patient more frequently for the possibility of an altered anticoagulant response. This is important because if adjustments in warfarin dosage were made on the basis of cholestyramine interference and then the cholestyramine was discontinued, the warfarin dosage also would have to be decreased accordingly, i.e., based on the patient's prothrombin time.

Selected Reading

Morefield, E.M., Feldkamp, J.R., Peck, G.E., White, J.L., and Hem, S.L.: Preformulation Information for Suspensions. *Int. J. Pharmaceutics*, 34:263–265, 1987.

Omotosho, J.A., Whateley, T.L., Law, T.K., and Florence, A.T.: The Nature of the Oil Phase and the Release of Solutes from Multiple (w/o/w) Emulsions. *J. Pharm. Pharmacol.*, 38:865–870, 1986.

Notes

1. The area of particle technology has come to be known as *micromeritics*.
2. From a therapeutic standpoint, small particle size is perhaps of greater importance in the formulation of parenteral and ophthalmic suspensions than in the preparation of oral suspensions. In the injection of a suspension, drug particles below 10 microns in size are reported to produce considerably less pain and tissue irritation than drug particles of greater dimension. Also, a suspension intended for injection must have a reasonable "syringeability," that is, the ability to flow freely through the bore of the hypodermic needle. Ophthalmic suspensions are similarly less irritating to the tissues when the dispersed phase is finely divided. As mentioned in Chapter 4, drug particle size can have a bearing on the therapeutic efficacy or effectiveness of a drug preparation.
3. Heyd, A. and Dhabhar, D.: Particle Shape Effect on Caking of Coarse Granulated Antacid Suspensions. *Drug & Cosmetic Industry*, 125:42, 1979.
4. *Oral Liquid Pharmaceuticals:* Wilmington, DE, ICI Americas Inc., 1975.
5. Allen, L.V.: Prednisone Oral Suspension. *U.S. Pharmacist*, 14:84, 1989.
6. Bhargava, H.N., Narurkar, A. and Lieb, L.M.: Using Microemulsions for Drug Delivery. *Pharm. Tech.*, 11:46, 1987.
7. Griffin, W.C.: *J. Soc. Cosmetics Chemists*, 1:311, 1949; *ibid*, 5:1, 1954.
8. A micron, μ, is one-thousandth of a millimeter; a millimicron, $m\mu$, is one thousandth of a micron or one-millionth of a millimeter.
9. From the Greek, meaning "to change by touching."
10. Hansten, P.D. and Horn, J.R.: *Drug Interactions.* 6th Ed., Philadelphia, Lea & Febiger, 1989, p. 80.

CONSIDERED IN this chapter are important pharmaceutical dosage forms that have the common characteristic of being prepared to be sterile; that is, free from contaminating microorganisms. Among these sterile dosage forms are the various small- and large-volume injectable preparations, irrigation fluids intended to bathe body wounds or surgical openings, dialysis solutions, biological preparations as vaccines, toxoids, antitoxins, blood replenishment products, and some products of recombinant DNA technology. Sterility in these preparations is of utmost importance because they are placed in direct contact with the internal body fluids or tissues where infection can easily arise. Ophthalmic preparations which are also prepared to be sterile will be discussed separately in Chapter 10.

Injections

Injections are sterile, pyrogen-free preparations intended to be administered parenterally. The term *parenteral* refers to the injectable routes of administration. The term has its derivation from the Greek words *para* and *enteron*, meaning outside of the intestine, and denotes routes of administration other than the oral route. *Pyrogens* are fever-producing organic substances arising from microbial contamination and are responsible for many of the febrile reactions which occur in patients following intravenous injection. Pyrogens and the determination of their presence in parenteral preparations will be discussed later in this chapter. In general, the parenteral routes of administration are undertaken when rapid drug action is desired, as in emergency situations, when the patient is uncooperative, unconscious, or unable to accept or tolerate medication by the oral route, or when the drug itself is ineffective by other routes. With the exception of insulin injections, which are commonly *self*-administered by diabetic patients, most injections are administered by the physician, his assistant, or nurse in the course of medical treatment. Thus injections are employed mostly in the hospital, extended care facility, and clinic and less frequently in the home. An exception would be in *home health care* programs in which health professionals pay scheduled visits to patients in their homes, providing needed treatment, including intravenous medications. These programs enable patients who do not require or are unable to pay for more expensive hospitalization to remain in the familiar surroundings of their homes while receiving appropriate medical care. The pharmacist supplies injectable preparations to the physician and nurse, as required for their use in the institutional setting, clinic, office, or home health care program.

Perhaps the earliest injectable drug to receive official recognition was the hypodermic morphine solution which appeared first in the 1874 addendum to the 1867 British Pharmacopeia, and later, in 1888 in the first edition of the National Formulary of the United States. Today, there are literally hundreds of drugs and drug products available for parenteral administration.

Interesting historical accounts of the origin and development of injection therapy may be found in the references cited.[1,2,3]

Parenteral Routes of Administration

Drugs may be injected into almost any organ or area of the body, including the joints (*intra-articular*), a joint-fluid area (*intrasynovial*), the spinal column (*intraspinal*), into spinal fluid (*intrathecal*), arteries (*intra-arterial*), and in an emergency, even into the heart (*intracardiac*). However, most commonly injections are performed into a vein (*intravenous, I.V.*), into a muscle (*intramuscular, I.M.*), into the skin (*Intradermal, I.D., intracutaneous*), or under the skin (*subcutaneous, S.C., Sub-Q, S.Q., hypodermic, "Hypo."*) (Fig. 8–1).

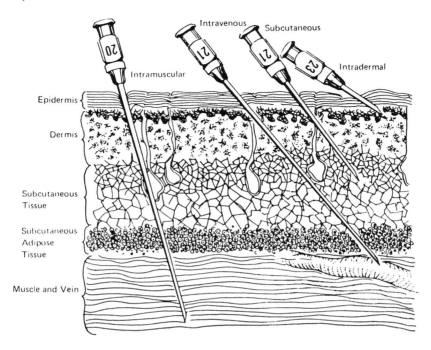

Fig. 8–1. *Routes of parenteral administration. Numbers on needles indicate size or gauge of needle based on outside diameter of needle shaft. (Turco, S. and King, R.E., Sterile Dosage Forms: Their Preparation and Clinical Applications. 3rd Ed., Courtesy of Lea & Febiger, 1987.)*

Intravenous Route

The intravenous injection of drugs had its scientific origin in 1656 in the experiments of Sir Christopher Wren, architect of St. Paul's Cathedral and amateur physiologist. Using a bladder and quill for a syringe and needle, he injected wine, ale, opium, and other substances into the veins of dogs and studied their effects. Intravenous medication was first given to man by Johann Daniel Major of Kiel in 1662, but was abandoned for a period because of the occurrence of thrombosis and embolism in the patients so treated. The invention of the hypodermic syringe toward the middle of the 19th century created a new interest in intravenous techniques and toward the turn of the century, intravenous administration of solutions of sodium chloride and glucose became popular. Today, the intravenous administration of drugs is a routine occurrence in the hospital, although there are still recognized dangers associated with the practice. Thrombus and embolus formation may be induced by intravenous needles and catheters, and the possibility of particulate matter in parenteral solutions poses concern for those involved in the development, administration, and use of intravenous solutions.

Intravenously administered drugs provide rapid action compared to other routes of administration and because drug absorption is not a factor, optimum blood levels may be achieved with the accuracy and immediacy not possible by other routes. In emergency situations, the intravenous administration of a drug may be a life-saving procedure because of the placement of the drug directly into the circulation and the prompt action which ensues. On the negative side, once a drug is administered intravenously, it cannot be retrieved. In the case of an adverse reaction to the drug, for instance, the drug cannot be easily removed from the circulation as it could, for example, by the induction of vomiting following the oral administration of the same drug.

Although most superficial veins are suitable for venipuncture, the veins of the antecubital area (situated in front of the elbow) are usually selected for direct intravenous injection. The veins in this location are large, superficial and easy to see and enter. Most clinicians insert the needle with the bevel facing upward, at the most acute angle possible with the vein, to ensure that the direction of flow of the injectable is that of the flow of the blood. Strict aseptic precautions must be taken at all times to avoid risk of infection. Not only are the injectable solutions sterile, the syringes and needles employed must also be sterilized and the point of entrance must be cleansed to reduce the chance of carrying bacteria from the skin into the blood via the needle.

Both small and large volumes of drug solutions may be administered intravenously. The use of 1000-mL containers of solutions for intravenous infusion is commonplace in the hospital. These solutions containing such agents as nutrients, blood extenders, electrolytes, amino acids, and other therapeutic agents are generally administered through an indwelling needle or catheter by continuous drip. The drip or flow rates may be adjusted by the clinician according to the needs of the patient. Generally, flow rates of 2 to 3 mL per minute are employed. For intravenous infusion, the needle or catheter is generally placed in the prominent veins of the forearm or leg and taped firmly to the patient so that it will not slip from place during infusion. The main hazard of intravenous infusion is the possibility of thrombus formation induced by the touching of the wall of the vein by the catheter or needle. Thrombi are more likely to occur when the infusion solution is of an irritating nature to the biologic tissues. A *thrombus* is a blood clot formed within the blood vessel (or heart) due usually to a slowing of the circulation or to an alteration of the blood or vessel wall. Once such a clot circulates, it becomes an *embolus,* carried by the blood stream until it lodges in a blood vessel, obstructing it, and resulting in a blockage or occlusion referred to as an *embolism.* Such an obstruction may be a critical hazard to the patient, depending upon the site and severity of the obstruction.

Intravenously administered drugs ordinarily must be in aqueous solution; they must mix with the circulating blood and not precipitate from solution. Such an event could lead to thrombus formation and the subsequent blockage of blood passage. An intravenously delivered fat emulsion (INTRALIPID, KabiVitrum) has gained acceptance for use as a source of calories and essential fatty acids for patients requiring parenteral nutrition for extended periods of time (usually for more than 5 days). The product contains up to 20% soybean oil

emulsified with egg yolk phospholipids, in a vehicle of glycerin in water for injection. The emulsion is administered via a peripheral vein or by central venous infusion.[4]

Naturally, the intravenous route is utilized in the administration of blood transfusions and it also serves as the point of exit in the removal of blood from patients for diagnostic work and for obtaining blood from donors.

Intramuscular Route

Intramuscular injections of drugs provide drug effects that are less rapid, but generally of greater duration than those obtained from intravenous administration. Aqueous or oleaginous solutions or suspensions of drug substances may be administered intramuscularly. Depending upon the type of preparation employed, the absorption rates may vary widely. Generally it would be expected that drugs in solution would be more rapidly absorbed than those in suspension and that drugs in aqueous preparations would be more rapidly absorbed than when in oleaginous preparations. The physical type of preparation employed is based on the properties of the drug itself and on the therapeutic goals desired.

Intramuscular injections are performed deep into the skeletal muscles. The point of injection should be as far as possible from major nerves and blood vessels. Injuries to patients from intramuscular injection usually are related to the point at which the needle entered and where the medication was deposited. Such injuries include paralysis resulting from neural damage, abscesses, cysts, embolism, hematoma, sloughing of the skin, and scar formation.

In adults, the upper outer quadrant of the gluteus maximus is the most frequently used site for intramuscular injection. In infants, the gluteal area is small and composed primarily of fat, not muscle. What muscle there is is poorly developed. An injection in this area might be presented dangerously close to the sciatic nerve, especially if the child is resisting the injection and squirming or fighting. Thus, in infants and young children, the deltoid muscles of the upper arm or the midlateral muscles of the thigh are preferred. An injection given in the upper or lower portion of the deltoid would be well away from the radial nerve. The deltoid may also be used in adults, but the pain is more noticeable here than in the gluteal area. If a series of injections are to be given, the injection site is usually varied. To be certain that a blood vessel has not been entered, the clinician may aspirate slightly on the syringe following insertion of the needle to observe if blood enters the syringe. Usually, the volume of medication which may be conveniently administered by the intramuscular route is limited; generally a maximum of 5 mL is administered intramuscularly in the gluteal region and 2 mL in the deltoid of the arm.

The Z-Track Injection technique is useful for intramuscular injections of medications that stain upper tissue, e.g., Imferon, or those that irritate tissue, e.g., Valium, by sealing these medications in the lower muscle. Because of its staining qualities, Imferon, for example, must be injected only into the muscle mass of the upper outer quadrant of the buttock. The skin is displaced laterally prior to injection, then the needle is inserted and syringe aspirated, and the injection performed slowly and smoothly. The needle is then withdrawn and the skin released. This creates a "Z" pattern that blocks infiltration of medication into the subcutaneous tissue. The injection is 2 to 3 inches deep, and a 19- to 20-gauge needle is utilized. To further prevent any staining of upper tissue, usually one needle is used to withdraw the iron dextran from its ampul, and then replaced with another for the purposes of the injection.

Intradermal Route

A number of substances may be effectively injected into the corium, the more vascular layer of the skin just beneath the epidermis. These substances include various agents for diagnostic determinations, desensitization, or immunization. The usual site for intradermal injection is the anterior surface of the forearm. A short ($\frac{3}{8}$ in.) and narrow gauge (23- to 26-gauge) needle is usually employed. The needle is inserted horizontally into the skin with the bevel facing upward. The injection is made when the bevel just disappears into the corium. Usually only about 0.1 mL volumes may be administered in this manner.

Subcutaneous Route

The subcutaneous route may be utilized for the injection of small amounts of medication. The injection of a drug beneath the surface of the skin is usually made in the loose interstitial tissues of the outer surface of the upper arm, the anterior surface of the thigh, and the lower portion of the abdomen. The site of injection is usually rotated when injections are frequently given, e.g., daily insulin injections. Prior to injection, the skin at the injection site should be thoroughly cleansed. The maximum amount of medication that can be comfortably injected subcutaneously is about 1.3 mL and amounts greater than 2 mL will most likely cause painful pressure. Syringes with up to 3 mL capacities and utilizing needles with 24 to 26 gauges are used for subcutaneous injections. These needles will have cannula lengths that vary between $\frac{3}{8}$ inch to 1 inch. Most typically, subcutaneous insulin needles are between 25 to 28 gauge with needle length between $\frac{3}{8}$ to $\frac{5}{8}$ inch. Upon insertion, if blood appears in the syringe a new site should be selected.

Drugs which are irritating or those which are present in thick suspension form may produce induration, sloughing, or abscess formation and may be painful to the patient. Such preparations should be considered not suitable for subcutaneous injection.

Official Types of Injections

According to the USP, injections are separated into five distinct types, generally defined as follows:

1. Medicaments or solutions, or emulsions suitable for injection, bearing titles of the form, "_____ *Injection*." (Ex: Insulin Injection, USP)
2. Dry solids or liquid concentrates containing no buffers, diluents, or other added substances, and which, upon the addition of suitable solvents, yield solutions conforming in all aspects to the requirements for injections, and which are distinguished by titles of the form, "*Sterile* _____" (Ex: Sterile Ampicillin Sodium, USP)
3. Preparations the same as those described in (2) except that they contain one or more buffers, diluents, or other added substances, and which are distinguished by titles of the form, "_____ *for Injection*" (Ex: Methicillin Sodium for Injection, USP)
4. Solids which are suspended in a suitable fluid medium and which are not to be injected intravenously or into the spinal canal, distinguished by titles of the form, "*Sterile* _____*Suspension*." (Ex: Sterile Dexamethasone Acetate Suspension, USP)

5. Dry solids, which, upon the addition of suitable vehicles, yield preparations conforming in all respects to the requirements for Sterile Suspensions, and which are distinguished by titles of the form, *"Sterile _____for Suspension."* (Ex: Sterile Ampicillin for Suspension, USP)

The form into which a given drug is prepared for parenteral use by the manufacturer depends upon the nature of the drug itself, with respect to its physical and chemical characteristics, and also upon certain therapeutic considerations. Generally, if a drug is unstable in solution, it may be prepared as a dry powder intended for reconstitution with the proper solvent at the time of its administration, or it may be prepared as a suspension of the drug particles in a vehicle in which the drug is insoluble. If the drug is unstable in the presence of water, that solvent may be replaced in part or totally by a solvent in which the drug is stable. If the drug is insoluble in water, an injection may be prepared as an aqueous suspension or as a solution of the drug in a suitable nonaqueous solvent, such as a vegetable oil. If an aqueous solution is desired, a water-soluble salt form of the insoluble drug is frequently prepared to satisfy the required solubility characteristics. Aqueous or blood-miscible solutions may be injected directly into the blood stream. Blood-immiscible liquids, e.g., oleaginous injections and suspensions, can interrupt the normal flow of blood within the circulatory system, and their use is generally restricted to other than intravenous administration. The onset and duration of action of a drug may be somewhat controlled by the chemical form of the drug used, the physical state of the injection (solution or suspension), and the vehicle employed. Drugs that are very soluble in body fluids generally have the most rapid absorption and onset of action. Thus, drugs in aqueous solution have a more rapid onset of action than do drugs in oleaginous solution. Drugs in aqueous suspension are also more rapid acting than drugs in oleaginous suspension due to the greater miscibility of the aqueous preparation with the body fluids after injection and the subsequent more rapid contact of the drug particles with the body fluids. Oftentimes more prolonged drug action is desired to reduce the necessity of frequently repeated injections. These long-acting types of injections

are commonly referred to as "repository" or "depot" types of preparations.

The solutions and suspensions of drugs intended for injection are prepared in the same general manner as was discussed previously in this text for oral solutions (Chapter 6) and oral suspensions (Chapter 7), with the following differences:

1. Solvents or vehicles used must meet special purity and other standards assuring their safety by injection.
2. The use of added substances, as buffers, stabilizers, and antimicrobial preservatives, fall under specific guidelines of use and are restricted in certain parenteral products. The use of coloring agents is strictly prohibited.
3. Parenteral products are always sterilized and meet sterility standards and must be pyrogen-free.
4. Parenteral solutions must meet compendial standards for particulate matter.
5. Parenteral products must be prepared in environmentally controlled areas, under strict sanitation standards, and by personnel specially trained and clothed to maintain the sanitation standards.
6. Parenteral products are packaged in special hermetic containers of specific and high quality. Special quality control procedures are utilized to ensure their hermetic seal and sterile condition.
7. Each container of an injection is filled to a volume in slight excess of the labeled "size" or volume to be withdrawn. This excess permits the ease of withdrawal and administration of the labeled volumes.
8. There are restrictions over the volume of injection permitted in multiple-dose containers and also a limitation over the types of containers (single-dose or multiple-dose) which may be used for certain injections.
9. Specific labeling regulations apply to injections.
10. Sterile powders intended for solution or suspension immediately prior to injection are frequently packaged as *lyophilized* or freeze-dried powders to permit ease of solution or suspension upon the addition of the solvent or vehicle.

Solvents and Vehicles for Injections

The most frequently used solvent in the large scale manufacture of injections is *Water for In-*

jection, USP. This water is purified by distillation or by reverse osmosis and meets the same standards for the presence of total solids as does *Purified Water, USP,* not more than 1 mg per 100 mL Water for Injection, USP and may not contain added substances. Although water for injection is not required to be sterile, it must be pyrogen-free. The water is intended to be used in the manufacture of injectable products which are to be sterilized after their preparation. Water for injection should be stored in tight containers at temperatures below or above the range in which microbial growth occurs.[5] Water for injection is intended to be used within 24 hours following its collection. Naturally, the water should be collected in sterile and pyrogen-free containers. The containers are usually glass or glass-lined.

Sterile Water for Injection, USP is water for injection which has been sterilized and packaged in single-dose containers of not greater than 1-liter size. As water for injection, it must be pyrogen-free and may not contain an antimicrobial agent or other added substance. This water may contain a slightly greater amount of total solids than water for injection due to the leaching of solids from the glass-lined tanks during the sterilization process. This water is intended to be used as a solvent, vehicle or diluent for already-sterilized and packaged injectable medications. In use, the water is aseptically added to the vial of medication to prepare the desired injection. For instance, a suitable injection may be prepared from the dry powder, Sterile Ampicillin Sodium, USP, by the aseptic addition of sterile water for injection.

Bacteriostatic Water for Injection, USP is sterile water for injection containing one or more suitable antimicrobial agents. It is packaged in prefilled syringes or in vials containing not more than 30 mL of the water. The container label must state the name and proportion of the antimicrobial agent(s) present. The water is employed as a sterile vehicle in the preparation of small volumes of injectable preparations. Because of the presence of antimicrobial agents the water must only be used in parenterals that are administered in small volumes. Its use in parenterals administered in large volume is restricted due to the excessive and perhaps toxic amounts of the antimicrobial agents which would be injected along with the medication. Generally, if volumes of greater than 5 mL of solvent are required, sterile water for injection

rather than bacteriostatic water for injection is preferred. In using bacteriostatic water for injection, due regard must also be given to the chemical compatibility of the bacteriostatic agent(s) present with the particular medicinal agent being dissolved or suspended.

Sodium Chloride Injection, USP is a sterile isotonic solution of sodium chloride in Water for Injection. It contains no antimicrobial agents. The sodium and chloride ion contents of the injection are approximately 154 mEq of each per liter. The solution may be used as a sterile vehicle in preparing solutions or suspensions of drugs for parenteral administration.

Bacteriostatic Sodium Chloride Injection, USP is a sterile isotonic solution of sodium chloride in Water for Injection. It contains one or more suitable antimicrobial agents which must be specified on the labeling. Sodium chloride is present at 0.9% concentration to render the solution isotonic. For the reasons noted previously for bacteriostatic water for injection, this solution may not be packaged in containers greater than 30 mL in size. When this solution is used as a vehicle, care must be exercised to assure the compatibility of the added medicinal agent with the preservative(s) present as well as with the sodium chloride. Further, USP labeling requirements demand that the label state, "Not for Use in Newborns." This new labeling statement was the result of problems encountered with neonates and the toxicity of the bacteriostat, i.e., benzyl alcohol.

Ringer's Injection, USP is a sterile solution of sodium chloride, potassium chloride, and calcium chloride in water for injection. The three agents are present in concentrations similar to that found in physiologic fluids. The solution is employed as a vehicle for other drugs, or alone as an electrolyte replenisher and fluid extender. *Lactated Ringer's Injection, USP* has different quantities of the same three salts in Ringer's Injection and contains sodium lactate. This injection is a fluid and electrolyte replenisher and a systemic alkalizer.

Nonaqueous Vehicles

Although an aqueous vehicle is generally preferred for an injection, its use may be precluded in a formulation due to the limited water solubility of a medicinal substance or its susceptibility to hydrolysis. When such physical or chemical factors limit the use of a wholly aqueous vehicle, the pharmaceutical formulator must turn to one or more nonaqueous vehicles.

The selected vehicle must be nonirritating, nontoxic in the amounts administered, and nonsensitizing. Like water, it must not exert a pharmacologic activity of its own, nor may it adversely affect the activity of the medicinal agent. In addition, the physical and chemical properties of the solvent or vehicle must be considered, evaluated, and determined to be suitable for the task at hand before it may be employed. Among the many considerations are the solvent's physical and chemical stability at various pH levels, its viscosity, which must be such as to allow ease of injection (syringeability), its fluidity, which must be maintained over a fairly wide temperature range, its boiling point, which should be sufficiently high to permit heat sterilization, its miscibility with body fluids, its low vapor pressure to avoid problems during heat sterilization, and its constant purity or ease of purification and standardization. There is no single solvent that is free of limitations, and thus the cross-consideration and the assessment of each solvent's advantages and disadvantages help the formulator determine the most appropriate solvent for use in a given preparation. Among the nonaqueous solvents presently employed in parenteral products are fixed vegetable oils, glycerin, polyethylene glycols, propylene glycol, alcohol, and a number of lesser used agents as ethyl oleate, isopropyl myristate, and dimethylacetamide. These and other nonaqueous vehicles may be used provided they are safe in the amounts administered and do not interfere with the therapeutic efficacy of the preparation or with its response to prescribed assays and tests.

The USP specifies restrictions on the fixed vegetable oils which may be employed in parenteral products. For one thing, they must remain clear when cooled to 10°C to ensure the stability and clarity of the injectable product upon storage under refrigeration. The oils must not contain mineral oil or paraffin, as these materials are not absorbed by body tissues. The fluidity of a vegetable oil generally depends upon the proportion of unsaturated fatty acids, such as oleic acid, to saturated acids, such as stearic acid. Oils to be employed in injections must meet officially stated requirements of iodine number and saponification number.

Although the toxicities of vegetable oils are generally considered to be relatively low, some patients exhibit allergic reactions to specific oils. Thus, when vegetable oils are employed in parenteral products, the label must state the specific oil present. The most commonly used fixed oils in injections are corn oil, cottonseed oil, peanut oil, and sesame oil. Castor oil and olive oil have been used on occasion.

By the selective employment of solvent or vehicle, a pharmacist can prepare injectable preparations as solutions or suspensions of a medicinal substance in either an aqueous or nonaqueous vehicle. For the most part, oleaginous injections are administered intramuscularly. Some examples of official injections employing oil as the vehicle are presented in Table 8–1.

Added Substances

The USP permits the addition of suitable substances to the official preparations intended for injection for the purpose of increasing their stability or usefulness, provided the substances are not interdicted in the individual monographs and are harmless in the amounts administered and do not interfere with the therapeutic efficacy of the preparation or with specified assays and tests. Many of these added substances are antibacterial preservatives, buffers, solubilizers, antioxidants, and other pharmaceutical adjuncts. Agents employed solely for their coloring effect are strictly prohibited in parenteral products.

The USP requires that one or more suitable substances be added to parenteral products that are packaged in multiple-dose containers, to prevent the growth of microorganisms regardless of the method of sterilization employed, unless otherwise directed in the individual monograph or unless the injection's active ingredients are themselves bacteriostatic. Such substances are used in concentrations that prevent the growth of or kill microorganisms in the preparations. Because many of the usual preservative agents are toxic when given in excessive amounts or irritating when parenterally administered, special care must be exercised in the selection of the appropriate preservative agents. For the following preservatives, the indicated maximum limits prevail for use in a parenteral product unless otherwise directed: for agents containing mercury and the cationic, surface-active compounds, 0.01%; for agents like chlorobutanol, cresol, and phenol, 0.5%; for sulfur dioxide as an antioxidant, or for an equivalent

Table 8–1. Examples of Some Injections in Oil

Injection	Oil	Category
Dimercaprol Injection	Peanut	Antidote to arsenic, gold and mercury poisoning
Estradiol Cypionate Injection	Cottonseed	Estrogen
Estradiol Valerate Injection	Sesame or Castor	Estrogen
Estrone Injection	Sesame	Estrogen
Hydroxyprogesterone Caproate Injection	Sesame	Progestin
Progesterone in Oil Injection	Sesame	Progestin
Testosterone Cypionate Injection	Cottonseed	Androgen
Testosterone Enanthate Injection	Sesame	Androgen

amount of the sulfite, bisulfite, or metabisulfite of potassium or sodium, 0.2%.

In addition to the stabilizing effect of the additives, the air within an injectable product is frequently replaced with an inert gas, such as nitrogen, to enhance the stability of the product by preventing chemical reaction between the oxygen in the air and the drug.

Methods of Sterilization

The term *sterilization*, as applied to pharmaceutical preparations, means the complete destruction of all living organisms and their spores or their complete removal from the preparation. Five general methods are used for the sterilization of pharmaceutical products:

1. Steam sterilization
2. Dry-heat sterilization
3. Sterilization by filtration
4. Gas sterilization
5. Sterilization by ionizing radiation

The method used in attaining sterility in a pharmaceutical preparation is determined largely by the nature of the preparation and its ingredients. However, regardless of the method used, the resulting product must pass a test for sterility as proof of the effectiveness of the method and the performance of the equipment and the personnel.

Steam Sterilization

Steam sterilization is conducted in an autoclave and employs steam under pressure. It is recognized as the method of choice in most cases where the product is capable of withstanding such treatment (Fig. 8–2).

Most pharmaceutical products are adversely affected by heat and cannot be heated safely to the temperature required for dry-heat sterilization (about 170°C). When moisture is present, bacteria are coagulated and destroyed at a considerably lower temperature than when moisture is absent. In fact, bacterial cells with a large percentage of water are generally killed rather easily. Spores, which contain a relatively low percentage of water, are comparatively difficult to destroy. The mechanism of microbial destruction in moist heat is thought to be by denaturation and coagulation of some of the organism's essential protein. It is the presence of the hot moisture within the microbial cell that permits destruction at relatively low temperature. Death by dry heat is thought to be by the dehydration of the microbial cell followed by a slow burning or oxidative process. Because it is not possible to raise the temperature of steam above 100°C under atmospheric conditions, pressure is employed to achieve higher temperatures. It

Fig. 8–2. *Autoclaving of intravenous electrolyte solutions. (Courtesy of Abbott Laboratories.)*

should be recognized that the temperature, not the pressure, is destructive to the microorganisms and that the application of pressure is solely for the purpose of increasing the temperature of the system. Time is another important factor in the destruction of microorganisms by heat. Most modern autoclaves have gauges to indicate to the operator the internal conditions of temperature and pressure and a timing device to permit the desired exposure time for the load. The usual steam pressures, the temperatures obtainable under these pressures, and the approximate length of time required for sterilization after the system reaches the indicated temperatures are as follows:

10 pounds pressure (115.5°C), for 30 minutes
15 pounds pressure (121.5°C), for 20 minutes
20 pounds pressure (126.5°C), for 15 minutes.

As can be seen, the greater the pressure applied, the higher the temperature obtainable and the less the time required for sterilization.

The temperature at which most autoclaves are routinely operated is usually 121°C, as measured at the steam discharge line running from the autoclave. It should be understood that the temperature attained in the chamber of the autoclave must also be reached by the interior of the load being sterilized, and this temperature must be maintained for an adequate time. The penetration time of the moist heat into the load may vary with the nature of the load, and the exposure time must be adjusted to account for this latent period. For example, a solution packaged in a thin-walled 50 mL ampul may reach a temperature of 121°C in from 6 to 8 minutes after that temperature is registered in the steam discharge line, whereas 20 minutes or longer may be required to reach that temperature within a solution packaged in a completely filled thick-walled 1000-mL glass bottle. An estimate of these latent periods must be added to the total time in order to ensure adequate exposure times. Because this sterilization process depends upon the presence of moisture and an elevated temperature, air is removed from the chamber as the sterilization process is begun, because a combination of air and steam yields a lower temperature than does steam alone under the same condition of pressure. For instance, at 15 pounds pressure the temperature of saturated steam is 121.5°C, but a mixture of equal parts of air and steam will reach only about 112°C.

In general, this method of sterilization is applicable to pharmaceutical preparations and materials that can withstand the required temperatures and are penetrated by, but not adversely affected by, moisture. In sterilizing aqueous solutions by this method, the moisture is already present, and all that is required is the elevation of the temperature of the solution for the prescribed period of time. Thus solutions packaged in sealed containers, as ampuls, are readily sterilized by this method. The method is also applicable to bulk solutions, glassware, surgical dressings, and instruments. It is not useful in the sterilization of oils, fats, oleaginous preparations, and other preparations not penetrated by the moisture or the sterilization of exposed powders that may be damaged by the condensed moisture.

Dry-Heat Sterilization

Dry-heat sterilization is usually carried out in sterilizing ovens specifically designed for this purpose. The ovens may be heated either by gas or electricity and are generally thermostatically controlled.

Because dry heat is less effective in killing microorganisms than is moist heat, higher temperatures and longer periods of exposure are required. These must be determined individually for each product with consideration to the size and type of product and the container and its heat distribution characteristics. In general, individual units to be sterilized should be as small as possible, and the sterilizer should be loaded in such a manner as to permit free circulation of heated air throughout the chamber. Dry-heat sterilization is usually conducted at temperatures of 160° to 170°C for periods of not less than 2 hours. Higher temperatures permit shorter exposure times for a given article; conversely, lower temperatures require longer exposure times. For example, if a particular chemical agent melts or decomposes at 170°C, but is unaffected at 140°C, the lower temperature would be employed in its sterilization, and the exposure time would be increased over that required to sterilize another chemical that may be safely heated to 170°C.

Dry-heat sterilization is generally employed for substances that are not effectively sterilized by moist heat. Such substances include fixed oils, glycerin, various petroleum products such as petrolatum, liquid petrolatum (mineral oil), and paraffin and various heat-stable powders such as zinc oxide. Dry-heat sterilization is also an effective method for the sterilization of glassware and surgical instruments. Dry-heat sterilization is the method of choice when dry apparatus or dry containers are required, as in the handling or packaging of dry chemicals or nonaqueous solutions.

Sterilization by Filtration

Sterilization by filtration, which depends upon the physical removal of microorganisms by adsorption on the filter medium or by a sieving mechanism, is used for the sterilization of heat-sensitive solutions. Medicinal preparations sterilized by this method are required to undergo severe validation and monitoring since the effectiveness of the filtered product can be greatly influenced by the microbial load in the solution being filtered (Fig. 8–3).

Historically available bacterial filters have included (1) test-tube shaped filters called "filter candles" which are made of compressed infusorial earth (Berkefeld and Mandler filters); (2) filter candles made of unglazed porcelain (Pasteur-Chamberland, Doulton, and Selas filters); (3) disks of compressed asbestos fastened in a special holder in the filtration apparatus (Seitz, and Swinney filters); (4) glass Buchner-type funnel with a fused fritted glass holder (Millipore). In practice, the filter, its accessories, and the receiving vessel must all be rendered sterile by suitable means; then the solution to be ster-

ilized is passed through the filter as rapidly as possible (using positive pressure at the non-sterile end of the system or suction at the receiving end, if necessary) and collected in the sterile receiving vessel. This method of sterilization demands rigid adherence to aseptic technique. The apparatus must be thoroughly inspected prior to its use for cracks or breaks that may render it ineffective as a bacterial filter.

Today, commercially available filters are produced with a variety of pore-size specifications. It would be well to mention briefly one type of these modern filters, the Millipore filters (Fig. 8–4).[6] Millipore filters are thin plastic membranes of cellulosic esters with millions of pores per square inch of filter surface. The pores are made to be extremely uniform in size and occupy approximately 80% of the filter membrane's volume, the remaining 20% being the solid filter material. This high degree of porosity permits flow rates much in excess of other filters having the same particle-retention capability. Millipore filters are made from a variety of polymers to provide membrane characteristics required for the filtration of almost any liquid or gas system. Also, the filters are made of various pore sizes to meet the selective filtration requirements of the operator. They are available in pore sizes from 14 to 0.025 μm. For comparative purposes, the period that ended the last sentence is approximately 500 μm in size. The size of the smallest particle visible to the naked

Fig. 8–3. *Sterilization by filtration. An eight-head bottle-filling machine using three large sterilizing filters for sterile filling of bottles in large scale pharmaceutical production. (Courtesy of Millipore Corporation.)*

Fig. 8–4. *Membrane filters act as microporous screens that retain all particles and microorganisms larger than the rated pore size on their surface. (Courtesy of Millipore Corporation.)*

Fig. 8–5. *Luer-Lock syringe adapted with a MILLEX Filter Unit and hypodermic needle. (Courtesy of Millipore Corporation.)*

eye is about 40 μm, a red blood cell is about 6.5 μm, the smallest bacteria, about 0.2 μm, and a polio virus, about 0.025 μm.

Although the pore size of a bacterial filter is of prime importance in the removal of microorganisms from a liquid, there are other factors such as the electrical charge on the filter and that of the microorganism, the pH of the solution, the temperature, and the pressure or vacuum applied to the system.

The major advantages of bacterial filtration include its speed in the filtration of small quantities of solution, its ability to sterilize effectively thermolabile materials, the relatively inexpensive equipment required, and the complete removal of living and dead microorganisms as well as other particulate matter from the solution. The disadvantages are less numerous and apply mainly to certain filters which have a tendency to absorb some active ingredients from the solution being filtered (infusorial earth) and to impart an alkalinity to the solution being filtered (asbestos filters). These disadvantages have largely been obviated through the use of the membrane filters. One serious disadvantage to the use of bacterial filters is the possibility of a flaw in the construction of the filter and thus some uncertainty of sterility, a circumstance not true of methods involving dry- or moist-heat sterilization in which the procedures are just about guaranteed to give effective sterilization. Also, filtration of large volumes of liquids would require more time, particularly if the liquid were viscous, than would, say, steam sterilization. In essence, the bacterial filters are use-

ful when heat cannot be used and also for small volumes of liquids.

Bacterial filters may be used conveniently and economically in the community pharmacy to filter extemporaneously prepared solutions (as ophthalmic solutions) that are required to be sterile (Figs. 8–5 and 8–6).

Gas Sterilization

Some heat-sensitive and moisture-sensitive materials can be sterilized much better by exposure to ethylene oxide or propylene oxide gas than by other means. These gases are highly flammable when mixed with air but can be employed safely when properly diluted with an inert gas such as carbon dioxide or a suitable fluorinated hydrocarbon. Such mixtures are commercially available.

Sterilization by this process requires specialized equipment resembling autoclaves, and many combination steam autoclaves-ethylene oxide sterilizers are commercially available. Greater precautions are required for this method of sterilization than for some of the others, because the variables—for instance, time, temperature, gas concentration, and humidity—are not as firmly quantitated as those of dry-heat and steam sterilization. In general, sterilization with gas is enhanced, and the exposure time required is reduced, by increasing the relative humidity of the system (to about 60%) and by increasing the exposure temperature (to between 50 and 60°C). If the material being sterilized cannot tolerate either the moisture or the elevated temperature, exposure time will have to be increased. Generally, sterilization with ethylene oxide gas requires from 4 to 16 hours of exposure. Ethylene oxide is thought

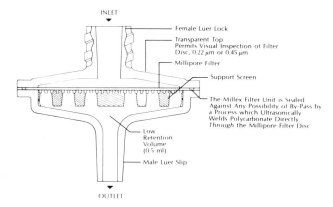

Fig. 8–6.   *Cutaway showing composition of the MILLEX filter unit. (Courtesy of Millipore Corporation.)*

to function as a sterilizing agent by its interference with the metabolism of the bacterial cell.

The great penetrating qualities of ethylene oxide gas make it a useful sterilizing agent in certain special applications, as in the sterilization of medical and surgical supplies and appliances such as catheters, needles, and plastic disposable syringes in their final plastic packaging just prior to shipment. The gas is also used to sterilize certain heat-labile enzyme preparations, certain antibiotics, and other drugs, with tests being performed to assure of the absence of chemical reaction or other deleterious effects on the drug substance.

Sterilization by Ionizing Radiation

Techniques are available for the sterilization of some types of pharmaceuticals by gamma rays and by cathode rays, but the application of such techniques is limited because of the highly specialized equipment required and the effects of irradiation on products and their containers.

The exact mechanism by which irradiation sterilizes a drug or preparation is still subject to investigation. One of the proposed theories involves an alteration of the chemicals within or supporting the microorganism to form deleterious new chemicals capable of destroying the cell. Another theory proposes that vital structures of the cell, such as the chromosomal nucleoprotein, are disoriented or destroyed. It is probably a combination of irradiation effects that causes the cellular destruction, which is complete and irreversible.

Regardless of the method of sterilization employed, pharmaceutical preparations required

to be sterile must undergo sterility tests to confirm the absence of microorganisms. The USP contains monographs and standards for biologic indicators of a sterilization process. A *biologic indicator* is a characterized preparation of specific microorganisms resistant to a particular sterilization process. They may be utilized to monitor a sterilization cycle and/or to periodically revalidate the process. Biologic indicators are generally of two main forms. In one, spores are added to a carrier, as a strip of filter paper, packaged to maintain physical integrity while allowing the sterilization effect. In the other, the spores are added to representative units of the product being sterilized, with sterilization assessed based on these samples. In steam sterilization, spores of suitable strains of *Bacillus stearothermophyilus* are commonly employed because of their resistance to this mode of sterilization. In dry-heat, or ethylene oxide sterilization, spores of a subspecies of *Bacillus subtilis* are commonly used. In sterilization by ionizing radiation, spores of suitable strains of *Bacillus pumilus* have been utilized.

The effectiveness of thermal sterilization procedures has been quantified through the determination and calculation of *F value* to express the time of thermal death. *Thermal death time* is defined as the time required to kill a particular organism under specified conditions. The F_0, at a particular temperature *other than 121°C*, is the time, in minutes, required to provide the lethality equivalent to that provided at 121° for a stated time.

Although heat distribution in an autoclave chamber is usually rapid with 121°C obtained nearly instantaneously throughout the autoclave, the product being sterilized may not achieve identical conditions due to a variety of factors of heat transfer, including the thermal conductivity of the packaging components, the viscosity and density of the product, the viscosity and density of the product, container proximity, passage of steam around containers and other variables. F values may be computed from biologic data derived from the rate of destruction of known numbers of microorganisms, as shown in the following equation:*

$$F_0 = D_{121} (Log\ A - Log\ B)$$

where

D_{121} = the time required for a one-log reduction in the microbial population exosed to a temperature of 121°C

A = the initial microbial population

B = the number of microorganisms that survive after a defined heating time.

Pyrogens and Pyrogen Testing

As indicated earlier, *pyrogens* are fever-producing organic substances arising from microbial contamination and responsible for many of the febrile reactions which occur in patients following injection. The causative material is thought to be a lipopolysaccharide from the outer cell wall of the bacteria and endotoxins. Because the material is thermostable, it may remain in water even after sterilization by autoclaving or by bacterial filtration.

Manufacturers of water for injection may employ any suitable method for the removal of pyrogens from their product. Because pyrogens are organic substances, one of the more common means of facilitating their removal is by oxidizing them to easily eliminated gases or to nonvolatile solids, both of which are easily separated from water by fractional distillation. Potassium permanganate is usually employed as the oxidizing agent, with its efficiency being increased by the addition of a small amount of barium hydroxide serving to impart alkalinity to the solution and to make nonvolatile barium salts of any acidic compounds that may be present. These two reagents are added to water that has previously been distilled several times, and

*Akers, M.J., Attia, I.A., and Avis, K.E.: Understanding and Utilizing F_0 Values. *Pharm. Tech.*, 11:44–48, 1987.

the distillation process is repeated with the chemical-free distillate being collected under strict aseptic conditions. When properly conducted, this method results in a highly purified, sterile, and pyrogen-free water. However, in each instance the official pyrogen test must be performed for assurance of the absence of these fever-producing materials.

PYROGEN TEST. The USP Pyrogen Test utilizes healthy rabbits that have been properly maintained in terms of environment and diet prior to performance of the test. Normal, or "control" temperatures are taken for each animal to be used in the test. These temperatures are used as the base for the determination of any temperature increase resulting from the injection of a test solution. In a given test, rabbits are used whose temperatures do not differ by more than one degree from each other and whose body temperatures are considered to be unelevated. A synopsis of the procedure of the test is as follows.

Render the syringes, needles, and glassware free from pyrogens by heating at 250°C for not less than 30 minutes or by other suitable method. Warm the product to be tested to 37°C ± 2°C.

Inject into an ear vein of each of three rabbits 10 mL of the product per kg of body weight, completing each injection within 10 minutes after the start of administration. Record the temperature at 1, 2, and 3 hours subsequent to the injection.

If no rabbit shows an individual rise in temperature at 0.6°C or more above its respective control temperature, and if the sum of the three individual maximum temperature rises does not exceed 1.4°C, the material under examination meets the requirements for the absence of pyrogens. If any rabbits show a temperature rise of 0.6°C or more, or if the sum of the temperature rises exceeds 1.4°C, repeat the test using five other rabbits. If not more than three of the eight rabbits show individual rises in temperature of 0.6°C or more, and if the sum of the eight temperature rises does not exceed 3.7°C, the material under examination meets the requirements for the absence of pyrogens.

In recent years, it has been shown that an extract from the blood cells of the horseshoe crab *(Limulus polyphemus)* contains an enzyme and protein system that coagulates in the presence of low levels of lipopolysaccharides. This discovery has led to the development of the *Limulus* amebocyte lysate (LAL) test for the presence of bacterial endotoxins. The USP Bacterial Endotoxins Test utilizes LAL and is considered generally more sensitive to endotoxin than the rabbit test. The FDA has endorsed the test as a replacement for the rabbit test.[8]

The Preparation of Parenteral Products

Once the formulation for a particular parenteral product is determined, including the selection of the proper solvents or vehicles and additives, the production pharmacist must follow rigid aseptic procedures in preparing the injectable products. In most manufacturing plants the area in which parenteral products are made is maintained bacteria-free through the use of ultraviolet lights, a filtered air supply, sterile manufacturing equipment, such as flasks, connecting tubes, and filters, and sterilized work clothing worn by the personnel in the area (Fig. 8–7).

In the preparation of parenteral solutions, the required ingredients are dissolved according to good pharmaceutical practice either in water for injection, in one of the alternate solvents, or in a combination of solvents. The solutions are then usually filtered until sparkling clear through a membrane-type filter. After filtration, the solution is transferred as rapidly as possible and with the least possible exposure into the final containers. The product is then sterilized, preferably by autoclaving, and samples of the finished product are tested for sterility and pyrogens. In instances in which sterilization by autoclaving is impractical due to the nature of the ingredients, the individual components of the preparation that are heat or moisture labile may be sterilized by other appropriate means and added aseptically to the sterilized solvent or to a sterile solution of all of the other components sterilizable by autoclaving.

Suspensions of drugs intended for parenteral use may be prepared by reducing the drug to a very fine powder with a ball mill, micronizer, colloid mill, or other appropriate equipment and then suspending the material in a liquid in which it is insoluble. It is frequently necessary to sterilize separately the individual components of a suspension before combining them, as frequently the integrity of a suspension is destroyed by autoclaving. Autoclaving of a parenteral suspension may alter the viscosity of the product, thereby affecting the suspending ability of the vehicle, or change the particle size of the suspended particles, thereby altering both

Fig. 8–7. *Sterile filling of vials. (Courtesy of Wyeth Laboratories.)*

the pharmaceutic and the therapeutic characteristics of the preparation. If a suspension remains unaltered by autoclaving, this method is generally employed to sterilize the final product. Because parenterally administered emulsions, which are dispersions or suspensions of a liquid throughout another liquid, are generally destroyed by autoclaving, an alternate method of sterilization must be employed for this type of injectable.

Some injections are packaged as dry solids rather than in conjunction with a solvent or vehicle due to the instability of the therapeutic agent in the presence of the liquid component. These dry powdered drugs are packaged as the sterilized powder in the final containers to be reconstituted with the proper liquid prior to use, generally to form a solution or less frequently a suspension. The method of sterilization of the powder may be dry heat or another method that is appropriate for the particular drug involved. Examples of sterile drugs prepared and packaged *without* the presence of pharmaceutical additives as buffers, preservatives, stabilizers, tonicity agents, and other substances include:

Sterile Ampicillin Sodium
Sterile Bacitracin
Sterile Ceftizoxime Sodium
Sterile Ceftazidime Sodium
Sterile Cefuroxime Sodium
Sterile Kanamycin Sulfate
Sterile Nafcillin Sodium
Sterile Penicillin G Benzathine
Sterile Streptomycin Sulfate
Sterile Tetracaine Hydrochloride
Sterile Tetracycline Hydrochloride
Sterile Tobramycin Sulfate

Antibiotics are prepared industrially in large fermentation tanks (Fig. 8–8).

Those sterile drugs formulated *with* pharmaceutical additives and intended to be reconstituted prior to injection include the following:

Cephradine for Injection
Cyclophosphamide for Injection
Dactinomycin for Injection
Erythromycin Lactobionate for Injection
Hyaluronidase for Injection
Hydrocortisone Sodium Succinate for Injection
Mitomycin for Injection
Nafcillin Sodium for Injection
Oxytetracycline Hydrochloride for Injection

Fig. 8–8. *Fermentation tank in the preparation of antibiotics. (Courtesy of Schering-Plough.)*

Penicillin G Potassium for Injection
Vinblastine Sulfate for Injection

In certain instances, a liquid is packaged along with the dry powder for use at the time of reconstitution (Fig. 8–9). This liquid is sterile and may contain some of the desired pharmaceutical additives as the buffering agents. More frequently, the solvent or vehicle is not provided along with the dry product, but the labeling on the injection generally lists suitable solvents. Sodium chloride injection or sterile water for injection are perhaps the most frequently employed solvents used to reconstitute dry-packaged injections. The dry powders are packaged in containers large enough to permit proper shaking with the liquid component when the latter is aseptically injected through the container's rubber closure during its reconstitution. To facilitate the dissolving process, the dry powder is prevented from caking upon standing by the appropriate means including its preparation by lyophilization (Fig. 8–10).[8] Powders so treated form a honeycomb, lattice structure that is rapidly penetrated by the liquid, and solution is rapidly effected because of the large surface area of powder exposed.

Several manufacturers now ship to the hospital pharmacy reconstituted intravenous antibiotic solutions, e.g., cefazolin sodium, in the frozen state. When thawed these nonpyrogenic solutions are stable for a finite amount of time, e.g., reconstituted cefazolin is stable for 24 hours at room temperature and for 96 hours refrigerated (5°C). The product is packaged in a small plastic bag for piggy-back use in intravenous administration to the patient.

Fig. 8–9. *The Mix-O-Vial shown above is a combination vial containing dry ingredients in the bottom compartment and a liquid diluent in the top compartment, separated by a specially formulated center seal. The bottom compartment can either be liquid filled, frozen and dried to make a lyophilized product, or it may be powder filled. The top diluent contains a preservative and may or may not contain one or more active ingredients.*

To use the vial, the dust cover is removed (as shown above), pressure is applied with the thumb to the top plunger which dislodges the center seal and the vial is shaken until the solution is effected. The top of the plunger is then swabbed with a disinfectant; the syringe needle inserted through the target circle on the plunger and the contents of the vial withdrawn into the syringe.

The Mix-O-Vial offers stability of product (until it is activated), convenience, fast operation and safety as regards the right drug with the proper diluent in the correct proportions. (Courtesy of The Upjohn Company.)

Packaging, Labeling, and Storage of Injection

Containers for injections, including the closures, must not interact physically or chemically with the preparation so as to alter its strength or efficacy (Fig. 8–11). If the container is made of glass, it must be clear and colorless or of a light amber color to permit the inspection of its contents. The type of glass suitable and preferred for each parenteral preparation is usually stated in the individual monograph. Injections are placed either in single-dose containers or in multiple-dose containers (Figs. 8–12 through 8–14). By definition:

Single-dose Container—A single-dose container is a hermetic container holding a quantity of sterile drug intended for parenteral administration as a single dose, and which when opened cannot be re-sealed with assurance that sterility has been maintained.

Multiple-dose Container—A multiple-dose container is a hermetic container that permits withdrawal of successive portions of the contents without changing the strength, quality, or purity of the remaining portion.

Single-dose containers, commonly called *ampuls* (Fig. 8–15), are sealed by fusion of the glass container under aseptic conditions (Figs. 8–16 and 8–17). The glass container is made so as to have a neck portion that may be easily separated from the body of the container without fragmentation of the glass. After opening, the contents of the ampul may be drawn into a syringe with a hypodermic needle. Once opened, the ampul cannot be resealed, and any unused portion may not be retained and used at a later time, since the contents would have questionable sterility. Some injectable products are packaged in pre-filled syringes, with or without special administration devices (Figs. 8–12, 8–18, 8–19, 8–20). The types of glass for parenteral product containers have already been pointed out in Chapter 4, and the student should recall that Types I, II, and III are suitable for parenteral products, with Type I being the most resistant to chemical deterioration. The type of glass to be used as the container for a particular injection is indicated in the individual monograph for that preparation.

One of the prime requisites of solutions for parenteral administration is clarity. They should be sparkling clear and free of all particulate matter, that is, all of the mobile, undissolved substances which are unintentionally present. Included are such contaminants as dust, cloth fibers, glass fragments, material leached from the glass or plastic containers or seals, and any other material which may find its way into the product during its manufacture or administration, or develop during storage.

To prevent the entrance of unwanted particles into parenteral products, a number of precautions must be taken during the manufacture, storage, and use of the products. During manufacture, for instance, the parenteral solution is

Fig. 8–10. *Antibiotic lyophilizers. (Courtesy of Abbott Laboratories.)*

Fig. 8–11. *Testing compatibility of rubber closures with the solution with which they are in contact. (Courtesy of Abbott Laboratories.)*

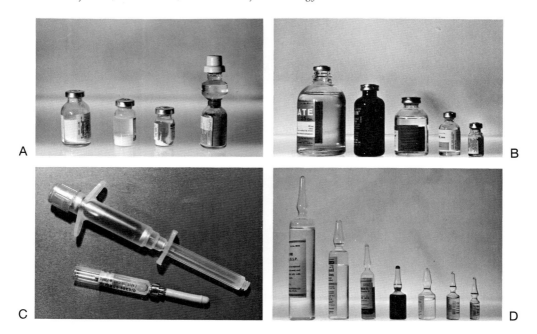

Fig. 8–12. *Examples of packaging of injectable products. A. Multiple-dose vials of suspensions and dry powders for reconstitution. B. Vials of solutions, including one of light-protective glass. C. Unit dose, disposable syringes. D. Various sizes of ampuls.*

Fig. 8–13. *A typical vial used for sterile injectable products. It is made from Type I (borosilicate) glass. The rubber closure has been specially selected as regards compatibility with the product, desirable physical characteristics, etc. The overseal holds the closure in place and provides a means for ready access to the contents of the vial. (Courtesy of the Upjohn Company.)*

Fig. 8–14. *Example of a 100 mL single-dose vial for intravenous infusion in ready-to-use (RTU) form. (Courtesy of Searle Pharmaceuticals, Inc.)*

Fig. 8–15. *Ampul, before filling and sealing. (Courtesy of Owens Illinois.)*

usually final filtered before being placed into the parenteral containers. The containers are carefully selected to be chemically resistant to the solution being added and of the highest available quality to minimize the chances of container components being leached into the solution. It has been recognized for some time, that some of the particulate matter found in parenteral products is generated from leached material from the glass or plastic containers. Once the container is selected for use, it must be carefully cleaned to be free of all extraneous matter (Fig. 8–21). During container-filling, extreme care must be exercised to prevent the entrance of air-borne dust, lint or other contaminants into the container. The provision of filtered and directed air flow in production areas is useful in reducing the likelihood of contamination. Laminar flow hoods have been developed which allow for the draft-free flow of clean, filtered air over the work area. These hoods are commonly found in the hospital setting for both the manufacture and the incorporation of additives into parenteral and ophthalmic products (Fig. 8–22). The personnel involved in the manufacture of parenterals must be made acutely aware of the importance of cleanliness and aseptic techniques. They are provided uniforms made of monofilament fabrics that do not shed lint. They wear face hoods,

caps, gloves, and disposable shoe covers to prevent contamination (Fig. 8–23).

After the containers are filled and hermetically sealed, they are visually (Fig. 8–24) or automatically (Fig. 8–25) inspected for particulate matter. Usually an inspector passes the filled container past a light source with a black background to observe for mobile particles. Particles of approximately 50 μm in size may be detected in this manner. Reflective particles, such as fragments of glass, may be visualized in smaller size, about 25 μm in size. Other methods are used to detect particulate matter smaller than that which may be detected by the unaided eye including microscopic examinations as well as the use of sophisticated equipment as the Coulter Counter which electronically counts particles present in a sample presented to it. Once past the inspection following production the product may be labeled. Prior to its use, however, the pharmacist should inspect each parenteral solution dispensed for evidence of particulate matter.

Although the total significance of injecting or infusing parenteral solutions containing particulate matter into a patient has not been ascertained, it is apparent that particulate matter has the potential of inducing thrombi and vessel blockage and depending upon the chemical composition of the particles the additional potential for introducing into the patient chemical agents which are undesired and possibly toxic.

In formulating a single-dose parenteral product, the pharmacist must consider not only the physicochemical aspects of the drug, but also the intended therapeutic use of the product itself. Some single-dose preparations are prepared to be administered rapidly in small volumes, but other preparations are allowed to drip slowly into the circulatory system over a period of hours. Most small-volume parenterals are formulated so that a convenient amount of solution, say 0.5 to 2 mL, contains the usual dose of the drug although larger volumes of more diluted solutions are frequently administered intravenously and intramuscularly. Generally, several strengths of injections of a given drug are marketed to permit a wider dosage selection by the physician without being wasteful of the drug as would be the case if he administered only part of a given single-dose parenteral solution. The large-volume, single-dose preparations generally are those solutions used to expand the blood volume or to replenish nu-

Fig. 8–16.   *Ampul filling. (Courtesy of Abbott Laboratories.)*

Fig. 8–17.   *Ampul sealing. (Courtesy of Abbott Laboratories.)*

Fig. 8–18.   *Operation of a TUBEX filling machine. (Courtesy of Wyeth Laboratories.)*

Fig. 8–19.   *The Tubex Injector. The ribbed collar and plunger rod securely hold a glass sterile cartridge-needle unit. Each pre-filled unit contains a dose of medication with an attached sterile needle. After administration, the cartridge-needle unit is discarded; the Injector is reusable. (Courtesy of Wyeth-Ayerst Laboratories.)*

Fig. 8–20.   *Diagram of the BUSHER Automatic Injector, utilized by patients who find it difficult to administer medication by self-injection. (Courtesy of Becton, Dickinson and Company.)*

Fig. 8–21.   *Production line in the preparation of vials for sterilization and filling. (Courtesy of Schering-Plough.)*

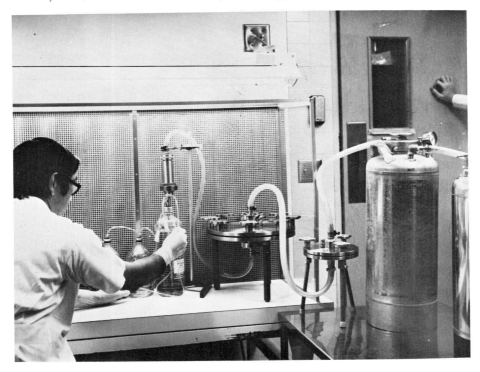

Fig. 8–22. *Hyperalimentation solutions being prepared in a laminar flow hood using Millipore sterilizing filtration in the hospital pharmacy. (Courtesy of Millipore Corporation.)*

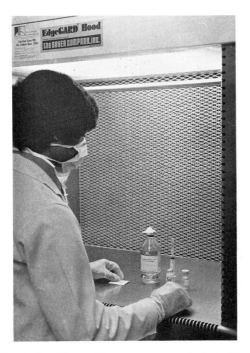

Fig. 8–23. *Pharmacist preparing a parenteral admixture in a laminar flow hood.*

Fig. 8–24. *Inspection of parenteral fluid for particulate matter. (Courtesy of Schering-Plough.)*

Fig. 8–25. *The AUTOSKAN automatic inspection machine which detects the presence of particulate matter in injectables with a television camera and electronics, and automatically rejects them from the production line. (Courtesy of Lakso Company, Inc.)*

trients or electrolytes and are given by slow intravenous drip. However, in no instance may a single-dose parenteral container permit the withdrawal and administration of greater than 1000 mL. In addition, preparations intended for intraspinal, intracisternal, or peridural administration must be packaged only in single-dose containers as a precaution against contamination.

Frequently in the hospital, a physician may order an additional agent to be placed in a large-volume parenteral solution for infusion. In these instances, the person filling such an order must be certain that aseptic conditions are employed and that the additive is compatible with the contents of the original large volume parenteral solution. Care must also be exercised not to introduce particulate matter into the solution. Many pharmaceutical companies have developed special devices for the aseptic transfer of pharmaceutical additives to large volume parenterals. An ordinary sterile needle and syringe, preferably affixed with a filtering device, may be effectively employed to transfer solutions from one parenteral product to another (Fig. 8–26). Many hospital pharmacies have established well controlled *I.V. additive* or *admix-*

ture programs to assure additive-solution compatibility, safety and efficacy.

Multiple-dose containers are affixed with rubber or plastic closures to permit the penetration of a hypodermic needle without the removal or destruction of the closure. Upon withdrawing the needle from the container, the closure reseals and protects the contents from airborne contamination. The needle may be inserted to withdraw a portion of the prepared liquid injection, or it may be used to introduce a solvent or vehicle to a dry powder intended for injection. In either instance, the sterility of the injection may be maintained so long as the needle itself is sterile at the time of entry into the container. It should be recalled that unless otherwise indicated in the monograph, multiple-dose injectables are required to contain added antibacterial preservatives. Also, unless otherwise specified, multiple-dose containers are not permitted to allow the withdrawal of greater than 30 mL in order to limit the number of penetrations made into the closure and thus protect against loss of sterility. The limited volume also guards against an excessive amount of antibacterial preservative being inadvertently coadministered with the drug when unusually large doses of an injection are required, in

Fig. 8–26. *Utilization of a filter syringe for the aseptic addition of an additive to a large volume parenteral solution. (Courtesy of Millipore Corporation.)*

Table 8–2. Recommended Overages for Official Parenteral Products

Labeled Size, mL	Excess Volume for Mobile Liquids, mL	Excess Volume for Viscous Liquids, mL
0.5	0.10	0.12
1.0	0.10	0.15
2.0	0.15	0.25
5.0	0.30	0.50
10.0	0.50	0.75
20.0	0.60	0.90
30.0	0.80	1.20
50.0 or more	2%	3%

The labels on containers of parenteral products must state: (1) the name of the preparation; (2) for a liquid preparation, the percentage content of drug or the amount of drug present in a specified volume, or for a dry preparation, the amount of active ingredient present and the volume of liquid to be added to the dry preparation to prepare a solution or suspension; (3) the route of administration; (4) a statement of storage conditions and an expiration date; (5) the name of the manufacturer or distributor; (6) the manufacturing lot number, which when referred to indicates all manufacturing processes for that preparation. Injections for veterinary use are labeled to that effect. Preparations intended to be used as dialysis, hemofiltration or irrigation solutions should meet the requirements for injections, except those relating to volume present in the containers, and should bear a statement indicating that the solution is not intended for use by intravenous infusion. All containers appropriately labeled should allow a sufficient area of the container to remain free of label for its full length or circumference to permit inspection of the contents. Any injection which upon visual inspection reveals particulate matter other than normally suspended material should be discarded.

Each individual monograph for the official injection states the type of container (single-dose and/or multiple-dose) permitted for the injection, the type of glass preferred for the container, exemptions, if any, to usual package-size limitations, and any special storage instructions. Most injections prepared from chemically pure medicinal agents are stable at room temperature and may be stored without special concern or conditions. However, most biological

which case a non-preserved single-dose preparation is advisable. The usual multiple-dose container contains about ten usual doses of the injection, but quantity may vary greatly with the individual preparation and manufacturer.

Because it is impossible in practice to transfer the entire volume of a single-dose container or the last dose in a multiple-dose container into a hypodermic syringe, a slight excess in volume of the contents of ampuls and vials over the labeled "size" or volume of the package is permitted. Table 8–2 presents the recommended "overages" permitted by the USP to allow the withdrawal and administration of the labeled volumes.

products—insulin injection and the various vaccines, toxoids, toxins, and related products—are usually stored under refrigeration. Reference should be made to the individual monograph to find the proper storage temperature for a particular injection.

Available Injections

There are hundreds of injections on the market of various medicinal agents. Tables 8–3 and 8–4 present some examples of those packaged in small-volume and large-volume containers, the latter for intravenous infusion.

Small Volume Parenterals

Table 8–3 presents some commonly employed injections given in small volume. Some of these injections are solutions and others suspensions.

Among the most used of the small volume injections are the various insulin preparations described below and presented in Table 8–5. Insulin, the active principle of the pancreas gland, is primarily concerned with the metabolism of carbohydrates, but also influences protein and fat metabolism. Insulin facilitates the cellular uptake of glucose and its metabolism in liver, muscle, and adipose tissue. It increases the uptake of amino acids and inhibits the breakdown of fats and the production of ketones. Insulin is administered to patients having abnormal or absent pancreatic beta cell function to restore glucose metabolism and maintain satisfactory carbohydrate, fat, and protein metabolism. It is used in the treatment of *diabetes mellitus,* in instances in which the condition cannot be controlled satisfactorily by dietary regulation alone or by oral hypoglycemic drugs. Insulin may also be used to improve the appetite and increase the weight in selected cases of nondiabetic malnutrition and is frequently added to intravenous infusions.

Insulin is administered by needle or jet injection (Figs. 8–27, 8–28, and 8–29). A system for the nasal administration of insulin is presently under study.[9]

Insulin Injection (Regular)

Insulin Injection is a sterile aqueous solution of insulin. Commercially, the solution is prepared from beef or pork pancreas or both or through biosynthetic means (Human Insulin), discussed in the next section. The source must be stated on the labeling. In 1980, purified pork insulin [Iletin II, pork (Lilly)] became available for individuals allergic to or otherwise adversely affected by the mixed pork-beef product. The first insulin developed for clinical use was an amorphous insulin. This type has since been replaced by a more purified crystalline insulin composed of zinc-insulin crystals which produces a clear aqueous solution. Until recently, insulin injection ("regular insulin") had been produced at a pH of 2.8 to 3.5. This was necessary, because particles formed in the vial when the pH was increased above the acid range. However, recent changes in the manufacturing methods resulting in the production of insulin of greater purity has allowed for the preparation of insulin injection having a neutral pH. The neutralized product has been shown to exhibit greater stability than the acidic product.

Insulin injection is prepared to contain 40, 100, or 500 USP Insulin Units in each mL.[10] The labeling must state the potency, in USP Insulin Units in each mL and the expiration date, which must not be later than 24 months after the date of distribution from the manufacturer's storage. As an added precaution against the inadvertent use of the incorrect strength of insulin by the patient during self-administration of the drug, the package colors vary, depending upon the strength of the insulin. For instance, all insulins (of the various types) containing 40 units per mL, have red in their package design, 100 units per mL have orange, and the 500 units per mL preparation has brown with diagonal white stripes. U-500 insulin is indicated for patients with a marked insulin requirement (more than 200 units per day) because a large unit/dose may be administered subcutaneously in a small volume.

Insulin injection is a colorless to straw-colored solution, depending upon its concentration; that containing 500 Units per mL is straw-colored. It is substantially free from turbidity. A small amount of glycerin (1.4 to 1.8%) is added for stability and 0.1 to 0.25% of either phenol or cresol is added for preservation. Insulin remains stable if stored in a cold place, preferably the refrigerator. Freezing should be avoided, as this reduces potency.

The various insulin preparations differ as to their rapidity of action (onset of action) after injection, their peak of action, and their duration of action (Table 8–5). Insulin injection, be-

Table 8–3. Examples of Some Injections Usually Packaged and Administered in Small Volume

Injection	Physical Form	Category and Comments
Aminophylline Injection	solution	Smooth muscle relaxant; usually administered as an IV admixture as a bronchodilator in treating asthma, emphysema, congestive heart failure and other conditions.
Butorphanol Tartrate Injection	solution	Narcotic Agonist-Antagonist Analgesic; administered IM or IV for relief of moderate to severe pain and as a preoperative or preanesthesia medication.
Cimetidine HCl Injection	solution	Histamine H_2 antagonist; administered IM or IV for patients with pathological hypersecretory conditions or intractable ulcers.
Dexamethasone Sodium Phosphate Injection	solution	Glucocorticoid; administered IM or IV for cerebral edema and unresponsive shock. Also used intra-articular, intralesional or soft tissue for joints, bursae, and ganglia.
Digoxin Injection	solution	Cardiotonic given IM or IV with highly individualized and monitored dosage.
Dihydroergotamine Mesylate Injection	solution	Alpha-adrenergic blocking agent specific in migraine, given IM or IV.
Furosemide Injection	solution	Loop diuretic; administered IM or IV [slowly] for edema or acute pulmonary edema.
Heparin Sodium Injection	solution	Anticoagulant administered IV or SubQ. as indicated by prothrombin time determination.
Histamine Phosphate Injection	solution	Diagnostic aid given SubQ. in the testing of gastric secretion capacity.
Hydromorphone HCl Injection	solution	Narcotic analgesic used for the relief of moderate to severe pain; administered subcutaneously or IM or by slow IV injection.
Interferon alpha-2a Injection	solution	A protein product prepared by recombinant-DNA technology. Indicated for use in the treatment of hairy cell leukemia in persons 18 years of age or older; administered subcutaneously or IM.
Isoproterenol HCl Injection	solution	Adrenergic (bronchodilator) given IM, SubQ., or IV.
Lidocaine HCl Injection	solution	Cardiac depressant given IV as an antiarrhythmic; also as a local anesthetic, epidurally, by infiltration, and in peripheral nerve block.
Magnesium Sulfate Injection	solution	Electrolyte; administered by IM or direct IV injection, IV infusion, or in other IV infusions for hyperalimentation therapy, mild magnesium deficiency, or severe hypomagnesemia.
Meperidine HCl Injection	solution	Narcotic analgesic given IM or SubQ.
Metoclopramide Monohydrochloride Injection	solution	Gastrointestinal stimulant; administered slowly as an IV admixture for the prevention of chemotherapy-induced emesis.
Morphine Sulfate Injection	solution	Narcotic analgesic.
Nalbuphine HCl Injection	solution	Narcotic Agonist-Antagonist Analgesic; administered SC, IM or IV for relief of moderate to severe pain and for preoperative analgesia.
Naloxone HCl Injection	solution	A narcotic antagonist which prevents or reverses the effects of opioids including respiratory depression, sedation and hypotension; administered IV, IM, or subcutaneously.
Oxytocin Injection	solution	Oxytocic, given IM or IV obstetrically for the therapeutic induction of labor.

Table 8–3.   Continued

Injection	Physical Form	Category and Comments
Phenytoin Sodium Injection	solution	Anticonvulsant; administered IM [erratic absorption] as a prophylactic dosage for neurosurgery or IV [slowly] for status epilepticus.
Phytonadione Injection	dispersion	Vitamin K (prothrombogenic) employed in hemorrhagic situations. An aqueous emulsion of phytonadione, a viscous liquid.
Procaine Penicillin G Injection	suspension	Anti-infective; administered IM for moderately severe infections due to penicillin-G sensitive microorganisms.
Prochlorperazine Edisylate Injection	solution	Antidopaminergic; administered IM or IV for control of severe nausea and vomiting associated with adult surgery.
Propranolol HCl Injection	solution	A beta-adrenergic receptor blocking agent indicated in the management of hypertension. Oral dosage (tablets) is usual; intravenous administration is reserved for life-threatening arrhythmias or those occurring under anesthesia.
Sodium Bicarbonate Injection	solution	Electrolyte; administered IV, either undiluted or diluted in other IV fluids for cardiac arrest and in less urgent forms of metabolic acidosis.
Verapamil HCl Injection	solution	Calcium channel blocking agent; administered as a slow IV injection over at least 2 minutes for supraventricular tachyarrhythmias

Table 8–4.   Examples of Some Injections Administered in Large Volume by Intravenous Infusion[1]

Injection	Usual Contents	Category and Comments
Dextrose Injection, USP	2.5, 5.0, 10, 20% dextrose, and other strengths	Fluid and nutrient replenisher.
Dextrose and Sodium Chloride Injection, USP	Dextrose varying from 2.5 to 25% and sodium chloride from 0.11 (19 mEq sodium) to 0.9% (154 mEq sodium)	Fluid, nutrient, and electrolyte replenisher.
Fructose Injection, USP	10% fructose	Fluid replenisher and nutrient.
Mannitol Injection, USP	5, 10, 15, 20 and 25% mannitol	Diagnostic aid in renal function determinations; diuretic.
Protein Hydrolysate Injection, USP	3.5, 5, 7, and 10% protein hydrolysate with or without varying proportions of dextrose, fructose, glycerin and electrolytes.	Fluid and nutrient replenisher.
Ringer's Injection, USP	0.86% sodium chloride, 0.03% potassium chloride, and 0.033% calcium chloride	Fluid and electrolyte replenisher.
Lactated Ringer's Injection, USP	2.7 mEq calcium, 4 mEq potassium, 130 mEq sodium and 2.45 g lactate per liter	Systemic alkalizer; fluid and electrolyte replenisher.
Sodium Chloride Injection, USP	0.9% sodium chloride	Fluid and electrolyte replenisher; isotonic vehicle.

[1]These solutions may be administered in volumes of 1 liter or more, alone, or with other drugs added.

Table 8–5. Insulin Preparations*

Product	Source	Strength, Insulin Units/mL	Onset	Peak (In Hours)	Duration
Regular Insulins					
Iletin I Regular (Lilly)	beef-pork	U-40, U-100	0.5–1	2–5	6–8
Regular (Squibb-Novo)	pork	U-40, U-100	0.5–1	2–5	6–8
Actrapid (Squibb-Novo)	pork	U-100	0.5–1	2–5	6–8
Velosulin (Nordisk)	pork	U-100	0.5–1	2–5	6–8
Iletin II Regular (Lilly)	pork	U-100, U-500	0.5–1	2–5	6–8
Iletin II Regular (Lilly)	beef	U-100	0.5–1	2–5	6–8
Humulin R (Lilly)	human†	U-100	0.5	2–4	6–8
Humulin BR [buffered, regular (Lilly)]	human	U-100	0.5	2–4	6–8
Novolin R (Squibb-Novo)	human, semisynthetic	U-100	0.5	2.5–5	8
Velosulin (Nordisk-USA)	pork	U-100	0.5	1–3	8
Zinc Suspension, Prompt					
Iletin I Semilente (Lilly)	beef-pork	U-40, U-100	1–2	3–8	10–16
Semitard (Squibb-Novo)	pork	U-100	0.5–1.5	2–10	12–16
Semilente (Squibb-Novo)	beef	U-100	0.5–1.5	2–10	12–16
Isophane Suspension (NPH)					
Iletin I NPH (Lilly)	beef-pork	U-40, U-100	1–2	6–12	18–26
NPH (Squibb-Novo)	beef	U-40, U-100	1–1.5	8–12	24
NPH (Squibb-Novo)	pork	U-100	1–1.5	4–12	24
Iletin II NPH (Lilly)	pork	U-100	1–2	6–12	18–26
Iletin II NPH (Lilly)	beef	U-100	1–2	6–12	18–26
Insulatard (Nordisk)	pork	U-100	1–1.5	8–12	24
Humulin N (Lilly)	human†	U-100		see below‡	
Novolin N (Squibb-Novo)	human, semisynthetic	U-100	1.5	4–12	24
Insulatard, human (Nordisk-USA)	human, semisynthetic	U-100	1.5	4–12	24
Isophane/Regular					
Mixtard (Nordisk)	pork	U-100	0.5–1		24
Novolin 70/30 (Squibb-Novo)	human	U-100	0.5–1	2–12	24
Zinc Suspension (Lente)					
Iletin I Lente (Lilly)	beef-pork	U-40, U-100	1–3	6–12	18–26
Lente (Squibb-Novo)	beef	U-40, U-100	1–2.5	8–12	24
Lentard (Squibb-Novo)	beef-pork	U-100	1–2.5	8–12	24
Monotard (Squibb-Novo)	pork	U-100	1–2.5	8–12	24
Iletin II Lente (Lilly)	pork	U-100	1–3	6–12	18–26
Iletin II Lente (Lilly)	beef	U-100	1–3	6–12	18–26
Humulin L (Lilly)	human	U-100	1–3	6–12	18–24
Novolin L (Squibb-Novo)	human, semisynthetic	U-100	2.5	4–15	22
Protamine Zinc Suspension					
Iletin I PZI (Lilly)	beef-pork	U-40, U-100	4–6	14–24	26–36
Iletin II PZI (Lilly)	pork	U-100	4–6	14–24	26–36
Iletin II PZI (Lilly)	beef	U-100	4–6	14–24	26–36
Zinc Suspension, Extended					
Iletin I Ultralente (Lilly)	beef-pork	U-40, U-100	4–6	14–24	28–36
Ultralente (Squibb-Novo)	beef	U-100	4–8	10–30	36
Ultratard (Squibb-Novo)	beef	U-100	4–8	10–30	36

*Adapted from Drug Information Newsletter, vol. 13, No. 4, 1987, Drug Information Center, Pharmacy Department, and Department of Pharmacology, Medical College of Georgia, and College of Pharmacy, University of Georgia.

†Recombinant DNA origin.

‡Human insulin may have a slightly faster onset of action and somewhat shorter duration of action than others in group.

Fig. 8–27. *The Medi-Jector II, an example of a jet injection device. The jet injection method utilizes pressure rather than a needle in providing the subcutaneous distribution of an injectable medication. The device shown can be used with U-100 insulin or a combination of insulins and can deliver 2 to 100 units in half-unit increments. (Courtesy of Derata Corporation.)*

Fig. 8–28. *Examples of insulin syringes calibrated in Units. (Courtesy of Becton, Dickinson and Company.)*

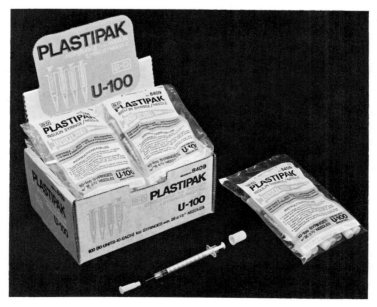

Fig. 8–29. *Example of packaging of disposable sterile insulin syringes and needles. (Courtesy of Becton, Dickinson and Company.)*

ing a solution, is categorized as a prompt-acting insulin preparation. Insulin preparations that are suspensions are slower acting. Only insulin injection may be administered intravenously; all others, as well as insulin injection, are normally given subcutaneously, usually ½ to 2 hours before a meal so that its physiological effects will parallel the absorption of glucose. The dosage is individually determined, with the usual dosage range being 5 to 100 USP Units. The insulin injection containing 500 units per mL is employed in insulin coma therapy and in cases of insulin resistance requiring very large doses.

It is important to emphasize at this point that the pharmacist plays a vital role in the education of the diabetic patient, particularly as it relates to the proper use of insulin. The insulin dosage should always be checked to ensure it is correct. Because it is a solution, Regular Insulin can be used in emergency situations, i.e., ketoacidosis, to effect a rapid decrease in blood glucose levels. However, with the exception of diabetic ketoacidosis, it is rare for a patient to ever require a dose of Regular Insulin greater than 25 units. Typically, diabetic patients combine Regular Insulin with a modified insulin, i.e., NPH, to provide daily coverage using two injections, i.e., morning, late-afternoon. So it is important that the patient understand how much of each to use and know in what order these should be mixed in the insulin syringe. The unmodified insulin, i.e., Regular Insulin, is drawn up first into the syringe.

In an institutional setting the pharmacist must make sure written insulin orders are correctly transcribed or transmitted. Errors in insulin dosage have occurred because of allied health professional error. Written orders for 6 U of insulin have been interpreted to mean 60 units, an order for 4 U has been read as 4 cc. Each of these occurred because the abbreviation "U" for units was read as a zero or a cc.

The patient should be instructed to rotate the site of insulin injections on a continual basis. Rotation of the site will help to avoid the development of lipohypertrophy, a buildup of fibrous tissue. Otherwise, if there is continual injection into one site, the tissue becomes spongy and avascular. The avascular nature of the site perpetuates the problem because the skin becomes anesthetized and the injection is not felt. This is a particular problem with children who continue to use the same site and do not realize that the absorption of insulin from this site becomes erratic and uncontrollable. Numerous brochures are available from manufacturers of diabetic supplies that demonstrate the appropriate rotation of insulin injection sites over the entire body.

Another encountered problem with insulin injection is the development of lipodystrophy. Generally, this problem appears within 2 months to 2 years following the beginning of insulin therapy and occurs predominantly in women and children. The etiology of the problem has been ascribed to the injection of refrigerated insulin (not giving enough time for it to warm up prior to injection), to a failure to rotate the injection site and to insulin impurities. The result is the formation of a subcutaneous indentation or "pothole" caused by a wasting or atrophy of the lipid tissue. It appears that the greater purity of current insulins significantly have decreased this problem, and a marked improvement in existing atrophic areas has been demonstrated by the injection of highly purified pork or human insulin directly into or on the periphery of the atrophic areas.

Prior to use, the patient should be instructed to carefully inspect the insulin. Regular Insulin, a solution should appear clear, while the other insulins which are suspensions should appear cloudy. With the insulins that are suspensions the patient should be instructed how to prepare the insulin, i.e., the vial is rotated slowly between the palms of the hands several times, prior to drawing the insulin into the syringe. This avoids frothing and bubble formation which would result in an inaccurate dose of insulin. The patient should not shake the insulin vial.

Proper storage should also be encouraged for insulins. These preparations should be stored in a cool place or a refrigerator. The patient should be warned to avoid having the insulin come into contact with extremes of temperature, i.e., freezing [overnight in the car during the wintertime], heat [glove compartment of a car, direct sunlight]. If this occurs, it is preferred that the patient discard the insulin and get a new bottle. Any bottle of insulin that appears "frosted" or "clumped" should be returned to the pharmacy where the purchase took place. Lastly, the patient should use the insulin in a timely fashion, but not beyond the expiration date indicated on the insulin vial.

Human Insulin

Biosynthetic human insulin was the first drug product developed through recombinant DNA techniques to receive approval by the federal Food and Drug Administration for marketing. This product, HUMULIN, Lilly, became available in 1983. It is produced by utilizing a special nondisease-forming laboratory strain of *Escherichia coli* and recombinant DNA technology. A recombined plasmid DNA coding for human insulin is introduced into the bacteria, and it is then cultured by fermentation to produce the A and B chains of human insulin. These A and B chains are freed and purified individually before they are linked by the specific disulfide bridges to form human insulin. The insulin produced is chemically, physically, and immunologically equivalent to insulin derived from the human pancreas. The biosynthetic insulin is free of contamination with *E. coli* peptides, and, is also free of the pancreatic peptides that are present as impurities in insulin preparations derived from animal pancreatic extraction. These latter impurities include proinsulin and proinsulin intermediates, glucagon, somatostatin, pancreatic polypeptide, and vasoactive intestinal peptide.

Pharmacokinetic studies in some normal subjects and clinical observations in patients indicate that formulations of human insulin have a slightly faster onset of action and a slightly shorter duration of action than their purified pork insulin counterparts. Two formulations of human insulin were initially marketed: Neutral Regular Human Insulin (HUMULIN R, Lilly) and NPH Human Insulin (HUMULIN N, Lilly). Other forms have since been added as shown in Table 8–5. Semisynthetic human insulin (e.g. NOVOLIN R, Squibb-Novo) is structurally identical to the insulin produced by the human pancreas. A naturally occurring enzyme is used as a process that converts pork insulin into human insulin. By this enzymatic transpeptidation process the amino acid alanine in pork insulin is selectively substituted by the amino acid threonine thus forming the human insulin molecule. Neutral Regular human insulin consists of zinc-insulin crystals in solution. It has a rapid onset-of-action and a relatively short duration-of-action (6 to 8 hours). NPH human insulin is a turbid preparation that is intermediate-acting, with a slower onset-of-action and longer duration-of-action (slightly less than 24 hours) than regular human insulin.

Human insulins should be stored as other insulins, in a cold place, preferably a refrigerator. Freezing should be avoided.

Isophane Insulin Suspension (NPH Insulin)

Isophane Insulin Suspension is a sterile suspension, in an aqueous vehicle buffered with dibasic sodium phosphate to between pH 7.1 and 7.4, of insulin prepared from zinc-insulin crystals modified by the addition of protamine so that the solid phase of the suspension consists of crystals composed of insulin, zinc, and protamine. Protamine is prepared from the sperm or the mature testes of fish belonging to the genus *Oncorhynchus* and others. As mentioned earlier during the discussion of the aqueous insulin solutions, suspensions of insulin with a pH on the alkaline side are inherently of a longer duration of action than those preparations that are solutions. Insulin is most insoluble at pH 7.2.

The rod-shaped crystals of isophane insulin suspension should be approximately 30 micrometers in length and the suspension free from large aggregates of crystals following moderate agitation. This is necessary for the insulin suspension to pass freely within the needle used in injection and for the absorption of the drug from the site of injection to be consistent from one manufactured batch of injection to another. When a portion of the suspension is examined microscopically, the suspended matter is largely crystalline with only traces of amorphous material. The official injection is required to contain glycerin and phenol for stability and preservation. The specified expiration date occurring in the labeling is 24 months after the immediate container was filled by the manufacturer. The suspension is packaged in multiple-dose containers having not less than 10 mL of injection. Each mL of the injection contains

40 or 100 units of insulin per mL of suspension. The suspension is best stored in a refrigerator, but freezing must be avoided.

As indicated earlier, isophane insulin suspension is an intermediate-acting insulin preparation administered as required mainly as hormonal replacement in diabetes mellitus. The usual dosage range subcutaneously is 10 to 80 USP Units.

The "NPH" used in some product names stands for "Neutral Protamine Hagedorn," since the preparation is about neutral (pH about 7.2), contains protamine, and was developed by Hagedorn. The term "isophane" is based on the Greek: *iso* and *phane*, meaning "equal" and "appearance" and refers to the equivalent balance between the protamine and insulin.

Insulin Zinc Suspension

Insulin for Insulin Zinc Suspension is modified by the addition of zinc chloride so that the suspended particles consist of a mixture of crystalline and amorphous insulin in a ratio of approximately 7 parts of crystals to 3 parts of amorphous material. The sterile suspension is in an aqueous vehicle buffered to pH 7.2 to 7.5 with sodium acetate. In treating insulin with zinc chloride, it is possible to obtain both crystalline and amorphous zinc insulin. The amorphous form has the most prompt hypoglycemic effect, since the particles are the smallest and are absorbed into the system more rapidly after subcutaneous injection than are the zinc insulin crystals. Also, the larger the crystals the less prompt and the longer-acting will be the insulin suspension. By combining the crystalline and amorphous forms into one preparation, an intermediate-acting suspension is obtained. As noted in Table 8–5, the time-activity of insulin zinc suspension is only slightly different than that for isophane insulin suspension. The advantage of the former is that no additional foreign protein (other than the insulin) is present, such as protamine, which may produce local sensitivity reactions. Also, it may be combined as desired with either of the following two suspensions to produce an insulin preparation having the time-activity characteristics that most closely meet the desires and requirements of the individual patient. Suspensions available contain 40 and 100 USP Insulin Units per mL packaged in 10-mL vials. The individual crystalline and amorphous particles may be seen microscopically, with the crystals being predomi-

nantly between 10 to 40 μm in maximum dimension and the amorphous particles no greater than 2 μm in maximum dimension.

In addition to the sodium acetate as a buffer, the suspension contains about 0.7% sodium chloride for tonicity and 0.10% methylparaben for preservation. The expiration date of the suspension is 24 months after the immediate container was filled. The suspension must be stored in a refrigerator with freezing being avoided. As with all such preparations, the dose depends upon the individual needs of the patient, but generally ranges between 10 and 80 USP Units.

Extended Insulin Zinc Suspension

Extended insulin zinc suspension is a sterile suspension of zinc insulin crystals in an aqueous medium buffered to between pH 7.2 and 7.5 with sodium acetate. Present also are 0.7% sodium chloride for tonicity and 0.1% methylparaben for preservation. Because the suspended matter is composed solely of zinc insulin crystals, which are slowly absorbed, this preparation is classified as a long-acting insulin preparation. Because of the compatibility between the preparations, this suspension may be mixed with either insulin zinc suspension or prompt insulin zinc suspension to achieve the proper time-activity requirements of an individual patient. The usual dosage range is 10 to 80 USP Units. The suspension is commercially available in 10-mL vials providing either 40 or 100 USP Insulin Units per mL. The suspension must be stored in a refrigerator with freezing being avoided. Under proper storage conditions, the expiration date of the injection is not later than 24 months after the immediate container was filled.

Prompt Insulin Zinc Suspension

The sterile suspension of insulin in Prompt Insulin Zinc Suspension is modified by the addition of zinc chloride so that the solid phase of the suspension is amorphous. The maximum dimension of the shapeless particles of zinc insulin must not exceed 2 micrometers. The suspension is available in 40 or 100 USP Insulin Units per mL in vials of 10 mL. This preparation has the same pH and additives as extended insulin zinc suspension, and they may be mixed as desired to achieve a preparation having the desired time-activity characteristics. This is a rapid-acting insulin preparation. It must be stored in a refrigerator and not permitted to freeze. Its expiration date is not greater than 24 months after the immediate container was filled.

Protamine Zinc Insulin Suspension

Protamine Zinc Insulin Suspension is a sterile suspension of insulin modified by the addition of zinc chloride and protamine. Because of a larger proportion of both zinc and protamine in this preparation, it has a much less prompt onset of action and a longer duration of action than does isophane insulin suspension, which also contains zinc and protamine. This suspension is stabilized and preserved with about 1.6% of glycerin and either 0.20% of cresol or 0.25% of phenol. It is packaged in containers having either 40 or 100 USP Units per mL. It has an expiration date of not later than 24 months after the immediate container was filled.

Insulin Infusion Pumps

Newly developed insulin infusion pumps allow patients to achieve and maintain blood glucose at near-normal levels on a *constant basis.* Continuous infusion of insulin through use of these pumps eliminates the need for the patient to self-administer daily injections of insulin. This provides patient convenience, better patient compliance, and control over the disease. The main objective of pump therapy is the strict control of the blood glucose level between 70 to 140 mg/dl. This is the primary way to avoid complications in diabetic patients, such as gangrene and diabetic retinopathy.

Early insulin infusion pumps were large bedside units, used mainly in hospitals. Today, portable, battery-operated, and programmable units are available. These systems utilize microcomputers to regulate the flow of insulin from a syringe attached to a catheter (usually 18 gauge) connected to a 27- to 28-gauge needle inserted in the patient. The insulin may be delivered subcutaneously, intravenously, or intraperitoneally.

Patients who use infusion pumps for the continuous subcutaneous administration of insulin may develop hard nodules at the site of injection. Some patients may demonstrate nodules that are tender, develop a rock-hard consistency, and take several months to subside. Although the cause of this nodule formation is unknown, a change in insulin may be beneficial. Speculation as to the cause centers around the development of local trauma or hematoma formation with a subsequent local inflammatory response, stimulation of fibroblast replacement, or dystrophic calcification. The need to rotate sites of injection on a several day basis cannot be overemphasized. For additional information on infusion pumps, the reader is directed to the footnote reference at the end of this chapter.[11]

Large Volume Parenterals (LVP's)

Common examples of large volume parenterals in use today are presented in Table 8–4. These solutions are generally administered by intravenous infusion to replenish body fluids, electrolytes, or to provide nutrition. They are usually administered in volumes of 100 mL to liter amounts and more per day by slow intravenous drip with or without controlled-rate infusion systems (Fig. 8–30). Because of the large volumes administered, these solutions must not contain bacteriostatic agents or other pharmaceutical additives. They are packaged in large single-dose containers (Figs. 8–31 and 8–32).

As indicated previously, therapeutic additives as electrolytes, vitamins, and antineoplastics are frequently incorporated into large volume parenterals for coadministration to the patient. It is the responsibility of the pharmacist to be knowledgeable of the physical and chemical compatibility of the additive in the solution in which it is placed. Obviously, an incompatible combination which results in the formation of insoluble material or which affects the efficacy or potency of the therapeutic agent of the vehicle is not acceptable.

Large volume parenteral solutions are employed in *maintenance therapy* for the patient entering or recovering from surgery, or for the patient who is unconscious and unable to obtain fluids, electrolytes, and nutrition orally. The solutions may also be utilized in *replacement therapy* in patients who have suffered a heavy loss of fluid and electrolytes.

MAINTENANCE THERAPY. When a patient is being maintained on parenteral fluids for only several days, simple solutions providing adequate amounts of water, dextrose, and small amounts of sodium and potassium generally suffice. When patients are unable to take oral nutrition or fluids for slightly longer periods, say 3 to 6 days, solutions of higher caloric content may be used. In instances in which oral feeding must be deferred for periods of weeks or longer, total parenteral nutrition must be implemented to provide all of the essential nutrients to minimize

Fig. 8–30. *Accurate delivery of intravenous fluids and medications by use of a controlled rate infusion system (CRIS) for the drug vial and a volumetric infusion pump for the intravenous fluids. (Courtesy of Eli Lilly and Company.)*

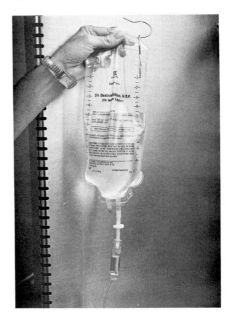

Fig. 8–31. *Intravenous solution packaged in pliable plastic.*

Fig. 8–32. *Examples of peritoneal dialysis and irrigation fluids.*

tissue break-down and to maintain normalcy within the body. Total nutrient admixtures (TNA) include all substrates necessary for nutritional support, e.g., carbohydrates, protein, fat, electrolytes, trace elements, that are usually mixed in a single plastic intravenous bag for more convenient administration. When using TNA, the pharmacist must consider the order of substrate mixing, differentiate between various brands of substrate and their physical-chemical properties, determine the type of plastic bag system that is most appropriate to use, determine whether (and by what mode) the TNA should be filtered prior to infusion, determine how the product should be stored, and assess any potential complications that might arise with the use of this method of administering nutritional products. For example, the use of "standard" total parenteral nutrition plastic bags may result in the leaching out of plasticizer into the solution, and be potentially injurious to the patient.

REPLACEMENT THERAPY. In instances in which there is a heavy loss of water and electrolytes, as in severe diarrhea or vomiting, greater than usual amounts of these materials may be initially administered and then maintenance therapy provided.

WATER REQUIREMENT. In normal individuals, the daily water requirement is that amount needed to replace normal and expected losses. Water is lost daily in the urine, feces, skin and from respiration. The normal daily requirement of water for adults is about 25 to 40 mL/kg of body weight, or an average of about 2,000 mL per square meter of body surface area.[12] Nomograms for the determination of body surface area from body height and weight are presented in Chapter 2, Figure 2–7. Children and small adults need more water per pound of body weight than do larger adults; water requirements correlate more closely with body surface area than with weight. However, in the newborn, the volume administered in the first week or two should be about half that calculated from body surface area.

In water replacement therapy for adults, 70 mL of water per kg per day may be required in addition to the maintenance water requirements; a badly dehydrated infant may require even a greater proportion.[12] Thus, a 50-kg patient may require 3500 mL for replacement plus 2400 mL for maintenance. In order to avoid the consequences of fluid overload, especially in elderly patients, and those with renal or cardiovascular disorders, monitoring of blood pressure is desirable.

Because water administered intravenously as such may cause the osmotic hemolysis of red blood cells, and, since a patient who requires water generally requires nutrition and/or electrolytes, the parenteral administration of water is generally as a solution with dextrose or electrolytes in which the solution has sufficient tonicity (sodium chloride equivalency) to protect the red blood cells from hemolyzing.

ELECTROLYTE REQUIREMENT. Potassium, the primary intracellular cation, is particularly important for normal cardiac and skeletal muscle function. The usual daily intake of potassium is about 100 mEq and the usual daily loss is about 40 mEq. Thus, any replacement therapy should include a minimum of 40 mEq plus the amount needed to replace additional losses. Potassium can be lost through excessive perspiration, repeated enemas, trauma (such as severe burns), uncontrolled diabetes, diseases of the intestinal tract, surgical operations, and the use of such medications as thiazide diuretics. People who suffer from poor nutrition, those using very low-calorie diet products, and victims of anorexia nervosa or acute alcoholism also may have low potassium levels, i.e., hypokalemia, because they are not taking in enough of the mineral. Symptoms of potassium loss include a weak pulse, faint heart sounds, falling blood pressure, and generalized weakness. Severe loss of potassium can lead to death. Too much potassium is not a good thing, either. An excess may cause diarrhea, irritability, muscle cramps, and pain. Hyperkalemia can be caused by kidney failure or consuming excess amounts of potassium-rich foods. Prescribed potassium supplements, potassium-sparing diuretic therapy, and the indiscriminate use of over-the-counter salt-substitute products have also been implicated to induce hyperkalemia.

In cases of severe potassium deficiency, electrolyte replacement through the intravenous administration of potassium is usually employed. The pharmacist who receives a prescription for intravenous potassium chloride must be careful and check the amount of potassium chloride in the prescription and the infusion rate at which the drug is to be administered to the patient. The usual additive dilution of potassium chloride is 40 mEq/liter of intravenous fluid. The maximum desirable concentration is 80 mEq/liter of potassium chloride, although severe emergencies may dictate greater concentrations. The maximum infusion rate should not exceed 40 mEq per hour with a maximum 24-hour dose not exceeding 400 mEq of potassium chloride. Because of its potent ECG effects, when infused it is wise to monitor the patient's ECG, and to check the patient's serum potassium level after the first 50 to 100 mEq of potassium chloride are administered.

Sodium, the principal extracellular cation, is vital to maintain normal extracellular fluids. Average daily intake of sodium is 135 to 170 mEq (8 to 10 g of sodium chloride). The body is able to conserve sodium when this ion is lost or removed from the diet. When there is sodium loss or a deficit, the daily administration of 3 to 5 g of sodium chloride (51 to 85 mEq of sodium) should prevent a negative sodium balance.[12] A low sodium level in the body may result from excessive sweating, the use of certain diuretics, or diarrhea. Fatigue, muscle weakness, apprehension, and convulsions are among the symptoms of excessive sodium loss. Sodium concentrations can increase when a person does not drink enough water, especially in hot weather, or if kidney function is impaired. Dry, sticky mucous membranes, flushed skin, elevated body temperature, lack of tears, and thirst are among the symptoms of sodium excess. In about 20% of individuals who suffer from high blood pressure, sodium has been implicated as a causative factor. Chloride, the principal anion of the extracellular fluid is usually paired with sodium. Chloride is also important for muscle contraction, balancing the fluid levels inside and outside the cells, and maintaining the acid-base balance of the extracellular fluid. An adequate supply of chloride is necessary to prevent bicarbonate, the second most prevalent anion, from tipping the acid-base balance to the alkaline side. (In 1979, a lack of chloride in a brand of infant formula caused metabolic alkalosis in babies who had been exclusively fed that formula. As a result of this episode, Congress passed the Infant Formula Act of 1980, which spells out the nutrients that must be in formulas and establishes quality control procedures for the manufacture of these infant foods.) Although other electrolytes and minerals as calcium, magnesium, and iron are lost from the body, they generally are not required during short-term parenteral therapy.

CALORIC REQUIREMENTS. Generally patients requiring parenteral fluids are given 5% dextrose to reduce the caloric deficit that usually occurs in patients undergoing maintenance or replacement therapy. The use of dextrose also minimizes ketosis and the breakdown of protein. Basic caloric requirements may be estimated by body weight; in the fasting state, the average daily loss of body protein is approximately 80 g/day for a 70 kg man. Daily ingestion of at least 100 g of glucose reduces this loss by half.

PARENTERAL HYPERALIMENTATION. This is the infusion of large amounts of basic nutrients sufficient to achieve active tissue synthesis and growth. It is employed in the long-term intravenous feeding of protein solutions containing high concentrations of dextrose (approximately 20%), electrolytes, vitamins, and in some instances insulin. Among the components utilized in parenteral nutrition solutions are the following, listed in quantities commonly provided per liter of fluid. The individual components and amounts administered to a patient would vary depending upon the patient's needs.

Electrolytes:

Sodium	25 mEq
Potassium	20 mEq
Magnesium	5 mEq
Calcium	5 mEq
Chloride	30 mEq
Acetate	25 mEq
Phosphate	18 mM

Vitamins:

Vitamin A	3300 I.U.
Vitamin D	200 I.U.
Vitamin E	10 I.U.
Vitamin C	100 mg
Niacin	40 mg
Vitamin B_2	3.6–4.93 mg
Vitamin B_1	3–3.35 mg
Vitamin B_6	4–4.86 mg
Pantothenic Acid	15 mg
Folic Acid	400 mcg
Vitamin B_{12}	5 mcg
Biotin	60 mcg

Amino Acids: Essential Amino Acids

L-Isoleucine	590 mg
L-Leucine	770 mg
L-Lysine acetate	870 mg
(free base	620 mg)
L-Methionine	450 mg
L-Phenylalanine	480 mg
L-Threonine	340 mg
L-Tryptophan	130 mg
L-Valine	560 mg

Nonessential Amino Acids

L-Alanine	600 mg
L-Arginine	810 mg
L-Histidine	240 mg
L-Proline	950 mg

L-Serine   500 mg
Aminoacetic Acid   1.19 g

The large proportion of dextrose increases the caloric value of the solution, while keeping the volume required to be administered to a minimum. The solutions are administered slowly through a large vein, such as the superior vena cava. The superior vena cava is accessed through the subclavian vein, which is located immediately beneath the clavicle and near to the heart. This permits the rapid dilution of the concentrated hyperalimentation fluid and minimizes the risk of tissue or cellular damage due to the hypertonicity of the solution.

The following abbreviations may be used in the hospital in describing the desired order for parenteral nutrition:

TCPN (Total Central Parenteral Nutrition)
PCPN (Partial Central Parenteral Nutrition)
TPPN (Total Peripheral Parenteral Nutrition)

PPPN (Partial Peripheral Parenteral Nutrition)

ENTERAL NUTRITION. As appropriate, hospitalized and home care patients may be provided their nutritional needs through *enteral* rather than *parenteral* means. Enteral nutrition utilizes nasogastric, gastrostomy and transpyloric routes for the feeding of nutritional support products. These products are formulated to contain a variety of vitamins, minerals, carbohydrates, proteins, fats and caloric requirements to meet the specific needs of patients. While parenteral feeding is appropriate for short-term use in a hospital or long-term care facility, or when the gastrointestinal tract is unable to absorb nutrients, enteral feeding is preferable whenever possible. It is just as effective as a source of nutrients, less expensive than parenteral feeding, and has a low potential to cause serious complications.

Specific enteral products are selected according to the patient type they serve. For example,

Table 8–6. Preparations for Blood Replenishment

Preparation	Description
Whole Blood	Whole human blood is blood that has been drawn from selected human donors under rigid aseptic precautions. It contains citrate ion or heparin as an anticoagulant. The collected blood is stored at temperatures between 1°C and 10°C, held constant within a 2°C range. The expiration date is not later than 21 days after the date of collection when citrate ion is used as the anticoagulant and not greater than 48 hours if heparin is used. The blood is usually contained in 1 unit (500 mL) volumes and administered by intravenous infusion first making certain of the compatibility of the donor's and recipient's blood.
Red Blood Cells	This is whole human blood from which the plasma has been removed. The plasma may be removed from the cells by centrifugation within 6 days following the collection of the whole human blood. The blood cells are stored at the same temperatures as whole human blood, or they may be stored frozen at −65°C. The frozen blood may be stored for as long as 3 years but must be used within 24 hours following removal from the freezing temperature and placement in 1°C to 10°C conditions.
Human Albumin	This is a sterile preparation of serum albumin obtained by fractionating blood from healthy human donors. Not less than 96% of the protein must be albumin. It is a solution containing in each 100 mL either 25 g of serum albumin osmotically equivalent to 500 mL of normal human plasma, or 5 g equivalent to 100 mL of normal human plasma. It is administered as a blood-volume supporter by intravenous infusion, generally in volumes equivalent to 25 to 75 g of albumin daily. The expiration date ranges from 3 to 10 years, depending upon the conditions of storage.
Plasma Protein Fraction	This is a sterile solution of selected proteins derived from the blood plasma of adult human donors. It contains approximately 5 g of protein per 100 mL of which 83 to 90% is albumin, the remainder is alpha and beta globulins. It is generally administered in volumes of 250 to 500 mL (sometimes up to 1500 mL) as a blood volume supporter. Its expiration date is between 3 and 5 years, depending upon conditions of storage.

a requirement for less than 2000 calories per day, or increased protein typically involves an elderly, bedfast patient who is not physically active. This level of support is also advocated for postsurgical patients, and those who suffer from infection or fractured bones. While requiring fewer calories, these individuals still need normal nutrients, including protein. Such products as Ensure HN, Sustacal, and Osmolite HN are appropriate in this circumstance. Alternatively, most persons fall within the 2000 to 3000 calorie per day category, inclusive of patients with poor appetite or those suffering from cancer. The last category of patients are those with daily caloric needs which exceed 3000 calories. These individuals usually have high protein losses from severe trauma, e.g., burns, sepsis, multiple trauma. As in the first example there are numerous products for the latter two patient categories.

The pharmacist can be helpful in the selection of these products because these do differ in the amount of their carbohydrate, fat, and protein content, and in fiber. Further, these products differ in taste and consumer acceptability criteria, e.g., "mouth feel," cost. Pharmacists may encounter consumers who wish to self-administer an enteral product. If the intent is to supplement calories or protein in an otherwise healthy individual who simply wishes to assure a balanced dietary intake, a complete formula can be recommended. However, if it is intended to help a person regain weight which has been lost unexpectedly, the individual should be instead referred to a doctor. Sudden weight loss may indicate a serious pathologic problem requiring medical attention.

BLOOD REPLENISHMENT PREPARATIONS. Table 8–6 describes the official products used in the replenishment of blood, namely whole human blood, human red blood cells, normal human serum albumin, and human plasma protein fraction. In collecting human blood from donors for the purpose of preparing transfusions of the whole blood or the blood cells, care must be taken to prevent the blood from clotting. The following official solutions are used for this purpose.

Anticoagulant Citrate Dextrose Solution, USP (ACD Solution)

Anticoagulant citrate dextrose solution is a sterile solution of citric acid, sodium citrate, and dextrose in water for injection. The solution is prepared by dissolving the ingredients, filtering the solution until clear, and then transferring the liquid to suitable containers and sterilizing. The final product must be pyrogen free. It may not contain bacteriostatic agents.

Two formulas are given in the USP for the preparation of the solution and are designated Solution A and Solution B:

	Solution A	Solution B
Citric Acid	7.3 g	4.4 g
Sodium Citrate (dihydrate)	22.0 g	13.2 g
Dextrose (monohydrate)	24.5 g	14.7 g
Water for Injection, a sufficient quantity to make	1000 mL	1000 mL

Solution B contains the ingredients in approximately the same ratio as Solution A, but is only about 60% as concentrated. In practice, either 75 mL of Solution A or 125 mL of Solution B are employed in the preservation of 500 mL of whole blood. When the solution is packaged, the label must indicate the number of mL required per 100 mL of blood.

The solution prevents the coagulation of blood by virtue of the citrate ion's ability to bind the calcium ions of the blood to form a nonionizing calcium citrate complex, thereby preventing the calcium ions from participating in the clotting mechanism which is rendered ineffective by its absence. The dextrose adds sufficient tonicity to the solution to prevent the osmotic hemolysis of the erythrocytes during storage.

The solution is commercially available prepackaged in transfusion bottles that are only partially filled by the solution. For example, a 500-mL bottle containing 100 mL of Solution B would be suitable for the entry and preservation of 400 mL of whole blood. During collection, the blood-solution mixture is swirled gently and stored continuously in a refrigerator perferably between 1° and 10°C. Under these conditions blood may be stored safely for 21 days (Fig. 8–33). Prior to its administration as a blood transfusion, the mixture is made uniform by gentle swirling and is then injected intravenously without warming, using sterile equipment.

Anticoagulant Citrate Phosphate Dextrose Solution (CPD Solution)

This is a sterile solution of citric acid, sodium citrate, sodium biphosphate and dextrose in water for injection. It is used in the proportion

Fig. 8–33. *Blood storage in the blood bank.*

of 70 mL of solution for each 500 mL of whole blood as an anticoagulant. This solution is less acid than the ACD solution (pH 5 to 6 for CPD vs. pH 4.5 to 5.5 for ACD) and this is thought to be of some advantage in preserving the red blood cell. The solution is also more nearly isotonic to the red blood cell and is considered better able to maintain the red cell membrane under physiological conditions. An additional solution, Anticoagulant Citrate Phosphate Dextrose Adenine Solution, is official in the USP. Adenine is present for the purpose of prolonging the survival rate of erythrocytes during storage and following transfusion.

Anticoagulant Heparin Solution

Heparin sodium is used in the preparation of this anticoagulant solution. Heparin sodium is a mixture of active principles having the property of prolonging the clotting of blood. The substance is usually obtained from the lungs, intestinal mucosa or other suitable tissues of animals used for food by man. The potency of heparin is based on USP Heparin Units and must meet the requirements of not less than 120 such units per mg when derived from lungs and 140 such units per mg when derived from other tissues. The anticoagulant heparin solution contains 2250 Units per 30 mL, the amount of so-lution required to stabilize each 500 mL of whole blood.

Biologics

In pharmacy, the broad term *biologics* refers to such pharmaceutical products as vaccines, toxins, toxoids, antitoxins, immune serums, blood derivatives, immunologic diagnostic aids, and other related preparations. The usual intent of the term is to describe materials of biologic origin having *immunologic* effects. In the modern context, immunologic agents may be of biologic and non-biologic origin, as cyclosporine. With current immunologic research and combined with the new biotechnologies, many new immunologic agents will be forthcoming in the future. There is some interest in abandoning the term "biologics" in favor of the term "immunologics."[13] The term "immunobiologics" includes both antigenic substances, as vaccines and toxoids, and antibody-containing preparations, as globulins and antitoxins, from human or animal donors. For the most part, biologics are administered by injection (a notable exception being the oral type of polio vaccine), and for this reason they are presented in this chapter.

Biologics are produced by manufacturers licensed to do so in accordance with the terms of the federal Public Health Service Act of 1944, and each product must meet the specified standards of the Bureau of Biologics of the federal Food and Drug Administration. Generally, each lot of a biologic product must pass rigid control requirements before it may be distributed for general use.

Biologics intended to be administered by injection are packaged and labeled in the same manner as other injections. In addition, however, the label of a biological product must include the name under which the product is licensed under the Public Health Service Act; the name, address, and license number of the manufacturer; the lot number; the expiration date; the recommended individual dose for multiple-dose containers; the preservative used and the amount; the amount of product in the container; the recommended storage temperature; and any other necessary information to assure the safe and effective use of the product.

With a few exceptions most biologics are stored in a refrigerator at between 2° C and 8° C, and freezing is avoided. In many instances it is

Table 8–7. Examples of Official Biologic Products

Biologic Product	Nature of Contents	Route of Administration[1]	Use
Vaccines and Vaccine Combinations			
BCG Vaccine, USP	Dried, living culture of the bacillus Calmette-Guerin strain of *Mycobacterium tuberculosis* var. *bovis*.	Intradermal	Active immunizing agent (tuberculosis)
Cholera Vaccine, USP	Suspension of killed cholera vibrios *(Vibrio comma)*.	Subcutaneous or intramuscular	Active immunizing agent
Diphtheria and Tetanus Toxoids and Pertussis Vaccine, USP	Suspension of killed pertussis bacilli *(Bordetella pertussis)* in a mixture of diphtheria toxoid and tetanus toxoid.	Subcutaneous or intramuscular	Active immunizing agent
Diphtheria and Tetanus Toxoids and Pertussis Vaccine Adsorbed, USP	Suspension of the precipitate obtained after treating a mixture of diphtheria and tetanus toxoids and pertussis vaccine with alum, aluminum hydroxide, or aluminum phosphate.	Intramuscular	Active immunizing agent
Influenza Virus Vaccine, USP	Aqueous suspension of inactivated influenza virus prepared from extra-embryonic fluid of influenza virus-infected chick embryo. May contain an adsorbant such as calcium phosphate or protamine.	Intramuscular or subcutaneous	Active immunizing agent
Measles Virus Vaccine Live, USP	Live measles virus grown on cultures of either chicken embryo tissue or canine renal tissue.	Subcutaneous	Active immunizing agent
Measles, Mumps, and Rubella Virus Vaccine Live, USP	Combination of viruses grown on either chicken or duck embryo tissue.	Subcutaneous	Active immunizing agent
Measles and Rubella Virus Vaccine Live, USP	Live viral vaccine with the measles virus grown on chicken embryo tissue and the rubella virus on duck embryo tissue.	Subcutaneous	Active immunizing agent
Mumps Virus Vaccine Live, USP	Sterile suspension of live mumps virus prepared in the chick embryo primary cell tissue culture.	Subcutaneous	Active immunizing agent
Pertussis Vaccine, USP	Suspension of killed pertussis bacilli *(Bordetella pertussis)*.	Subcutaneous	Active immunizing agent
Plague Vaccine, USP	Suspension of killed plague bacilli *(Pasteurella pestis)*.	Intramuscular or subcutaneous	Active immunizing agent
Poliovirus Vaccine, Inactivated, USP	Suspension of inactivated poliomyelitis virus of Types 1, 2, and 3, grown separately in primary cultures of monkey kidney tissue and combined after inactivation.	Intramuscular or subcutaneous	Active immunizing agent
Live Oral Poliovirus Vaccine, USP	A preparation of one or a combination of the three types of live, attenuated polioviruses, grown separately in primary cultures of monkey kidney tissue.	Oral	Active immunizing agent

Table 8–7. Continued

Biologic Product	Nature of Contents	Route of Administration[1]	Use
Rabies Vaccine, USP	A preparation in liquid or dried form of killed fixed virus of rabies, obtained from brain tissue of rabbits or from duck embryo that have been infected with the virus.	Subcutaneous	Active immunizing agent
Rubella Virus Vaccine Live, USP	Live rubella (German measles) virus grown on duck embryo or rabbit kidney tissue.	Subcutaneous	Active immunizing agent
Rubella and Mumps Viral Vaccine Live, USP	Combination of rubella virus grown on cultures of duck embryo tissue and mumps virus grown on chicken embryo tissue.	Subcutaneous	Active immunizing agent
Smallpox Vaccine, USP	A liquid or dried form of living virus of vaccinia that has been grown in the skin of a vaccinated bovine calf or in membranes of a chick embryo.	Percutaneous	Active immunizing agent
Typhoid Vaccine, USP	Suspension of killed typhoid bacilli (*Salmonella typhosa*).	Subcutaneous	Active immunizing agent
Yellow Fever Vaccine, USP	Dried, frozen, attenuated strain of living yellow fever virus prepared by culturing the virus in the living embryo of the domestic fowl, separating, and freeze-drying.	Subcutaneous	Active immunizing agent
Toxoids			
Diphtheria Toxoid, USP	Solution of the formaldehyde-treated products of the growth of the diphtheria bacillus *Corynebacterium diphtheriae*).	Intramuscular or subcutaneous	Active immunizing agent
Diphtheria Toxoid Adsorbed, USP	Suspension of diphtheria toxoid (as above) precipitated or adsorbed by the addition of alum, aluminum hydroxide, or aluminum phosphate.	Intramuscular or subcutaneous	Active immunizing agent
Diphtheria and Tetanus Toxoids, USP	Solution of mixed diphtheria toxoid and tetanus toxoid.	Intramuscular or subcutaneous	Active immunizing agent
Diphtheria and Tetanus Toxoids Adsorbed, USP	Suspension prepared by mixing adsorbed diphtheria toxoid and adsorbed tetanus toxoid.	Intramuscular or subcutaneous	Active immunizing agent
Tetanus Toxoid, USP	Solution of formaldehyde-treated products of growth of the tetanus bacillus (*Clostridium tetani*).	Subcutaneous	Active immunizing agent
Tetanus Toxoid Adsorbed, USP	Suspension of tetanus toxoid precipitated or adsorbed by the addition of alum, aluminum hydroxide, or aluminum phosphate.	Intramuscular or subcutaneous	Active immunizing agent
Tetanus and Diphtheria Toxoids Adsorbed for Adult Use, USP	Suspension of adsorbed tetanus toxoid and absorbed diphtheria toxoid.	Intramuscular	Active immunizing agent

Table 8–7. Continued

Biologic Product	Nature of Contents	Route of Administration[1]	Use
Antitoxins			
Botulism Antitoxin, USP	Solution of refined and concentrated proteins, chiefly globulins, containing antitoxin obtained from the blood serum or plasma of healthy horses immunized against the toxins produced by both type A and B strains of *Clostridium botulinum.*	Intramuscular or intravenous	Passive immunizing agent
Tetanus Antitoxin, USP	Solution of the refined and concentrated proteins, chiefly globulins, containing antitoxic antibodies obtained from the blood serum or plasma of a healthy animal, usually the horse, that has been immunized against tetanus toxoid or toxin.	Intramuscular or subcutaneous (prophylactic) or intravenous (therapeutic)	Passive immunizing agent
Toxins			
Diphtheria Toxin for Schick Test, USP	Solution of the toxic products of growth of the diphtheria bacillus *(Corynebacterium diphtheriae).*	Intradermal	Diagnostic aid (dermal reactivity indicator)
Serums and Globulins			
Antirabies Serum, USP	Solution containing antiviral substances from the blood serum or plasma of a healthy animal, usually the horse, that has been immunized against rabies by means of vaccine.	Intramuscular	Passive immunizing agent
Iodinated I 125 Albumin Injection, USP	Isotonic solution containing radio-iodinated (125_I) normal human serum albumin.	Intravenous	Diagnostic aid (blood volume determination)
Iodinated I 131 Albumin Injection, USP	Isotonic solution containing radio-iodinated (131_I) normal human serum albumin.	Intravenous	Diagnostic aid (blood volume determination; intrathecal scanning)
Anti-A Blood Grouping Serum, USP	Agglutinates human red cells containing B-agglutinogens.	. . .	Diagnostic aid (in vitro)
Anti-Rh Typing Serums, USP	Derived from human blood having specific Rh antibodies.	. . .	Diagnostic aid (in vitro)
Human Globulin, USP	Solution of globulins containing many antibodies normally present in adult human blood. Each lot is derived from an original plasma or serum pool representing venous or placental blood from at least 1000 individuals.	Intramuscular	Passive immunizing agent (infectious hepatitis, poliomyelitis, rubella, rubeola, varicella)
Vaccinia Immune Globulin, USP	Sterile solution of globulins from blood plasmas of human donors who have been immunized with vaccinia virus smallpox vaccine.	Intramuscular	Passive immunizing agent

Table 8–7.   Continued

Biologic Product	Nature of Contents	Route of Administration[1]	Use
Pertussis Immune Globulin, USP	Solution of globulins derived from the blood plasma of adult human donors who have been immunized with pertussis vaccine.	Intramuscular	Passive immunizing agent
Tetanus Immune Globulin, USP	Solution of globulins derived from the blood plasma of adult human donors who have been immunized with tetanus toxoid.	Intramuscular	Passive immunizing agent

Miscellaneous Biologic Products

Antivenin (Crotalidae) Polyvalent, USP	A preparation derived by drying a frozen solution of specific venon-neutralizing globulins obtained from the serum of healthy horses immunized against venoms of four species of pit vipers, *Crotalus atrox, C. adamanteus, C. terrificus,* and *Bothrops atrox.*	Intramuscular or intravenous	To neutralize the toxic effects of venoms of crotalids native to North, Central, and South America
Histoplasmin, USP	Liquid concentrate of the soluble growth products developed by the fungus *Histoplasma capsulatum* when grown in the mycelial phase on a synthetic medium.	Intradermal	Diagnostic aid (histoplasmosis)
Plasma Protein Fraction, USP	Solution of selected proteins derived from the blood plasma of adult human donors. It contains about 5% of protein, about 85% of which is albumin, the remainder alpha and beta globulins.	Intravenous	Blood-volume supporter
Tuberculin, USP	Solution of the concentrated, soluble products of growth of the tubercle bacillus, *Mycobacterium tuberculosis.* (Old Tuberculin), or, a soluble partially purified product of growth of the tubercle bacillus prepared in a special liquid medium free from protein (Purified Protein Derivative, PPD).	Intradermal	Diagnostic aid (tuberculosis)

[1]The doses to be administered and the schedule of doses vary widely, depending upon the patient's age, exposure, previous record of immunizations, etc.

not the biologic substance that is harmed by freezing, but rather the container which may be broken through the freezing and expansion of an aqueous vehicle so that some of the product is lost. The expiration date for biological products varies with the product and the storage temperatures employed. Generally, most biological products have an expiration date of a year or longer after the date of manufacture or issue. Biologics must be dispensed in their original containers in order to avoid contamination and deterioration. They are sterile when packaged and are injected by aseptic techniques.

As indicated by the listings in Table 8–7, some biologics are diagnostic aids, others are prophylactic, and some are therapeutic. Although it is not within the scope of this book to undertake a discussion of immunity, some brief definitions may assist in the understanding of the use of the official products presented. Also, it is not the intent here to discuss the detailed methods of preparation for these biologics, and only brief descriptions of the products are given. If additional information is desired, the student is encouraged to read other references.

IMMUNITY—The power of the body to resist and overcome infection.

NATURAL, INNATE, OR NATIVE IMMUNITY—A constitutional attribute of individuals who because of race, species specificity, endocrine balance, and other factors may be resistant to a particular toxic agent. It is something with which they are born and is not acquired through the use of biologics.

ACQUIRED IMMUNITY—A specific immunity that may be actively acquired (active immunity) or passively acquired (passive immunity).

ACTIVE IMMUNITY—Specific immunity developed in an individual in response to the introduction of antigenic substances into his body. This may occur by natural means, as by infection, in which case it is termed *naturally acquired active immunity,* or it may be developed in response to the administration of a specific vaccine or toxoid, in which case it is termed *artificially acquired active immunity.* In either case, the body builds up its own defenses in response to the antigen.

PASSIVE IMMUNITY—Immunity developed by the introduction of already formed antibodies into the body to combat the specific antigen. If the antibodies are passed to the individual naturally, as by the placental transfer of antibodies from the mother to the fetus, the term *naturally acquired passive immunity* applies. However, if the antibodies are passed on to the individual through the injection of a specific antitoxin, the immunity is referred to as *artificially acquired passive immunity.* Passive immunity is not long-lasting.

VACCINES—Agents administered primarily for prophylactic action in the development of active immunity (acquired). Vaccines may contain living, attenuated (weakened), or killed viruses; killed rickettsia; or killed bacteria.

TOXOIDS—Toxins modified and detoxified by the use of moderate heat and chemical treatment so that the antigenic properties remain. They are employed for the development of active immunity.

TOXINS—Poisonous bacterial products that act as antigens and cause the human body to develop specific antibodies to combat their presence. Most toxins are used for diagnostic purposes to determine the susceptibility of the patient to the disease caused by the toxin-containing organism.

ANTITOXINS—Substances prepared from the blood of animals, usually horses, which have been immunized by repeated injections of specific bacterial toxins. The resulting antitoxins produce passive immunity, or they may be used for curative purposes for persons already known to be infected by the specific antigen.

ANTISERUMS—Serums prepared in the same manner as the antitoxins, except that bacteria or viruses are injected into the animal to stimulate the production of specific antibodies. The antibody-rich blood serum may be employed to produce passive immunity.

HUMAN IMMUNE SERUMS AND GLOBULINS—Serums containing the specific antibodies obtained from the blood of humans and produced as a result of having had the specific disease or having been immunized against it with a specific biologic product. They provide passive immunity.

A recommended immunization schedule for infants and children is presented in Table 8–8.

According to the National Childhood Vaccine Injury Act of 1986, health care-providers who administer certain vaccines and toxoids are required to record permanently and to report ad-

Table 8–8.   Recommended Immunization Schedule[1]

Age	Immunizations
2 months	diphtheria, pertussis, tetanus,[2] polio[3]
4 months	DPT, TOPV
6 months	DPT
15 months	mumps, measles, rubella[4], DPT, TOPV
18 months	Hemophilus b Polysaccharide Vaccine
4–6 years	DPT, TOPV
14–16 years	Td[5] and every 10 years thereafter

[1]Adapted from *Morbidity and Mortality Weekly Report,* Centers for Disease Control, *38*:210, 1989.

[2]May be given combined as DPT: Diphtheria (pediatric) toxoid, tetanus toxoid, and pertussis vaccine.

[3]Usually given as TOPV: trivalent live oral polio vaccine, adsorbed.

[4]May be given as the combined vaccine: MMR.

[5]Combined tetanus and diphtheria (adult) toxoids for anyone over the age of 6.

verse effects resulting from the use of one of the biologic products.[14] Among the products included in the law are diphtheria and tetanus toxoids and pertussis vaccine (DTP), pertussis vaccine, measles, mumps and rubella vaccines, tetanus and diphtheria toxoids, and poliovirus vaccines, both live and inactivated. The health-care provider who observes an adverse effect must permanently record the findings in the patient's medical record and report the incident to the U.S. Department of Health and Human Services as well as to local and state health authorities. Reporting of the adverse effects includes such conditions as anaphylactic shock, encephalitis, and seizures.

Processes of the New Biotechnology

The term *biotechnology* encompasses any technique that uses living organisms (e.g., microorganisms) in the production or modification of materials or products. Today, recombinant DNA (rDNA) and monoclonal antibody (MAb) technologies are providing exciting opportunities for new pharmaceutical product development and approaches to the diagnosis, prevention, and treatment of diseases. Many products of the new biotechnology are or will be administered by injection and thus this subject matter is included in this chapter. The material presented is only briefly introduced here, as the

field of pharmaceutical biotechnology constitutes an extensive area of study beyond the scope of this text.

Recombinant DNA (rDNA)

DNA, *deoxyribonucleic acid,* has been called "the substance of life." It is DNA that constitutes genes, allowing cells to reproduce and maintain life. Of the over a million kinds of plants and animals known today, no two are exactly alike; however, the similarity within families is the result of genetic information stored in cells, duplicated, and passed from cell to cell and from generation to generation. It is DNA that provides this continuity.

DNA was first isolated in 1869, its chemical composition determined in the early 1900s, and by the 1940s, it had been proven that the genes within cell chromosomes are made of DNA.[15,16] It was not until the 1950s, when James D. Watson and Francis H.C. Crick postulated the structure of DNA, that biologists began to comprehend the molecular mechanisms of heredity and cell regulation. Watson and Crick described their model of DNA as a double helix, two strands of DNA coiled about itself like a spiral staircase.[15] We now know that the two strands of DNA are connected by the bases adenine, guanine, cytosine, and thymine (A, G, C, and T). The order or arrangement of these bases within the two strands of DNA comprise a specific gene for a specific trait. A typical gene has hundreds of bases that are always arranged in pairs. When A occurs on one strand, T occurs opposite it on the other; G pairs with C.[16] A gene is a segment of DNA that has a specific sequence of these chemical base pairs. The pattern constitutes the DNA message for maintaining cells and organisms and building the next generation. To create a new cell, or a whole new organism, DNA must be able to duplicate or "clone" itself. This is done through the unwinding and separation of the two strands and the subsequent attachment to each of new bases from within the cell according to the A-T/C-G rule.[16] The result is two new double strands of DNA, each of the same structure and conformation.

DNA also plays an essential role in the production of proteins needed for cellular maintenance and function. DNA is translated to messenger RNA (*ribonucleic acid*), which contains instructions for the production of the 20 amino acids from which all proteins are made.[16] Amino acids can be arranged in vast number of combinations to produce hundreds of thousands of different proteins. In essence, a cell is a miniature assembly plant for the production of thousands of proteins. A single *E. coli* bacterium is capable of making about 2000 proteins.[15]

Through the process of recombinant DNA technology, scientists can utilize nonhuman cells (as a special strain of *E. coli*) to manufacture proteins identical to those produced in human cells. Recombinant DNA is defined as the hybrid DNA produced by joining pieces of DNA from different sources. The process of joining segments of DNA from different organisms for a specific purpose, permits the ability to direct the synthesis of specific products from selected host cells.[17] This process has enabled scientists to produce molecules that are naturally present in the human body in large quantities previously difficult to obtain from human sources. For example, approximately 50 cadaver pituitary glands were required to treat a single growth hormone-deficient child for 1 year until DNA-produced growth hormone became available through the new technology.[18] Further, the biosynthetic product is more free of viral contamination than the previous cadaver-source of the hormone. Human growth hormone and insulin were the first recombinant DNA products to become available for patient use.

DNA probe technology is a new tool utilized to diagnose disease. It utilizes small pieces of DNA to search a cell for viral infection or for genetic defects. DNA probes have application in testing for infectious disease, cancer, genetic defects, and disease susceptibility. Using DNA probes, scientists have acquired the capability of locating a disease-causing gene, which, in turn, can lead to the development of replacement therapies.[19] In producing a DNA probe, the initial step involves the synthesis of the specific strand of DNA with the sequence of nucleotides which matches that of the gene being investigated.[15] For instance, if the intent is to test for a particular virus, the DNA strand is developed to be identical to one in the virus. The second step is to tag the synthetic gene with a dye or radioactive isotope. When introduced into a specimen, the synthetic strand of DNA acts as a probe, searching for a matching or complementary strand. When located, the two hybridize, or join together.[15] When the probe is bound to the virus, the dye reveals the location of the viral gene. If a radioactive isotope was employed on the synthetic DNA strand, it binds to the viral strand of DNA, and can reveal the virus through X-ray technology.

Monoclonal Antibodies (MAbs)

Monoclonal antibodies are purified antibodies produced by a single source or clone of cells. These are utilized in diagnostics, therapy, immunology, and research. Monoclonal antibodies are engineered to recognize and bind to a single specific antigen. Thus, when administered, a monoclonal antibody will target a particular protein or cell having the specific matching antigenic feature. When coupled with a drug molecule, radioactive isotope or toxin, a monoclonal antibody can target the desired cells or tissues with great precision.[20]

The specificity of monoclonal antibodies is utilized in diagnostics, such as in home pregnancy-test kits and ovulation-predicting kits. The monoclonal antibodies detect the presence of endogenous hormones in the urine to establish the test results. They are also being utilized in detecting allergies, anemia, heart disease, and many infectious diseases, as hepatitis, AIDS-related cytomegalovirus, streptococcal infections, gonorrhea, syphilis, herpes, and chlamydia.[15] When linked with radioisotopes or with anticancer drugs, monoclonal antibodies can be utilized to diagnose and treat malignant tumors.

Prior to 1975, when hybridoma technology was fully developed, antibodies for diagnostic, therapeutic, or research use were obtained from the blood of humans or animals. The antibodies, produced through the body's immune system in response to the presence of foreign substances of antigens, were obtained through separation from the blood. It has been difficult to obtain pure antibodies specific to a particular antigen. Today, antibodies are generated in large quantities by laboratory grown hybridomas or hybrid cells. In making monoclonal antibodies, an animal is immunized with the foreign substance or antigen which will yield the antibody desired. The antibody-producing cells are removed and mixed with myeloma cells under conditions that promote cell fusion. The resulting hybrid cells grow indefinitely and produce monoclonal antibodies in large quantities.[15,19]

Products of Biotechnology

The following descriptions and Table 8–9 provide examples of products of biotechnology that have been approved by the FDA or are being developed for submission for approval.[21]

ANTICOAGULANTS/THROMBOLYTIC AGENTS. Inappropriate or unnecessary clotting of the blood is responsible for more deaths than cancer. The body's own clot-dissolving process begins with formation of the enzyme plasmin. Substances that activate plasmin are found in the body only in minute amounts. As a result of biotechnology, sufficient quantities of these substances are available and are being developed.

COLONY STIMULATING FACTORS. The production of white blood cells is controlled by proteins called colony stimulating factors (CSFs). Cancer chemotherapy and inherited disorders are among the causes of low white blood counts, which lower resistance to infection. CSFs are being investigated as a way not only to counteract low white blood cell counts generally, but also to produce specific types of white blood cells. In addition, there is thought that CSFs can stimulate the body to produce additional bone marrow as well as cause some cancer cells to stop dividing.

DISMUTASES. Dismutase, an enzyme, is important in organ transplantation and in treating heart attack when tissues have been deprived of blood for a short time. When the blood flow is restored to the transplanted organ or to the heart muscle after a clot is dissolved, the cells in the organ can be damaged by the excessively oxygen-rich blood. Dismutases prevent this "reperfusion injury" by allowing the oxygen-deprived tissues to recover their normal state in a more orderly manner.

ERYTHROPOIETIN (EPO). Kidney disease often impairs the body's ability to produce this hormone, causing anemia, a deficiency in red blood cell production. Frequent blood transfusions or restoration of the missing hormone, EPO, can add more red blood cells to correct chronic anemia. Since transfusions may expose those who receive them to infectious agents, such as hepatitis, EPO may provide major gains in safety and efficiency. Through genetic engineering, it is now possible to obtain EPO in large amounts, a development of great importance to the 225,000 Americans who rely on kidney dialysis machines. Further, since EPO can cause a tenfold increase in red cell production, it is possible that blood banks may be turned into blood farms.

HUMAN GROWTH HORMONE. Our growth is regulated by human growth hormone (hGH) secreted by the pituitary gland. A child whose body produces insufficient hGH will be limited to an adult height of about 4 feet. It is estimated that as many as 15,000 American children suffer from hGH deficiency. Beginning in the late 1950s, such children were treated with hGH extracted from cadaver pituitaries. This not only was extraordinarily expensive, but exposed the children to the risk of infection from viral contamination of the hormone. Now, genetic engineering technology makes available pure supplies of hGH.

HUMAN INSULIN. Human insulin is derived from two sources: (a) recombinant DNA biotechnology, with *E. coli* genetically engineered to produce it, and (b) through an alteration of pork insulin. In the biosynthetic process, the production involves the separate syntheses by *E. coli* of the A-chain and B-chain of insulin. The two chains may then be chemically linked to form human insulin. However, since 1986 human insulin has been produced by a single fermentation step within the hybrid bacteria to produce proinsulin, which is then cleaved enzymatically to yield human insulin. Semisynthetic human insulin is produced through the enzymatic transpeptidation of alanine with threonine, at position 30 on the B-chain of pork insulin. The resulting product is chemically identical to human insulin.

INTERFERON. In 1957 it was discovered that a glycoprotein naturally produced by the cells apparently could interfere with the ability of a virus to reproduce after it invaded the body. By the mid-1970s it appeared that this protein, interferon, might also curtail the spread of certain types of cancer. The use of recombinant DNA techniques provided sufficient interferon for continued research. While much more needs to be learned about the interferons, they hold great promise. The alpha group has proved effective against hairy cell leukemia, once a lethal disease. It normalizes blood counts and controls tumor growth in 90% of patients.

INTERLEUKINS. In the 1960s it was discovered that interleukin, a natural substance occurring in the body, transmits signals between types of while blood cells or leukocytes. While the full therapeutic potential of the interleukins is only beginning to be explored, interleukin-2 has been used to fight cancer. A patient's T-cells, specialized white blood cells involved in ridding the body of diseased cells, are exposed to the interleukin outside of the patient's body to activate them against the cancer. The activated T-cells are then given back to the patient, where they are much more effective in finding and destroying the cancer cells.

MONOCLONAL ANTIBODIES. Antibodies, often referred to as the body's missile defense system, are large protein molecules produced by white blood cells. They seek out and destroy harmful foreign substances. Such foreign cells are recognized by telltale surface proteins, called antigens. After the invader has been destroyed, the antibodies remain in the blood on instant alert should a similar antigen arrive. Antibodies also are useful in matching donors and recipients in organ transplantation, in blood typing, and in measuring and identifying hormones, toxins, and various antigens in blood and fluids. In addition to their extraordinary diagnostic capability, monoclonals can be used alone for a pinpoint attack on a cancerous cell or to act against cancerous cells remaining after conventional chemotherapy. They can also be enlisted as porters (adjuvants or adjuncts) to transport drugs, toxins or radioactive particles to such cells.

PEPTIDES. Proteins are made of amino acids linked together to form peptide chains. As more amino acids are combined, the chain of the peptide becomes longer. At a certain point, when about 40 or 50 amino acids are joined together, the peptide becomes a protein. Thus, peptides and proteins only differ by the length of their amino acid chain. The body often uses peptides as special messenger substances for specific purposes such as increasing heart beat or body temperature and turning on or off a cell which secretes an important substance. Because peptides are smaller, they travel around the body more efficiently than larger proteins. Scientists have discovered that only portions of a protein are involved in biologic activity. By making the peptide portion of the protein which shows biologic activity, a number of peptide drugs have been developed.

TUMOR NECROSIS FACTOR. As far back as the 1700s, a few physicians noted that a regression of cancer sometimes accompanied an infection. In 1975 it was learned that, in response to some bacterial infections, the body produces peptides that permit cells to transmit signals to one another. One such intercellular messenger, tumor necrosis factor (TNF), triggers the deployment of immune defenses that can destroy tumors. By damaging the blood vessels that nourish the tumor, it is, in effect, starved to death.

VACCINES. When a virus or other germ invades the body, the immune system produces antigens to protect it by attaching to the protein coat on the surface of the virus. Genetic engineering allows large-scale production of the protein components of a virus. A vaccine using only the protein coat of the virus will still activate antigen production to neutralize the real full virus. The "protein coat" vaccine is incapable of reproducing like the virus and therefore cannot cause the disease.

Other Injectable Products—Pellets or Implants

Pellets or implants are sterile, small, usually cylindrical-shaped solid objects about 3.2 mm in diameter and 8 mm in length, prepared by compression and intended to be implanted subcutaneously for the purpose of providing the continuous release of medication over a prolonged period of time. The pellets, which are implanted under the skin (usually of the thigh or abdomen) with a special injector or by surgical incision, are used for potent hormones. Their implantation provides the patient with an economical means of obtaining long-lasting effects (up to many months after a single implantation) and obviates the need for frequent parenteral or oral hormone therapy. The implanted pellet, which may contain 100 times the amount of drug given by other routes of administration, slowly dissolves under the skin to release the drug to the tissues for absorption into the general circulation.

Pellets must not contain any binder, diluent, or excipient in order to permit total dissolution and absorption of the pellet from the site of implantation. The following are examples of pellets for implantation.

Desoxycorticosterone Acetate Pellets

Desoxycorticosterone acetate pellets usually contain 125 mg of desoxycorticosterone acetate, an adrenocortical hormone (the usual intramuscular dose of desoxycorticosterone acetate is 1 mg).

Estradiol Pellets

Estradiol pellets usually contain 10 and 25 mg of estrogen estradiol (the usual single oral or parenteral dose of estradiol is about 250 mcg).

Testosterone Pellets

Testosterone pellets usually contain 75 mg of testosterone (the usual dose of testosterone is 10 mg buccally, 25 mg intramuscularly, and 300 mg by implantation). Four tablets usually are implanted for prolonged androgenic effects of the drug.

Table 8–9. Examples of Products of Biotechnology, Approved or In Development[21]

Category/Product	Use/Indication
Anticoagulants/Thrombolytic Agents	
Prourokinase	Heart attack
Tissue Plasminogen Activator (TPA)	Acute myocardial infarction, deep vein thrombosis, acute stroke, pulmonary embolism
Colony Stimulating Factors	
Granulocyte Macrophage/Colony Stimulating Factor	Chemotherapy effects, AIDS, leukemia, aplastic anemia, bone marrow transplants, Hodgkin's disease
Dismutases	
Superoxide dismutase	Reperfusion injury as it applied to acute myocardial infarction, renal transplantation
Erythropoietins	
Eprex erythropoietin	Dialysis anemia, chronic renal failure, AIDS, chronic disease anemias, pre- and post-surgical use
Human Growth Hormones	
Human Growth Hormone	Human growth deficiency in children
Human Insulin	Insulin deficiency
Interferons	
Interferon-alpha	Genital warts, genital herpes, hairy cell leukemia
Interferon-alpha2a	AIDS-related Kaposi's sarcoma, chronic myelogenous leukemia, renal cell carcinoma
Interferon-alpha2b	Kaposi's sarcoma, malignant melanoma, multiple myeloma, superficial bladder cancer, upper respiratory infections, chronic myelogenous leukemia, basal cell carcinoma
Recombinant Human Interferon-beta	AIDS, ARC, multiple sclerosis, cancer
Interferon-gamma	Rheumatoid arthritis, renal cell carcinoma, venereal warts, cancers (small-cell lung, melanoma, colorectal)
Interleukins	
Interleukin-2	Cancer immunotherapy
Recombinant Human Interleukin-2	Cancer immunotherapy
Monoclonal Antibodies	
MAb	Renal-allograft rejection, lung cancer, septic shock, colorectal cancer, pancreatic cancer, ovarian cancer, breast cancer
Anti-platelet MAb	Anti-platelet prevention of blood clots
Peptides	
Atrial peptide (injectable)	Acute congestive heart failure
Pentigetide (aerosol)	Asthma
Pentigetide (injectable)	Allergic rhinitis
Pentigetide (nasal spray)	Allergic rhinitis
Pentigetide (ophthalmic)	Allergic conjunctivitis
T-cell Modulatory Peptide	Auto-immune diseases
Tumor Necrosis Factors	
Tumor Necrosis Factor	Cancer
Vaccines	
Hepatitis B Vaccine	Hepatitis B
Conjugative Vaccine for *Haemophilis influenzae*	*Haemophilus influenzae* type B
Cancer Vaccine	Malignant melanoma
Other Products	
Thymosin Alpha-1	Hepatitis vaccine adjuvant, chronic active Hepatitis B
Factor VIII:C	Hemophilia
Recombinant Factor VIII	Hemophilia
Epidermal Growth Factor	Eye surgery, wound healing

Table 8–10.   Examples of Irrigation Solutions

Solution	Description
Acetic Acid Irrigation, USP	This solution is employed topically to the bladder as a 0.25% solution for irrigation. It has a pH of between 2.9 and 3.3 and is employed during urologic procedures. It is administered to wash blood and surgical debris away while maintaining suitable conditions for the tissue and permitting the surgeon an unobstructed view.
Neomycin and Polymyxin B Sulfates Solution for Irrigation, USP	This solution is employed as a topical antibacterial in the continuous irrigation of the bladder.
Ringer's Irrigation, USP	This solution contains sodium chloride, potassium chloride, and calcium chloride in purified water, in the same proportions, as is present in Ringer's Injection. The solution is sterile and pyrogen-free. It is used topically as an irrigation and must be labeled "not for injection."
Sodium Chloride Irrigation, USP	This solution contains 0.9% sodium chloride which is isotonic with body fluids. The solution is employed topically to wash wounds and into body cavities where absorption into the blood is not likely. The solution may also be employed rectally as an enema; for simple evacuation, 150 mL is usually employed and for colonic flush, 1500 mL may be used.
Sterile Water for Irrigation, USP	This is water for injection that has been sterilized and suitably packaged. The label must state "for irrigation only" and "not for injection." The water must not contain any antimicrobial or other added agent.

Irrigation and Dialysis Solutions

Solutions for irrigation of body tissues and for dialysis resemble parenteral solutions in that they are subject to the same stringent standards. The difference is in their use. These solutions are not injected into the vein, but employed outside of the circulatory system. Since they are generally used in large volumes, they are packaged in large volume containers, generally of the screw-cap type which permits the rapid pouring of the solution.

Irrigation Solutions

Irrigation solutions are intended to bathe or wash wounds, surgical incisions, or body tissues. Examples are presented in Table 8–10.

Dialysis Solutions

Dialysis may be defined as a process whereby substances may be separated from one another in solution by taking advantage of their differing diffusibility through membranes. *Peritoneal dialysis* solutions, allowed to flow into the peritoneal cavity, are used to remove toxic substances normally excreted by the kidney. In cases of poisoning or kidney failure, or in patients awaiting renal transplants, dialysis is an emergency life-saving procedure. Solutions are commercially available containing dextrose as a major source of calories, vitamins, minerals, electrolytes, and amino acids or peptides as a source of nitrogen. The solutions are made to be hypertonic (with dextrose) to plasma to avoid absorption of water from the dialysis solution into the circulation. The peritoneal cavity, containing the hypertonic fluid, acts as a semipermeable membrane and allows for the flow of undesired elements into the peritoneal dialysis fluid which is removed by peritoneal tube to collection vessels.

Hemodialysis is employed to remove toxins from the blood. In this method, the arterial blood is shunted through a polyethylene catheter through an artificial dialyzing membrane bathed in an electrolyte solution. Following the dialysis, the blood is returned to the body circulation through a vein.

Various dialysis solutions are available commercially and the pharmacist may be called upon to provide them or to make adjustments in their composition.

Selected Reading

America's Immunization Schedule for Wiping Out Disease. *J. Am. Pharm.*, NS22:35–47, 1982.

Avis, K.E., and Akers, M.J.: *Sterile Preparation for the Hospital Pharmacist.* Ann Arbor, MI, Ann Arbor Science Publishers, 1982.

Best, C.H.: The History of Insulin. *Diabetes,* 11:495–503, 1962.

Brodsky, F.M.: Monoclonal Antibodies as Magic Bullets. *Pharm. Res.,* 5:1, 1988.

Campbell, R.K.: The New Purified Insulins. *J. Am. Pharm.,* NS21:21–24, 1981.

Current Problems and Innovations in Intravenous Drug Delivery. *Am. J. Hosp. Pharm.,* 44:2528–2559, 1987.

Cutie, M.R.: Effects of Cold and Freezing Temperatures on Pharmaceutical Dosage Forms. *Drug & Cosmetic Ind.,* 126:40, 1980.

Davis, N.M.: A Call for Insulin Medication Errors (editorial). *Hosp. Pharm.,* 20:73, 1985.

Grabenstein, J.D.: Pharmacists and Immunizations: Advocating Preventive Medicine. *Am. Pharm.,* NS28:25–33, 1988.

Gehres, R.W. Lasell, P., and Spencer, M.R.: Insulin Infusion Pumps. *U.S. Pharmacist,* 7:62–68, 1982.

Hochstein, H.D.: The LAL Test versus the Rabbit Pyrogen Test for Endotoxin Detection. *Pharm. Tech.,* 11:123–129, 1987.

"Humulin," Product Information, Indianapolis, Eli Lilly and Company, 1983.

Johnson, C., Cloyd, J., and Rapp, R.P.: Parenteral Hyperalimentation. *Drug Intell. Clin. Pharm.,* 9:493–499, 1975.

Kay, A.A.: The Selection and Evaluation of Package Components for Parenteral Products. *Pharm. Tech.,* 6:54–61, 1982.

Lawson, D.H., and Henry, D.A.: Drug Therapy Reviews: Intravenous Fluid Therapy. *Am. J. Hosp. Pharm.,* 34:1332, 1977.

Managing Viral Diseases—Two Centuries of Progress. *J. Am. Pharm.,* NS22:36–44, 1983.

O'Donnell, J.T., and Baumgartner, T.G., eds.: Nutrition. *J. Pharm. Pract.,* 1:73–153, 1988.

Pehling, G.B., and Gerich, J.E.: Comparison of Plasma Insulin Profiles after Subcutaneous Administration of Insulin by Jet Spray and Conventional Needle Injection in Patients with Insulin-Dependent Diabetes Mellitus. *Mayo Clin. Proc.,* 59:751–754, 1984.

Popovich, N.G.: The New Role of the Pharmacist in the Management of Diabetes Mellitus. Boehringer Manheim Diagnostics. Indianapolis, IN, 1985.

Pray, W.S.: IV Fluid Administration Sets. *US Pharmacist,* 13(3):6–17, 1988.

Pray, W.S.: IV Update: Selection of an IV Fluid Container. *US Pharmacist,* 13(4):6–13, 1988.

Pray, W.S.: Preparation of IV Admixtures. *US Pharmacist,* 13(5):6–18, 1988.

Pray, W.S.: Small Volume Parenterals: Ampuls and Vials. *US Pharmacist,* 13(6):1–11, 1988.

Pray, W.S.: Preparation of Antibiotic Solutions for Intermittent IV Injection. *US Pharmacist,* 13(9):1–5, 1988.

Recombinant DNA and Biosynthetic Human Insulin, A Source Book, Eli Lilly and Company, 1981.

Skyler, J.S.: Human Insulin of Recombinant DNA Origin: Chemical Potential. *Diabetes Care,* 5:181–186, 1982.

Tami, J.A., Parr, M.D., and Thompson, J.S.: The Immune System. *Am. J. Hosp. Pharm.,* 43:2483, 1986.

Tami, J.A., Parr, M.D., Brown, S.A., and Thompson, J.S.: Monoclonal Antibody Technology. *Am. J. Hosp. Pharm.,* 43:2816, 1986.

Trissel, L.A.: *Handbook on Injectable Drugs,* 3rd ed. Bethesda, MD, American Society of Hospital Pharmacists, 1983.

Turco, S., and King, R.E.: *Sterile Dosage Forms: Their Preparation and Clinical Applications,* 3rd ed. Philadelphia, Lea & Febiger, 1987.

Valenta, L., and Elias, A.N.: Insulin-induced lipodystrophy in diabetic patients resolved with treatment with human insulin. *Ann. Intern. Med.,* 102:790–791, 1985.

Vemuri, S.: The Formulation of Parenteral Products. *Drug & Cosmetic Industry,* 124:48, 1979.

Notes

1. Van Itallie, P.H.: The Rugged Beginnings of Injection Therapy, *Pulse of Pharmacy* (Wyeth Laboratories), 19:3–17, 1965.

2. Griffenhagen, G.B.: The History of Parenteral Medication. *Bull. Parenteral Drug Assoc.,* 16:12, 1962.

3. Groves, M.J.: Perspectives on the Use of Parenteral Solutions. *Parenteral Products,* London, William Heinemann Medical Books, 1973, pp. 1–14.

4. Hirsch, J.D., and Bradley, D.L.: Clinical Applications of 20% Fat Emulsions. *Current Perspectives in the Use of Lipid Emulsion,* Johnston, I.D.A., (ed.) Lancaster (England), MTP Press, Ltd., 1983, pp. 11–14.

5. For each species of bacteria there is a temperature at which it is in every way most active (optimum-growth temperature) and temperatures above (maximum-growth temperature) or below (minimum-growth temperature) which the organism is inactive. At temperatures below the minimum-growth temperature, bacteria cease to develop, but most species are not killed by cold. Bacteriologists successfully keep many cultures alive in the ordinary refrigerator (2–15°C) for several days or weeks. Indeed, many organisms will survive for weeks frozen in ice and will grow normally again when the ice melts. High temperatures are much more injurious to microorganisms than are cold temperatures. If any bacterium is heated above its maximum-growth temperature to a sufficient degree and for sufficient length of time, it will be killed. Although thermal death temperature may range between 30°C for cold-loving organisms and 90°C for heat-loving organisms, nearly all nonsporeforming bacteria when exposed in aqueous media to temperatures of 60 to 75°C are killed within 30 minutes. (Burdon, K.L., and Williams, R.P.: *Microbiology,* 5th ed. New York, Macmillan, 1964, pp. 145–158.)

6. Millipore Filter Corporation, Bedford, Massachusetts.

7. McCullough, K.Z.: Process Control: In Process and Raw Materials Testing Using LAL. *Pharm. Tech.,* 12:40–48, 1988.

8. Lyophilization, a process also known as "freeze drying," involves the removal of water from products in the frozen state at extremely low pressures. The process is generally used to dry prod-

ucts that are thermolabile and would be destroyed or otherwise adversely affected by heat-drying.

9. Nazlin, California Biotechnology, Inc.

10. Effective on March 24, 1980, the FDA decertified U-80 insulin thereby removing it from the marketplace. The move resulted from the increased use by physicians and patients of U-100 insulin and eliminated one source of patient confusion and error. With the changeover from U-80 to U-100, patients were able to measure the medication more accurately and inject a smaller volume for the same effect. U-100 insulin has been proposed as a replacement for the U-40 insulin as well, to make it the single strength for home-use by the patient.

11. Kwan, J.W.: High-Technology I.V. Infusion Devices. *Am. J. Hosp. Pharm.*, 46:320–335, 1989.

12. Vidt, D.G.: Use and Abuse of Intravenous Solutions. *JAMA*, 232:533, 1975.

13. Grabenstein, J.D.: Don't say "biologics" if you mean "immunologics." *Am. J. Hosp. Pharm.*, 45:1941, 1988.

14. *Morbidity and Mortality Weekly Report*, Centers for Disease Control, 37:197, 1988.

15. *A Progress Report on Biotechnology*. 2nd ed. Nutley NJ, Hoffman-LaRoche, 1986.

16. *Genetic Engineering: A Natural Science*. St. Louis, MO, Monsanto, 1984.

17. Stewart, G.A.: Biotechnology: An Introduction. *Am. Pharm.*, NS26:31, 1986.

18. Technology Forges a Revolution in Drug Therapy. *The Consultant Pharmacist*. 1:91, 1986.

19. Bagley, J.L.: Biotech. *Am. Druggist*, 195:57, 1986.

20. High-tech Drugs to Burst on Pharmacy Scene. *Drug Topics*, 130:38, 1986.

21. Reproduced from: Biotechnology Products in Development. Pharmaceutical Manufacturers Association, 1988.

9 | *Transdermal Drug Delivery Systems, Ointments, Creams, Lotions, and Other Preparations*

THIS CHAPTER includes drug delivery systems and dosage forms which are intended to be applied to the skin. Ointments, creams, transdermal drug delivery systems, lotions, topical solutions and tinctures represent the most frequently used dermatologic dosage forms; however, other preparations as pastes, liniments, powders, and aerosols are also commonly used.

Preparations are applied to the skin either for their physical effects, that is, for their ability to act as skin protectants, lubricants, emollients, drying agents, etc., or for the specific effect of the medicinal agent(s) present. Preparations sold over-the-counter frequently contain mixtures of medicinal substances used in the treatment of such conditions as minor skin infections, itching, burns, diaper rash, insect stings and bites, athlete's foot, corns, calluses, warts, dandruff, acne, psoriasis, and eczema. Skin applications which require a prescription generally contain a single medicinal agent intended to counter a specific diagnosed condition.

Although it is generally desirable in treating skin diseases for the drug in the medicated application to penetrate past the surface and into the skin, it is not generally the intent (except for transdermal medicated systems) that the medication enter the general circulation. However, once past the epidermis, a drug substance finds itself in proximity to blood capillaries feeding the subcutaneous tissues (see Fig. 9–1), and absorption into the general circulation is not unlikely. In fact, such absorption commonly results after topical application of certain preparations as evidenced by detectable blood levels of the drug and the urinary excretion of the drug or its metabolic products. Fortunately, most of the materials employed for nonsystemic topical use are sufficiently nontoxic in the amounts absorbed so that the effects of absorption are generally unrecognized by the patient.

Percutaneous Absorption

The absorption of substances from outside the skin to positions beneath the skin, including entrance into the blood stream, is referred to as *percutaneous absorption*. In general, the percutaneous absorption of a medicinal substance present in a transdermal therapeutic system, or in a dermatological preparation such as a liquid, gel, ointment, cream, or paste depends not only upon the physical and chemical properties of the medicinal substance but also upon its behavior when placed in the pharmaceutical vehicle and upon the condition of the skin. It is well known that although a pharmaceutical vehicle may not penetrate the skin to any great extent nor actually carry the medicinal substance through the skin, the vehicle does influence the rate and degree of penetration of a medicinal agent, and the degree and rate vary with different drugs and with different vehicles. Therefore each drug substance-vehicle combination must be examined individually for percutaneous absorption and therapeutic efficacy.

The Skin

Upon the surface of the skin is a film of emulsified material composed of a complex mixture of sebum, sweat, and desquamating horny layer, the latter from the layer of dead epidermal cells, termed the "horny layer" or the "stratum corneum," and situated directly beneath the emulsified film. Beneath the horny layer in order is a "barrier layer," the living epidermis or the stratum germinativum, and the dermis or true skin.

Blood capillaries and nerve fibers rise from the subcutaneous fat tissue into the dermis and

Fig. 9–1. *Stratified organization of the skin. (Pillsbury, D.M. and Heston, Charles, L.: A Manual of Dermatology. 2nd Ed., Courtesy of W.B. Saunders Co., 1979.)*

up to the epidermis. Sweat glands present in the subcutaneous tissue yield their products by way of sweat ducts which find their way to the surface of the skin. Sebaceous (oil) glands and hair follicles originating in the dermis and subcutaneous layers also find their way to the surface and are revealed as ducts and hairs respectively.

Penetration of the Skin by Drugs

Drugs may penetrate intact skin after topical application through the walls of the hair follicles, through the sweat glands or the sebaceous glands, or between the cells of the horny layer. Naturally, broken or abraded skin is easily en-

tered by applied substances, but such penetration does not really constitute true percutaneous absorption.

If the skin is intact, the main route for the penetration of drug is generally through the epidermal layers, rather than through the hair follicles or the gland ducts, because the surface area of the latter is rather minute compared to the area of skin containing neither of these anatomical elements. The film covering the horny layer is not generally continuous and presents no real resistance to penetration. Because the composition of the film varies with the proportion of sebum and sweat produced and the degree of their removal through washing and sweat evaporation, the film is not a true barrier to drug transfer, because it has no definite composition, thickness, or continuity.

The percutaneous absorption of a drug generally results from the direct penetration of the drug through the stratum corneum, a 10 to 15 μm thick layer of flat, partially desiccated, non-living tissue which forms the skin's outermost surface.[1,2] The stratum corneum is composed of approximately 40% protein (mainly keratin) and 40% water, with the balance being lipid, principally as triglycerides, free fatty acids, cholesterol, and phospholipids. The lipid content is concentrated in the extracellular phase of the stratum corneum and forms to a large extent the membranes surrounding the cells. The lipid component is considered the factor directly responsible for low penetration of drug through the stratum corneum. Once through the stratum corneum, drug molecules may then pass through the deeper epidermal tissues and into the dermis. When the drug reaches the vascularized dermal layer, it becomes available for absorption into the general circulation.

The stratum corneum, being keratinized tissue, behaves as a semipermeable artificial membrane, and drug molecules penetrate by passive diffusion. Thus, the rate of drug movement across this skin layer is dependent on the drug concentration in the vehicle, its aqueous solubility, and its oil/water partition coefficient between the stratum corneum and the vehicle. Substances that possess both aqueous and lipid solubility characteristics are good candidates for diffusion through the stratum corneum as well as through the epidermal and dermal layers.

Although the skin has been divided histologically into the stratum corneum, the living epidermis, and the dermis, collectively it can be considered a laminate of barriers. Permeation of this laminate can occur by diffusion via:[3]

1. *trans*cellular penetration (across the cells)
2. *inter*cellular penetration (between the cells)
3. transappendageal penetration (via hair follicles, sweat and sebum glands, and pilosebaceous apparatus).

Factors Affecting Percutaneous Absorption

Among the factors playing a part in the percutaneous absorption of drugs are the nature of the drug itself, the nature of the vehicle, the condition of the skin, and the presence of mois-ture. Although general statements applicable to all possible combinations of drug, vehicle, and skin condition are difficult to draw, the consensus of the majority of research findings may be summarized as follows.[4]

1. The drug incorporated in an appropriate vehicle must interface the skin surface in sufficient concentration.
2. Drug concentration is an important factor. Generally, the amount of drug percutaneously absorbed per unit of surface area per time interval increases as the concentration of the drug substance in the vehicle is increased.
3. More drug is absorbed through percutaneous absorption when the drug substance is applied to a larger surface area.
4. The drug substance should have a greater physicochemical attraction to the skin than to the vehicle in which it is presented in order for the drug to leave the vehicle in favor of the skin.
5. Some degree of solubility of the drug substance in both oil and water is thought to be essential for effective percutaneous absorption. In essence, the aqueous solubility of a drug determines the concentration presented to the absorption site and the partition coefficient strongly influences the rate of transport across the absorption site. Solutes with molecular weights below 800 to 100 with adequate solubility in mineral oil and water (>1 mg/mL) can permeate skin.
6. Drug absorption appears to be enhanced from vehicles that easily cover the skin surface, mix readily with the sebum, and bring the drug into contact with the tissue cells for absorption.
7. Vehicles that increase the amount of moisture imbibed by the skin generally favor the percutaneous absorption of drugs. Oleaginous vehicles act as moisture barriers through which the sweat from the skin cannot pass, and the skin therefore remains occluded, generally resulting in an increased hydration of the skin beneath the vehicle.
8. The hydration of the skin is one of the most important factors in percutaneous absorption. The hydration of the stratum corneum appears to increase the rate of passage of certain substances that penetrate the skin.

Increased absorption is probably due to the softening of the tissue and the consequent "sponging" effect with an increase in the size of the pores, allowing a greater flow of substances, large and small, through them.

9. Hydration of the skin is influenced not only by the type of vehicle (e.g., oleaginous) but also by the absence or presence of a bandage (and the type) over the medicated application. In general, bandaging a nonocclusive application, such as a water-miscible vehicle, will enhance the moisturizing effect of the skin through the inhibition of the evaporation of the sweat and thereby enhance absorption. An occlusive bandage is more effective in this regard than a loosely woven, nonocclusive one.

10. In general, the amount of rubbing in or inunction of the topical application will have a bearing on the amount of drug absorbed; the longer the period of inunction, the greater the absorption.

11. Percutaneous absorption appears to be greater when the drug is applied to skin with a thin horny layer than with one that is thick. Thus, the site of application may have a bearing on the degree of drug absorption, with the absorption from calloused or thickened sites as the palms of the hands and soles of the feet being comparatively slow. Studies have shown that skin in the postauricular area is more permeable to drugs than is skin from the back, chest, forearm, or thigh.[2] In addition to thickness, the properties of the stratum corneum vary at different body sites including differences in number of cell layers, stacking of cells, size of cells, and amount of surface lipid.

12. Generally, the longer the period of time the medicated application is permitted to remain in contact with the skin, the greater will be the absorption. However, changes in the hydration of the skin during the application period or the saturation of the skin with the drug could preclude significant additional absorption with increasing time.

These general statements on percutaneous absorption apply to skin in the normal state. In injury to the skin or in disease states of varying dimension, differences in drug absorption will occur. Quite clearly, skin that has been abraded, cut, or broken will permit drugs, and for that matter other foreign substances, to gain direct access to the subcutaneous tissues.

The intrinsic permeability of skin shows little variation from a few hours after birth to extreme old age; the ultrastructure of the stratum corneum in a newborn infant is indistinguishable from that of an adult.[2] However, blood levels of drug following topical application may be higher in infants than in adults due to a greater body surface to volume ratio. There is little, if any, difference between the permeability characteristics of human male and female skin. Differences in the drug permeability of skin of different races has not been unequivocally demonstrated.

Percutaneous Absorption Enhancers

There is a continuing interest among pharmaceutical scientists to identify substances that can enhance the percutaneous absorption of therapeutic agents. It is often difficult to determine whether materials used to enhance absorption do so by directly influencing the stratum corneum or by enhancing drug release from the formulation to the skin. However, a number of agents have been credited with enhancing skin penetration including dimethylsulfoxide (DMSO), dimethylacetamide, dimethylformamide, alcohol, acetone, propylene glycol, and polyethylene glycol.[2,5] Proposed mechanisms of action for percutaneous absorption enhancers are: the reduction of the resistance of the stratum corneum by altering its physicochemical properties; alteration of the hydration of the stratum corneum; effecting a change in the structure of the lipids and lipoproteins in the intercellular channels, through solvent action or denaturation; and carrier mechanisms in the transport of ionizable drugs.[2,5]

Transdermal Drug Delivery Systems

Transdermal drug delivery systems are designed to support the passage of drug substances from the surface of the skin, through its various layers, and into the systemic circulation (Fig. 9–2). Physically, these systems are sophisticated patches as shown in Figures 9–3 through 9–9, outlined in Table 9–1, and described as follows.

There are two basic types of transdermal dos-

Fig. 9–2. *Depiction of a four-layered therapeutic transdermal system showing the continuous and controlled amount of medication released from the system, permeating the skin and entering the systemic circulation. (Courtesy of Alza Corporation.)*

ing systems: (1) *those that control* the rate of drug delivery to the skin, and (2) *those that allow the skin to control* the rate of drug absorption. The second type is useful for drugs for which there is a wide range of plasma concentration over which the drug is effective, but not toxic. For these drugs, transdermal dosage forms may be developed of various sizes and drug concentrations, with the physician increasing the dose and blood level of the drug by increasing the size of the transdermal application until the desired effect is obtained. However, for many drugs, it is important to control more closely and predictably the rate of drug delivery and percutaneous absorption. In these instances, drug delivery systems have been developed that control the rate of drug delivery to the skin for subsequent absorption. Effective transdermal drug delivery systems of this type deliver uniform quantities of drug to the skin over a period of time. The amounts of drug delivered per unit of time are determined to be less than that which is "absorbable" by varied types of skin, and thus, the drug delivery system, and not the skin, controls the amount of drug entering the circulation.

Included among the design features and objectives of rate-controlling transdermal drug delivery systems are the following:[6-9]

1. Deliver the drug substances at a controlled rate, to the intact skin of patients, for absorption into the systemic circulation.
2. The system should possess the proper physicochemical characteristics to permit the ready release of the drug substance and facilitate its partition from the delivery system into the stratum corneum.
3. The system should occlude the skin to ensure the one-way flux of the drug substance.
4. The transdermal system should have a therapeutic advantage over other dosage forms and drug delivery systems.
5. The system's adhesive, vehicle, and active agent should be nonirritating and nonsensitizing to the skin of the patient.
6. The patch should adhere well to the patient's skin and its physical size and appearance and placement on the body should not be a deterrent to use.
7. The system should not permit the proliferation of skin bacteria beneath the occlusion.

Among the advantages of transdermal drug delivery systems are the following:

1. Avoids gastrointestinal drug absorption difficulties caused by gastrointestinal pH, enzymatic activity, drug interactions with food, drink, or other orally administered drugs.
2. Substitutes for oral administration of medication when that route is unsuitable, as in instances of vomiting and/or diarrhea.
3. Avoids *first-pass effect*, that is, the initial pass of a drug substance through the systemic and portal circulation following gastrointestinal absorption (thereby possibly avoiding the drug's deactivation by digestive and liver enzymes).
4. Avoids the risks and inconveniences of parenteral therapy and the variable absorption and metabolism associated with oral therapy.
5. Provides the capacity for multiday therapy with a single application, thereby improving patient compliance over use of other dosage forms requiring more frequent dose administration.
6. Extends the activity of drugs having short half-lives through the reservoir of drug present in the therapeutic delivery system and its controlled release characteristics.
7. Provides capacity to terminate drug effect rapidly (if clinically desired) by removal of drug application from the surface of the skin.
8. Provides ease of rapid identification of the medication in emergencies (e.g., nonresponsive, unconscious, or comatose patient).

Among the disadvantages of transdermal drug delivery systems are the following:

1. The transdermal route of administration is unsuitable for drugs that irritate or sensitize the skin.
2. Only relatively potent drugs are suitable candidates for transdermal delivery due to the natural limits of drug entry imposed by the skin's impermeability.
3. Technical difficulties are associated with: the adhesion of the systems to different skin types and under various environmental conditions, and, the development of rate-controlling drug delivery features which are economically feasible and therapeutically advantageous for more than a few drug substances.

Examples of Transdermal Systems in Use

The first transdermal therapeutic system designed to control the delivery of drug to the skin for absorption was developed in 1980 by Alza Corporation. This system was designed to deliver the drug, scopolamine, to the skin behind the ear for systemic absorption in the control of nausea and vomiting associated with motion sickness (Fig. 9–3). Scopolamine has a narrow range of plasma concentration within which it is effective. Dosing levels and intervals which cause peaks and valleys to occur in blood level concentrations of the drug are more likely to produce side effects than when the drug is administered in a steady-state manner. The transdermal drug delivery system which has been developed provides the steady-state drug delivery over a 72 hour (3-day) period. The system obviates the oral route which yields unpredictable absorption, and, utilizes a lower dose which minimizes the incidence of side effects. The system, marketed as Transderm-Scōp by CIBA, is a circular flat adhesive patch designed for the continuous release of scopolamine through a rate-controlling microporous membrane.

The Transderm-Scōp system is a 0.2 mm thick patch having the following four layers:[10] (1) a backing layer of tan-colored, aluminized polyester film; (2) a drug reservoir of scopolamine, mineral oil, and polyisobutylene; (3) a microporous polypropylene membrane that controls the rate of delivery of scopolamine from the system to the skin surface; and (4) an adhesive formulation of mineral oil, polyisobutylene, and scopolamine. Prior to use, a protective peel strip

Fig. 9–3. *The Transderm Scōp (scopolamine) disc provides protection from the nausea and vomiting of motion sickness. (Courtesy of Alza Corporation and CIBA Pharmaceutical Company.)*

of siliconized polyester which covers layer 4 is removed.

The patch is 2.5 cm² in area and contains 1.5 mg of scopolamine. The system is designed to deliver 0.5 mg scopolamine, at an approximately constant rate to the systemic circulation, over the 3-day lifetime of the system. An initial priming dose of 200 mcg of scopolamine, released from the adhesive layer of the system, saturates the skin binding sites for scopolamine and rapidly brings the plasma concentration to the required steady-state level. The continuous controlled release of scopolamine from the drug reservoir through the rate-controlling membrane maintains the plasma level constant. The microporous membrane releases the scopolamine from the drug-reservoir at a rate less than the skin's capability for absorption and thus, the membrane, not the skin, controls the delivery of the drug into the circulation. Because of the small size of the patch, the system is unobtrusive, convenient, and well-accepted by the patient. Patients should be advised to place the adhesive disk behind the ear about 4 hours before travel. Only one disk should be worn at a time and may be kept in place for up to 3 days. If continued treatment is desired, the first disk should be removed and discarded, and a fresh disk placed behind the second ear. The most common side effects encountered are dryness of the mouth and/or drowsiness. However, it is known that anticholinergics like scopolamine can also interfere with orientation, cognition and memory, and may cause disruption of global function, i.e., delirium, particularly in the geriatric population. The elderly have a relative deficiency of brain acetylcholine, which can increase their susceptibility to disruption in function because of central-acting anticholinergic drugs. Therefore, the use of transdermal scopolamine, even in low doses, should be with caution.

A second example of a drug used in transdermal drug delivery systems is nitroglycerin. A number of nitroglycerin-containing systems have been developed, including: Deponit (Wyeth-Ayerst), Minitran (3M Riker), Transderm-Nitro (CIBA), Nitro-Dur (Key), Nitrocine (Schwarz Pharma), and Nitrodisc (Searle). As indicated in Table 9–1, these products contain sufficient nitroglycerin to maintain drug delivery for 24 hours.

Nitroglycerin is a drug substance utilized widely in the prophylactic treatment of angina. The drug has a relatively low dose, short plasma half-life, high-peak plasma levels and inherent side-effects when taken sublingually (a popular route for its administration). It is rapidly metabolized by the liver when taken orally, which contributes to its low bioavailability by this route. For these reasons, nitroglycerin is a drug which has been advantageously administered by the transdermal route.

The various commercially available products control the rate of drug delivery to the systemic circulation through a rate-controlling membrane, and/or through controlled drug-release from the drug matrix (the drug-reservoir of the system). One of these products, Transderm-Nitro (CIBA), is similar in design to the Transderm-Scōp system, and is depicted in Figures 9–4 to 9–6. The system is a flat unit designed to provide controlled release of nitroglycerin through a semipermeable membrane continuously for 24 hours following application to intact skin. The Transderm-Nitro system comprises four layers:[11] (1) a tan-colored backing layer (aluminized plastic) that is impermeable to nitro-

glycerin (important since nitroglycerin is a volatile substance which could be lost unless protected); (2) a drug reservoir containing nitroglycerin adsorbed on lactose, colloidal silicon dioxide, and silicone medical fluid; (3) an ethylene/vinyl acetate copolymer membrane that is permeable to nitroglycerin; and (4) a layer of hypoallergenic silicone adhesive. Prior to use, a protective peel strip is removed from the adhesive surface (Fig. 9–5).

When the Transderm-Nitro system is applied to the skin, nitroglycerin is absorbed continuously through the skin into the systemic circulation. This results in active drug reaching the target organs (heart, extremities) before being inactivated by the liver. One-fifth of the total nitroglycerin in the system is delivered transdermally to the patient over 24 hours; the remainder serves as the thermodynamic energy source to release the drug and remains in the system. The rated release of drug is dependent upon the area of the system; 0.5 mg nitroglycerin is delivered in vivo for every cm^2 of system size. Systems are rated to release in vivo 2.5, 5, 10 and 15 mg of nitroglycerin over 24 hours in patch sizes of 5, 10, 20, and 30 cm^2 respectively.

Other nitroglycerin transdermal infusion systems have their own unique construction and features. Nitro-Dur (Key) contains 2% of nitroglycerin in a gel-like matrix composed of glycerin, water (purified), lactose, polyvinyl alcohol, povidone and sodium citrate to provide a continuous source of the active ingredient. The transdermal system is available in dosage sizes of 5, 10, 15, 20, and 30 cm^2, containing 20, 40, 60, 80 and 120 mg of nitroglycerin, respectively. Nitro-Dur has a rated release in vivo of approximately 0.5 mg/cm^2/24 hours. Each unit is sealed in a polyester-foil-polyethylene laminate as shown in Figure 9–7.[12] The bandage portion consists of a non-woven, heat sealable, microporous tape.

When the Nitro-Dur system is applied to the skin, nitroglycerin is absorbed continuously through the skin into the systemic circulation. The Nitro-Dur matrix is in a highly kinetic equilibrium state. Dissolved nitroglycerin molecules are constantly exchanging with adsorbed nitroglycerin molecules bound to the surfaces of the suspended lactose crystals. Sufficient nitroglycerin is adsorbed to the lactose in each matrix to maintain nitroglycerin in the fluid phase (aqueous glycerol) at a stable but saturated level (5 mg nitroglycerin/cm^2 matrix). When the matrix is applied to the surface of the skin, nitroglyc-

Table 9–1.   Examples of Transdermal Drug Delivery Systems[10-17]

Therapeutic Agent	Product	Design/Contents	Comments
Clonidine	Catapres-TTS (Boehringer Ingelheim)	Four-layered patch: (1) a backing layer of pigmented polyester film; (2) drug reservoir of clonidine, mineral oil, polyisobutylene, and colloidal silicon dioxide; (3) a microporous polypropylene membrane controlling the rate of drug delivery, and (4) an adhesive formulation of agents noted in (2) above.	Transdermal therapeutic systems designed to deliver a therapeutic dose of the antihypertensive clonidine at a constant rate for 7 days, permitting once-a-week dosing. TTS generally applied to hairless or shaven areas of upper arm or torso.
Estradiol	Estraderm (CIBA)	Four-layered patch: (1) a transparent polyester film; (2) drug reservoir of estradiol and alcohol gelled with hydroxypropyl cellulose; (3) an ethylene-vinyl acetate copolymer membrane, and (4) an adhesive formulation of light mineral oil and polyisobutylene.	Transdermal system designed to release 17β-estradiol continuously. The transdermal patch is generally applied twice weekly over a cycle of 3 weeks with dosage frequency adjusted as required. The patch is generally applied to the abdomen, alternating sites with each application.
Nitroglycerin	Deponit (Wyeth-Ayerst)	Nitroglycerin in a matrix of lactose, plasticizer, polyisobutylene, and aluminized plastic.	Transdermal therapeutic systems designed to provide controlled release of nitroglycerin continuously for a 24-hour period. Patches are generally applied to hairless or shaven inner part of upper arm, shoulders, or chest; never to distal part of extremities. Each application is rotated to a slightly different skin area to avoid irritation.
	Minitran (3M Riker)	Nitroglycerin in a hypoallergenic acrylate-based polymer adhesive sealed in a foil/polymer film laminate. The patch is transparent when applied.	
	Nitrocine (Schwarz Pharma)	Nitroglycerin in a laminated matrix of polyvinyl chloride/polyvinyl acetate copolymer, di-(2-ethylhexyl)phthalate, isopropyl palmitate, colloidal silicon dioxide, aluminum foil laminate, polyethylene foam and acrylic adhesive.	
	Nitrodisc (Searle)	Microseal Drug Delivery system consisting of a solid, nitroglycerin-impregnated polymer bonded to a flexible, nonsensitizing adhesive bandage. Inactive ingredients are lactose, isopropyl palmitate, mineral oil, polyethylene glycol, water, silicone rubber, plasticizers, aluminum foil laminate, polyethylene foam, and acrylic adhesive.	

Table 9–1. Continued

Therapeutic Agent	Product	Design/Contents	Comments
Nitroglycerin (cont.)	Nitro-Dur (Key)	Nitroglycerin in a gel-like matrix composed of glycerin, water, lactose, polyvinyl alcohol, povidone and sodium citrate sealed in a polyester-foil-polyethylene laminate.	
	Transderm-Nitro (CIBA)	Four-layered patch: (1) backing layer of aluminized plastic; (2) drug reservoir containing nitroglycerin adsorbed on lactose, colloidal silicon dioxide, and silicone medical fluid, (3) an ethylene/vinyl acetate copolymer membrane; and (4) silicone adhesive.	
Scopolamine	Transderm Scōp (CIBA)	Four-layered patch: (1) backing layer of aluminized polyester film; (2) drug reservoir of scopolamine, mineral oil, and polyisobutylene; (3) a microporous polypropylene membrane for rate delivery of scopolamine; and (4) adhesive of polyisobutylene, mineral oil, and scopolamine.	Transdermal therapeutic system for continuous release of scopolamine over a 3-day period as required for the prevention of nausea and vomiting associated with motion sickness. The patch is placed behind the ear. When repeated administration is desired, the first patch is removed and the second patch placed behind the other ear.

Fig. 9–4. *The Transderm-Nitro Transdermal Therapeutic System (CIBA). The patch delivers nitroglycerin through the skin directly into the blood stream for 24 hours. Transderm-Nitro is used to treat and prevent angina. The system consists of a water-resistant backing layer, a reservoir of nitroglycerin, followed by a semipermeable membrane to control precisely and predictably the release of medicine, and an adhesive layer to hold the system onto the skin. The adhesive layer also contains an initial priming dose of nitroglycerin to insure prompt release and absorption of the medication. (Courtesy of CIBA Pharmaceutical.)*

Fig. 9–5. (A, B). *The Transderm-Nitro patch (CIBA). Prior to applying to the skin, a plastic liner is removed exposing the adhesive side of the patch. Transderm-Nitro delivers nitroglycerin at a constant and predetermined rate through the skin directly into the bloodstream. The patch is designed to provide 24-hour protection against angina attacks. (Courtesy of Alza Corporation and CIBA Pharmaceutical Company.)*

Fig. 9–6. *The Minitran (nitroglycerin) Transdermal Delivery System, a transparent nitroglycerin patch for use in treating angina. The Minitran patch is thin, flexible, and adheres well to the skin. (Courtesy of 3M Riker.)*

erin molecules migrate from solution in the matrix, by diffusion, to solution in the skin. To make up for the molecules lost to the body, there is a shift of equilibrium in the matrix such that more molecules of nitroglycerin leave the crystals than are adsorbed from solution. When balance is restored, the solution is again at a saturated level. Thus, the crystals of lactose act as a "reservoir" of drug to maintain drug saturation in the fluid phase. The Nitro-Dur matrix, in turn, acts as a saturated "reservoir" for diffusive drug input through the skin.[13]

In bioavailability studies, transdermal absorption of nitroglycerin from the gel-like matrix achieved steady rate venous plasma levels comparable to that of sublingual nitroglycerin and maintained these levels for 24 hours. Therapeutic effect is achieved within 30 minutes after application of the unit, and persists about 30 minutes after removal of the unit.[12,13]

The Nitrodisc (Searle) system consists of a solid, nitroglycerin-impregnated polymer bonded to a flexible, non-sensitizing adhesive bandage. Nitrodisc provides constant and controlled drug delivery over a uniform skin surface area for 24 hours (Fig. 9–8).

Similar to Key's Nitro-Dur system, the core of the Nitrodisc system is a polymeric matrix

1. FOIL COVERSTRIP
2. DRUG MATRIX
3. RELEASE LINER
4. FOIL BASEPLATE
5. MICROPOROUS TAPE
6. ABSORBENT PAD
7. OCCLUSIVE OVERLAY

Fig. 9–7. *The Nitro-Dur Transdermal Infusion System, depicting the construction of the product. (Courtesy of Key Pharmaceuticals, Inc.)*

from which the nitroglycerin is released. However, the matrix of the Nitrodisc system is a solid silicone-based polymer rather than a gel-like matrix. The manufacturing process for the system involves mixing the nitroglycerin and a silicone polymer together as liquids and allowing the polymer to "cure," thereby forming the drug-impregnated solid matrix.

The Nitrodisc system is applied to the skin as a flexible, nonsensitizing foam adhesive bandage. It is available in two strengths which release either 5 mg or 10 mg of nitroglycerin during a 24-hour period. The 5 mg/24 hour system contains 16 mg nitroglycerin over an 8 cm² releasing surface. The 10 mg/24 hours system contains 32 mg nitroglycerin over a 16 cm² releasing surface.

In clinical studies, transdermal absorption of nitroglycerin from Nitrodisc occurred in a continuous and well-controlled manner for a minimum of 24 hours. Therapeutic plasma levels were attained within 1 hour after the application of the pad and remained in the therapeutic range for 24 hours. Plasma levels of nitroglycerin were still detectable 30 minutes after removal of the system.[14]

Fig. 9–8. *Example of the product package of the Nitrodisc transdermal nitroglycerin system. The 5 mg/24 hour system contains 16 mg of nitroglycerin over an 8 cm² releasing surface. (Courtesy of Searle Pharmaceuticals, Inc.)*

Patients should be given explicit instructions regarding the use of transdermal systems. Generally, these patches are placed on the chest, with the back, upper arms or shoulders being used as alternatives. The site selected should be free of hair, clean and dry so that the patch adheres with no difficulty. The use of the extremities below the knee or elbow should be discouraged as should those areas that are abraded or have lesions, cuts, etc. The patient should understand that physical exercise and elevated ambient temperatures, e.g., sauna, may increase the absorption of the nitroglycerin. Further, patients must be told to remove the old patch when the new patch is applied. Because patient preference plays a role in therapy success, the patient should be asked occasionally by the pharmacist about a product's ease of application and removal, adhesiveness, comfort, size, and appearance of the patch. If patient difficulty is encountered with any of these, the patient should be told to discuss this with his/her physician so that the patient can be converted to an acceptable patch that encourages compliance.

In 1985, the first *transdermal therapeutic* system for hypertension, Catapres TTS (Boehringer Ingelheim), was marketed. The drug present, clonidine, lends itself to the transdermal delivery system because of its lipid solubility, high volume of distribution, and therapeutic effectiveness in low plasma concentrations. The product, developed jointly by Alza Corporation and Boehringer-Ingelheim provides 7 days of continuous antihypertensive therapy. The product is designed as a four-layered patch to provide the controlled release of clonidine in fixed amounts that yields constant blood levels. The system is 0.2 mm thick with surface areas of 3.5, 7.0, or 10.5 cm^2.[15] The amount of drug released is proportional to the area of the system used. The four areas of the system are: (1) a backing layer of pigmented polyester film; (2) a drug reservoir of clonidine, mineral oil, polyisobutylene, and colloidal silicon dioxide; (3) a microporous polypropylene membrane that controls the rate of delivery of clonidine from the system to the skin surface; (4) an adhesive formulation of clonidine, mineral oil, polyisobutylene, and colloidal silicon dioxide. Prior to use, a protective peel strip of polyester that covers layer 4 is removed.

The 3.5, 7.0 and 10.5 cm^2 systems available respectively deliver 0.1, 0.2, and 0.3 mg clonidine per day. To ensure constant release of drug over 7 days, the total drug content of the system is greater than the total amount of drug delivered. The energy source of drug release derives from the concentration gradient existing between a saturated solution of drug in the system and the much lower concentration prevailing in the skin. Clonidine flows in the direction of the lower concentration at a constant rate, limited by the rate-controlling membrane, so long as a saturated solution is maintained in the drug reservoir.[15]

Following system application to intact skin, clonidine in the adhesive layer saturates the skin sites below the system. Clonidine from the drug reservoir then begins to flow through the rate-controlling membrane and the adhesive layer of the system into the systemic circulation via the capillaries beneath the skin. Therapeutic plasma clonidine levels are achieved 2 to 3 days after initial application of the system. Application of a new system to a fresh skin site at weekly intervals continuously maintains therapeutic plasma concentrations of clonidine. If the patch is removed and not replaced with a new system, therapeutic plasma clonidine levels will persist for about 8 hours and then decline slowly over several days. Over this time period, blood pressure returns gradually to pretreatment levels. If the patient experiences localized skin irritation before completing 7 days of use, the system may be removed and replaced with a new one applied on a fresh skin site.[15]

Another drug developed for transdermal delivery is the estrogen, estradiol. The Estraderm (CIBA) transdermal system (Fig. 9–9) is designed to release 17β-estradiol through a rate-limiting membrane continuously upon application to intact skin.[16] Two systems (10 or 20 cm^2) provide delivery of 0.05 or 0.1 mg estradiol per day via skin of average permeability.

The Estraderm system comprises four layers: (1) a transparent polyester film, (2) a drug reservoir of estradiol and alcohol gelled with hydroxypropyl cellulose, (3) an ethylene-vinyl acetate copolymer membrane, and (4) an adhesive formulation of light mineral oil and polyisobutylene. A protective liner of siliconized polyethylene terephthalate film is attached to the adhesive surface and is removed before the system can be used.[16]

Estradiol is indicated for the treatment of moderate-to-severe vasomotor symptoms as-

Fig. 9–9. *An estrogen skin patch, marketed under the brand name Estraderm (CIBA, Estradiol Transdermal System), is transparent and about the size of a silver dollar. It contains 17-beta estradiol, which is identical to the estrogen produced naturally prior to menopause. In releasing small amounts of estrogen at a relatively constant and controlled rate directly into the bloodstream, the patch closely mimics the natural levels of estrogen produced in premenopausal women. (Courtesy of Alza Corporation and CIBA Pharmaceutical Company.)*

sociated with menopause; female hypogonadism; female castration; primary ovarian failure; and atrophic conditions caused by deficient endogenous estrogen production, such as atrophic vaginitis and kraurosis vulva.

Orally administered estradiol is rapidly metabolized by the liver to estrone and its conjugates, giving rise to higher circulating levels of estrone than estradiol. In contrast, the skin metabolizes estradiol only to a small extent. Therefore, transdermal administration produces therapeutic serum levels of estradiol with lower circulating levels of estrone and estrone conjugates, and requires smaller total doses than does oral therapy. Research has demonstrated that postmenopausal women receiving either transdermal or oral therapy will obtain the desired therapeutic effects from both dosage forms, e.g., lower gonadotropin levels, lower percentages of vaginal parabasal cells, decreased excretion of calcium, and lower calcium-to-creatinine ratio. Studies have also demon-

strated that systemic side effects from oral estrogens can be reduced by using the transdermal dosage form. Because estradiol has a short half-life (~1 hour), transdermal administration of estradiol allows a rapid decline in blood levels after the transdermal system is removed, e.g., in a cycling regimen.[16]

Therapy is usually administered on a cyclic schedule (e.g., 3 weeks of therapy followed by 1 week without) especially in women who have not undergone a hysterectomy. The transdermal system is generally applied to the abdominal skin twice weekly. The woman should be told to place the adhesive side of the patch on a clean dry area of the skin, preferably the abdomen. The system should be applied immediately after opening the pouch and removing the protective liner. The woman should press the patch firmly in place with the palm of the hand for at least 10 seconds and make sure that good contact has been obtained around the edges of the patch. The patch should not be applied to the breast or the waistline because tight clothing may damage or dislodge the system. The area selected should not be oily, damaged, or irritated. The woman should understand the need to remove the old patch when a new patch is applied, and to rotate the application site with an interval at least of 1 week between applications to a particular body area.

A transdermal patch for local application has been introduced for the treatment of viral wart infections. Trans-Ver-Sal (Minnetonka) contains 15% salicylic acid in a vehicle consisting primarily of karaya, a substance known for its nonirritating and self-adhesive properties (in ostomy therapy). The system is designed to be applied topically to a wart and provide constant and controlled release of the salicylic acid over an 8-hour treatment period. Each pad is covered with a polyethylene moisture barrier, which creates a desired occlusive effect.

The product is available in two pad sizes, i.e., 6 mm and 12 mm. Preferably the pad is applied at bedtime. The patient should clean the affected area, and then smooth the wart surface as much as possible with the provided cleaning file. The pharmacist should instruct the patient to lift a pad from the clear strip laminate in which it is contained, leaving the top plastic film in place. If the pad is too large for the wart, the patient should trim it to a size that will cover only the wart surface. Prior to application of the pad the patient should wet the wart with a drop of warm water, while ensuring that surrounding healthy skin remains dry. This enhances penetration of the salicylic acid into the wart. With the plastic film side facing up, the patient should apply the sticky bottom side onto the wart. Lastly, the patient uses a strip of tape that is provided to hold the pad in place. The pad is removed by the patient the next morning and discarded. The patient then continues using the Trans-Ver-Sal as the doctor has indicated.

Technology of Transdermal Delivery Systems

Examples of the configuration and composition of transdermal drug delivery systems are described in the text, presented in Table 9–1, and shown in Figures 9–3 through 9–9. Technically, transdermal drug delivery systems may be categorized into two types, monolithic and membrane-controlled systems.

Monolithic systems incorporate a drug matrix layer between backing and frontal layers (Fig. 9–7). The drug-matrix layer is composed of a polymeric material in which the drug is dispersed. The polymer matrix controls the rate at which the drug is released for percutaneous absorption. The matrix may be of two types; that is, with or without an excess of drug with regard to its equilibrium solubility and steady-state concentration gradient at the stratum corneum.[17,18] In types having no excess, drug is available to maintain the saturation of the stratum corneum only as long as the level of drug in the device exceeds the solubility limit of the stratum corneum. As the concentration of drug in the device diminishes below the skin's saturation limit, the transport of drug from device to skin gradually declines.[18,19] In monolithic systems that have an excess amount of drug persent in the matrix, a drug reserve is present to assure continued drug saturation at the stratum corneum. In these instances, the rate of drug decline is less than in the type designed with no drug reserve. Nitro-Dur (Key) and Nitrodisc (Searle) are examples of monolithic systems.

In the preparation of monolithic systems, the drug and the polymer are dissolved or blended together, cast as the matrix, and dried.[17] The gelled matrix may be produced in sheet or cylindrical form, with individual dosage units cut and assembled between the backing and frontal layers. Most transdermal drug delivery systems are designed to contain an excess of drug and thus drug-releasing capacity *beyond the time frame* recommended for replacement. This as-sures continuous drug availability and absorption as used patches are replaced on schedule with fresh ones.

Membrane-controlled transdermal systems are designed to contain a drug reservoir, usually in liquid or gel form, a rate-controlling membrane, and backing, adhesive, and protecting layers (Fig. 9–4). Transderm-Nitro (CIBA) and Transderm-Scōp (CIBA) are examples of this technology. Membrane-controlled systems have the advantage over monolithic systems in that as long as the drug solution in the reservoir remains saturated, the release rate of drug through the controlling membrane remains constant.[18] In membrane systems, a small quantity of drug is frequently placed in the adhesive layer to initiate prompt drug absorption and pharmacotherapeutic effects upon skin placement. Membrane-controlled systems may be prepared by preconstructing the delivery unit, filling the drug reservoir, and sealing, or by a process of lamination, which involves a continuous process of construction, dosing, and sealing. Some steps in the production of transdermal drug delivery systems are shown in Figures 9–10 through 9–12.

In summary, either the drug delivery device or the skin may serve as the rate-controlling mechanism in drug transport from transdermal systems. For example, if the drug is delivered to the stratum córneum at a rate less than the absorption capacity, the *device* is the controlling factor. If, on the other hand, the drug is delivered to the skin area to saturation, the *skin* is the controlling factor to the rate of drug absorption. Thus, in actuality, the rate of drug transport in all transdermal systems, monolithic and membrane, are controlled by either artificial or natural (skin) membranes.

In addition to the drugs currently incorporated into transdermal delivery devices, many others are under study, including: cardiovascular drugs, as isosorbide dinitrate; beta blockers, as timolol and propranolol; antihistamines, as chlorpheniramine; cholinergics, as physostigmine; analgesics, as fentanyl; and, nicotine, as a smoking deterrent.

Ointments

Ointments *(unguents)* are semisolid preparations intended for external application. Those intended for application to the eye are specially prepared and are termed *ophthalmic ointments*.

Fig. 9–10. *Measured dose for reservoir, placed on web prior to sealing into the transdermal delivery system. (Courtesy of CIBA Pharmaceutical Company.)*

Fig. 9–11. *Placing transdermal therapeutic system in pressure tester for seal test. (Courtesy of CIBA Pharmaceutical Company.)*

Fig. 9–12. *A rotary die-cutting pressure executes the final step in manufacturing Transderm Scōp systems prior to packaging. (Courtesy of Alza Corporation.)*

They will be taken up in the next chapter. Ointments may be medicated or nonmedicated, the latter type being commonly referred to as *ointment bases* and used as such for their emollient or lubricating effect or used as vehicles in the preparation of medicated ointments.

Ointment Bases

Ointment bases are classified into four general groups: (1) hydrocarbon bases, (2) absorption bases, (3) water-removable bases, and (4) water-soluble bases.

Hydrocarbon Bases

Hydrocarbon bases (oleaginous bases) are water-free, and aqueous preparations may be incorporated into them only in small amounts and then with difficulty. Hydrocarbon bases are used chiefly for their emollient effect. They are retained on the skin for prolonged periods, do not permit the escape of moisture from the skin to the atmosphere, and are difficult to wash off. As such they act as occlusive dressings. They do not "dry out" or change noticeably upon aging.

Petrolatum

Petrolatum, USP, is a mixture of semisolid hydrocarbons obtained from petroleum. Pet-

rolatum is an unctuous mass, varying in color from yellowish to light amber. It melts at temperatures between 38°C and 60°C. It may be used alone or in combination with other agents as an ointment base.

Synonyms: Yellow Petrolatum: Petroleum Jelly
Commercial Product: Vaseline (Chesebrough)

White Petrolatum

White Petrolatum, USP, is petrolatum that has been decolorized. It differs only in this respect to petrolatum and is used for the same purpose. White petrolatum is more esthetically acceptable to a patient than petrolatum. In addition, because of its occlusive, nonwater-washable characteristics, white petrolatum is particularly useful to treat diaper rash (impervious to urine and protects the baby's skin) and dry skin (helps the skin retain moisture).

Synonym: White Petroleum Jelly
Commercial Product: White Vaseline (Chesebrough)

Yellow Ointment

Each 100 g of Yellow Ointment, USP, contains 5 g of yellow wax and 95 g of petrolatum. **Yellow Wax,** is the purified wax obtained from the honeycomb of the bee *(Apis mellifera)*.

Synonym: Simple Ointment

Mineral Oil

Mineral Oil is a mixture of liquid hydrocarbons obtained from petroleum. It is useful as a levigating substance to wet and to incorporate solid substances, e.g., salicylic acid, zinc oxide, into the preparation of ointments that consist of oleaginous bases as their vehicle.

Synonym: Liquid Petrolatum

Absorption Bases

Absorption bases may be of two types: (1) those that permit the incorporation of aqueous solutions, resulting in the formation of water-in-oil emulsions (e.g. *Hydrophilic Petrolatum* and *Anhydrous Lanolin*) and (2) those that are already water-in-oil emulsions *(emulsion bases)* that permit the incorporation of small, additional quantities of aqueous solutions (e.g. *Lanolin* and *Cold Cream)*. These bases are useful as emollients although they do not provide the degree of occlusion afforded by the oleaginous bases. Like the oleaginous bases, absorption bases are not easily removed from the skin with water washing. They are also useful pharmaceutically to incorporate aqueous solutions of drugs, e.g., sodium sulfacetamide, into oleaginous bases. For example, an aqueous solution may be first incorporated into the absorption base, and then this mixture added into the oleaginous base. In doing this, an equivalent amount of oleaginous base in the formula is replaced by the absorption base. The classic example of this is in the preparation of occlusive ointment dosage forms of water-soluble drugs, e.g., gentamicin sulfate, for ophthalmic therapy.

Hydrophilic Petrolatum

Hydrophilic Petrolatum is composed of cholesterol, stearyl alcohol, white wax, and white petrolatum. It has the ability to absorb water, with the formation of a water-in-oil emulsion. Aquaphor is a highly-refined variation of Hydrophilic Petrolatum and because it can absorb up to 3 times its weight in water, it has proven useful to pharmacists who have to incorporate extemporaneously a water-soluble drug into an oleaginous base.

Anhydrous Lanolin

Anhydrous Lanolin may contain no more than 0.25% of water. Anhydrous Lanolin is insoluble in water, but mixes without separation with about twice its weight of water. The incorporation of water results in the formation of a water-in-oil emulsion. Although its rancid odor is offensive, this base finds particular use as a vehicle for the application of compound tincture of benzoin and sucrose to treat decubitus ulcers, i.e., bedsores. The extemporaneous product is rolled onto the lesion with the use of a cotton swab.
Synonym: Refined Wool Fat

Lanolin

Lanolin is a semisolid, fatlike substance obtained from the wool of sheep (*Ovis aries*). It is a water-in-oil emulsion that contains between 25 and 30% water. Additional water may be incorporated into lanolin by mixing.
Synonym: Hydrous Wool Fat

Cold Cream

Cold Cream is a semisolid, white, water-in-oil emulsion prepared with cetyl esters wax, white wax, mineral oil, sodium borate, and purified water. The sodium borate combines with the free fatty acids present in the waxes to form sodium soaps that act as the emulsifiers. Cold cream is employed as an emollient and ointment base. Eucerin Creme is a water-in-oil emulsion of petrolatum, mineral oil, mineral wax, wool wax, alcohol and bronopol. It is frequently prescribed as a vehicle for the delivery

of lactic acid and glycerin to treat dry skin. Further, the presence of water in the base is useful because the occlusive external phase traps the water onto the skin and enhances skin moisturization.

Water-Removable Bases

Water-removable bases are oil-in-water emulsions that are capable of being washed from skin or clothing with water. For this reason, they are frequently referred to as "water-washable" ointment bases. These bases, which resemble creams in appearance, may be diluted with water or with aqueous solutions. From a therapeutic viewpoint, they have the ability to absorb serous discharges in dermatologic conditions. Certain medicinal agents may be better absorbed by the skin when present in a base of this type than in other types of bases.

Hydrophilic Ointment

Hydrophilic Ointment as the name indicates, is "water-loving." It contains sodium lauryl sulfate as the emulsifying agent, with stearyl alcohol and white petrolatum representing the oleaginous phase of the emulsion and propylene glycol and water representing the aqueous phase. Methylparaben and propylparaben are used to preserve the ointment against microbial growth. The ointment is employed as a water-removable vehicle for medicinal substances.

Water-Soluble Bases

Unlike water-removable bases, which contain both water-soluble and water-insoluble components, water-soluble bases contain only water-soluble components. Like water-removable bases, however, water-soluble bases are water washable. Water-soluble bases are commonly referred to as "greaseless" because of the absence of any oleaginous materials. Because they soften greatly with the addition of water, aqueous solutions are not effectively incorporated into these bases. Rather, they are better used for the incorporation of nonaqueous or solid substances.

Polyethylene Glycol Ointment

The general formula for this base calls for the combining of 400 g of polyethylene glycol 3350 (a solid) and 600 g of polyethylene glycol 400 (a liquid) to prepare 1000 g of base. However, if a firmer ointment is required, the formula may be altered to permit up to equal parts of the two ingredients. If 6 to 25% of an aqueous solution is to be incorporated into the base, the substitution of 50 g of the polyethylene glycol 3350 with an equal amount of stearyl alcohol would be advantageous to render the final product more firm.

Polyethylene glycols are polymers of ethylene oxide and water represented by the formula $HOCH_2(CH_2OCH_2)_nCH_2OH$. The chain length may be varied to achieve polymers having desired viscosity and physical (liquid, semisolid, or solid) form.

Selection of the Appropriate Base

The selection of the base to use in the formulation of an ointment depends upon the careful assessment of a number of factors, including (a) the desired release rate of the particular drug substance from the ointment base, (b) the desirability for enhancement by the base of the percutaneous absorption of the drug, (c) the advisability of occlusion of moisture from the skin by the base, (d) the short-term and long-term stability of the drug in the ointment base, and (e) the influence, if any, of the drug on the consistency or other features of the ointment base. All of these factors, and others, must be weighed one against the other to find the most suitable base. It should be understood that no ointment base is ideal nor possesses all of the desired attributes. For instance, for a drug that hydrolyzes rapidly, a hydrocarbon base would provide the greatest stability, even though from a therapeutic standpoint another base might be preferred. The idea is to find the base that provides the majority of the most desired attributes.

Besides the physical-chemical factors that play a role in the selection of a base, patient factors also play an important role in a base's selection. The condition of the patient's skin, e.g., weeping (oozing) or dry, may dictate an ointment or a cream dosage form. For example, the old rule in dermatology that is still practiced is that if a patient's skin is dry—wet it. If it is wet—dry it. Thus, for example, if a patient's skin is dry, an occlusive ointment base that will retain moisture would be preferable. Therefore, pharmacists must realize that ointment bases and cream bases are not necessarily interchangeable, and that a dermatologist is using the effects of the ointment base as much as the active ingredient within the product to treat the patient's condition.

Preparation of Ointments

Both on a large and a small scale, ointments are prepared by two general methods: (1) incorporation and (2) fusion. The method for a particular preparation depends primarily upon the nature of the ingredients.

Incorporation

In the incorporation method, the components of the ointment are mixed together by various means until a uniform preparation has been attained. On a small scale, as in the extemporaneous compounding of prescriptions, the pharmacist may mix the components of an ointment in a mortar with a pestle, or he may employ a spatula and an ointment slab (a large glass or porcelain plate) to rub the ingredients together. Some glass ointment slabs are of ground glass to permit greater friction in the rubbing process. Some pharmacists utilize nonabsorbent parchment papers that are large enough to cover the working surface and have the advantage of being disposable, eliminating much of the time-consuming chore of cleaning the ointment slab.

INCORPORATION OF SOLIDS. When preparing an ointment by spatulation, the pharmacist generally works the ointment with a stainless steel spatula with a long, broad blade and periodically removes the accumulation of ointment on the larger spatula with a smaller spatula. If the components of an ointment are reactive with the metal of the spatula (as for example, phenol), hard rubber spatulas may be used. The ointment is prepared by thoroughly rubbing and working the components together on the hard surface with the spatula until the product is smooth and uniform. Generally the ointment base is placed on one side of the working surface, and the powdered components, previously reduced to fine powders and thoroughly blended in a mortar, are placed on the other. Then a portion of the powder is mixed with a portion of the base until uniform, and the process is repeated until all portions of the powder and base are combined. The portions of prepared ointment are then combined and thoroughly blended by continuous movement of the spatula over and through the combined portions of ointment.

When only a small portion of powder is to be added, it may be added in its entirety to a small portion of ointment base. After the two have been thoroughly mixed, another portion is added to this mixture, the process being repeated as in the "geometric method" of diluting until all of the ointment base has been incorporated.

Frequently it is desirable to reduce the particle size of any solid material before incorporation into the ointment base so that the final product will not be gritty. This may be done by *levigating* the powder by mixing it in a vehicle in which it is insoluble to make a smooth dispersion of the material. Most commonly the solid substance is mixed with a levigating agent that is compatible with the base, e.g., mineral oil, glycerin, and then with a portion of the ointment base, using an amount of levigating agent about equal to the material to be levigated, and a mortar and pestle to accomplish the reduction of particle size as well as the dispersion of the substance. After levigation, the dispersion is incorporated with the remainder of the base by spatulation or by using the mortar and pestle.

Solid materials soluble in a common solvent that will affect neither the stability of the drug nor the efficacy of the product may first be dissolved in that solvent, e.g., dissolve salicylic acid crystals in alcohol, and then the solution added to the ointment base by spatulation or by mixing in a mortar and pestle. Generally, the mortar and pestle is preferred when large volumes of liquid are added since the liquid is more captive in the mortar than on an ointment slab.

INCORPORATION OF LIQUIDS. Liquid substances or solutions of drugs, as described above, are added to an ointment only after due consideration of the ointment's nature. For instance, an aqueous solution or preparation would be added with difficulty to an oleaginous ointment, except in very small amounts. However, water-absorbable or hydrophilic ointment bases would be quite suitable for the absorption and incorporation of the aqueous solution. Frequently when adding an aqueous preparation to a base that is hydrophobic in character, the pharmacist replaces a portion of the base with a hydrophilic base, incorporates the solution in the latter, and then mixes the product with the original base. It should be understood, however, that all bases, even if hydrophilic, have their limits of capacity; additional amounts of water render them too soft or semiliquid. Oint-

Fig. 9–13. *Day ointment roller mill. Standards of fineness and smoothness require that no grains of material be visible under a ten-power microscope after passage through this machine. (Courtesy of Eli Lilly and Company.)*

ments must be semisolid, and sometimes pharmacists may find it necessary to use a drug concentrate or solid dosage form in adding a drug to an ointment base.

Alcoholic solutions of small volume usually may be added quite well to oleaginous vehicles or emulsion bases. Other liquid materials, for instance, natural balsams, are incorporated into ointment bases with difficulty. It is customary to mix a balsam such as Peru balsam with an equal portion of castor oil before incorporating it into the base. This procedure reduces the surface tension of the balsam and provides for the even distribution of the balsam throughout the vehicle.

On a large scale, mechanical ointment roller mills force coarsely formed ointments through moving stainless steel rollers, resulting in the formation of products that are smooth and uniform in composition and texture (Fig. 9–13). Prior to passage through the mills, the ointment may be coarsely prepared in powerful ointment and paste mixers. Small ointment mills are available for the production of small batches of product, and pharmacies that routinely prepare medicated applications find these small mills useful additions to their equipment.

Fusion

By the fusion method, all or some of the components of an ointment are combined by being melted together and cooled with constant stirring until congealed. Those components not melted are generally added to the congealing mixture as it is being cooled and stirred. Naturally, heat-labile substances and any volatile components are added last when the temperature of the mixture is low enough not to cause decomposition or volatilization of the components. Many substances are added to the congealing mixture in solution, others are added as insoluble powders generally levigated with a portion of the base. On a small scale, the fusion process may be conducted in a porcelain dish or glass beaker; on a large scale, it is generally carried out in large steam-jacketed kettles. Once congealed, the ointment may be passed through an ointment mill (in large-scale manufacture) or rubbed with a spatula or in a mortar (in small-scale preparation) to ensure a uniform texture.

Many medicated ointments and ointment bases containing such components as beeswax, paraffin, stearyl alcohol, and high molecular weight polyethylene glycols, which do not lend themselves well to mixture by incorporation, are prepared by fusion. In preparing an ointment with these types of materials by fusion, it is generally found that the melting points of the individual components are quite varied; therefore, the temperatures required to achieve fusion may also vary from formula to formula. In a given formula, if the item having the highest melting point is melted first and the other components are added to this hot liquid, all of the components will be subjected to this high temperature, irrespective of their own individual melting points, and generally a temperature higher than necessary will have to be employed to achieve fusion. Either by melting the component having the lowest melting point first and adding the components of higher melting points in order of their individual melting points or by melting all of the components together very slowly, a lower temperature is usually sufficient to achieve fusion. This is apparently due to the solvent action exerted by the first melted component on the other components, and if the process is allowed to proceed by using only slowly rising temperatures, the fusion process does not generally require the high temperature normally required to melt the individual component having the highest melting point.

In the preparation of ointments having an emulsion type of formula, the general method of manufacture involves a melting process as well as an emulsification process. Usually, the water-immiscible components such as the oil and waxes are melted together in a steam bath to about 70° to 75°C. Meantime, an aqueous solution of all of the heat-stable, water-soluble components is being prepared in the amount of purified water specified in the formula and heated to the same temperature as the oleaginous components. Then the aqueous solution is slowly added, with constant stirring (usually with a mechanical stirrer), to the melted oleaginous mixture, the temperature is maintained for 5 to 10 minutes to prevent crystallization of waxes, and then the mixture is slowly cooled with the stirring continued until the mixture is congealed. If the aqueous solution were not the same temperature as the oleaginous melt, there would be solidification of some of the waxes upon the addition of the colder aqueous solution to the melted mixture.

Preservation of Ointments

Even though they may not be designed to be sterile, topical preparations are subject to considerations of microbial content.[20] It is particularly important that the presence of *Pseudomonas aeruginosa* and *Staphylococcus aureus* be determined and controlled in topical products. Product contamination by these organisms could induce an infectious response in a patient. Some topical products are manufactured to be sterile through the use of microbial filtration of the vehicle, aseptic manufacturing processes, and the filling of containers under laminar-flow hoods. However, the majority of topical products are not intended to be sterile and do not undergo such aseptic procedures, but must still meet acceptable limits for microbial content. Certain preparations, because of the processes involved in their manufacture and/or the nature of their components, may encourage or may discourage microbial contamination and growth. As is the case in the manufacture of all pharmaceutical products, strict adherence to hygienic practices is vital to minimize both the type and number of microorganisms which may be present in a product.

Semisolid pharmaceutical preparations, as ointments, frequently require the addition of chemical antimicrobial preservatives to the formulation to inhibit the growth of contaminating microorganisms. These preservatives include p-hydroxybenzoates, phenols, benzoic acid, sorbic acid, quaternary ammonium salts and other compounds. Semisolid preparations utilizing bases which contain or hold water support microbial growth to a greater extent than those which have little moisture, and thus constitute the greater problem of preservation.

Semisolid preparations must also be protected through proper packaging and storage from the destructive influences of air, light, moisture, and heat, and the possible chemical interactions between the preparation and the container.

Packaging and Storage of Ointments

Ointments are usually packaged either in jars or in tubes. The jars may be made of glass, uncolored, colored green, amber, or blue, or opaque and porcelain-white. Plastic jars are also in use. Opaque and colored-glass containers are useful for ointments containing drugs that are light-sensitive. The tubes are made of tin or of plastic, some of them co-packaged with special tips when the ointment is to be used for rectal, ophthalmic, vaginal, aural, or nasal application. Tubes of ointments for ophthalmic use are most commonly packaged in small, tin or plastic collapsible tubes holding about ⅛ oz (about 3.5 g) of ointment. Tubes of ointments for topical use are more frequently of 5 g to 30 g size. Jars for ointments may vary in size from as little as one half ounce to one pound or more.

Ointment jars may be filled on a small scale by the pharmacist by packaging the weighed amount of ointment into the jar by means of a flexible spatula and forcing the ointment down and along the sides of the jar to avoid the entrapment of air. In packing an ointment jar, the idea is to attain a level surface of ointment high enough to be near the top of the jar, but not so high as to touch the lid when it is placed on the jar. Through the adept use of the spatula, some pharmacists place a "curl" in the center of the surface of the ointment. Ointments prepared by fusion may be poured directly into the ointment jars for congealing within the jar. These oint-

ments normally assume a finished look. In the large-scale manufacture of ointments, pressure fillers force a specified amount of an ointment into a jar.

Tubes are generally filled by pressure fillers from the open back end (opposite end from the cap end) of the tube (Fig. 9–14), which is then closed and sealed. Ointments prepared by fusion may be poured directly into the tubes. On a small scale, as in the extemporaneous filling of an ointment tube by the community pharmacist, the tube may be filled manually[21] or with a small scale filling machine (Fig. 9–15).

Industrially, automatic tube-filling, closing, crimping, labeling and packaging machines are used for the large-scale production of tube-filled ointments (Figs. 9–16 to 9–18).

Tube-filled ointments predominate over jar-filled ointments primarily because they are more convenient for the patient, with less handling and mess resulting. Also, ointments in tubes are less exposed to air and to potential contaminants and are therefore likely to be more stable and to remain efficacious for longer periods of time than ointments packaged in jars.

Most ointments must be stored at temperatures below 30°C to prevent the softening and even the liquefying of the base.

Creams

Creams are defined as "viscous liquid or semisolid emulsions of either the oil-in-water or the water-in-oil type." Creams are usually employed as emollients or as medicated applications to the skin.

The term cream is widely used in the pharmaceutical and cosmetic industry, and many of the commercial products referred to as creams may not actually conform to the above definition. Many products that are creamy in appearance but do not have an emulsion-type base are commonly called creams.

So-called "vanishing creams" are generally oil-in-water emulsions containing large percentages of water and stearic acid. After application of the cream, the water evaporates leaving behind a thin residue film of the stearic acid.

Many patients and physicians prefer creams to ointments. For one thing, they are generally easier to spread, and, in the case of creams of the oil-in-water emulsion-type, easier to remove than many ointments. Pharmaceutical manufacturers frequently market their topical prep-

Fig. 9–14.   *Empty tubes being prepared for filling. (Courtesy of Abbott Laboratories.)*

Fig. 9–15.   *Example of a small-scale fully automatic filling and crimping machine for collapsible metal tubes. The capacity of the machine is up to 60 units per minute. (Courtesy of Chemical and Pharmaceutical Industry Co.)*

Fig. 9–16. *Arenco tube-filling machine automatically fills 125 tubes a minute with proper amount, tightens cap, orients each tube by electric eye so that label faces forward, then closes and crimps the end. (Courtesy of Eli Lilly and Company.)*

Fig. 9–17. *This glaminate tube filler loads, fills, crimps, codes, and cuts 2-gram, tubes of topical cream. (Courtesy of Lederle Laboratories.)*

Fig. 9–18. *Industrial scale tube labeling machinery. (Courtesy of Eli Lilly and Company.)*

arations in both cream and ointment bases to satisfy the preference of the patient and physician.

Creams are packaged and preserved in the same manner as discussed previously for ointments. Table 9–2 presents examples of some dermatologic ointments and creams.

Pastes

Pastes, like ointments, are intended for external application to the skin. They differ from ointments primarily in that they generally contain a larger percentage of solid material and as a consequence are thicker and stiffer than ointments. Because of their large percentage of solids, pastes are generally more absorptive and less greasy than ointments prepared with the same components.

Pastes are prepared similarly to ointments. However, when a levigating agent is to be used to render the powdered component smooth, a portion of the base is often used rather than a liquid like mineral oil that would soften the paste.

Because of the stiffness and absorptive qual-

ities of pastes, they remain in place after application with little tendency to soften and flow and are therefore effectively employed to absorb serous secretions from the site of application. Pastes are therefore preferred over ointments for acute lesions that have a tendency toward crusting, vesiculation, or oozing. However, because of their stiffness and impenetrability, pastes are not generally suited for application to hairy parts of the body.

Among the pastes in use today are Triamcinolone Acetonide Dental Paste, an anti-inflammatory preparation applied topically to the oral mucous membranes and Zinc Oxide Paste.

Zinc Oxide Paste

Zinc Oxide Paste is prepared by levigating and then mixing 25% each of zinc oxide and starch with white petrolatum. The product is very firm and difficult to manipulate with a spatula. It is capable of absorbing moisture to a much greater extent than zinc oxide ointment and is employed as an astringent and protectant. The paste also frequently serves as a ve-

Table 9–2. Examples of Dermatologic Ointments and Creams by Therapeutic Category

Preparation	Corresponding Commercial Product	Usual Percentage of Active Ingredient	Comments
Adrenocortical Steroids			
Betamethasone Valerate Cream and Ointment	Valisone Cream & Ointment (Schering)	0.1% (ointment) and 0.01%, and 0.1% (cream)	These preparations are indicated for the relief of the inflammatory manifestations of corticosteroid responsive dermatoses. They are usually applied to affected skin areas once to three times a day.
Diflorasone Cream and Ointment	Florone Cream and Ointment (Dermik)	0.05%	
Fluocinolone Acetonide Cream and Ointment	Synalar Cream & Ointment (Syntex)	0.025% and 0.01% (cream) and 0.025% (ointment)	
Flurandrenolide Ointment	Cordran Ointment (Dista)	0.025% and 0.05%	
Hydrocortisone Acetate Cream and Ointment	Cortaid Cream and Ointment (Upjohn)	0.5%	
Hydrocortisone Ointment	Cortril Ointment (Pfizer)	1%	
Triamcinolone Acetonide Cream and Ointment	Aristocort Ointment (Lederle); Aristocort Cream (Lederle)	0.1% and 0.5% (ointment) and 0.1%, 0.025%, and 0.5% (cream)	
Adrenocorticoid/Antifungal Combination			
Betamethasone and Clotrimazole Cream	Lotrisone (Schering)	0.05%/1%	Useful for the relief and treatment of inflammatory and pruritic manifestations of corticosteroid-responsive dermatoses that could be complicated by fungal overgrowth.
Antiacne Drugs			
Tretinoin Cream	Retin-A (Ortho)	0.05%, 0.1%	A derivative of vitamin A that is used for the topical treatment of acne vulgaris. It is also approved as a preventive measure for skin aging.
Antiaginal Drug			
Nitroglycerin Ointment	Nitrostat (Parke-Davis)	2%	Reduces the workload of the heart by smooth muscle relaxation of peripheral arteries and veins. It is applied by using a specially designed dose-measuring applicator
Antibacterial/Anti-infective			
Bacitracin Ointment	Baciguent Ointment (Upjohn)	500 units/g	These antibiotic preparations are used in the treatment of skin infections due to susceptible organisms amenable to local treatment.
Gentamicin Sulfate Cream and Ointment	Garamycin Cream and Ointment (Schering)	0.1%	
Neomycin Sulfate Ointment	Myciguent Ointment (Upjohn)	0.5%	
Nystatin Cream and Ointment	Mycostatin Cream and Ointment (Squibb)	10,000 units/g	

Table 9–2. Continued

Preparation	Corresponding Commercial Product	Usual Percentage of Active Ingredient	Comments
Mafenide Cream	Sulfamylon (Winthrop)	8.5%	A sulfonamide derivative with bacteriostatic properties against many gram-negative and gram-positive organisms. It is used as adjunctive therapy of second and third degree burns.
Meclocycline Sulfosalicylate Cream	Meclan (Ortho)	1%	Topical tetracycline derivative for the treatment of inflammatory acne.
Mupirocin Ointment	Bactroban (Beecham)	2%	Antibacterial agent that possesses activity against organisms most frequently encountered in common, primary bacterial skin infections.
Antieczematic/Antipsoriatics			
Anthralin Ointment	Anthra-Derm (Dermik)	0.1, 0.25, 0.5, and 1.0%	Anthralin inhibits enzyme metabolism. Used in treating psoriasis.
Antifungals			
Nystatin Ointment	Mycostatin Ointment (Squibb)	100,000 units/g	An antifungal antibiotic for cutaneous and mucocutaneous mycotic infections.
Miconazole Nitrate Cream	Micatin (Ortho)	2%	For cutaneous candidiasis and treatment of tinea infections caused by *Trichophyton sp.*
Naftidine HCl	Naftin (Herbert)	1%	
Tolnaftate Cream	Tinactin Cream (Schering)	1%	For topical treatment of tinea pedis, tinea cruris, tinea corporis and tinea manuum.
Antineoplastic			
Fluorouracil Cream	Efudex Cream (Roche)	5%	For treatment of multiple actinic or solar keratoses.
Anesthetics (Local)			
Benzocaine Cream	Various	1% and 5%	Applied to skin to relieve pain and itching of sunburn, insect bites, etc.
Cyclomethycaine Sulfate Cream and Cyclomethycaine Sulfate Ointment	Surfacaine Cream and Ointment (Lilly)	0.5% (cream) and 1% (ointment)	
Dibucaine Cream and Ointment	Nupercainal Cream and Ointment (CIBA)	0.5% (cream) and 1% (ointment)	

Table 9–2.   Continued

Preparation	Corresponding Commercial Product	Usual Percentage of Active Ingredient	Comments
Astringent/Protectant			
Zinc Oxide Ointment	Various	20%	In the extemporaneous preparation of Zinc Oxide Ointment, 20% of zinc oxide is levigated with mineral oil, and the mixture incorporated into white ointment. The ointment is employed topically as an astringent and protective in various skin conditions.
Depigmenting Agents			
Hydroquinone Cream	Eldopaque Cream (Elder)	2% and 4%	Used in the temporary bleaching of hyperpigmented skin blemished due to freckles, old age spots, and cholasma.
Monobenzone Ointment	Benoquin Ointment (Elder)	20%	
Scabicides			
Lindane Cream	Kwell Cream (Reed and Carnrick)	1%	Used in the treatment of scabies and infestations with head lice and crab lice.
Crotamiton Cream	Eurax Cream (Westwood)	10%	For eradication of scabies and symptomatic treatment of pruritus.
Sunscreening Agent			
Dioxybenzone and Oxybenzone Cream	Solbar Cream (Person & Covey)	3% each of dioxybenzone and oxybenzone	Protects the skin against burning effects of the sun's ultraviolet rays.

hicle for other medicinal substances, e.g., anthralin therapy for psoriasis.

Synonym: Lassar's Plain Zinc Paste

Lotions

Lotions are liquid preparations intended for external application to the skin. Most lotions contain finely powdered substances that are insoluble in the dispersion medium and are suspended through the use of suspending agents and dispersing agents. Other lotions have as the dispersed phase liquid substances that are immiscible with the vehicle and are usually dispersed by means of emulsifying agents or other suitable stabilizers. Most commonly the vehicles of lotions are aqueous. Depending upon the nature of the ingredients, lotions may be prepared in the same manner as suspensions, emulsions, or solutions.

Lotions are intended to be applied to the skin for the protective or therapeutic value of their constituents. Their fluidity permits rapid and uniform application over a wide surface area. Lotions are intended to dry on the skin soon after application, leaving a thin coat of their medicinal components on the skin's surface.

Because the dispersed phase of lotions tends to separate from the vehicle upon standing, they should be shaken vigorously before each use to redistribute any separated matter. Containers of lotions should be labeled to instruct the patient to shake thoroughly before use and also to use externally only.

Examples of medicated lotions are presented in Table 9–3. Those lotions of particular pharmaceutical interest are discussed as follows.

Calamine Lotion

Calamine Lotion contains 8% each of zinc oxide and calamine, the latter composed primarily

Table 9–3. Examples of Medicated Lotions

Lotion	Corresponding Commercial Product	Percentage Strength of Active Constituent in Commercial Lotion	Category and Comments
Ammonium Lactate Lotion	Lac-Hydrin	12%	Promotes hydration and removal of excess keratin dry skin and hyperkeratotic conditions.
Benzoyl Peroxide	Various	5%; 5.5%; 10%	Demonstrates an antibacterial activity against *Propionibacterium acnes*, the predominant organism in sebaceous comedones that cause acne vulgaris.
Betamethasone Dipropionate Lotion, USP	Diprosone Lotion (Schering)	0.05% betamethasone diproprionate	Glucocorticoid indicated for the relief of inflammatory manifestations of corticosteroid-responsive dermatoses.
Betamethasone Valerate Lotion, USP	Valisone Lotion (Schering)	0.1% betamethasone	Glucocorticoid employed as an anti-inflammatory agent.
Calamine Lotion, USP	. . .	8% each of calamine and zinc oxide	Topical protectant. See text for additional discussion.
Clotrimazole Lotion, USP	Lotrimin Lotion (Schering)	1% clotrimazole	Indicated for the topical treatment of dermal infections tinea pedis, tinea cruris, and tinea corporus.
Flurandrenolide Lotion, USP	Cordran Lotion (Dista)	0.05% flurandrenolide	Adrenocortical steroid. Anti-inflammatory agent.
Lindane Lotion, USP	Kwell Lotion (Reed & Carnrick)	1% gamma benzene HCl	Pediculicide; scabicide. Applied topically to the skin once or twice a week. Contact with eyes or mucous membranes should be avoided.
Hydrocortisone Lotion, USP	Cort-Dome Lotion (Miles)	0.125 to 1.0% hydrocortisone	Adrenocortical steroid. Topical anti-inflammatory agent.
Permethrin Rinse	Nix (Burroughs-Wellcome)	1%	A synthetic pyrethroid which is active against lice, i.e., pediculosis.
Selenium Sulfide Lotion	Selsun (Abbott) and Selsun Blue (Ross)	1% (Selsun Blue) and 2.5% (Selsun) of selenium sulfide	Anti-fungal; antiseborrheic. Used principally in the treatment of dandruff and seborrheic dermatitis. Contact with the eyes should be avoided.
Urea Lotion	Aquacare (Herbert)	2%; 10%	Promotes hydration and removal of excess keratin dry skin and hyperkeratotic conditions.

of zinc oxide with a small amount of ferric oxide, which gives calamine its characteristic pink color. In the preparation of the lotion, the two powders are levigated with a small portion of glycerin, the mixture being gradually diluted with a combination of bentonite magma and calcium hydroxide solution and the product made to volume with additional calcium hydroxide solution.

The bentonite magma is used to suspend the zinc oxide and calamine; however, on standing the powders do settle. Calamine is categorized as a protectant and is useful in relieving the itching and pain of sunburn, insect bites, and other minor skin irritations. The pink color helps disguise the presence of the lotion on the skin. Calamine lotion must be thoroughly shaken before use.

"Phenolated calamine lotion" contains 1% of liquefied phenol in calamine lotion. Because phenol has anesthetic as well as antiseptic activity, it enhances the antipruritic action of the lotion. Like the plain calamine lotion, it must be shaken thoroughly before use. To maintain the phenol concentration, the container must be tightly closed.

Topical Solutions and Tinctures

Examples of solutions and tinctures intended for application to the skin are presented in Tables 9–4 and 9–5. As shown in these tables, the majority of these preparations are used as anti-infective agents.

Generally, the topical solutions employ an aqueous vehicle, whereas the topical tinctures characteristically employ an alcoholic vehicle. As required, co-solvents or adjuncts to enhance stability or the solubility of the solute are employed.

Most topical solutions and tinctures are prepared by simple solution of the solutes in the solvent. However, certain solutions are prepared by chemical reaction and these in particular are discussed later in this section. Of the tinctures for topical use, one, Compound Benzoin Tincture is prepared by maceration (see Chapter 13) of the natural components in the solvent; the others are prepared by simple solution.

Because of the nature of the active constituents or the solvents, many of the topical solutions and tinctures are self-preserved. Those that are not may contain suitable preservatives.

Topical solutions and tinctures should be packaged in containers that make them convenient to use. Those that are used in small volume, as the anti-infectives, are usually packaged in glass bottles having an applicator tip as a part of the cap assembly, or in plastic squeeze bottles which deliver the medication in drops. Many of the anti-infective solutions and tinctures contain a dye to delineate the area of application to the skin. In contrast to aqueous solutions, when the alcoholic tinctures are applied to abraded or broken skin, they cause a stinging sensation.

All medication intended for external use should be clearly labeled "FOR EXTERNAL USE ONLY" and kept out of the reach of youngsters.

In addition to their listing in Table 9–4, the following topical solutions are discussed because of their particular pharmaceutic interest.

Aluminum Acetate Topical Solution

The solution is colorless and has a faint acetous odor and a sweetish, astringent taste. It is widely applied topically as an astringent wash or wet dressing after dilution with 10 to 40 parts of water. It is frequently used as an ingredient in various types of dermatological preparations, as lotions, creams, and pastes. Commercial premeasured tablets and packets of powders are available for the preparation of this solution. Synonym: Burow's Solution

Aluminum Subacetate Topical Solution

The requirement for the amount of acetic acid differentiates Aluminum Acetate Topical Solution from Aluminum Subacetate Topical Solution. In the latter solution the ratio of aluminum oxide to acetic acid is 1:2.35, whereas in aluminum acetate topical solution the ratio is 1:3.52. Aluminum subacetate topical solution is the stronger solution and is used in the preparation of the aluminum acetate topical solution.

The solution, diluted first with 20 to 40 parts of water, is used externally as an astringent wash and wet dressing (modified Burow's Solution).

Calcium Hydroxide Topical Solution

Calcium hydroxide topical solution, commonly referred to as *limewater*, must contain not less than 140 mg of $Ca(OH)_2$ in each 100 mL of solution. Calcium hydroxide is less soluble in

Table 9–4. Examples of Solutions Applied Topically to the Skin

Solution	Corresponding Commercial Product	Percent Active Constituent in Commercial Solution	Vehicle	Category and Comments
Aluminum Acetate Topical Solution	. . .	5%	aqueous	Astringent. See text for additional discussion.
Aluminum Subacetate Topical Solution	. . .	Approximately 2.45% aluminum oxide and 5.8% acetic acid	aqueous	Astringent. See text for additional discussion.
Calcium Hydroxide Topical Solution (Limewater)	. . .	0.14%	aqueous	Astringent. See text for additional discussion.
Chlorhexidine Gluconate Solution	Hibiclens (Stuart)	4%		Used topically as a skin wound and general skin cleanser, a surgical scrub, and preoperative skin preparation. Effectiveness encompasses gram-positive and gram-negative bacteria such as *Pseudomonas aeruginosa*.
	Peridex Rinse (Procter & Gamble)	0.12%		For the treatment of gingivitis as characterized by gingival redness and swelling, including bleeding upon probing.
Clindamycin Phosphate Topical Solution	Cleocin T (Upjohn)	1%	isopropyl alcohol/water	Used in treatment of acne vulgaris.
Clotrimazole Topical Solution	Lotrimin Solution (Schering)	1%	PEG 400	Antifungal
Coal Tar Topical Solution (Liquor Carbonis Detergens; LCD)	. . .	20%	alcoholic	Antieczematic; antipsoriatic. See text for additional discussion.
Erythromycin Topical Solution	Eryderm (Abbott)	2%	polyethylene glycol/acetone/alcohol	Used in treatment of acne vulgaris.
Fluocinolone Acetonide Topical Solution	Synalar Solution (Syntex)	0.01%	propylene glycol	Adrenocortical steroid (topical anti-inflammatory)
Fluorouracil Topical Solution	Efudex Topical Solution (Roche)	2 and 5%	propylene glycol	Antineoplastic (actinic keratoses).
Hydrogen Peroxide Topical Solution	. . .	3%	aqueous	Topical anti-infective. See text for additional discussion.
Minoxidil Solution	Rogaine (Upjohn)	2%		Long-term topical treatment of male pattern baldness by stimulating hair regrowth.
Povidone-Iodine Topical Solution	Betadine Solution (Purdue Frederick)	7.5 and 10%	aqueous	Topical anti-infective. See text for additional discussion.
Thimerosal Solution	Merthiolate Solution (Lilly)	0.1%	alcohol-acetone	Local anti-infective. See text for additional discussion.
Tolnaftate Topical Solution	Tinactin Solution (Schering)	1%	polyethylene glycol	Topical anti-fungal.

Table 9–5. Examples of Tinctures Applied Topically to the Skin

Tincture	Corresponding Commercial Product	Percent Active Constituent in Commercial Tincture	Vehicle	Category and Comments
Green Soap Tincture	. . .	65%	alcohol	Detergent. Also contains 2% lavender oil as perfume.
Iodine Tincture	. . .	2%	alcohol-water	Topical anti-infective. See text for additional discussion.
Compound Benzoin Tincture	. . .	10% benzoin; 2% aloe; 8% storax; 4% tolu balsam	alcohol	Topical protectant. Prepared by maceration of the ingredients in alcohol. See text for additional discussion.
Thimerosal Tincture	Merthiolate Tincture (Lilly)	0.1%	ethylene diaminemonoethanolamine alcohol-acetone-water	Topical anti-infective. See text for additional discussion.

hot than in cold water, and, in the preparation of this solution cool purified water is employed as the solvent. The solution is intended to be saturated with solute, and to ensure saturation, an excess of calcium hydroxide, 300 mg for each 100 mL of solution to be prepared, is agitated with the purified water vigorously and repeatedly during a period of 1 hour. After this time, the excess calcium hydroxide is allowed to settle and remain at the bottom of the container. This permits the solution to remain saturated should a portion of the dissolved solute at the solution's surface react with the carbon dioxide of the air to form insoluble calcium carbonate:

$$Ca(OH)_2 + CO_2 \rightarrow CaCO_3 + H_2O$$

The calcium carbonate settles to the bottom of the container and by appearance is indistinguishable from the remaining excess of calcium hydroxide. The calcium hydroxide reserve dissolves as calcium is removed from solution in the form of the carbonate and in this way continually maintains the saturation of the solution. After the solution stands for an appreciable length of time, the undissolved material in the bottom of the container is composed of varying proportions of calcium hydroxide and calcium carbonate. Because of the uncertainty of the residue's composition, additional quantities of calcium hydroxide solution may not be pre-

pared by adding more purified water to the solution.

The solution should be stored in well-filled, tightly stoppered containers to deter the absorption of carbon dioxide and should be kept in a cool place to maintain an adequate concentration of dissolved solute. Only the clear supernatant liquid is dispensed. This is best accomplished by the use of a siphoning apparatus assembled so as to avoid the entrainment of the residue in the siphoning tubes.

The solution is categorized as an astringent. For this purpose it is generally employed in combination with other ingredients in dermatological solutions and lotions to be applied topically.

Synonyms: Lime Water; Liquor Calcis

Coal Tar Topical Solution

Coal tar topical solution is an alcoholic solution containing 20% of coal tar and 5% of polysorbate 80. It is prepared by mixing the coal tar with two and a half times its weight of washed sand, adding the polysorbate 80 and most of the alcohol, and then macerating the mixture for 7 days in a closed vessel with frequent agitation followed by filtration and adjustment to the proper volume with alcohol. The final alcoholic content is between 81 and 86% ethyl alcohol.

Coal tar (pix carbonis) is a nearly black, viscous liquid having a characteristic naphthalenelike odor and a sharp, burning taste. It is the tar obtained as a by-product during the destructive distillation of bituminous coal. It is slightly soluble in water and partially soluble in most organic solvents, including alcohol. In the preparation of the official solution, the coal tar is mixed with the sand in order to distribute it mechanically and create a large surface area of tar exposed to the solvent action of the alcohol. During the period of maceration, or soaking, the alcohol-soluble components of the tar dissolve, leaving the undissolved portion clinging to the sand. Filtration removes the sand and the insoluble tar components from the solution. The container in which the solution was prepared should be rinsed with alcohol, and the washings should be passed through the filter paper in the adjustment of the final volume of the solution.

In the extemporaneous compounding of prescriptions and in the therapeutic application of this preparation onto the skin, the solution is frequently mixed with aqueous preparations or simply diluted with water. Because coal tar is only slightly soluble in water, in instances such as this it would separate from the solution were it not for the presence of the polysorbate 80 in the preparation. This agent, commercially available as Tween 80 (ICI Americas) and as other brandname products, is an oily liquid that is a nonionic surfactant. It is quite effective in dispersing the water-insoluble components of coal tar upon its admixture with an aqueous preparation.

Coal tar is a local antieczematic. The solution is used in the external treatment of a wide variety of chronic skin conditions after dilution with about 9 volumes of water, or in combination with other agents in various lotions, ointments, or solutions.

Synonyms: Liquor Carbonis Detergens: Liquor Picis Carbonis; LCD

Hydrogen Peroxide Topical Solution

Hydrogen peroxide topical solution contains between 2.5 and 3.5% (w/v) of hydrogen peroxide, H_2O_2. Suitable preservatives, totaling not more than 0.05%, may be added.

One method of preparation involves the action of either phosphoric acid or sulfuric acid on barium peroxide:

$$BaO_2 + H_2SO_4 \rightarrow BaSO_4 + H_2O_2$$

Another method involves the electrolytic oxidation of a cold solution of concentrated sulfuric acid to form persulfuric acid, which when hydrolyzed liberates hydrogen peroxide:

$$2H_2SO_4 \rightarrow H_2S_2O_8 + H_2$$

$$H_2S_2O_8 + 2H_2O \rightarrow H_2O_2 + 2H_2SO_4$$

A solution prepared by this method usually contains about 30% of hydrogen peroxide and is capable of liberating 100 times its volume of oxygen. A solution of this strength is commonly referred to as "100 volume peroxide." The dilute solution, which contains about 3% hydrogen peroxide and liberates 10 times its volume of oxygen, may be prepared from the concentrated solution.

The solution is a clear, colorless liquid that may be odorless or may have the odor of ozone. It usually deteriorates upon long standing with the formation of oxygen and water. Preservative agents, as acetanilide, which have been found to retard the solution's decomposition are usually added in the amount stated above. Decomposition is enhanced by light and by heat, and for this reason the solution should be preserved in tight, light-resistant containers, preferably at a temperature not exceeding 35°C (95°F). The solution is also decomposed by practically all organic matter and other reducing agents and reacts with oxidizing agents to liberate oxygen and water; metals, alkalies, and other agents can catalyze its decomposition.

Hydrogen peroxide solution is categorized as a local anti-infective for use topically on the skin and mucous membranes. Its germicidal activity is based on the release of nascent oxygen on contact with the tissues. However, because of the short duration of this release, the chief value of the preparation in the reduction of infection is probably its ability to cleanse wounds by mechanical action through the effervescence and frothing caused by the release of oxygen.

Synonym: "Peroxide"

Chlorhexidine Gluconate Solution

Since 1957 chlorhexidine gluconate has been employed extensively as a broad spectrum antiseptic in clinical and veterinarian medicine. Its spectrum encompasses gram-positive and gram-negative bacteria, including *Pseudomonas aeruginosa*. In a concentration of 4% (Hibiclens, Stuart) it is used as a surgical scrub, hand wash and as a skin wound and general skin cleanser. Procedures are established for all of these purposes to maximize the effectiveness of the chlorhexidine. Experience has demonstrated that irritation, dermatitis and/or photosensitivity associated with the topical use of chlorhexidine are rare.

In 1987, the FDA and the Council of Dental Therapeutics of the American Dental Association approved chlorhexidine gluconate, 0.12% (Peridex, Procter & Gamble) as the first prescription only antiplaque/antigingivitis drug with antimicrobial activity. When used as a mouth rinse, microbiologic sampling of plaque has shown a reduction of aerobic and anaerobic bacteria, ranging from 54 to 97% through 6 months of use. The oral rinse should be used twice daily for 30 seconds, morning and night after toothbrushing. Usually a 15 mL dose of undiluted solution is used, and expectorated after rinsing. The most common side effect of chlorhexidine is the formation of an extrinsic yellow-brown stain on the teeth and tongue, after only a few days use. The amount of stain that appears is dependent upon the concentration of chlorhexidine and individual susceptibility. Increased consumption of tannin containing substances, e.g., tea, red wine, port wine, will increase the level of discoloration. The developed stain can be periodically removed with a dental prophylaxis.

Povidone-Iodine Topical Solution

The agent povidone-iodine is a chemical complex of iodine with polyvinylpyrrolidone, the latter agent being a polymer having an average molecular weight of about 40,000. The povidone-iodine complex contains approximately 10% of available iodine and slowly releases it when applied to the skin.

The preparation is employed topically as a surgical scrub and nonirritating antiseptic solution with its effectiveness directly attributable to the presence and the release of iodine from the complex.

Commercial Product: Betadine Solution (Purdue Frederick)

Thimerosal Topical Solution

Thimerosal is a water-soluble, organic, mercurial, antibacterial agent used topically for its bacteriostatic and mild fungistatic properties. It is used mainly to disinfect skin surfaces and as an application to wounds and abrasions. In certain instances it has been applied to the eye, nose, throat, and urethra in dilutions of 1:5000. It is also used as a preservative for various pharmaceutical preparations, including many vaccines and other biological products.

Thimerosal Topical Solution contains 0.1% thimerosal. Also present are ethylenediamine solution and sodium borate to maintain the alkalinity (usually pH 9.8 to 10.3) required for the solution's stability. Monoethanolamine is used as an additional stabilizer. The solution is affected by light and must be maintained in light-resistant containers.

Commercial Product: Merthiolate Solution (Lilly)

Topical Tinctures

Examples of tinctures for topical application to the skin are presented in Table 9–5. Those of particular pharmaceutic interest are discussed briefly as follows.

Iodine Tincture

Iodine tincture is prepared by dissolving 2% of iodine crystals and 2.4% of sodium iodide in an amount of alcohol equal to half the volume of tincture to be prepared and then diluting the solution to volume with sufficient purified water. The sodium iodide reacts with the iodine to form sodium triiodide:

$$I_2 + NaI \rightleftharpoons NaI_3$$

This reaction prevents the formation of ethyl iodide from the interaction between iodine and the alcohol, which would result in the loss of the antibacterial activity of the tincture. An added benefit of the triiodide form of iodine is its water solubility which is important should the tincture, which contains between 44 and 50% alcohol, be diluted with water during use.

The tincture is a popular local anti-infective agent applied topically to the skin in general household first-aid procedures. The reddish-brown color, which produces a stain on the skin, is useful in delineating the application over the affected skin area.

The tincture should be stored in tight containers to prevent loss of alcohol.

Compound Benzoin Tincture

Compound benzoin tincture is prepared by the maceration in alcohol of 10% of benzoin and lesser amounts of aloe, storax, and tolu balsam totaling about 24% of starting material. The drug mixture is best macerated in a wide-mouthed container, since it is difficult to introduce storax, a semi-liquid, sticky material into a narrow-mouthed container. Generally, it is advisable to weigh the storax in the container in which it will be macerated to avoid possible loss through a transfer of the material from one container to another.

The tincture is categorized as a protectant. It is used to protect and toughen skin in the treatment of bedsores, ulcers, cracked nipples, and fissures of the lips and anus. It is also commonly used as an inhalant in bronchitis and other respiratory conditions, one teaspoonful commonly being added to a pint of boiling water. The volatile components of the tincture travel with the steam vapor and are inhaled by the patient. Because of the incompatibility of the alcoholic tincture and water, mixture of the two produces a milky product with some separation of resinous material. Alcohol or acetone may be used as necessary to remove the residue from the vaporizer after use.

Compound tincture of benzoin serves as a delivery vehicle for podophyllum in the treatment of venereal warts. It is imporant that podophyllum not be systemically absorbed after application because the drug can effect peripheral neuropathy characterized by paresthesias, loss of sensation and loss of deep tendon reflexes in the extremities, in addition to neuropathy involving the central nervous system, e.g., lethargy, confusion, coma. Secondly, the podophyllum is teratogenic and should be administered only when the risk to benefit ratio is extremely low in a pregnant woman suffering from venereal warts. Thus, the nonocclusive compound tincture of benzoin is preferred to the occlusive flexible collodion.

Compound benzoin tincture is best stored in tight, light-resistant containers. Exposure to direct sunlight or to excessive heat should be avoided.

The tincture originated in the fifteenth or sixteenth century and through the years probably has acquired more synonyms than any other official preparation. A few of these are indicated as follows.

Synonyms: Friar's Balsam; Turlington's Drops; Persian Balsam; Swedish Balsam; Jerusalem Balsam; Wade's Drops; Turlington's Balsam of Life.

Thimerosal Tincture

The same general remarks made during the discussion of Thimerosal Topical Solution apply to Thimerosal Tincture except that sodium chloride and sodium borate are absent from the tincture and the vehicle of the tincture is composed of water, acetone, and about 50% alcohol. A number of metals, notably copper, cause the decomposition of the tincture, and for this reason it must be manufactured and stored in glass or suitably resistant containers. Monoethanolamine and ethylenediamine are used as stabilizers in the official solution and tincture and are thought to be effective because of their chelating action on traces of metallic impurities that may be present at the time of preparation or may later gain access to the preparation.

The commercial preparation is colored orange red and has a greenish fluorescence. The red stain it leaves on the skin defines the area of application. The preparation is a commonly used household antiseptic for application topically on the skin in abrasions and cuts and also in the preoperative preparation of patients for surgery.

Commercial Product: Merthiolate Tincture (Lilly)

Liniments

Liniments are alcoholic or oleaginous solutions or emulsions of various medicinal substances intended for external application to the skin generally with rubbing. Liniments with an alcoholic or hydroalcoholic vehicle are useful in instances in which rubefacient, counterirritant, or penetrating action is desired; oleaginous liniments are employed primarily when massage is desired. By their nature, oleaginous liniments are less irritating to the skin than alcoholic liniments. Liniments are not generally applied to skin areas that are broken or bruised because excessive irritation might result. The vehicle for a liniment should therefore be selected on the basis of the type of action desired (rubefacient, counterirritant, or just massage) and also on the solubility of the desired components in the various solvents. For oleaginous liniments, the solvent may be a fixed oil such as almond oil, peanut oil, sesame oil, or cottonseed oil or a volatile substance such as wintergreen oil or turpentine, or it may be a combination of fixed and volatile oils.

All liniments should bear a label indicating

that they are suitable only for external use and must never be taken internally. Liniments that are emulsions or that contain insoluble matter must be shaken thoroughly before use to ensure an even distribution of the dispersed phase, and for these preparations a "Shake Well" label is indicated. Liniments should be stored in tight containers.

Depending upon their individual ingredients, liniments are prepared in the same manner as solutions, emulsions, or suspensions, as the case may warrant.

There are presently no official liniments.

Collodions

Collodions are liquid preparations composed of pyroxylin dissolved in a solvent mixture usually composed of alcohol and ether with or without added medicinal substances. Pyroxylin (soluble gun cotton, collodion cotton) is obtained by the action of a mixture of nitric and sulfuric acids on cotton and consists chiefly of cellulose tetranitrate. It has the appearance of raw cotton when dry but is harsh to the touch. It is frequently available commercially moistened with about 30% alcohol or other similar solvent.

One part of pyroxylin is slowly but completely soluble in 25 parts of a mixture of 3 volumes of ether and 1 volume of alcohol. It is also soluble in acetone and glacial acetic acid. Pyroxylin is precipitated from solution in these solvents upon the addition of water. Pyroxylin, like collodions, is exceedingly flammable and must be stored away from flame in well-closed containers, protected from light.

Collodions are intended for external use. When applied to the skin with a fine camel's hair brush or glass applicator, the solvent rapidly evaporates, leaving a filmy residue of pyroxylin. This provides an occlusive protective coating to the skin, and when the collodion is medicated, it leaves a thin layer of that medication firmly placed against the skin. Naturally, collodions must be applied to dry tissues to effect adhesion to the skin's surface. The products must be clearly labeled "For External Use Only" or with words of similar effect.

Collodion

Collodion is a clear or slightly opalescent, viscous liquid prepared by dissolving pyroxylin (4% w/v) in a 3:1 mixture of ether and alcohol. The resulting solution is highly volatile and

flammable and should be reserved in tight containers at a temperature not exceeding 30°C remote from fire.

The product is capable of forming a protective film on application to the skin and the volatilization of the solvent. The film is useful in holding the edges of an incised wound together. However, its presence on the skin is uncomfortable due to its inflexible nature. The following product, which is flexible, has greater appeal when a nonpliable film is not required.

Flexible Collodion

Flexible collodion is prepared by adding 2% of camphor and 3% of castor oil to collodion. The castor oil renders the product flexible, permitting its comfortable use over skin areas that are normally moved, such as fingers and toes. The camphor makes the product waterproof. Physicians frequently apply the coating over bandages or stitched incisions to make them waterproof and to protect them from external stress.

Salicylic Acid Collodion

Salicylic acid collodion is a 10% solution of salicylic acid in flexible collodion. It is used for its keratolytic effects, especially in the removal of corns from the toes. Similar preparations are marketed as Compound W (Whitehall) and Freezone (Whitehall). Patients who use these products should be advised about their proper use. The product should be applied one drop at a time onto the corn or wart allowing time to dry before the next drop is added. Because salicylic acid can be irritating to normal, healthy skin every attempt must be made to ensure application directly onto the corn or wart. A useful preventive measure is to line the adjacent healthy skin with some white petrolatum prior to application of the product. Lastly, proper tightening and storage of the product after use is an absolute necessity because of the volatility of the vehicle.

Glycerogelatins

Glycerogelatins may be described as plastic masses intended for topical application and containing gelatin, glycerin, and water, in addition to any added medicinal substance. In dermatologic practice, such medicinal substances as zinc oxide, salicylic acid, resorcinol, and other appropriate agents may be added. Glycerogelatins are melted prior to application, cooled to only slightly above body temperature, and applied to the affected area with a fine brush. After application, the glycerogelatin hardens, is usually covered with a bandage, and is allowed to remain in place for periods up to 6 weeks and longer as is necessary.

Unless otherwise specified, glycerogelatins contain 10% of the medicinal substance prepared according to the formula:

Medicinal Substance	100 g
Gelatin	150 g
Glycerin	400 g
Purified Water	350 g
To make about	1000 g

In preparing a glycerogelatin, the gelatin is first softened in the purified water, being stirred when added, then allowed to stand for about 10 minutes after which time the mixture is heated in a steam bath until the gelatin is dissolved. The medicinal substance is mixed first with the glycerin (either dissolving in it or being dispersed by it) and then with the gelatin solution, the glycerogelatin being stirred until it congeals.

Zinc Gelatin

Zinc Gelatin is a firm, plastic mass containing 10% zinc oxide in a glycerogelatin base. It is used mainly for the treatment of varicose ulcers because of its ability to form a pressure bandage known as a "gelatin boot." The mass is softened on a water bath before being applied to the skin with a soft brush. This coating is then covered with a bandage and allowed to remain in place for up to 6 weeks, depending upon the degree of serous discharge from the lesion. Synonym: Zinc Gelatin Boot.

Plasters

Plasters are solid or semisolid adhesive masses spread upon a suitable backing material and intended for external application to a part of the body to provide prolonged contact at that site. Among the backing materials used are paper, cotton, felt, linen, muslin, silk, moleskin, or plastic. The plasters are adhesive at body temperature and may be used to provide protection or mechanical support (nonmedicated plasters) or to provide localized or systemic effects (medicated plasters). The backings onto which the masses are placed are cut into dif-

ferent shapes appropriate to the contour and the extent of the body surface to be covered. Commonly used are back plasters, chest plasters, breast plasters, kidney plasters, and corn plasters. Common adhesive tape was formerly official under the title "Adhesive Plaster," the use of this material being well known.

Today, most plasters are prepared industrially. The adhesive material in many of the commercially available plasters consist of either a rubber base or a synthetic resin material.

One plaster in general use is Salicylic Acid Plaster.

Salicylic Acid Plaster

Salicylic Acid Plaster is a uniform mixture of salicylic acid in a suitable base spread on a backing material and is intended to be placed on areas requiring the removal of horny layers of skin. The preparation is employed typically as corn plasters for the toes. The horny layers of skin are removed by virtue of the keratolytic action of salicylic acid. The usual concentration of salicylic acid in the plaster is 10 to 40%.

The effectiveness of these plasters is considerably enhanced when the patient soaks the corn or callus in warm water for a period of time, e.g., 15 to 30 minutes, prior to application of the plaster. Skin hydration enhances the penetration of the salicylic acid into the corn or the callus. Complete removal of the corn or the callus is not always essential because partial removal may provide needed comfort to the patient. Therefore, the FDA restricts the application of over-the-counter salicylic acid disks, pads or plasters to five treatments over a period of not more than 14 days for corns and calluses. Lastly, the patient should be instructed on the proper cutting of the plaster to conform to the size of the corn or callus.

Powders for Application to the Skin

Nonmedicated and medicated powders are frequently applied to the skin. The use of plain talcum powder is common as a topical dusting powder to prevent skin irritation and chafing. Medicated powders are often employed to combat such conditions as diaper rash and athlete's foot.

Powders for topical use are prepared in the same manner as has been described previously in Chapter 5. Powders for use on the skin are generally packaged in paper, metal, or plastic containers having a sifter-type cap. Some commercial powders are also packaged in plastic squeeze bottles in aerosol containers.

Some popular commercial medicated powders in use today include: Tolnaftate (Tritin, Scholl's) and Miconazole Nitrate (Micatin, Ortho) for athete's foot, Zinc Undecylenate and Undecylenic Acid (Cruex, Pharmacraft) for jock itch, Methylbenzethonium Chloride (Diaparene, Glenbrook) for diaper rash, and Polymyxin B Sulfate and Zinc Bacitracin (Polysporin, Burroughs-Wellcome) for infection prophylaxis in minor skin abrasions. These are generally used in conjunction with corresponding anti-fungal solutions, tinctures, creams or ointments.

Topical Aerosols

Aerosol packages for topical use on the skin are prepared in the same manner as discussed in Chapter 12. Common aerosols used topically include the anti-infective agents: povidone-iodine, tolnaftate and thimerosal; the adrenocortical steroids: betamethasone dipropionate and valerate, dexamethasone, and triamcinolone acetonide; and the local anesthetic dibucaine hydrochloride.

The use of topical aerosols provides to the patient a means of applying the drug in a convenient manner. The preparation may be applied to the desired surface area without the use of the fingertips, thus making the procedure less messy than with most other types of topical preparations. Among the disadvantages to the use of topical aerosols are the difficulty in applying the medication to a small area and the greater expense associated with the aerosol package.

Topical Gels

As described previously in Chaper 7, gels are *semisolid systems* consisting of dispersions of small or large molecules in a liquid vehicle rendered jelly-like through the action of an added substance, as carboxymethylcellulose. A number of topically used drugs are available as gels and are gaining widespread appeal. Examples of such drugs and drug products are: erythromycin and benzoyl peroxide topical gel [Benzamycin Topical Gel (Dermik Laboratories)]; clindamycin topical gel [Cleocin T Topical Gel (Upjohn)], and benzoyl peroxide gel [Desquam-

E Emollient Gel (Westwood)] used in the control and treatment of acne vulgaris; hydroquinone gel [Solaquin Forte Gel (Elder)], a bleach for hyperpigmented skin; salicylic acid gel [Keralyt Gel (Westwood)], a keratolytic; and desoximetasone gel [Topicort Gel (Hoechst-Roussel)], an anti-inflammatory and antipruritic agent.

Tapes and Gauzes

The USP contains monographs setting the standards for a number of topical dressings, including the following:

Adhesive Tape—defined as "fabric and/or film evenly coated on one side with a pressure sensitive adhesive mixture." Standards are set for sterility of those tapes which are labeled to be sterile, as well as for the dimensions, tensile strength, and adhesive strength of the sterile and nonsterile tapes.

Flurandrenolide Tape—this is adhesive-type tape having flurandrenolide impregnated in the adhesive material. The tape is applied as an anti-inflammatory adrenocortical steroid once or twice daily.

Absorbent Gauze—this is cotton or a mixture of cotton and Rayon in the form of a plain woven cloth. Official standards are set for thread count, length, width, weight, absorbency as well as sterility for absorbent gauze that has been rendered sterile.

Gauze Bandage—this is one continuous piece of absorbent gauze, tightly rolled in various widths and lengths and substantially free from loose threads and ravelings. Standards are set for width, length, weight, absorbency, thread count, as well as for sterility for those products labeled to be sterile.

Adhesive Bandage—this is a compress of four layers of absorbent or other suitable material, affixed to a film of fabric coated with a pressure-sensitive adhesive substance. Adhesive bandage is sterile and is protected by a suitable removable covering.

Petrolatum Gauze—this is absorbent gauze saturated with white petrolatum. This gauze is sterile. It is prepared by adding molten, sterile, white petrolatum to dry, sterile absorbent gauze, previously cut to size, ratio of 60 g of petrolatum to each

20 g of gauze. Standards are set for packaging, labeling, and sterility.

Zinc Gelatin Impregnated Gauze—this is absorbent gauze impregnated with zinc gelatin. The gauze is used as a topical protectant.

Miscellaneous Preparations for Topical Application to the Skin

Rubbing Alcohol

Rubbing Alcohol contains about 70% of ethyl alcohol by volume, the remainder consisting of water, denaturants with or without color additives and perfume oils, and stabilizers. In each 100 mL it must contain not less than 355 mg of sucrose octaacetate or 1.4 mg of denatonium benzoate, bitter substances that discourage accidental or abusive oral ingestion. The denaturants employed in rubbing alcohol are according to the Internal Revenue Service, U.S. Treasury Department, Formula 23-H, which is composed of 8 parts by volume of acetone, 1.5 parts by volume of methyl isobutyl ketone, and 100 parts by volume of ethyl alcohol. The use of this denaturant mixture makes the separation of ethyl alcohol from the denaturants a virtually impossible task with ordinary distillation apparatus. This discourages the illegal removal and use as a beverage of the alcoholic content of rubbing alcohol.

The product is volatile and flammable and should be stored in tight containers remote from fire. It is employed as a rubefacient externally and as a soothing rub for bedridden patients, a germicide for instruments, and a skin cleanser prior to injection.

Synonym: Alcohol Rubbing Compound.

Isopropyl Rubbing Alcohol

Isopropyl Rubbing Alcohol is about 70% by volume of isopropyl alcohol, the remainder consisting of water with or without color additives, stabilizers, and perfume oils. It is used externally as a rubefacient and soothing rub. This preparation and a commercially available 91% isopropyl alcohol solution are commonly employed by diabetic patients in preparing needles and syringes for hypodermic injections of insulin and for disinfecting the skin.

Hexachlorophene Liquid Cleanser

The commercial product [pHisoHex (Winthrop)] is an antibacterial sudsing emulsion containing a colloidal dispersion of hexachlorophene 3% (w/w) in a stable emulsion consisting of entsufon sodium (a synthetic detergent), petrolatum, lanolin cholesterols, methylcellulose, polyethylene glycol, polyethylene glycol monostearate, lauryl myristyl diethanolamide, sodium benzoate and water.

The preparation is a bacteriostatic cleansing agent. It cleanses the skin thoroughly and has bacteriostatic action against staphylococci and other gram-positive bacteria. Cumulative antibacterial action develops with repeated use. The preparation is indicated for use as a surgical scrub and a bacteriostatic skin cleanser.

Hexachlorophene may be absorbed through the skin and its use should be discontinued if signs of absorption (CNS irritation) or sensitivity (dermatoses) occur. Care must be exercised particularly when used on infants and children.

General Considerations in the Application of Topical Medications

Although differences in bioavailability or skin penetration are not a problem associated with a majority of topical products, in the recent past there has been research that has demonstrated differences in bioavailability between topical corticosteroids. Skin penetration is crucial for certain diseases of the skin, e.g., psoriasis, corticosteroid-responsive dermatoses, and vasoconstrictor assay procedures have demonstrated that differences exist in bioavailability between topical ointments and creams which possess an active ingredient in identical strengths. The ability of topical corticosteroids to induce vasoconstriction in normal intact human skin has been used by pharmaceutical companies to predict clinical potency, and more recently by the US FDA to judge the equivalence of generic topical corticosteroids and their brandname counterparts. Clinical trials have substantiated the predictive value of the vasoconstrictor assays.

With topical corticosteroid therapy, bioavailability or penetration into the skin is important. In an effort to enhance this penetration into the skin, particularly for those conditions, e.g., psoriasis, which may be amenable to corticosteroid therapy, a dermatologic patch has been developed, i.e., Actiderm (Squibb). The patient applies the corticosteroid product and then places the dermatologic patch over it. The patch remains in place for 48 hours and then is removed.

The benefit of the patch is that it keeps the steroid in intimate contact with the skin, enhances penetration of the steroid into the skin by its occlusiveness and decreases the number of applications necessary, i.e., from four to six applications of drug over 2 days to only one application. Further, when compared to plastic wrap or other occlusive alternatives, the Actiderm system is less conspicuous.

When considering brand interchange of a topical steroid product, the pharmacist must be aware that when one product with the same active ingredient and strength is substituted for another, the products may contain adjuvants which differ. Occasionally, an allergic response in a patient may be traced to the adjuvants.

Topical dosage forms, e.g., ointments, creams, are expensive and it is important that the pharmacist ensure the patient use these to maximum benefit. Before these are applied the affected area and adjacent healthy skin should be cleansed with soap and water, unless otherwise directed by the physician or directions on the package. This area should be dried thoroughly before application of the medicine. The patient should gently massage the medicine into the affected area as directed by the prescription.

Creams and ointments should be applied as a thin film onto the skin and spread evenly. Overuse, in general, will merely waste the medication. When using a solution, the patient should place two or three drops at most onto the area and gently massage these to cover the desired area. Powder dosage forms are sprinkled liberally on all areas of need, and for athlete's foot sprinkled into the shoes and socks as well.

How extensive the application of a topical product should be is really a function of the problem being treated. For example, when treating acne vulgaris with a topical product, it is important that patients realize that they should apply the product to the whole face, neck and back, and not merely to just the lesions alone. Application to the entire face is thought to "nip in the bud" forming comedones.

After application of the medicine, especially if it was applied with clean fingertips, the patient should cleanse his/her hands with soap and water. Inadvertent application of contaminated fingertips having residual drug, e.g., benzoyl peroxide, onto mucous membranes, e.g., mouth, eyes, nose, could be quite painful and bothersome.

For any topical product, patients should understand that symptoms should improve within a certain time frame, and that if symptoms persist beyond this time or if irritation develops, they should discontinue use and contact their physician. Patients should also understand not to apply any product to severely broken or abraded skin.

A question that will arise with topical products is the necessity of a bandage or covering. Whenever possible, with the exception of the need for an occlusive dressing with a corticosteroid drug, the wound should be medicated and left open to the atmosphere.

Selected Reading

Barr, M.: Percutaneous Absorption. *J. Pharm. Sci.*, 51:395–409, 1962.

Black, C.D.: Transdermal Drug Delivery Systems. *U.S. Pharm.*, 7:49, 1982.

Cleary, G.W.: *Transdermal Concepts and Perspectives.* Miami, FL, Key Pharmaceuticals, 1982.

Fara, J.W.: Short- and Long-term Transdermal Drug Delivery Systems. *Pharm. Tech.* "Drug Delivery Systems," 1983, pp. 33–40.

Friedman, S.J.: Management of Psoriasis Vulgaris with a Hydrocolloid Occlusive Dressing. *Arch. Dermatol.*, 123:1046–1052, 1987.

Hirschmann, J.V.: Topical Antibiotics in Dermatology. *Arch. Dermatol.*, 124:1691–1700, 1988.

Hien, N.G., Prawer, S.E., and Katz, H.J.: Facilitated Wound Healing Using Transparent Film Dressing Following Mohs Micrographic Surgery. *Arch. Dermatol.*, 124:903–906, 1988.

Idson, B.: Percutaneous Absorption. *J. Pharm. Sci.*, 64:901–924, 1975.

Shaw, J.E., and Chandrasekaran, S.K.: Controlled Topical Delivery of Drugs for Systemic Action. *Drug Metabolism Rev.*, 8:223, 1978.

Walters, K.A.: Percutaneous Absorption and Transdermal Therapy. *Pharm. Tech.*, 10:30–42, 1986.

Notes

1. Black, C.D.: Transdermal Drug Delivery Systems. *U.S. Pharm.*, 1:49, 1982.

2. Walters, K.A.: Percutaneous Absorption and Transdermal Therapy. *Pharm. Tech.*, 10:30–42, 1986.

3. Cleary, G.W.: *Transdermal Concepts and Perspectives.* Miami, FL, Key Pharmaceuticals, 1982.

4. Adapted largely from Barr, M.: Percutaneous Absorption. *J. Pharm. Sci.*, 51:395–409, 1962; Idson, B.: Percutaneous Absorption., *J. Pharm. Sci.* 64:901–924, 1975; and Fara, J.W.: Short- and Long-term Transdermal Drug Delivery Systems. *Pharm. Tech. Drug Delivery Systems*, 1983, pp. 33–40.

5. Idson, B.: Percutaneous Absorption Enhancers. *Drug & Cosmetic Ind.*, 137:30, 1985.
6. Cleary, G.W.: *Transdermal Concepts and Perspectives*. Miami, FL, Key Pharmaceuticals, 1982.
7. Fara, J.W.: Short- and Long-term Transdermal Drug Delivery Systems. *Pharm. Tech. Drug Delivery Systems*, 1983, pp. 33–40.
8. Black, C.D.: Transdermal Drug Delivery Systems. *U.S. Pharmacist*, 7:49, 1982.
9. Shaw, J.E. and Chandrasekaran, S.K.: Controlled Topical Delivery of Drugs for Systemic Action. *Drug Metabolism Rev.*, 8:223, 1978.
10. *Transderm-Scōp* (professional literature). Summit, NJ, CIBA Pharmaceutical Company, 1989.
11. *Transderm-Nitro* (professional literature). Summit, NJ, CIBA Pharmaceutical Co., 1989.
12. *Nitro-Dur* (professional literature). Miami, FL, Key Pharmaceuticals, 1989.
13. D.E. Magnuson, Personal communication, Key Pharmaceuticals, Miami, FL, 1983.
14. *Nitrodisc* (professional literature). Chicago, IL, Searle Pharmaceuticals, 1989.
15. *Catapres TTS* (professional literature). Ridgefield, CT, Boehringer Ingelheim Pharmaceuticals, 1989.
16. *Estraderm* (professional literature). Summit, NJ, CIBA Pharmaceutical Company, 1989.
17. Good, W.R.: Transdermal Drug Delivery Systems. Drug Delivery Systems. *Pharm. Tech.*, Aster Publishing Company, 1985, pp. 40–48.
18. Good, W.R.: Transdermal Drug-Delivery Systems. *Medical Device & Diagnostic Ind.*, 8:35–42, 1986.
19. Baker, R.W., and Farrant, J.: Patents in Transdermal Drug Delivery. Drug Delivery Systems. *Pharm. Tech.*, Aster Publishing Corporation, 1987, pp. 26–31.
20. Avallone, H.L.: Microbial Control of Topicals. *Pharm. Tech.*, 12:55–62, 1988.
21. Ansel, H.C.: Introduction to Pharmaceutical Dosage Forms. 4th Ed., Philadelphia, Lea & Febiger, 1985, p. 304.

10 | *Ophthalmic, Nasal, Otic, and Oral Preparations Applied Topically*

PREPARATIONS APPLIED topically to the eye, ear, nose, and oral cavity include many of the types of pharmaceutic dosage forms previously discussed as solutions, suspensions, and ointments. The purpose of this chapter is to identify more closely the types of dosage forms used with these sites of application and to define the purpose of special formulative components.

Ophthalmic Preparations

Drugs are applied to the eye for the localized effect of the medication on the surface of the eye or on its interior. Most frequently aqueous solutions are employed; however, suspensions, and ophthalmic ointments are also used. Recently, ophthalmic inserts, impregnated with drug, have been developed to provide for the continuous release of medication. These inserts are particularly useful for those drugs requiring frequent daytime and nighttime administration.

Because the capacity of the eye to retain liquid and ointment preparations is limited, they are generally administered in small volume. Liquid preparations are most frequently administered dropwise and ointments by the application of a thin ribbon of ointment to the lid margin. Larger volumes of liquid preparations may be used to flush or wash the eye.

The normal volume of tears in the eye is 7 μL. Whereas a nonblinking eye can accommodate a maximum of 30 μL of fluid, blinking eyes can hold only 10 μL. Excessive liquids, both normally produced and externally added, are rapidly drained from the eye. The usual single drop size of an instilled drug solution may be 50 μL (based on 20 drops/mL) and thus, much of the drop instilled may be lost. The ideal volume of drug solution to administer, based on eye capacity, would be 5 to 10 μL.[1] Since microliter dosing eye droppers are not generally available or used by patients, the loss of instilled medication using standard eye droppers is a common occurrence. If multiple drop therapy is desired, 5-minute intervals between drops is recommended.[1] This permits the buildup of drug in the corner while allowing for minimal loss through drainage. Sometimes, use of an ophthalmic solution of greater drug concentration can substitute for multiple drop therapy of a more dilute solution.

Thus, the effective "dose" of medication administered ophthalmically may be varied by the strength of medication administered, the volume administered, the retention time of the medication in contact with the surface of the eye and the frequency of administration. Although the local administration of medications to the eye is the main route of administration employed by the ophthalmologist in the treatment of diseases of the eye, other routes as oral and parenteral may also be used. The use of systemic antibiotic therapy to combat an intraocular infection is an example of this type of therapy.

Ophthalmic Solutions

Considerations in the preparation of ophthalmic solutions includes sterility, preservation, isotonicity, buffering, viscosity, and appropriate packaging.

Sterility and Preservation

All ophthalmic solutions should be sterile when dispensed, and whenever possible, a suitable preservative should be added to ensure sterility during the course of use. Ophthalmic solutions intended to be used during surgery or in the traumatized eye generally do not contain preservative agents, because these are irritating to the tissues within the eye. These solutions are usually packaged in single-dose containers and any unused solution discarded.

Although it is preferable that ophthalmic solutions be sterilized by autoclaving in the final container, the method employed, as always, is dependent upon the nature of the particular preparation. Certain drugs that are thermostabile in acid media may become thermolabile when buffered near the physiological pH range (about 7.4). If the higher pH is desired for the product, the unbuffered solution of the drug may first be autoclaved, and the buffering agents aseptically added later. With the exception of basic salts of weak acids such as sodium fluorescein or sodium sulfacetamide, solutions of most of the common ophthalmic drugs, prepared in a boric acid vehicle, can be safely sterilized at 121°C for 15 minutes as previously discussed in Chapter 8.

If necessary, a bacterial filter may be used to avoid the use of heat sterilization. Although bacterial filters work with a high degree of efficiency, they are not as trusted sterilizers as is the autoclave. The advantage of filtration, as was pointed out earlier, is the retention of all particulate matter, the removal of which is of prime importance in the manufacture and use of ophthalmic solutions. Figures 10–1 and 10–2 show filtration equipment which may be employed in the extemporaneous filtration of ophthalmic solutions.

Ophthalmic solutions to be used on eyes with intact corneal membranes may be packaged in multiple-dose containers. Even though sterile when dispensed, each of these solutions should contain a rapidly effective, topically nonirritating antibacterial agent or a mixture of such agents to prevent the growth of, or to destroy, microorganisms accidentally introduced into the solution when the container is opened during use. Suitable preservatives and their maximum concentrations for this purpose include (a) benzalkonium chloride, 0.013%; (b) benzethonium chloride, 0.01%; (c) chlorobutanol, 0.5%; (d) phenylmercuric acetate, 0.004%; (e) phenylmercuric nitrate, 0.004%; and, (f) thimerosal, 0.01%. Each of these has certain limitations with respect to stability, chemical compatibility with other formulative ingredients, and antibacterial activity. For example, chlorobutanol hydrolyzes and decomposes at autoclaving temperatures. Further, the hydrolysis of chlorobutanol may take place under moderate heat or slowly at room temperature with the formation of hydrochloric acid which not only may render the solution susceptible to microorganism growth but may change the pH of an unbuffered solution and affect the stability or the physiologic activity of the active ingredient. Benzalkonium chloride is one of the most reli-

Fig. 10–1. *Sterilization by filtration. The preparation of a sterile solution by passage through a syringe affixed with a microbial filter. (Courtesy of Millipore Corporation.)*

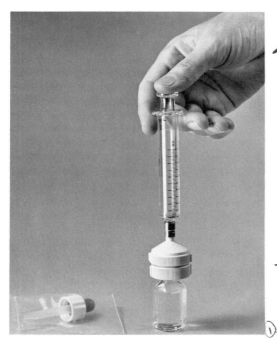

Fig. 10–2. *The preparation of a sterile ophthalmic solution by filtration. (Courtesy of Millipore Corporation.)*

able ophthalmic solution preservatives, because it has a broad antimicrobial spectrum of activity, but the pharmacist must be aware of its incompatibility with anionic drugs.

In concentrations tolerated by the tissues of the eye, all of the aforementioned preservative agents are ineffective against some strains of *Pseudomonas aeruginosa,* an organism that can invade an abraded cornea and cause ulceration and blindness. It has been found that a preservative mixture of benzalkonium chloride (0.01%) and 1000 USP Units of polymyxin B sulfate, the latter in each mL of solution, is effective against most resistant strains of *Pseudomonas* and is nonirritating to the eye. In some ophthalmic preparations a mixture of benzalkonium chloride (0.01%) and disodium ethylenediaminetetraacetate, 0.01 to 0.1%, is employed for the same purpose. The latter agent is a chelating agent for metals, having the ability to render the resistant strains of *Pseudomonas aeruginosa* more sensitive to the benzalkonium chloride.

Isotonicity Value

If a solution is placed within or behind a membrane that is permeable only to solvent molecules and not to solute molecules (a *semipermeable membrane*), a phenomenon called *osmosis* occurs as the molecules of solvent traverse the membrane. If the solution-filled membrane is placed in a solution of a higher solute concentration than its own, the solvent, which has free passage in either direction, passes into the more concentrated solution. It does this until an equilibrium is established on both sides of the membrane and an equal concentration of solute exists on the two sides. The pressure responsible for this movement is termed *osmotic pressure.*

The concentration of a solution with respect to osmotic pressure is concerned with the number of "particles" of solute in solution. That is, if the solute is a nonelectrolyte (as sucrose), the concentration of the solution will depend solely on the number of molecules present. However, if the solute is an electrolyte (as sodium chloride), the number of particles that it contributes to the solution will depend not only upon the concentration of the molecules present, but also on their degree of ionization. A chemical that is highly ionized will contribute a greater number of particles to the solution than will the same amount of a poorly ionized substance. The effect is that a solution with a greater number of particles, whether they be molecules or ions, has a greater osmotic pressure than does a solution having fewer particles.

Body fluids, including blood and lacrimal fluid, have an osmotic pressure corresponding to that of a 0.9% solution of sodium chloride. Thus, a sodium chloride solution of this concentration is said to be *isosmotic,* or having an equal osmotic pressure, with physiologic fluids. The term *isotonic,* meaning equal tone, is commonly used interchangeably with isosmotic although the former term must be used with reference to some body fluid, and isosmotic actually is a physical chemical term which compares the osmotic pressure of two liquids, one of which may or may not be a physiologic fluid. Solutions with a lower osmotic pressure than body fluids or a 0.9% sodium chloride solution are commonly referred to as *hypotonic,* whereas solutions having a greater osmotic pressure are termed *hypertonic.*

Theoretically, a hypertonic solution added to the body's system will have a tendency to draw water from the body tissues toward the solution in an effort to dilute and establish a concentration equilibrium. In the blood stream, a hypertonic injection could cause the *crenation* (shrinking) of blood cells; in the eye, the solution could cause the drawing of water toward the site of the topical application. Conversely, a hypotonic solution might induce the hemolysis of red blood cells, or the passage of water from the site of an ophthalmic application through the tissues of the eye.

In practice, the isotonicity limits of an ophthalmic solution in terms of sodium chloride, or its osmotic equivalent, may range from 0.6 to 2.0% without marked discomfort to the eye. As indicated, sodium chloride does not have to be used to establish the solution's osmotic pressure. Boric acid in a concentration of 1.9% produces the same osmotic pressure as does 0.9% sodium chloride. All of the ophthalmic solution's solutes, including the active ingredients, contribute to the osmotic pressure of the solution.

The calculations involved in preparing isosmotic solutions may be made in terms of data relating to the colligative properties of solutions.[2] Like osmotic pressure, the other colligative properties of solutions, namely, vapor pressure, boiling point, and freezing point, depend upon the number of particles in solution. These properties, therefore, are related, and a change in any one of them will be accompanied by corresponding changes in the others. Although any one of these properties may be used to determine isosmoticity, a comparison of freezing points between the solutions in question, is most used.

When 1 g molecular weight of a non-electrolyte, such as boric acid, is dissolved in 1000 g of water, the freezing point of the solution is about 1.86°C below the freezing point of pure water. By simple proportion, therefore, the weight may be calculated for any non-electrolyte that should be dissolved in each 1000 g of water to prepare a solution isosmotic with lacrymal fluid and blood serum, which have freezing points of −0.56°C.

Boric acid, for example, has a molecular weight of 61.8, and thus 61.8 g in 1000 g of water should produce a freezing point of −1.86°C. Therefore:

$$\frac{1.86(°C)}{0.52(°C)} = \frac{61.8 \text{ (g)}}{x \text{ (g)}}$$

$$x = 17.3 \text{ g}$$

Hence, 17.3 g of boric acid in 1000 g of water

theoretically should produce a solution isosmotic with tears and blood.

The calculation employed to prepare a solution isosmotic (with tears or blood) when using electrolytes is different than when the calculation is made for a non-electrolyte. Since osmotic pressure depends upon the number of particles, substances that dissociate have an effect that increases with the degree of dissociation; the greater the dissociation, the smaller the quantity required to produce a given osmotic pressure. If we assume that sodium chloride in weak solutions is about 80% dissociated, then each 100 molecules yield 180 particles, or 1.8 times as many particles as are yielded by 100 molecules of a non-electrolyte. This dissociation factor, commonly symbolized by the letter i, must be included in the proportion when we seek to determine the strength of an isosmotic solution of sodium chloride (molecular weight, 58.5):

$$\frac{1.86 \text{ (°C)} \times 1.8}{0.52 \text{ (°C)}} = \frac{58.5 \text{ (g)}}{x \text{ (g)}} \quad x = 9.09 \text{ g}$$

Therefore, 9.09 g of sodium chloride in 1000 g of water should make a solution isosmotic with blood or lachrymal fluid. As indicated previously, a 0.90% (w/v) sodium chloride solution is taken to be isosmotic (and isotonic) with the body fluids.

Simple isosmotic solutions, then, may be calculated by this general formula:

$$\frac{0.52 \times \text{molecular weight}}{1.86 \times \text{dissociation } (i)}$$

$$= \text{g of solute per 1000 g of water}$$

Although the i value has not been determined for every medicinal agent that might be named, the following values may be (generally) used:

Non-electrolytes and substances of slight dissociation:	1.0
Substances that dissociate into 2 ions:	1.8
Substances that dissociate into 3 ions:	2.6
Substances that dissociate into 4 ions:	3.4
Substances that dissociate into 5 ions:	4.2

Since 0.9% sodium chloride solution is considered to be isosmotic (and isotonic) with lacrymal fluid, other medicinal substances are compared with regard to their "sodium chloride equivalency." An often used rule states:[2]

> *quantities of two substances that are tonicic equivalents are proportional to the molecular weights of each multiplied by the i value of the other.*

Using the drug atropine sulfate as an example:
Molecular weight of sodium chloride = 58.5; $i = 1.8$
Molecular weight of atropine sulfate = 695; $i = 2.6$

$$\frac{695 \times 1.8}{58.5 \times 2.6} = \frac{1 \ (g)}{x \ (g)}$$

$x = 0.12$ g of sodium chloride represented by 1 g of atropine sulfate

Thus, the *sodium chloride equivalent* for atropine sulfate is 0.12 g. To put it one way, 1.0 g of atropine sulfate equals the "tonic effect" of 0.12 g of sodium chloride. To put it another way, atropine sulfate is 12% as effective as an equal weight of sodium chloride in contributing toward tonicity. When a combination of drugs is used in a prescription or formulation to be rendered isotonic, each agent's contribution to tonicity must be taken into consideration. For instance, consider the following prescription:

Atropine Sulfate	1%
Sodium Chloride	q.s. to isotonicity
Sterile Purified Water, ad	30.0 mL

To make the 30 mL isotonic with sodium chloride, 30 mL × 0.9% = 0.27 g or 270 mg of sodium chloride would be required. However, since 300 mg of atropine sulfate is to be present, its contribution to tonicity needs to be taken into consideration. Since the sodium chloride equivalent for atropine sulfate is 0.12, its contribution is calculated as follows:

$$0.12 \times 300 \ mg = 36 \ mg$$

Thus, 270 mg − 36 mg = 234 mg of sodium chloride would actually be required.

Table 10–1 presents an abbreviated list of sodium chloride equivalents. A more complete list may be found in pharmaceutical calculations or physical pharmacy textbooks.

As a convenience, the USP presents precalculated amounts of some common ophthalmic drugs which may be used to prepare isotonic solutions. Some of the drugs and the related values are presented in Table 10–2. The data shown are utilized in the following manner. One gram of each of the drugs listed, when added to purified water, will prepare the corresponding volume of an isotonic solution. For instance, 1 g of atropine sulfate will prepare 14.3 mL of isotonic solution. This solution may

Table 10–1. Some Sodium Chloride Equivalents

Substance	Molecular Weight	Ions	i	Sodium Chloride Equivalent
Atropine sulfate · H_2O	695	3	2.6	0.12
Benzalkonium chloride	360	2	1.8	0.16
Benzyl alcohol	108	1	1.0	0.30
Boric Acid	61.8	1	1.0	0.52
Chlorobutanol	177	1	1.0	0.18
Cocaine hydrochloride	340	2	1.8	0.17
Ephedrine sulfate	429	3	2.6	0.20
Epinephrine bitartrate	333	2	1.8	0.18
Ethylmorphine hydrochloride · $2H_2O$	386	2	1.8	0.15
Naphazoline hydrochloride	247	2	1.8	0.27
Physostigmine salicylate	413	2	1.8	0.14
Pilocarpine hydrochloride	245	2	1.8	0.24
Procaine hydrochloride	273	2	1.8	0.21
Scopolamine hydrobromide · $3H_2O$	438	2	1.8	0.13
Tetracycline hydrochloride	481	2	1.8	0.12
Zinc sulfate · $7H_2O$	288	2	1.4	0.16

Table 10–2. Isotonic Solutions Prepared from Common Ophthalmic Drugs*

Drug (1.0 g)	Volume of Isotonic Solution Yielded (mL)
Atropine Sulfate	14.3
Boric Acid	55.7
Chlorobutanol (hydrous)	26.7
Cocaine Hydrochloride	17.7
Colistimethate Sodium	16.7
Dibucaine Hydrochloride	14.3
Ephedrine Sulfate	25.7
Epinephrine Bitartrate	20.0
Eucatropine Hydrochloride	20.0
Fluorescein Sodium	34.3
Homatropine Hydrobromide	19.0
Neomycin Sulfate	12.3
Penicillin G Potassium	20.0
Phenylephrine Hydrochloride	35.7
Physostigmine Salicylate	17.7
Physostigmine Sulfate	14.3
Pilocarpine Hydrochloride	26.7
Pilocarpine Nitrate	25.7
Polymyxin B Sulfate	10.0
Procaine Hydrochloride	23.3
Proparacaine Hydrochloride	16.7
Scopolamine Hydrobromide	13.3
Silver Nitrate	36.7
Sodium Bicarbonate	72.3
Sodium Biphosphate	44.3
Sodium Borate	46.7
Sodium Phosphate (dibasic, heptahydrate)	32.3
Streptomycin Sulfate	7.7
Sulfacetamide Sodium	25.7
Sulfadiazine Sodium	26.7
Tetracaine Hydrochloride	20.0
Tetracycline Hydrochloride	15.7
Zinc Sulfate	16.7

*Adapted from USP XXII.

then be diluted with an isotonic vehicle to maintain the isotonicity while changing the strength of the active constituent in the solution to any desired level. For instance, if a 1% isotonic solution of atropine sulfate is desired, the 14.3 mL of isotonic solution containing 1 g of atropine sulfate would be diluted to 100 mL (1 g atropine sulfate in 100 mL = a 1% w/v solution) with an isotonic vehicle. By utilizing sterile drug, sterile purified water, a sterile isotonic vehicle, and aseptic techniques, a sterile product may be prepared. In addition to being sterile and isotonic, the diluting vehicles generally used are also buffered and contain suitable preservative to maintain the stability and sterility of the product.

Buffering

Buffers may be used in an ophthalmic solution for one or all of the following reasons: (1) to reduce discomfort to the patient, (2) to ensure drug stability, and (3) to control the therapeutic activity of the drug substance.

Normal tears, having a pH of about 7.4, possess some buffer capacity. The introduction of a medicated solution into the eye stimulates the flow of tears, which attempts to neutralize any excess hydrogen or hydroxyl ions introduced with the solution. Most drugs used ophthalmically, such as alkaloidal salts, are weakly acidic and have only weak buffer capacity. Normally, the buffering action of the tears is capable of neutralizing the ophthalmic solution and is thereby able to prevent marked discomfort. However, a few drugs—notably pilocarpine hydrochloride and epinephrine bitartrate—are quite acid and overtax the buffer capacity of the lacrimal fluid. For maximum comfort, an ophthalmic solution should have the same pH as the lacrimal fluid. However, this is not pharmaceutically possible, since at pH 7.4, many drugs are insoluble in water. Alkaloidal salts, for instance, are likely to precipitate as the free alkaloidal base at pH 7.4.

Most drugs, including many used in ophthalmic solutions, are most active therapeutically at pH levels which favor the undissociated molecule. However, the pH that permits greatest activity may also be the pH at which the drug is least stable. For this reason, a compromise pH is generally selected for a solution and maintained by buffers to permit the greatest activity while maintaining stability. The buffer system of an ophthalmic solution contributes to stability in another way by preventing an increase in the pH of the solution due to the normal leaching by the solution of alkali from the glass container.

The USP provides formulas for the preparation of buffer vehicles suitable for use for specific drugs. Included are the following:

BORIC ACID VEHICLE. This vehicle has a pH of slightly below 5.0. It is prepared by dissolving 1.9 g of boric acid in sufficient water to make 100 mL of solution. The vehicle is suitable for the water-soluble salts of the following medicinal agents: benoxinate, cocaine, dibucaine, phenylephrine, pilocarpine, piperocaine, procaine, proparacaine, tetracaine, and zinc.

ISOTONIC PHOSPHATE VEHICLE. This vehicle is

Table 10–3. Isotonic Phosphate Vehicle*

Monobasic Sodium Phosphate Solution, mL	Dibasic Sodium Phosphate Solution, mL	Resulting Buffer Solution, pH	Sodium Chloride Required for Isotonicity, g/100 mL
90	10	5.9	0.52
80	20	6.2	0.51
70	30	6.5	0.50
60	40	6.6	0.49
50	50	6.8	0.48
40	60	7.0	0.46
30	70	7.2	0.45
20	80	7.4	0.44
10	90	7.7	0.43
5	95	8.0	0.42

*From USP XXII.

adjusted for tonicity and provides a choice of pH ranging from 5.9 to 8.0. It is prepared through the use of two stock solutions, one containing 8.00 g of monobasic sodium phosphate (NaH_2PO_4) per liter, and the other containing 9.47 g of dibasic sodium phosphate (Na_2HPO_4) per liter, the weights being on an anhydrous basis. The stock solutions are utilized in proportions indicated in Table 10–3.

The vehicles listed in Table 10–3 are satisfactory for many ophthalmic drugs with the exception of pilocarpine, eucatropine, scopolamine and homatropine salts which show instability in the vehicle. The vehicle is used effectively as the diluent for ophthalmic drugs already in isotonic solution, as those prepared according to the method presented in Table 10–2. When drug substances are added directly to the isotonic phosphate vehicle, the solution becomes slightly hypertonic. Generally, this provides no discomfort to the patient. However, if such a solution is not desired, the appropriate adjustment can be made through calculated dilution of the vehicle with purified water.

Viscosity and Thickening Agents

Viscosity is a property of liquids that is closely related to the resistance to flow. The reciprocal of viscosity is *fluidity*. Viscosity is defined in terms of the force required to move one plane surface past another under specified conditions when the space between is filled by the liquid in question. More simply, it can be considered as a relative property with water as the reference material and all viscosities expressed in terms of the viscosity of pure water at 20°C. The viscosity of water is given as one centipoise (actually 1.0087 centipoise). A liquid material ten times as viscous as water at the same temperature has a viscosity of 10 centipoises. The centipoise, abbreviated cp. (*cps.* plural), is a more convenient term than the basic unit, the poise; one poise is equal to 100 centipoises.

Specifying the temperature is important because viscosity changes with temperature; generally, the viscosity of a liquid decreases with increasing temperature. The determination of viscosity in terms of poise or centipoise results in the calculation of *absolute* viscosity. It is sometimes more convenient to use the kinematic scale in which the units of viscosity are *stokes* and *centistokes* (1 stoke equals 100 centistokes). The kinematic viscosity is obtained from the absolute viscosity by dividing the latter by the density of the liquid at the same temperature:

$$\text{kinematic viscosity} = \frac{\text{absolute viscosity}}{\text{density}}$$

Using water as the standard, examples of some viscosities at 20°C are:

Ethyl alcohol —	1.19	cps
Olive oil —	100	cps
Glycerin —	400	cps
Castor oil —	1000	cps

Viscosity can be determined by any method that will measure the resistance to shear offered by the liquid. For ordinary liquids, it is customary to determine the time required for a given sample of the liquid to flow at a regulated temperature through a small vertical capillary tube and to compare this time with that required to perform the same task by the reference liquid. Many capillary tube viscosimeters have been devised, and nearly all are modifications of the Ostwald type. With an apparatus such as this, the viscosity of a liquid may be determined by the following equation:

$$\frac{\eta_1}{\eta_2} = \frac{\rho_1 t_1}{\rho_2 t_2}$$

where η_1 is the unknown viscosity of the liquid, η_2 is the viscosity of the standard, ρ_1 and ρ_2 are the respective densities of the liquids, and t_1 and t_2 are the respective flow times in seconds.

In the preparation of ophthalmic solutions, a suitable grade of methylcellulose or other thickening agent is frequently added to increase the viscosity and thereby aid in holding the drug in contact with the tissues so as to enhance the therapeutic effectiveness. Generally, methylcellulose of the 4000 cps viscosity type is used in concentrations of 0.25% and the 25 cps type at 1% concentration. Hydroxypropyl methylcellulose and polyvinyl alcohol are also used as thickeners in ophthalmic solutions. Occasionally a 1% solution of methylcellulose without medication is used as a tear replacement. Viscosity for ophthalmic solutions is considered optimal in the range of 15 to 25 cps.

Ocular Bioavailability[3]

The bioavailability of drugs administered to the eye is an important consideration. There are physiologic factors which can affect a drug's ocular bioavailability, including protein binding, drug metabolism, and lacrimal drainage. Protein-bound drugs are incapable of penetrating the corneal epithelium due to the size of the protein-drug complex. Because of the brief time in which an ophthalmic solution may remain present in the eye (due to lacrimal drainage) the protein binding of a drug substance could quickly negate its therapeutic value by rendering it unavailable for absorption. Normally, tears contain between 0.6 and 2.0% of protein content, but disease states (as uvetis) can raise these protein levels.

As in the case with other biological fluids, tears contain enzymes (such as lysozyme) capable of the metabolism degradation of drug substances. However, the full extent to which drug metabolism occurs in the precorneal area is uncertain at this time.

In addition to physiologic factors affecting ocular bioavailability, other factors, as the physicochemical characteristics of the drug substance, and product formulation are important. Because the cornea is a membrane barrier containing both lipophilic and hydrophilic layers, it is permeated most effectively by drug substances having both lipophilic and hydrophilic characteristics. Drugs which can exist in both the ionized state, as the weak bases pilocarpine, atropine, tetracaine, and others, permeate the membrane best. It is advantageous for corneal permeation to adjust the pH of the solution to increase the proportion of unionized drug in the instilled dose. As discussed in Chapter 3 of this text, weak bases become more unionized at pHs greater than their pKa, and, weak acids become more unionized at pHs less than their pKa. Drugs which are highly water-soluble do not readily permeate the cornea.

Suspensions of drugs and ophthalmic ointments mix with lacrimal fluids less readily than do solutions, and thus, remain in the cul-de-sac for longer periods of time, enhancing the bioavailability of the drug substance. Ophthalmic solutions of increased viscosity also remain in the cul-de-sac longer than solutions with lower viscosity.

Ophthalmic Suspensions

Ophthalmic suspensions are employed to a lesser extent than are ophthalmic solutions, however, as noted previously, suspensions may be used to increase the corneal contact time of a drug substance and thus provide a more sustained action. Ophthalmic suspensions may be required when the medicinal agent is insoluble in the desired vehicle or unstable in solution form.

Ophthalmic suspensions must possess the same characteristic of sterility as ophthalmic solutions, with proper consideration given also to preservation, isotonicity, buffering, viscosity and packaging. Additionally, ophthalmic suspensions must contain particles of such chemical characteristics and small dimensions that they are non-irritating to the eyes. The ophthalmic suspension must also be of such a quality that the suspended particles do not agglomerate into larger ones upon storage. The suspension must be shaken prior to use and the particles distributed uniformly throughout the vehicle.

Examples of ophthalmic solutions and suspensions are presented in Table 10–4.

Packaging and Use of Ophthalmic Solutions and Suspensions

Ophthalmic solutions and suspensions should be packaged so that they are easily administered and their sterility maintained. Usually they, being administered by drop, are packaged in glass or plastic containers with a dropper service. Some plastic packages contain a fixed, built-in dropper that releases the med-

Table 10–4. Examples of Some Ophthalmic Agents by Category

Ophthalmic Agent	*Corresponding Commercial Product*	*Concentration of Active Ingredient*	*Comments*
Adrenergic			
Epinephrine Bitartrate	Epitrate Ophthalmic Solution (Ayerst)	2%	Used in management of chronic simple (open angle) glaucoma.
Naphazoline HCl	Naphcon Forte Ophthalmic Solution (Alcon)	0.1%	Used as a topical ocular vasoconstrictor.
Phenylephrine HCl	Mydfrin Ophthalmic Solution (Alcon)	2.5%	Used as a vasoconstrictor and mydriatic.
Anesthetic			
Proparacaine HCl	Ophthaine Ophthalmic Solution (Squibb)	0.5%	Rapid acting local anesthetic.
Antiallergic Agent			
Cromolyn Sodium	Opticrom (Fisons)	4%	For treatment of allergic ocular disorders
Antibacterial			
Chloramphenicol	Ophthochlor Ophthalmic Solution (Parke-Davis)	0.5%	Used for superficial infections of the eye due to susceptible microorganisms.
Gentamicin Sulfate	Garamycin Ophthalmic Solution (Schering)	0.3%	
Tetracycline Hydrochloride	Achromycin Ophthalmic Suspension (Lederle)	1%	
Sulfacetamide Sodium	Sodium Sulamyd Ophthalmic Solution (Schering)	10 and 30%	Used in treatment of conjunctivitis, corneal ulcer, and superficial ocular infections due to susceptible microorganisms.
Anticholinergic			
Atropine Sulfate	Isopto Atropine Ophthalmic Solution (Alcon)	0.125 to 4%	Used to produce mydriasis and cycloplegia.
Homatropine HBr	Isopto Homatropine Ophthalmic Solution (Alcon)	2 and 5%	
Scopolamine HBr	Isopto Hyoscine Ophthalmic Solution (Alcon)	0.25%	
Tropicamide	Mydriacyl Ophthalmic Solution (Alcon)	0.5 and 1%	
Antiviral			
Trifluridine	Viroptic Ophthalmic Solution (Burroughs Wellcome)	1%	Indicated in the treatment of herpes simplex keratitis.
Artificial Tears			
Dextran 70, Hydroxypropyl Methylcellulose	Tears Naturale II (Alcon)	....	For relief of dry eyes
Astringent			
Zinc Sulfate	Zincfrin Ophthalmic Solution (Alcon)	0.25%	Used for relief of discomfort and congestion caused by minor irritations to the eyes, such as dust, fatigue, and allergies.

Table 10–4.   Continued

Ophthalmic Agent	Corresponding Commercial Product	Concentration of Active Ingredient	Comments
Anti-inflammatory			
Dexamethasone Sodium Phosphate	Decadron Phosphate Ophthalmic Solution (Merck Sharp & Dohme)	0.1%	Combats inflammation due to mechanical, chemical, or immunologic causes.
Antibacterial/Antiinflammatory Combinations			
Prednisolone Acetate and Sulfacetamide Solution	Metimyd Ophthalmic Suspension (Schering)	0.5% prednisolone acetate and 10% sulfacetamide solution	For steroid-responsive inflammatory ocular conditions where bacterial infection or a risk of bacterial ocular infection exists.
Neomycin Sulfate and Dexamethasone Sodium Phosphate	NeoDecadron Ophthalmic Solution (Merck Sharp & Dohme)	0.35% neomycin base equivalent and 0.1% dexamethasone	
Oxytetracycline and Hydrocortisone Acetate	Terra-Cortril Ophthalmic Suspension (Roerig) Suspension (Roerig)	0.5% oxytetracycline equivalent and 1.5% hydrocortisone acetate	
Beta-Adrenergic Blocking Agents			
Betaxolol HCl	Betoptic (Alcon)	0.5%	Used for ocular hypertension and chronic open-angle glaucoma.
Levobunolol HCl	Betagan Liquifilm (Allergen)	0.5%	
Timolol Maleate	Timoptic (MSD)	0.25%, 0.5%	Used in patients with chronic open-angle glaucoma and aphakic patients with glaucoma.
Cholinergic			
Carbachol Ophthalmic Solution	Isopto Carbachol Ophthalmic Solution (Alcon)	0.75 to 3%	Reduces intraocular pressure in open-angle or narrow-angle glaucoma.
Pilocarpine HCl Ophthalmic Solution	Isopto Carpine Ophthalmic Solution (Alcon)	0.25 to 10%	Used as a miotic in treating glaucoma, especially open-angle glaucoma. Also used to neutralize mydriasis following ophthalmoscopy or surgery.
Nonsteroidal Anti-inflammatory Agent			
Flurbiprofen Sodium	Ocufen	0.03%	For inhibition of intraoperative miosis. Unlabeled use includes topical treatment of inflammation after cataract surgery.

Fig. 10–3. *Commercial package of an ophthalmic solution in plastic container with built-in dropper device. (Courtesy of Alcon.)*

ication when held in the inverted position (Fig. 10–3). The patient must exercise care in protecting the ophthalmic preparation from contamination. Obviously the ophthalmic solution packaged with the fixed dropper is less likely to acquire airborne contaminants than the screw-type bottle which must be opened and the dropper removed when using. However, each type is subject to contamination during use, brought about by the touching of the tip of the dropper to the tissues or to airborne contaminants.

When selecting the packaging material it must be determined that the container does not interfere with the stability or efficacy of the preparation.

The prescribed amount of ophthalmic solution or suspension should be dropped quickly, but completely, into the eye without touching the dropper to the eye or surrounding tissue. In administering ophthalmic drugs, the eye dropper should be held above the eye, and, with one hand the patient should pull the lower eyelid down. The medicine is then dropped in the eye while the patient looks upward. The patient should remain in place with the eye open for approximately 30 seconds. After instillation of the drops, the patient should be instructed to not close eyes tightly or blink more often than usual (which could cause the loss of the medication from the eye). Any ophthalmic solution that contains particulate matter or appears the least bit cloudy should be discarded.

Ophthalmic solutions used as eye washes are generally copackaged with an eye cup which should be cleaned and dried thoroughly after and prior to each use.

The major types of drugs used ophthalmically are as follows:

Anti-inflammatory Agents: These agents combat inflammation of the eye. Most prominent among those employed topically are hydrocortisone, prednisolone, and dexamethasone salts.

Antibiotic/Antimicrobial Agents: Antibiotic/antimicrobial agents are used specifically to combat infection of the eye. They are frequently employed both systemically and locally for their effect. Among those applied topically to the eye are gentamicin, sulfacetamide, tetracycline and tobramycin.

Antiviral Agents: For viral infections, preparations of idoxuridine, trifluridine, or vidarabine are employed.

Astringents: These agents are generally used in the treatment of conjunctivitis. Most preparations for this purpose utilize zinc compounds, particularly zinc sulfate, as the astringent.

Beta-Adrenergic Blocking Agents: These are indicated for treatment of ocular hypertension and chronic open-angle glaucoma. Typical preparations include betaxolol HCl, levobunolol HCl, or timolol maleate.

Local Anesthetics: Local anesthetics allow for the relief of pain preoperatively, postoperatively, following trauma, and during ophthalmic examination. Among the local anesthetics used ophthalmically are benoxinate, proparacaine, and cocaine.

Local Antiseptics: Local antiseptics are employed topically to reduce microbial presence on the eye. Among the agents so employed are certain organic mercury compounds as ammoniated mercury (used primarily as an ophthalmic ointment), and silver nitrate.

Miotics: Miotics are used primarily in the therapy of glaucoma but have been utilized in other conditions as accommodative esotropia, convergent strabismus, and for the local treatment of myasthenia gravis. Many miotics may be absorbed systemically after instillation into the eye and may produce undesirable effects in some patients. Miotics reduce intraocular pressure associated with glaucoma. Among the miotics are pilocarpine, carbachol, echothiophate iodide, and demecarium bromide. In addition to the miotics, several other types of agents are employed in the treatment of glaucoma, including: carbonic anhydrase inhibitors, as acetazolamide (oral), and adrenergic agents, as epinephrine.

Mydriatics and Cycloplegics: Mydriatics allow examination of the fundus through the dilation of the pupil. The stronger mydriatics having a long duration of action are called *cycloplegics.* Among the mydriatics and cycloplegics are atropine, scopolamine, homatropine, cyclopentolate, naphazoline, cocaine, and tropicamide.

Topical Protectants: These solutions are employed as artificial tears or as a contact lens fluid. Examples of agents used in these solutions are methylcellulose and hydroxypropyl methylcellulose.

Vasoconstrictors: These are intended to soothe, refresh and remove redness due to minor eye irritation. Among these are naphazoline HCl, oxymetazoline HCl, and tetrahydrozoline HCl.

Proper Administration and Use of Eye Drops

Prior to the administration of an ophthalamic solution or suspension, the patient should be advised to wash his/her hands thoroughly with soap and water. If the drops are supplied with a dropper, the patient should inspect the dropper to make sure there are no chips or cracks at the end of it. If the drops are a cloudy suspension, the patient should be told to shake them for about 10 seconds.

The patient should position himself/herself either lying down or tilting the head back. The index finger of one hand should be used to gently pull downward the affected eye to form a pocket or cup. Without touching the dropper to the eye, the prescribed number of drops are then gently placed into the formed pocket. The patient should understand that if the drops are placed directly onto the eyeball (cornea), they may cause a stinging sensation. Once the drops have been instilled, the dropper should be returned to its original container and capped tightly. The dropper should not be rinsed or wiped off.

To allow the drops to remain in the eye and enhance efficacy, the patient should press his/her finger against the inner corner of the eye

for 1 minute. This prevents the medication from entering the tearduct and in the case of some drugs prevents systemic absorption from occurring if the drug product passes down the throat into the gastrointestinal tract. After instillation the patient should close the eye and wipe any excess liquid off with a tissue.

The patient should be advised about the correct number of drops to instill, the frequency of application and the duration of treatment necessary. The patient should also be advised to appropriately store the medicine, including out of the reach of children.

Ophthalmic Ointments

Ophthalmic ointments, in contrast to the dermatological ointments discussed in the previous chapter, must be sterile. They are either manufactured from sterilized ingredients and under rigid aseptic conditions, or they are sterilized following manufacture.

The ointment base selected for an ophthalmic ointment must be non-irritating to the eye and must permit the diffusion of the medicinal substance throughout the secretions bathing the eye. Ointment bases utilized for ophthalmics have a melting or softening point close to body temperature. In most instances, mixtures of petrolatum and liquid petrolatum (mineral oil) are utilized as the ointment base. Sometimes a water-miscible agent as lanolin is added. This permits water and water-insoluble drugs to be retained within the delivery system.

The medicinal agent is added to the ointment base either as a solution or as a finely micronized powder. The drug is then intimately mixed with the base, usually by milling.

After preparation the ophthalmic ointments are filled into previously sterilized tin or plastic ophthalmic tubes. These tubes are typically small, holding approximately 3.5 g of ointment, and fitted with narrow gauge tips which permit the expulsion of narrow bands of ointment (Fig. 10–4). This is convenient for placement of the ointment onto the margin of the eyelid, the usual site of application. This should be done without touching the applicator tip to the eye.

The primary advantage of an ophthalmic ointment over an ophthalmic solution is the increased ocular contact time of the drug. Studies have shown that the ocular contact time is two

Fig. 10–4. *Examples of ophthalmic product packaging. Liquids are in 5-mL and 15-mL plastic Drop-Tainer dispensers and ointments are in tubes containing 3.5 g of product. (Courtesy of Alcon.)*

to four times greater when ointments are used than when a saline solution is used.[4] One disadvantage to ophthalmic ointment use is the blurred vision which occurs as the ointment base melts and is spread across the lens.

Examples of ophthalmic ointments are presented in Table 10–5.

Proper Administration of Ophthalmic Ointments

Prior to administration the patient should be advised to wash the hands thoroughly with soap and water. To make this procedure easier, a patient may use a mirror or simply have another person administer the ointment. The ointment tube should be held between the thumb and the forefinger of the opposite hand, and place the tube as near as possible to the eyelid, without touching it. The remaining fingers of this hand should be braced against the cheek or nose. The patient then tilts the head back, and with the index finger of the opposite hand, the lower lid should be gently pulled downward to form a pocket or cup. A ribbon of medication is then placed into the lower lid. The patient should then blink gently and with a tissue wipe off any excess ointment from the eyelids and lashes. Lastly, the cap should be replaced onto the ointment tube.

The patient should be advised that when the ointment is instilled into the eye, blurred vision will occur and not to be alarmed. If the ointment is to be administered one time per day, it is preferable to do so at bedtime where vision impairment will be inconsequential. The patient should be advised about the frequency of application and the length of time the regimen is

to be followed. Lastly, it is important to emphasize that the ointment must be kept clean and every effort should be made to avoid touching the tip of the tube against the eye or anything else.

Ophthalmic Inserts

An innovative development in the delivery of medication to the eyes has been that of ophthalmic inserts. One such device, the OCUSERT system (Alza) is shown in Figure 10–5. The insert unit is designed to provide for the release of medication at predetermined and predictable rates permitting the elimination of frequent dosing by the patient, ensuring nighttime medication, and providing a better means of patient compliance.

The insert shown in Figure 10–5 is elliptical with dimensions of 13.4 by 5.7 mm and 0.3 mm in thickness. The insert is flexible and is a multilayered structure consisting of a drug-containing core surrounded on each side by a layer of copolymer membranes through which the drug diffuses at a constant rate (Fig. 10–6). The rate of drug diffusion is controlled by the polymer composition, the membrane thickness, and the solubility of the drug. The devices are sterile and do not contain preservatives.

Inserts containing pilocarpine have been found to be effective in glaucoma therapy.[5] After placement in the conjunctival sac, the inserts are designed to release medication at the desired rates over a 7-day period at which time they are removed and replaced with new ones. Other drugs such as adrenocortical steroids have been utilized in the system with similar effectiveness.[6]

Soft contact lenses, composed of various polymeric materials, have also been used as drug delivery systems with success.[4] Readers interested in the use, composition, and care of both conventional hard contact lenses and the soft contact lenses may wish to refer to the papers listed in the footnote.[7] A brief summary of contact lens solutions is presented below.

Contact Lens Solutions

In 1987 it was estimated that about 24 million Americans wore contact lens, and that the numbers will continue to grow. The growing popularity of contact lenses has promoted the development of new types of lenses and lens care

Table 10–5. Examples of Ophthalmic Ointments

Ophthalmic Ointment	Corresponding Commercial Product	Concentration of Active Ingredient	Category
Atropine Sulfate Ophthalmic Ointment	Atropine Sulfate Ophthalmic Ointment (Allergan)	0.5 and 1.0%	Parasympatholytic used to produce mydriasis for refraction.
Chloramphenicol Ophthalmic Ointment	Chloromycetin Ophthalmic Ointment (Parke Davis)	1%	Antibacterial
Dexamethasone Sodium Phosphate Ophthalmic Ointment	Decadron Phosphate Ophthalmic Ointment (Merck Sharp & Dohme)	0.05%	Anti-inflammatory adrenocortical steroid
Gentamicin Sulfate Ophthalmic Ointment	Garamycin Ophthalmic Ointment (Schering)	0.3%	Antibacterial
Neomycin Sulfate and Dexamethasone Sodium Phosphate Ophthalmic Ointment	NeoDecadron Ophthalmic Ointment (Merck Sharp & Dohme)	0.35% neomycin base and 0.05% dexamethasone phosphate equivalents	Antibacterial/anti-inflammatory
Polymyxin B—Bacitracin Ophthalmic Ointment	Polysporin Ophthalmic Ointment (Burroughs Wellcome)	polymyxin B sulfate, 10,000 units and bacitracin zinc, 500 units per g	Antimicrobial
Polymyxin B—Bacitracin—Neomycin Ophthalmic Ointment	Neosporin Ophthalmic Ointment (Burroughs Wellcome)	per g: polymyxin B sulfate, 5000 units; bacitracin, zinc, 400 units; neomycin sulfate, 5 mg	Antimicrobial
Prednisolone Acetate Sulfacetamide Sodium Ophthalmic Ointment	Metimyd Ophthalmic Ointment (Schering)	0.5% prednisolone acetate and 10% sulfacetamide sodium	Antibacterial/anti-inflammatory
Sulfacetamide Sodium Ophthalmic Ointment	Sodium Sulamyd Ophthalmic Ointment (Schering)	10 and 30%	Antibacterial
Sulfisoxazole Diolamine Ophthalmic Ointment	Gantrisin Ophthalmic Ointment (Roche)	4%	Antibacterial
Tetracycline HCl Ophthalmic Ointment	Achromycin Ophthalmic Ointment (Lederle)	1%	Antibacterial
Tobramycin Ophthalmic Ointment	Tobrex Ophthalmic Ointment (Alcon)	0.3%	Antibacterial
Vidarabine Ophthalmic Ointment	Vira-A-Ophthalmic Ointment (Parke Davis)	3%	Antiviral

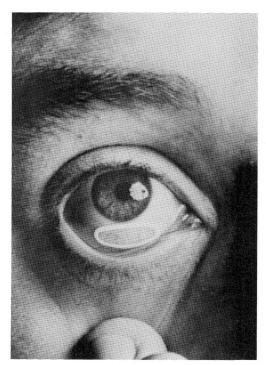

Fig. 10–5. *Ocusert Ocular Therapeutic Systems are thin, flexible wafers placed under the eyelid to provide a week's dosage of pilocarpine in the treatment of glaucoma. Ocusert systems cause less blurring of vision than pilocarpine eyedrops, which must be used 4 times daily. (Courtesy of Alza Corporation.)*

PILOCARPINE RESERVOIR

TRANSPARENT RATE CONTROLLING MEMBRANES

ANNULAR RING (SURROUNDS RESERVOIR OPAQUE WHITE FOR VISIBILITY IN HANDLING AND INSERTING SYSTEM)

Fig. 10–6. *Construction of the Ocusert Ocular Therapeutic System containing pilocarpine between transparent rate-controlling membranes. (Courtesy of Alza Corporation.)*

products. In the last decade, many different kinds of soft, hard and rigid gas permeable (RGP) lenses have been tested and marketed. Coupled with this growth has been the emergence of such products as contact lens cleaners and disinfectants.

For the pharmacist it is a responsibility to keep current and know the details of lens cleaning, disinfection, neutralization, rinsing and storage of all lenses. In addition, pharmacists must be knowledgeable about lens lubricating drops and up-to-date about the compatibilities and incompatibilities among all the products that a contact lens wearer might use.

The three basic types of contact lenses are classified by their chemical composition and physical properties, e.g., soft, hard, and rigid gas permeable (RGP).

Hard contact lenses provides durability and clear, crisp vision for the patient. These lenses are termed hard because they are made of a rigid plastic resin, polymethylmethacrylate (PMMA), and as a consequence many people have found them extremely uncomfortable to wear and tolerate. PMMA lenses are practically impermeable to oxygen and moisture (these absorb only about 0.5% water), a disadvantage to corneal epithelial respiration and to patient comfort. Care must be exercised to prevent the hard lens from resting directly on the corneal surface to protect the epithelial tissue from physical damage. To prevent such direct contact, solutions are used that wet the surface of the lens to provide a cushioning layer between the corneal epithelium and the inner surface of the lens.

Soft contact lenses were introduced in 1971 and have become extremely popular in comparison to hard lenses because they are much more comfortable. Soft lenses are made of a hydrophilic transparent plastic, hydroxyethylmethacrylate (HEMA) that contains between 30 and 80% water. This increased water content of the lens improves its permeability to oxygen. There are two types of soft contact lens: daily-wear and extended-wear. As each name suggests, daily-wear lenses must be removed at night before the wearer goes to sleep, whereas the extended-wear lenses are designed to be worn for more than 24 hours. Some of these lenses have been approved for up to 30 days of continuous wear, however, it is advised that a person not leave them in the eye for longer than 4 to 7 days at one time without removal for cleaning and disinfection. Long use without cleaning and disinfection can predispose the wearer to a serious eye infection.

Disposable soft lenses are now available and these do pose an advance for patients. Specifically, disposable lenses do not necessitate lens cleaning and disinfection after a week's wear. These are simply discarded and replaced with a new pair. The problem, however, is that the wearer may be tempted to wear these for longer than suggested with the distinct possibility that a serious eye infection may result. The success of disposable soft lenses will be coupled to a patient's ability to incur the higher cost to use them.

Rigid gas permeable (RGP) contact lenses take advantage of features of the soft and the hard contact lenses. These lenses are constructed of material that is oxygen-permeable but hydrophobic. Thus, they permit the transmission of oxygen through the lens more so than hard lenses, while still providing the durability and ease of handling that hard lenses provide. These lenses have the greater wearing comfort of the soft lenses and usually are intended for daily wear. Some of the newer "super-permeable" RGP lenses are for extended wear.

There are advantages and disadvantages associated with each type of contact lens. Hard contact lenses and RGP lenses provide strength and durability and relatively easy care regimens. These are easy to handle during insertion and removal. Further these are relatively resistant to the absorption of disinfectants, surfactant cleansers, and environmental contaminants. These lenses provide visual acuity superior to soft contact lenses, which is very important to some individuals. On the opposite side of the coin, hard contact lenses and RGP lenses require an adjustment period and may become dislodged or migrate in the eye.

Soft contact lenses are advantageous to wear for longer periods of time, and usually there is little adaptation time associated with them. These lenses make visual adjustment easier for the wearer when it is necessary to switch from contact lenses to eyeglasses. Lastly, soft lenses do not dislodge as easily nor fall out of the eye as readily as the hard contact lenses. Unfortunately, soft contact lenses provide a slight reduction in quality of vision and have a shorter life span. Furthermore, the wearer must ensure that the lenses not dry out because they are extremely fragile.

It is important that all contact lenses receive appropriate care in handling and maintenance to retain their shape and optical characteristics, and for their safe use. Wearers should be instructed in the techniques for the proper insertion and removal of the lenses from the eye, as well as in the methods for cleaning, sterilizing, and storing the lenses.

With the exception of disposable soft contact lenses, all soft lenses require a routine care program that includes (1) cleaning to loosen and remove lipid and protein deposits, (2) rinsing to remove the cleaning solution and material loosened by cleaning, and (3) disinfection to kill microorganisms. If these lenses are not maintained at proper intervals, they are prone to deposit build-up, discoloration, and microbial contamination. The moist, porous surface of the hydrophilic lens provides a perfect medium for the growth of bacteria, fungi, and viruses. Thus, disinfection is essential to prevent eye infections and microbial damage to the lens material.

Hard contact lenses require a routine care program that includes (1) cleaning to remove debris and deposits from the lens, (2) soaking the lens in a storage/disinfecting solution while not in use, and (3) wetting the lenses to decrease their hydrophobic characteristics.

To achieve the care needs of lenses there are several solutions employed as follows:
1. Wetting Solutions
2. Cleaning Solutions
3. Soaking Solutions
4. Combination Purpose Solutions

The pharmacist plays a key role in counseling patients about the use of these products as well as other over-the-counter drug products and legend medications. For example, oral medications which are excreted in tear fluid or discolor tears may also affect contact lenses. Most notably, rifampin (orange-colored tears) and sulfasalazine (yellow-colored tears) have been implicated to cause permanent lens staining. Also, those oral or topical drugs that can cause ocular side effects can potentially interfere with contact lens use. For example, drugs with anticholinergic effects, e.g., antihistamines, tricyclic antidepressants, decrease tear secretion and may cause lens intolerance and damage. Isotretinoin, prescribed for severe, recalcitrant acne, can induce marked dryness of the eye, so while acne therapy is being conducted it would be wise for the pharmacist to suggest to the patient to check with his/her ophthalmologist about the advisability to continue wearing contact lenses. Concern must also be expressed when patients are maintained on medicines that promote excessive lacrimation, e.g., reserpine, or ocular or eyelid edema, e.g., primidone, hydrochlorthiazide, chlorthalidone, which may interfere with lens wear.

When the lens wearer is prescribed an ophthalmic ointment, contact lenses should not be worn until the therapy is completed. These dosage forms are capable of discoloring the lens and can interfere with the optimal use of the lens.

It is possible that a lens wearer will consult a pharmacist about the advisability of an OTC ophthalmic product, e.g., topical vasoconstrictor, to relieve eye irritation or redness. These individuals should be counseled to consult their fitter if they experience sharp eye pain, excessive watering of the eyes, persistent irritation or inflammation of the eyes, sudden changes in vision or spectacle blur that does not clear up overnight. Spectacle blur is a phenomenon in which hard lenses worn for a number of hours cause corneal edema. This affects visual acuity from several minutes to hours after lens removal until the eye returns to normal.

It is useful if the pharmacist reinforces several general considerations in the care of contact lens products. Wearers should wash their hands thoroughly before and after handling the lens with a nonabrasive, noncosmetic soap. Wearers should not rub the eyes when the lens are in place, and if irritation develops, the lens should be removed until these symptoms subside. To avoid differences between products produced by different manufacturers it is preferable to use solutions made by the same manufacturer. Cleaning and storing of lenses should be performed in the appropriate solution for that purpose. Lenses should not be stored in tap water, nor should saliva be used to help reinsert a lens into the eye. Saliva is not sterile and contains numerous microorganisms, including *Pseudomonas aeruginosa*.

Because many lens wearers are young women between the ages of 18 to 24, it is appropriate for the pharmacist to counsel these woman with regard to cosmetic restriction. Many ophthalmologists advise lens wearers to purchase makeup in the smallest container. Once opened and the longer the container is around the greater the likelihood of bacterial contamination. Further, mascara and pearlized eye shadow should be avoided by women wearing hard lenses because particles of these can get into the eye, and even a small flake can cause much irritation and corneal damage is a possibility. Aerosol hairsprays should be used before the lens is inserted into the eye, and preferably applied in another room. Otherwise airborne particles could attach to the lens during its insertion into the eye and cause irritation. The lenses should be inserted prior to makeup application because oily substances on the fingertips can smudge the lenses when they are handled. For similar reasons, lenses should be removed before removing makeup.

Lastly, it is important that contact lens wearers get their eyes medically checked 3 times per year to make sure that no damage is occurring as a result of wearing contact lenses.

Products for Soft Contact Lenses

CLEANERS. Because of their porous composition, soft lenses tend to accumulate proteinaceous material which forms a film on the lens (decreasing clarity) and serves as a base for microbial growth. The two main categories of cleaners are *surfactants*, which emulsify accumulated oils, lipids and inorganic compounds, and *enzymatic cleansers*, which break down and remove protein deposits. Surfactant materials are utilized either within a mechanical washing device (Opti-Heat) or by simply placing several drops of the solution on the lens surface and gently rubbing the lens back and forth, either by placing the lens on the thumb and rubbing with the forefinger or by placing the lens in the palm of the hand and rubbing gently with a fingertip (about a 20 to 30 second procedure). The ingredients in these cleansers usually include a nonionic detergent, wetting agent, chelating agent, buffers, and preservatives.

Enzymatic cleaning is accomplished by soaking the lenses in a solution prepared from enzyme tablets. This procedure is recommended at least once per week or twice per month in conjunction with regular surfactant cleansing. These tablets contain either papain, pancreatin, or subtilisin, which causes the hydrolysis of protein to peptides and amino acids. Typically these are added to saline solution, but one solution can be prepared using 3% hydrogen peroxide, which combines enzymatic cleaning with disinfection. After the lenses have been soaked for the recommended length of time they should be thoroughly rinsed.

RINSING/STORAGE. Saline solutions for soft lenses should have a neutral pH and be isotonic with human tears, i.e., 0.9% sodium chloride. Besides rinsing the lenses, these solutions are used for storage because saline maintains their curvature and diameter, as well as optical power of the soft lenses. Further, it facilitates lens hydration and prevents the lens from drying out and becoming brittle.

Because they are used for storage, many saline solutions contain preservatives which, while inhibiting bacterial growth, can induce sensitivity reactions or eye irritation. Most notably, thiomersal has been implicated in this regard, and manufacturers have endeavored to create preservative-free saline solutions and package them in aerosol containers or unit-of-use vials. The use of salt tablets to prepare a normal saline solution is discouraged because of the potential of contamination and risk of serious eye infections, e.g., *Acanthamoeba* keratitis.

DISINFECTION AND NEUTRALIZATION. Disinfection can be accomplished by two methods, i.e., thermal (heat) and chemical (no heat). In the past both methods were equally popular, however, with the introduction of hydrogen peroxide systems for chemical disinfection, chemical disinfection has become more popular.

For thermal disinfection, the lenses are placed into a specially designed heating unit with saline solution. The solution is heated sufficiently to kill microorganisms, e.g., for 10 minutes at a minimum of 80°C. It is important that after disinfection the lenses be stored in the unopened case until ready to be worn. Further, the wearer must ensure that the lenses have been thoroughly cleaned prior to using heat disinfection. Otherwise, heating can hasten lens deterioration.

In years past chemical disinfection was conducted with products that contained thimerosal in combination with either chlorhexidine or a quaternary ammonium compound. Unfortunately, many wearers encountered sensitivity reactions and these products fell into disfavor. Subsequently, the introduction of hydrogen peroxide systems for chemical disinfection has revitalized this method of disinfection. It is thought that the "free radicals" chemically released from the peroxide react with the cell wall of the microorganisms. Further, the bubbling action of the peroxide is thought to promote the removal of any remaining debris on the lens.

To prevent eye irritation from residual peroxide after disinfection, it is necessary that the lenses be exposed to one of three types of neutralizing agents. These are the *catalytic type* (an enzyme catalase or a platinum disc), e.g., Lensept Neutralizer (CIBA Vision); a *reactive type* (such as sodium pyruvate or sodium thiosulfate), e.g., Rinsing and Neutralizing Solution (CooperVision); or the *dilution-elution* type, e.g., PureSept Disinfection Solution (Ross).

Chemical disinfection systems may come as two-solution systems, which use separate disinfecting and rinsing solutions, or one-solution systems, which use the same solution for rinsing and storage. It is important that the wearer realize that lenses must not be disinfected by heating when using these solutions.

Products for Hard Contact Lenses

CLEANERS. Hard lenses should be cleaned immediately after their removal from the eye. Otherwise, oils deposits, proteins, salts, cosmetics, tobacco smoke and airborne contaminants can build up, interfere with clear vision and possibly cause irritation. A surfactant cleaner is used by applying the solution or gel onto both surfaces of the lens, and then rubbing the lens in the palm of the hand with the index finger for about 20 seconds. The wearer should realize that too vigorous rubbing can cause scratching or warping of the lens.

SOAKING/STORAGE SOLUTIONS. Although some ophthalmologists advocate dry storage of PMMA lenses, most believe that these lenses should be stored in a soaking solution once they are removed from the eye. To be effective soaking solutions must contain sufficient concentration of disinfecting agent, usually 0.01% benzalkonium chloride and 0.01% edetate sodium, to kill surface bacteria. Overnight soaking is advantageous because it keeps the lenses wettable and the prolonged contact time helps to loosen deposits that remain after routine cleaning.

WETTING SOLUTIONS. These solutions contain surfactants to facilitate the hydration of the hydrophobic lens surface. Wetting solutions enable the tears of the eye to evenly spread across the lens surface by converting the hydrophobic surface of the lens to a temporary hydrophilic surface. These solutions also facilitate a cushion between the lens and the cornea and the eyelid. Typical ingredients include a viscosity-inducing agent, hydroxyethylcellulose, a wetting agent, such as polyvinyl alcohol, preservatives, such as benzalkonium chloride or edetate disodium, and buffering agents/salts to adjust the pH and maintain tonicity.

COMBINATION SOLUTIONS. These solutions serve as cleaning/soaking solutions, wetting/soaking solutions, or cleaning, soaking, and wetting solutions. While patient ease of use is improved with these, combination products may lower the effectiveness of the cleaning function if the concentration of cleaning solution is too low to adequately remove debris from the lens surface. These combination solutions should be reserved for those wearers who have a demonstrated need for simplification of the lens care process.

Products for Rigid Gas Permeable (RGP) Contact Lenses

Wearers of rigid gas permeable contact lenses should know to use only solutions that are compatible with this type of lens. These lenses generally follow the same regimen for care as hard contact lenses, except that specific solutions must be used for this type of lens. One of two cleaning methods may be used, i.e., hand washing or mechanical washing. In the first method, the lens may be cleaned by holding the concave side up in the palm of the hand. The lens should not be held between the fingers because the flexibility of the lens may inadvertently cause the lens to warp or turn inside out. Mechanical washing is advantageous because the possibility of the lens turning inside out or warping during cleaning is minimized.

After cleansing, the RGP lens should then be thoroughly rinsed and soaked in a wetting/soaking solution overnight. After soaking, the next morning the lens is rubbed with fresh wetting/soaking solution and then inserted into the eye. To facilitate removal of stubborn protein deposits, some opthalmologists recommend weekly cleaning with enzymatic, i.e., papain, cleaners.

Nasal Preparations

The vast majority of preparations intended for intranasal use contain adrenergic agents and are employed for their decongestant activity on the nasal mucosa. Most of these preparations are in solution-form, and are administered as nose drops or sprays; however, a few are available as nasal jellies. Examples of products for intranasal use are shown in Figure 10–7 and presented in Table 10–6.

Nasal Decongestant Solutions

Most nasal decongestant solutions are aqueous preparations, rendered isotonic to nasal fluids (approximately equivalent to 0.9% sodium chloride), buffered to maintain drug stability while approximating the normal pH range of the nasal fluids (pH 5.5 to 6.5), and stabilized and preserved as required. The antimicrobial preservatives used are the same as those used in preserving ophthalmic solutions. The concentration of adrenergic agent in the majority of nasal decongestant solutions is quite low, ranging from about 0.05 to 1.0%. Certain commercial solutions which are available for both pediatric and adult use, are generally available in two strengths, the pediatric strength being approximately one-half of the adult strength.

Nasal decongestant solutions are employed in the treatment of rhinitis of the common cold and for vasomotor and allergic rhinitis including hay fever, and for sinusitis. Their frequent use or their use for prolonged periods may lead to chronic edema of the nasal mucosa, i.e., *rhinitis medicamentosa*, aggravating the symptom that they are intended to relieve. Thus, they are best used for short periods of time (no longer than 3 to 5 days) with the patients advised not to exceed the recommended dosage and frequency of use.

The easiest but least comfortable approach to treat rebound congestion is to completely withdraw application of the topical vasoconstrictor. Unfortunately, this approach will promptly result in bilateral vasodilation with almost total nasal obstruction. A more acceptable method is to withdraw application of drug in only one nostril, and have the patient continue using the medication in the other nostril. Once the rebound congestion subsides in the drug-free nostril, about 1 to 2 weeks, a total withdrawal is then instituted. Another approach is the substitution of a topical saline solution or spray *in lieu* of the topical vasoconstrictor. This effectively keeps the nasal mucosa moist and provides psychologic assistance to patients who are dependent upon placing medication into their nostrils.

Most of the adrenergic drugs used in nasal decongestant solutions are synthetic compounds similar in chemical structure, pharma-

Fig. 10–7. *Examples of commercial packaging of nasal solutions, showing drop and spray containers, and nasal inhaler.*

Table 10–6. Examples of Some Commercial Nasal Preparations

Product Name	Manufacturer	Active Ingredient	Use/Indications
Afrin Nasal Spray and Afrin Nose Drops	Schering	oxymetazole HCl (0.05%)	Nasal adrenergic/decongestant
Beconase AQ Nasal Spray	Glaxo	beclomethasone diprorionate (0.042%)	Synthetic corticosteroid indicated for the relief of symptoms of seasonal or perennial allergic or vasomotor rhinitis
Diapid Nasal Spray	Sandoz	lopressin (0.185 mg/mL)	Antidiuretic; for control or prevention of diabetes insipidus due to deficiency of endogenous posterior pituitary antidiuretic hormone.
Nasalcrom Nasal Solution	Fisons	cromolyn sodium (4%)	Prevention and treatment of symptoms of allergic rhinitis
Nasalide Nasal Solution	Syntex	flunisolide (0.025%)	Indicated in the treatment of symptoms of seasonal or perennial rhinitis
Neo-Synephrine Nose Drops	Winthrop	phenylephrine HCl (0.125 to 1.0%)	Nasal adrenergic/decongestant
Neo-Synephrine II Long Acting Drops and Spray	Winthrop	xylometazoline HCl (0.1%)	Nasal adrenergic/decongestant
Ocean Solution Spray	Fleming	sodium chloride (0.65%)	To restore moisture and relieve dry, crusted and inflamed nasal membranes.
Privine HCl Nasal Solution	Ciba	naphazoline HCl (0.05 and 0.1%)	Nasal adrenergic/decongestant
Syntocinon Nasal Spray	Sandoz	oxytocin (40 units/mL)	Synthetic oxytocin hormone. Employed for initial milk let-down preparatory to breast feeding.
Tyzine Pediatric Nose Drops	Key	tetrahydrozoline HCl (0.05%)	Nasal adrenergic/decongestant

cologic activity, and side effects to the parent compound, naturally occurring epinephrine. Epinephrine as a pure chemical substance was first isolated from suprarenal gland in 1901 and was called both *Suprarenin* and *Adrenalin*. Synthetic epinephrine was prepared just a few years later.

Most solutions for nasal use are packaged in dropper bottles or in plastic spray bottles, usually containing 15 to 30 mL of medication. The products should be determined to be stable in the containers used and the packages tightly closed during periods of nonuse. The patient should be advised that should the solution become discolored or contain precipitated matter, it should be discarded.

The patient should also understand that there is a difference in the duration of the effect of topical decongestants. For example, phenylephrine should be used every 3 to 4 hours, whereas xylometazoline, which is longer acting, should only be used every 8 to 10 hours.

Decongestant Inhalers

Certain nasal decongestants may also be employed in the form of inhalants. For instance the drug propylhexedrine (Benzedrex, Menley & James) is a liquid which volatilizes slowly at room temperature. This quality enables it to be effective as an inhalant. The inhalers in which the drug is held contain cylindrical rolls of fibrous material impregnated with the volatile drug substance. The medication which has an amine-like odor is usually masked with added aromatic agents. The inhaler is placed in the nostril and vapor inhaled to relieve nasal congestion. As with the other nasal adrenergic agents, excessive or too frequent use can result in nasal edema and increased rather than decreased congestion.

The inhalers are effective so long as the volatile drug remains present. To insure that the drug does not escape during periods of nonuse, the caps on the inhalers should be tightly closed.

At this point it is relevant to mention that some future drug delivery systems will be through nasal administration. Insulin, for example, is one drug for which nasal administration is being investigated; this route has definite advantages over the traditional method of subcutaneous injection, which can be painful and bothersome to the patient.

Proper Administration and Use of Nasal Drops/Sprays

To minimize the possibility of contamination, the pharmacist should point out to the patient that the nasal product only be used by one person and kept out of the reach of children. If the nasal product is intended for a child the directions should be clear to the patient. If an over-the-counter product is used, the parent should note the directions on the label.

Prior to administration, the patient should blow the nose to clear the nostrils and wash his/her hands thoroughly with soap and water. For maximum penetration with drops, a patient should lie down on a flat surface, such as a bed, hanging the head over the edge, and then tilting the head back as far as comfortable. The prescribed number of drops are then gently placed into the nostrils, and to allow the medication to spread in the nose, the patient should remain in this position for a few minutes. After this, the dropper should be replaced in the bottle and tightened.

The patient should be advised to use the drops only as long as prescribed. Long-acting nasal drops, as mentioned, can cause rebound congestion so whenever possible, treatment should not extend beyond 5 days.

If a spray dosage form is utilized by the patient, basically the same suggestions apply with the exception that the patient should not lie on a flat surface. If this is performed there is a chance that the administration would be enhanced by the prone position. It is better to merely have the patient tilt the head back while standing and gently squeeze the medicine container to deliver the medication.

Certain nasal medications (e.g., Vancenase [beclomethasone diproprionate]) are available for administration through aerosol inhalers. A clever method for a patient to estimate the proportion of medication remaining in the inhaler is shown in Figure 10–8.

Topical Oral Preparations

A variety of medicinal substances are employed topically in the oral cavity for a number

Fig. 10–8. *An easy method of estimating the amount of Vancenase left in an inhaler. The canister is placed in a bowl of water and its position compared with the diagram shown. (Courtesy of Schering Corp.)*

of purposes and in a wide range of dosage forms. Among the drugs and preparations included in this group are the following:

Benzocaine—Topical anesthetic. Indicated for temporary relief of pain, soreness, and irritation in the mouth associated with teething, orthodontic appliances, new or poorly fitting dentures, and canker sores.

Camphorated Parachlorophenol—Dental anti-infective. A eutectic liquid composed of 65% camphor and 35% parachlorophenol, used in dentistry for the sterilization of deep root canals.

Carbamide Peroxide Topical Solution—Dental anti-infective. Acts as a chemomechanical cleansing and debriding agent through the release of bubbling oxygen. The commercial product (Gly-Oxide Liquid, Marion) contains 10% carbamide in flavored anhydrous glycerin.

Cetylpyridinium Chloride Solution and Cetylpyridinium Chloride Lozenges—Local anti-infective. Commercial counterparts (Cepacol Mouthwash/Gargle and Cepacol Lozenges, Lakeside) contain 1:2000 w/v and 1:1500 w/v of cetylpyridinium chloride respectively. Used primarily as a freshening mouth cleanser. Lozenges have benzyl alcohol present to act as a local anesthetic in soothing throat irritations.

Erythrosine Sodium Topical Solution and Erythrosine Sodium Soluble Tablets—Diagnostic aid (dental disclosing agent). Solution applied topically to the teeth to reveal plaque left by inadequate brushing. Tablets chewed for the same purpose and are not to be swallowed.

Eugenol—Dental analgesic. Applied topically to dental cavities and dental protectives. Eugenol is a pale yellow liquid having an aromatic odor of clove and a spicy taste.

Lidocaine Oral Spray—Topical dental anesthetic. Applied through metered spray in the amounts of 10 mg per spray; 20 mg per quadrant of gingiva and oral mucosa is usually employed. [Xylocaine Oral Spray (Astra)]

Nystatin Oral Suspension—Antifungal. May be employed for oral fungal infections by retaining in the mouth as long as possible before swallowing.

Saliva Substitutes—These contain electrolytes in a carboxymethylcellulose base and are indicated for the relief of dry mouth and throat in xerostomia.

Sodium Fluoride Oral Solution, and Sodium Fluoride Tablets—Dental caries prophylactic. Solution applied to the teeth or, when drinking water does not contain adequate fluoride, a dilute solution may be swallowed. Tablets containing 1.1 or 2.2 mg of sodium fluoride are chewed or swallowed as required.

Sodium Fluoride and Phosphoric Acid Gel and Sodium Fluoride and Phosphoric Acid Topical Solution—Dental caries prophylactic. Gel and solution applied to the teeth; each contains 1.23% of fluoride ion and 1% of phosphoric acid.

Triamcinolone Acetonide Dental Paste—Topical anti-inflammatory agent. Applied to the oral mucous membranes as a 0.1% paste.

Zinc Oxide-Eugenol Mixture—A temporary filling mix available over-the-counter, i.e., DenTemp, so that a consumer can prepare and use the mixture when a dental filling falls out or dislodges.

In addition to the above-named drugs and preparations, a host of other products for oral use are commercially available. Some of these products are medicated, as teething lotions and toothache drops, whereas others are used for hygienic purposes, as dentifrices, denture products, and many of the mouthwashes. Among the variety of products is a like variety of physical forms, as solutions, emulsions, ointments, pastes, aerosols, etc., with the manufacture of each following the same general procedures as has been previously outlined in this text. One type of dosage form for oral use, the lozenge, has not been previously described.

Lozenges

Lozenges, also called *troches*, are disk-shaped solid dosage forms containing a medicinal substance and generally flavoring and sweetening agents, intended to be dissolved slowly in the oral cavity for localized effects. Commercially, lozenges may be made by compression, using a tablet machine and large, flat punches. The tablet machines are operated at high compression to produce troches that are harder than ordinary tablets so that they slowly dissolve or disintegrate in the mouth. The use of adhesives such as mucilages or natural gums, added to effect the adhesion of the powders used, also contributes to the hardness of the resulting lozenges.

Medicinal substances that are heat stable may be prepared into hard, sugar candy lozenges by candy-making machines that process a warm, highly concentrated, flavored syrup as the base. These lozenges dissolve slowly, and because of their high sugar content are especially soothing to the throat. Most of the commercially available cough drops are of a hard candy base.

Historically, lozenges have been employed to relieve minor sore throat pain and irritation and have conveniently delivered topical anesthetics and antibacterials for this purpose, e.g., phenol, sodium phenolate, cetylpyridinium chloride. In recent years there has been an emergence of other lozenge/troche products. Clotrimazole and nystatin are marketed in troche dosage forms and intended to treat oropharyngeal candidiasis. Lozenge/troche dosage forms are also a covenient means to deliver drugs, e.g., dextromethorphan, phenylpropanolamine, and phenylephrine to treat cough and cold symptoms.

When patients are prescribed medications that employ the troche dosage form, the pharmacist should recommend that the patient allow the troche/lozenge to dissolve slowly in the mouth. Further, the intent of the product and the duration of treatment should be emphasized to the patient.

Ear Preparations

Ear preparations are sometimes referred to as *otic* or *aural* preparations. Solutions are most frequently used in the ear, with suspensions and ointments also finding some application. Ear preparations are usually placed in the ear canal by drops or in small amounts for the removal of excessive cerumen (ear wax) or for the treatment of ear infections, inflammation, or pain. Because the outer ear is a skin-covered structure and susceptible to the same dermatologic conditions as other parts of the body's surface, skin conditions which arise are treated using the variety of topical dermatological preparations previously discussed in Chapter 9.

Cerumen-Removing Preparations

Cerumen is a combination of the secretions of the sweat and sebaceous glands of the external auditory canal. The secretions, if allowed to dry, form a sticky semisolid which holds shed epithelial cells, fallen hair, dust and other foreign bodies that make their way into the ear canal. Excessive accumulation of cerumen in the ear may cause itching, pain, impaired hearing and is a deterrent to otologic examination. If not removed periodically, the cerumen may become impacted and its removal made more difficult and painful.

Through the years, light mineral oil, vegetable oils, and hydrogen peroxide have been commonly used agents to soften impacted cerumen for its removal. Recently, solutions of synthetic surfactants have been developed for their *cerumenolytic* activity in the removal of ear wax. One of these agents, triethanolamine polypeptide oleate-condensate, commercially formulated in propylene glycol, is used to emulsify the cerumen thereby facilitating its removal [Cerumenex Drops (Purdue Frederick)]. Another commercial product utilizes carbamide peroxide in glycerin/propylene glycol [Debrox Drops (Marion)]. On contact with the cerumen, the carbamide peroxide releases oxygen which disrupts the integrity of the impacted wax, allowing its easy removal.

In removing cerumen, the procedure usually involves placing the otic solution in the ear canal with the patient's head tilted at a 45° angle, inserting a cotton plug to retain the medication in the ear for 15 to 30 minutes, followed by gentle flushing of the ear canal with lukewarm water using a soft rubber ear syringe.

Anti-infective, Anti-inflammatory, and Analgesic Ear Preparations

Drugs used topically in the ear for their anti-infective activity include such agents as chloramphenicol, colistin sulfate, neomycin, polymyxin B sulfate, and nystatin, the latter agent used to combat fungal infections. These agents are generally formulated into ear drops (solutions or suspensions) in a vehicle of anhydrous glycerin or propylene glycol. These viscous vehicles permit maximum contact time between the medication and the tissues of the ear. In addition, their hygroscopicity causes them to draw moisture from the tissues thereby reducing inflammation and diminishing the moisture available for the life process of the microorganisms present. To assist in relieving the pain which frequently accompanies ear infections, a number of anti-infective otic preparations also contain analgesic agents as antipyrine and local anesthetics as lidocaine, dibucaine, and benzocaine.

Topical treatment of ear infections is frequently considered adjunctive, with concomitant systemic treatment with orally administered antibiotics also undertaken.

Liquid ear preparations of the anti-inflammatory agents hydrocortisone and dexamethasone sodium phosphate are prescribed for their effects against the swelling and inflammation which frequently accompany allergic and irritative manifestations of the ear as well as for the inflammation and pruritus which sometimes follow treatment of ear infections. In the latter instance, some physicians prefer the use of corticosteroids in ointment form, packaged in ophthalmic tubes. These packages allow the placement of small amounts of ointment in the ear canal with a minimum of waste. Many of the commercially available products used in this manner are labeled "eye-ear" to indicate their dual use.

Aside from the antibiotic-steroid combinations that are used to treat otitis externa, which is known synonymously as swimmer's ear, acetic acid (2%) in aluminum acetate solution and boric acid (2.75%) in isopropyl alcohol are used. These drugs help to re-acidify the ear canal and the vehicles serve to help dry the ear canal. By drying the ear canal, the growth medium for the offending microorganisms, usually *Pseudomonas aeruginosa*, is kept in check. Pharmacists may also be called upon to extemporaneously prepare a solution of acetic acid, 2 to 2.5% in rubbing alcohol (70% isopropyl alcohol or ethanol), propylene glycol or anhydrous glycerin. The source of the acetic acid can be glacial acetic acid but usually distilled white vinegar (5% acetic acid) is used. Boric acid, 2 to 5%, dissolved in either ethanol or propylene glycol has also been recommended for use in the ear. This substance, however, may be absorbed from broken skin and be toxic. Thus, its use is usually limited, especially in children with burst ear drums.

Pain in the ear frequently accompanies ear infection or inflamed or swollen ear tissue. Frequently, the pain is far out of proportion to the actual condition. Because the ear canal is so narrow, even a slight inflammation can cause intense pain and discomfort for the patient. Topical analgesic agents generally are employed together with internally administered analgesics, as aspirin, and other agents, as anti-infectives, to combat the cause of the problem.

Topical analgesics for the ear are usually solutions and frequently contain the analgesic antipyrine and the local anesthetic benzocaine in a vehicle of propylene glycol or anhydrous glycerin (e.g., Auralgan Otic Solution, Ayerst). Again, these hygroscopic vehicles reduce the swelling of tissues (and thus some pain) and the growth of microorganisms by drawing moisture from the swollen tissues into the vehicle. These preparations are commonly employed to relieve the symptoms of acute otitis media. Examples of some commercial otic preparations are presented in Table 10–7.

As determined on an individual product basis, some liquid otic preparations require preservation against microbial growth. When preservation is required, such agents as chlorobutanol (0.5%), thimerosal (0.01%), and combinations of the parabens are commonly used. Antioxidants, as sodium bisulfite, and other stabilizers are also included in otic formulations, as required.

Ear preparations are usually packaged in small (5 to 15 mL) glass or plastic containers with a dropper.

Pharmacists must be aware that there may be subtle differences in the formulation of otic drops that could be potentially bothersome to the patient. This is especially so as it relates to inactive or inert ingredient differences between formulations from manufacturers which are considered equivalent on the basis of active in-

Table 10–7. Examples of Some Commercial Otic Preparations

Product Name	Manufacturer	Active Ingredient	Vehicle	Use/Indications
Auralgan Otic Solution	Ayerst	antipyrine, benzo-caine	dehydrated glycerin	Acute otitis media
Cerumenex Drops	Purdue Frederick	triethanolamine polypeptide oleate-condensate	propylene glycol	Cerumenolytic agent to remove impacted ear-wax
Chloromycetin Otic	Parke-Davis	chloramphenicol	propylene glycol	Antiinfective
Cortisporin Otic Solution	Burroughs Wellcome	polymyxin B sulfate, neomycin sulfate, hydrocortisone	glycerin, propylene glycol, water for injection	Superficial bacterial infections
Debrox Drops	Marion	carbamide peroxide	anhydrous glycerin	Ear wax removal
PediOtic Suspension	Burroughs-Wellcome	Polymyxin B sulfate, neomycin sulfate, hydrocortisone	mineral oil, propylene glycol, water for injection	Superficial bacterial infections
Metreton Ophthalmic/Otic Solution	Schering	prednisolone sodium phosphate	aqueous	Antiinflammatory
Otobiotic Otic Solution	Schering	polymyxin B sulfate, hydrocortisone	propylene glycol, glycerin, water	Superficial bacterial infections
VoSol Otic Solution	Wallace	acetic acid	propylene glycol	Antibacterial/antifungal

gredient(s) and strength. For example, several generic suspension combinations of polymyxin B sulfate, neomycin sulfate and hydrocortisone have been shown to be more acidic, i.e., pH 3.0 to 3.5, compared to the standard brandname, i.e., Cortisporin Otic Suspension, which possesses a higher pH range, i.e., 4.8 to 5.1. Consequently, there is a risk that when the generic drops are legally substituted, a burning and stinging sensation can occur when the drops are introduced into the ear of young children, especially those with tympanostomies. Further, it has been demonstrated that with time, the pH of these formulations, including Cortisporin, becomes more acidic, e.g., pH 3.0. Thus, if stored on the shelf for a period of time, it is conceivable that if used again, the acidity could cause irritation to the ear canal. For this reason, Burroughs-Wellcome has specially formulated this antibiotic-hydrocortisone combination into a new suspension product, i.e., PediOtic, which has a minimum pH of 4.1, which is less acidic than the parent Cortisporin Otic Suspension.

Proper Administration and Use of Otic Drops

When ear drops are prescribed, it is important for the pharmacist to first determine how the drops are to be used. For example, ear wax removal drops should be instilled and then removed by the patient with an ear syringe. Alternatively, drops intended to treat external otitis infection are intended to be instilled and left in the ear.

The pharmacist should make sure the patient or parent understands that administration is intended for the ear and the frequency of application. To facilitate patient acceptance the pharmacist should point out that the bottle or container of medication should first be warmed in the hands, and if the product is a suspension, shaken prior to withdrawal into the dropper. The pharmacist should also explain the need to store the medication in a safe place out of the reach of children and away from extremes of temperature.

When instilled into the ear, to allow the drops to run in deeper, the earlobe should be held up and back. For a child, the earlobe should be held down and back. For convenience it is probably easier to have someone other than the patient to administer the drops.

Some ear drops by virtue of their formulation, i.e., low pH, may cause stinging upon administration. Thus, parents and children should be forewarned especially if a child, for example, has tympanostomy tubes in the ear. The patient should also understand the length, in days, to use the product. For antibiotic ear drops it is not necessary to finish the entire bottle because therapy could last 20 to 30 days depending upon the dosage regimen. Therefore, patients should be instructed to continue using the drops for 3 days beyond the time ear symptoms disappear. Products for otitis externa may take up to 7 to 10 days to demonstrate efficacy.

If a child is prone to develop ear infections as a result of swimming or showering, it might be advisable to recommend the parents to consult a physician for prophylactic medication to use during swimming season, and consider using form-fitting ear stopples that fit snugly in the ear when swimming or showering. Further, after the child emerges from the water or shower, the parents can be advised to use a home hair blow dryer on a low setting to dry out the ear. It will dry out the ear quickly without trauma. The dryer should not be placed too close to the child's ear.

Selected Reading

Akers, M.J.: Ocular Bioavailability of Topically Applied Ophthalmic Drugs. *J. Am. Pharm.*, NS23:33–36, 1983.

Engle, J.P.: Contact Lens Solutions. *Drug Topics*, 132:56–66, 1988.

Fraunfelder, F.T., and Hanna, D.: Ophthalmic Drug Delivery Systems. *Surv. Ophthalmol., 18:*292–297, 1974.

Grass, G.M., and Robinson, J.R.: Mechanisms of Corneal Drug Penetration I: In Vivo and In Vitro Kinetics. *J. Pharm. Sci.,* 77:3–14, 1988; *ibid.,* II, Ul-

trastructural Analysis of Potential Pathways for Drug Movement. *J. Pharm. Sci., 787:*15–33, 1988; Grass, G.M., Cooper, E.R., and Robinson, J.R., *ibid.,* III, Modeling of Molecular Transport. *J. Pharm. Sci.,* 77:24–26, 1988.

Hind, H.W., and Zuccaro, V.S.: *Pharmacist's Handbook of Contact Lenses and Contact Lens Solutions.* Sunnyvale, CA, Barnes-Hind, Inc., 1986.

Jurgens, R.W.: Ophthalmic Preservatives. *Drug & Cosmetic Ind., 118:*56, 1976.

MacKeen, D.L.: Contact Lens Solutions. *Am. Pharm.,* NS26:27–31, 1986.

Robinson, J.R., and Goshman, L.M.: Topical Drug Delivery Systems (Eye, Ear, Nose). *Pharmaceutics and Pharmacy Practice.* Edited by G.S. Banker and R.K. Chalmers. Philadelphia, J.B. Lippincott Co., 1982, pp. 312–352.

Notes

1. Akers, M.J.: Ocular Bioavailability of Topically Applied Ophthalmic Drugs. *J. Am. Pharm.,* NS23:33–36, 1983.

2. Adapted from Stoklosa, M.J., and Ansel, H.C.: *Pharmaceutical Calculations.* 7th Ed. Philadelphia, Lea & Febiger, 1980, pp. 196–211.

3. Adapted, in part, from Akers, M.J.: Ocular Bioavailability. *J. Am. Pharm.,* NS23:33–36, 1983.

4. Fraunfelder, F.T., and Hanna, C.: Drug Delivery Systems. *Surv. Ophthalmol., 18:*292–298, 1974.

5. Worthen, D.M., Zimmerman, T.J., and Wind, C.A.: An Evaluation of the Pilocarpine Ocusert. *Invest. Ophthalmol.,* 13:296–299, 1974.

6. Dohlman, C.H., Pavan-Langston, D., and Rose, J.: A New Ocular Insert Device for Continuous Constant-Rate Delivery of Medication to the Eye. *Ann. Ophthalmol.,* 4:823–832, 1972.

7. Hind, H.W., and Zuccaro, V.S.: *Pharmacist's Handbook of Contact Lenses and Contact Lens Solutions.* Sunnyvale, CA, Barnes-Hind, Inc., 1986; MacKeen, D.L.: Contact Lens Solutions. *Am. Pharm.,* NS26:27–31, 1986; Engle, J.P.: Contact Lens Solutions. *Drug Topics,* 132:56–66, 1988.

11 | Suppositories and Other Rectal, Vaginal, and Urethral Preparations

Suppositories

SUPPOSITORIES ARE solid dosage forms intended for insertion into body orifices where they melt, soften, or dissolve and exert localized or systemic effects.[1] Suppositories are commonly employed rectally, vaginally, and occasionally urethrally. They have various shapes and weights (Fig. 11–1). The shape and size of a suppository must be such that it is capable of being easily inserted into the intended body orifice without causing undue distension, and, once inserted, it must be retained for the appropriate period of time. Rectal suppositories are generally inserted with the fingers, but certain vaginal suppositories, particularly the vaginal "inserts" or vaginal tablets prepared by compression, may be inserted high in the vaginal tract with the aid of a special insertion appliance.

Generally, rectal suppositories are usually about 32 mm (1½ inches) in length, are cylindrical, and have one or both ends tapered. Some rectal suppositories are shaped like a bullet, a torpedo, or the little finger. Depending upon the density of the base and the medicaments present in the suppository, the weight of rectal suppositories may vary. The USP states that adult rectal suppositories weigh about 2 g when cocoa butter (theobroma oil) is employed as the suppository base. Rectal suppositories for use by infants and children are about half the weight and size of the adult suppositories and assume a more pencil-like shape. Vaginal suppositories, also called *pessaries,* are usually globular, oviform, or cone-shaped and weigh about 5 g when cocoa butter is the base. Again, depending upon the base and the individual manufacturer's product, the weights of vaginal suppositories may vary widely. Urethral suppositories, also called *bougies,* are slender, pencil-shaped suppositories intended for insertion

Fig. 11–1. *A. Close-up of a commercially prepared and packaged rectal suppository (Courtesy of Wyeth-Ayerst Laboratories); B. Examples of a variety of commercially available rectal and vaginal suppositories wrapped in paper, foil, and plastic.*

into the male or female urethra. Male urethral suppositories may be 3 to 6 mm in diameter and approximately 140 mm in length, although this may vary. When cocoa butter is employed as the base, these suppositories weigh about 4 g. Female urethral suppositories are about half the length and weight of the male urethral suppository, being about 70 mm in length and weighing about 2 g when of cocoa butter.

Local Action

Once inserted, the suppository base melts, softens, or dissolves, distributing the medicaments it carries to the tissues of the region. These medicaments may be intended for retention within the cavity for localized drug effects, or they may be intended to be absorbed for the exertion of systemic effects. Rectal suppositories intended for localized action are most frequently employed to relieve constipation or the pain, irritation, itching, and inflammation associated with hemorrhoids or other anorectal conditions. Antihemorrhoidal suppositories frequently contain a number of components, including local anesthetics, vasoconstrictors, astringents, analgesics, soothing emollients, and protective agents. A popular laxative, glycerin suppositories, promote laxation by the local irritation of the mucous membranes, probably by the dehydrating effect of the glycerin on those membranes. Vaginal suppositories or inserts intended for localized effects are employed mainly as contraceptives, antiseptics in feminine hygiene and as specific agents to combat an invading pathogen. Most commonly, the drugs employed are nonoxynol-9 for contraception, and trichomonacides to combat vaginitis caused by *Trichomonas vaginalis, Candida (Monilia) albicans,* and other microorganisms. Urethral suppositories may be used as antibacterials and as a local anesthetic preparative to urethral examination.

Systemic Action

For systemic effects, the mucous membranes of the rectum and vagina permit the absorption of many soluble drugs. Although the rectum is utilized quite frequently as the site for the systemic absorption of drugs, the vagina is not as frequently used for this purpose.

Among the advantages over oral therapy of the rectal route of administration for achieving systemic effects are these: (a) drugs destroyed or inactivated by the pH or enzymatic activity of the stomach or intestines need not be exposed to these destructive environments; (b) drugs irritating to the stomach may be given without causing such irritation; (c) drugs destroyed by portal circulation may bypass the liver after rectal absorption (drugs enter the portal circulation after oral administration and absorption); (d) the route is convenient for administration of drugs to adult or pediatric patients who may be unable or unwilling to swallow medication; and (e) it is an effective route in the treatment of patients with vomiting episodes.

Drugs administered rectally in the form of suppositories for their systemic effects include

(a) prochlorperazine and chlorpromazine for the relief of nausea and vomiting and as a tranquilizer; (b) oxymorphone HCl for narcotic analgesia; (c) ergotamine tartrate, for the relief of migraine syndrome and (d) indomethacin, a non-steroidal antiinflammatory analgesic and antipyretic.

Some Factors of Drug Absorption from Rectal Suppositories

The dose of a drug administered rectally may be greater than or less than the dose of the same drug given orally, depending upon such factors as the constitution of the patient, the physicochemical nature of the drug and its ability to traverse the physiologic barriers to absorption, and the nature of the suppository vehicle and its capacity to release the drug and make it available for absorption.

The factors affecting the rectal absorption of a drug administered in the form of a suppository may be divided into two main groups: (1) physiologic factors and (2) physicochemical factors of the drug and the base.[2]

Physiologic Factors

The human rectum is approximately 15 to 20 cm in length. When empty of fecal material, the rectum contains only 2 to 3 mL of inert mucous fluid. In the resting state, the rectum is non-motile; there are no villi or microvilli on the rectal mucosa. However, there is abundant vascularization of the submucosal region of the rectum wall with blood and lymphatic vessels.

Among the physiologic factors affecting drug absorption from the rectum are the colonic contents, circulation route, and the pH and lack of buffering capacity of the rectal fluids.

COLONIC CONTENT. When systemic effects are desired from the administration of a medicated suppository, greater absorption may be expected from a rectum that is void than from one that is distended with fecal matter. A drug will obviously have greater opportunity to make contact with the absorbing surface of the rectum and colon in the absence of fecal matter. Therefore, when deemed desirable, an evacuant enema may be administered and allowed to act before the administration of a suppository of a drug to be absorbed. Other conditions such as diarrhea, colonic obstruction due to tumorous growths, and tissue dehydration can all influence the rate and degree of drug absorption from the rectal site.

CIRCULATION ROUTE. Drugs absorbed rectally,

unlike those absorbed after oral administration, bypass the portal circulation during their first pass into the general circulation, thereby enabling drugs otherwise destroyed in the liver to exert systemic effects. The lower hemorrhoidal veins surrounding the colon receive the absorbed drug and initiate its circulation throughout the body, bypassing the liver. Lymphatic circulation also assists in the absorption of rectally administered drugs.

pH AND LACK OF BUFFERING CAPACITY OF THE RECTAL FLUIDS. Because rectal fluids are essentially neutral in pH (7–8) and have no effective buffer capacity, the form in which the drug is administered will not generally be chemically changed by the rectal environment.

The suppository base employed has a marked influence on the release of active constituents incorporated into it. While cocoa butter melts rapidly at body temperature, because of its immiscibility with fluids, it fails to release fat-soluble drugs readily. For systemic drug action, it is preferable to incorporate the ionized rather than the unionized form of a drug in order to maximize bioavailability. Although unionized drugs partition out of water-miscible bases such as glycerinated gelatin and polyethylene glycol more readily, the bases themselves tend to dissolve slowly and thus retard the release of the drug.

Physicochemical Factors of the Drug and Suppository Base

Physicochemical factors include such properties as the relative solubility of the drug in lipid and in water and the particle size of a dispersed drug. Physicochemical factors of the base include its ability to melt, soften, or dissolve at body temperature, its ability to release the drug substance, and its hydrophilic or hydrophobic character.

LIPID-WATER SOLUBILITY. The lipid-water partition coefficient of a drug (discussed in Chapter 3) is an important consideration in the selection of the suppository base and in anticipating drug release from that base. A lipophilic drug that is distributed in a fatty suppository base in low concentration has less of a tendency to escape to the surrounding aqueous fluids than would a hydrophilic substance present in a fatty base to an extent approaching its saturation. Water-soluble bases—for example, polyethylene glycols—which dissolve in the anorectal fluids, release for absorption both water-soluble and oil-

soluble drugs. Naturally, the more drug a base contains, the more drug will be available for potential absorption. However, if the concentration of a drug in the intestinal lumen is above a particular amount, which varies with the drug, the rate of absorption is not changed by a further increase in the concentration of the drug.

PARTICLE SIZE. For drugs present in the suppository in the undissolved state, the size of the particle will influence the amount released and dissolved for absorption. As indicated many times previously, the smaller the particle size, the more readily the dissolution of the particle and the greater the chance for rapid absorption.

NATURE OF THE BASE. As indicated earlier, the base must be capable of melting, softening, or dissolving to release its drug components for absorption. If the base interacts with the drug inhibiting its release, drug absorption will be impaired or even prevented. Also, if the base is irritating to the mucous membranes of the rectum, it may initiate a colonic response and prompt a bowel movement, negating the prospect of a thorough drug release and absorption.

In a study of the bioavailability of aspirin from five brands of commercial suppositories, it was shown that the absorption rates varied widely, and that even with the best product only about 40% of the dose was absorbed when the retention time in the bowel was limited to 2 hours. Thus, the absorption rates were considered exceedingly low, especially when compared to orally administered aspirin, and of dubious dependability.[3]

Because of the possibility of chemical and/or physical interactions between the medicinal agent and the suppository base, which could affect the stability and/or bioavailability of the drug, the absence of any drug interaction between the two agents should be ascertained prior to formulation or use.

Suppository Bases

Analogous to the ointment bases, suppository bases play an important role in the release of the medication they hold and therefore in the availability of the drug for absorption for systemic effects or for localized effects. Of course, one of the first requisites for a suppository base is that it remains solid at room temperature but softens, melts, or dissolves readily at body temperature so that the drug it contains may be made fully available soon after insertion. Certain bases are more efficient in drug release than others. For instance, cocoa butter (theobroma oil) melts quickly at body temperature, but because the resulting oil is immiscible with the body fluids, fat-soluble drugs tend to remain in the oil and have little tendency to enter the aqueous physiologic fluids. For water-soluble drugs incorporated into cocoa butter, the reverse is generally true, and good release results. Fat-soluble drugs seem to be released more readily from bases of glycerinated gelatin or polyethylene glycol, both of which dissolve slowly in body fluids. When irritation or inflammation is to be relieved, as in the treatment of anorectal disorders, cocoa butter appears to be the superior base because of its emollient or soothing, spreading action.

Classification of Suppository Bases

For most purposes, it is convenient to classify suppository bases according to their physical characteristics into two main categories and a third miscellaneous group: (1) fatty or oleaginous bases, (2) water-soluble or water-miscible bases, and (3) miscellaneous bases, generally combinations of lipophilic and hydrophilic substances.

FATTY OR OLEAGINOUS BASES. Fatty bases are perhaps the most frequently employed suppository bases, principally because cocoa butter is a member of this group of substances. Among the other fatty or oleaginous materials used in suppository bases are many hydrogenated fatty acids of vegetable oils such as palm kernel oil and cottonseed oil. Also, fat-based compounds containing compounds of glycerin with the higher molecular weight fatty acids, such as palmitic and stearic acids, may be found in fatty suppository bases. Such compounds as glyceryl monostearate and glyceryl monopalmitate are examples of this type of agent. The suppository bases in many commercial products employ various and varied combinations of these types of materials to achieve a base possessing the desired hardness under conditions of shipment and storage and the desired quality of submitting to the temperature of the body to release their medicaments. In some instances, suppository bases are prepared with the fatty materials emulsified or with an emulsifying agent present to prompt emulsification when the suppository makes contact with the aqueous body fluids. These types of bases are arbitrarily placed in the third, or "miscellaneous," group of suppository bases.

Cocoa Butter, USP, is defined as the fat obtained from the roasted seed of *Theobroma cacao*. At room temperature it is a yellowish, white solid having a faint, agreeable chocolate-like odor. Chemically, it is a triglyceride (combination of glycerin and one or different fatty acids) primarily of oleopalmitostearin and oleodistearin.[4] Because cocoa butter melts between 30° to 36°C, it is an ideal suppository base, melting just below body temperature and yet maintaining its solidity at usual room temperatures. However, because of its triglyceride content, cocoa butter exhibits marked *polymorphism*, or the property of existing in several different crystalline forms. Because of this, when cocoa butter is hastily or carelessly melted at a temperature greatly exceeding the minimum required temperature and then quickly chilled, the result is a metastable crystalline form (α crystals) with a melting point much lower than the original cocoa butter. In fact, the melting point may be so low that the cocoa butter will not solidify at room temperature. However, since the crystalline form represents a metastable condition, there is a slow transition to the more stable β form of crystals having the greater stability and the higher melting point. This transition may require several days. Consequently if suppositories that have been prepared by melting cocoa butter for the base do not harden soon after molding, they will be useless to the patient and a loss of time, materials, and prestige to the pharmacist. Cocoa butter must be slowly and evenly melted, preferably over a water bath of warm water, to avoid the formation of the unstable crystalline form and ensure the retention in the liquid of the more stable β crystals that will constitute nuclei upon which the congealing may occur during chilling of the liquid.

Substances such as phenol and chloral hydrate have a tendency to lower the melting point of cocoa butter when incorporated with it. If the melting point is lowered to such an extent that it is not feasible to prepare a solid suppository using cocoa butter alone as the base, solidifying agents like cetyl esters wax (about 20%) or beeswax (about 4%) may be melted with the cocoa butter to compensate for the softening effect of the added substance. However, the additions of hardening agents must not be so excessive as to prevent the melting of the base after the suppository has been inserted into the body, nor must the waxy material interfere with the therapeutic agent in any way so as to alter the efficacy of the product.

WATER-SOLUBLE AND WATER-MISCIBLE BASES. The main members of this group are bases of glycerinated gelatin and bases of polyethylene glycols.

The USP gives the following directions for the preparation of glycerinated gelatin suppositories:

Weigh the medicinal substance into a tared container, add purified water to make a total of 10 g, and dissolve or mix, depending upon the solubility of the medicinal substance. Add 70 g of glycerin, and mix. To the mixture add 20 g of granular gelatin, mix carefully to avoid incorporating air, and heat on a steam bath until the gelatin is dissolved. Pour the melted mixture into molds, and allow to congeal.

A glycerinated gelatin base is most frequently used in the preparation of vaginal suppositories, where the prolonged localized action of the medicinal agent is usually desired. The glycerinated gelatin base is slower to soften and mix with the physiologic fluids than is cocoa butter and therefore provides a more prolonged release.

Because glycerinated gelatin-based suppositories have a tendency to absorb moisture due to the hygroscopic nature of glycerin, they must be protected from atmospheric moisture in order for them to maintain their shape and consistency. Due also to the hygroscopicity of the glycerin, the suppository may have a dehydrating effect and be irritating to the tissues upon insertion. The water present in the formula for the suppositories minimizes this action; however, if necessary, the suppositories may be moistened with water prior to their insertion to reduce the initial tendency of the base to draw water from the mucous membranes and irritate the tissues.

Urethral suppositories may be prepared from a glycerinated gelatin base of a formula somewhat different from the one indicated above. For urethral suppositories, the gelatin constitutes about 60% of the weight of the formula, the glycerin about 20%, and the medicated aqueous portion about 20%. Urethral suppositories of glycerinated gelatin are much more easily inserted than suppositories with a cocoa butter base, owing to the brittleness of cocoa butter and its rapid softening at body temperature.

Polyethylene glycols are polymers of ethylene oxide and water, prepared to various chain lengths, molecular weights, and physical states. They are available in a number of molecular weight ranges, the more commonly used being polyethylene glycol 200, 400, 600, 1000, 1500, 1540, 3350, 4000, 6000, and 8000. The numerical designations refer to the average molecular weights of each of the polymers. Polyethylene glycols having average molecular weights of 200, 400, and 600 are clear, colorless liquids. Those having molecular weights of greater than 1000 are wax-like, white solids with the hardness increasing with an increase in the molecular weight. Various combinations of these polyethylene glycols may be combined by fusion, using two or more of the various types to achieve a suppository base of the desired consistency and characteristics.

Pharmacists have been called upon in recent years to prepare progesterone vaginal suppositories extemporaneously. These suppositories, used in premenstrual syndrome, are commonly prepared by molding using a polyethylene glycol base. Formulas for these suppositories are presented later in this chapter.

Polyethylene glycol suppositories do not melt at body temperature but rather dissolve slowly in the body's fluids. Therefore, the base need not be formulated to melt at body temperature. Thus it is possible, and in fact routine, to prepare suppositories from polyethylene glycol mixtures having melting points considerably higher than that of body temperature. Not only does this property permit a slower release of the medication from the base once the suppository has been inserted, but it also permits the convenient storage of these suppositories without need of refrigeration and without danger of their softening excessively in warm weather. Their solid nature also permits them to be inserted slowly without the fear that they will melt in the fingertips (as cocoa butter suppositories sometimes do). Because they do not melt at body temperature, but mix with mucous secretions upon their dissolution, polyethylene glycol-based suppositories do not "leak" from the orifice as do many cocoa butter-based suppositories. If the polyethylene glycol suppositories do not contain at least 20% of water to avoid the irritation of the mucous membranes after insertion, they should be dipped in water just prior to use. This procedure prevents moisture being drawn from the tissues after insertion and the "stinging" sensation.

MISCELLANEOUS BASES. In the miscellaneous group of bases are included those which are mixtures of the oleaginous and water-soluble or water-miscible materials. These materials may be chemical or physical mixtures. Some are preformed emulsions, generally of the w/o type, or they may be capable of dispersing in aqueous fluids. One of these substances is polyoxyl 40 stearate, a surface-active agent that is employed in a number of commercial suppository bases. Polyoxyl 40 stearate is a mixture of the monostearate and distearate esters of mixed polyoxyethylene diols and the free glycols, the average polymer length being equivalent to about 40 oxyethylene units. The substance is a waxy, white to light tan solid that is water-soluble. Its melting point is generally between 39°C and 45°C. Other surface active agents useful in the preparation of suppository bases also fall into this broad grouping. Mixtures of many fatty bases (including cocoa butter) with emulsifying agents capable of forming w/o emulsions have been prepared. These bases have the ability to hold water or aqueous solutions and are sometimes referred to as "hydrophilic" suppository bases.

Preparation of Suppositories

Suppositories are prepared by three methods: (1) *molding* from a melt, (2) *compression,* and (3) *hand rolling* and *shaping.* The method most frequently employed in the preparation of suppositories both on a small scale and on an industrial scale is molding.

Preparation by Molding

Basically, the steps in molding include (a) the melting of the base, (b) incorporating of any required medicaments, (c) pouring the melt into molds, (d) allowing the melt to cool and congeal into suppositories, and (e) removing the formed suppositories from the mold. Suppositories of cocoa butter, glycerinated gelatin, polyethylene glycol, and most other suppository bases are suitable for preparation by molding.

SUPPOSITORY MOLDS. Suppository molds are commercially available with the capability of producing individual or large numbers of suppositories of various shapes and sizes. Individual plastic suppository molds may be obtained to form a single suppository. Other molds, as

Fig. 11–2. *Partially opened suppository mold capable of producing 50 torpedo-shaped suppositories in a single molding. (Courtesy of Chemical and Pharmaceutical Industry Co., Inc.)*

those most commonly found in the community pharmacy, are capable of producing 6, 12, or more suppositories in a single operation (Fig. 11–2). Industrial molds produce hundreds of suppositories from a single batch (Figs. 11–3 and 11–4).

Molds in common use today are made from stainless steel, aluminum, brass, or plastic. The molds, which separate into sections, generally longitudinally, are opened for cleaning before and after the preparation of a batch of suppositories, closed when the melt is poured, and opened again to remove the cold, molded suppositories. Care must be exercised in cleaning the molds, as any scratches on the molding surfaces will take away from the desired smoothness of the resulting suppositories. Plastic molds are especially prone to scratching.

Although satisfactory molds are commercially available for the preparation of suitable rectal, vaginal, and urethral suppositories, if necessary in the extemporaneous preparation of suppositories, temporary molds may be successfully formed by pressing heavy aluminum foil about an object having the shape of the desired suppository, then carefully removing the object, and filling the shaped foil with the melt. For instance, glass stirring rods may be used to form molds for urethral suppositories, cylindrical pencils or pens may be used to form molds for rectal suppositories, and any cone-shaped object may be used to form vaginal suppositories.

LUBRICATION OF THE MOLD. Depending upon the formulation, suppository molds may require lubrication before the melt is poured to facilitate the clean and easy removal of the

Fig. 11–3. *Large, heated tanks for the preparation of the melt in the commercial production of suppositories by molding. (Courtesy of Wyeth-Ayerst Laboratories.)*

molded suppositories. Lubrication is seldom necessary when the suppository base is cocoa butter or polyethylene glycol, as these materials contract sufficiently on cooling within the mold to separate from the inner surfaces and allow their easy removal. Lubrication is usually necessary when glycerinated gelatin suppositories are prepared. A thin coating of mineral oil applied with the finger to the molding surfaces usually suffices to provide the necessary lubrication. It should be stressed, however, that any materials which might cause irritation to the mucous membranes should not be employed as a mold lubricant.

CALIBRATION OF THE MOLD. Each individual mold is capable of holding a specific volume of material in each of its openings. If the material is cocoa butter, the weight of the resulting suppositories will differ from the weight of suppositories prepared in the same mold with a mixture of polyethylene glycols as the base because of the difference in the densities of the materials. Similarly, any added medicinal agent would further alter the densities of the bases, and the weights of the resulting suppositories

would be different from those prepared with base material alone.

It is important that the pharmacist calibrate each of his suppository molds for the suppository bases that he generally employs (usually cocoa butter and a polyethylene glycol base) in order that he may prepare medicated suppositories each having the proper quantity of medicaments.

The first step in the calibration of a mold is to prepare molded suppositories from base material alone. After removal from the mold, the suppositories are weighed, and the total weight and the average weight of each suppository are recorded (for the particular base used). To determine the volume of the mold, the suppositories are then carefully melted in a calibrated beaker, and the volume of the melt is determined for the total number as well as for the average of one suppository.

DETERMINATION OF THE AMOUNT OF BASE REQUIRED. In his prescriptions for medicated suppositories to be prepared extemporaneously by the pharmacist, the prescribing physician generally indicates the amount of a medicinal sub-

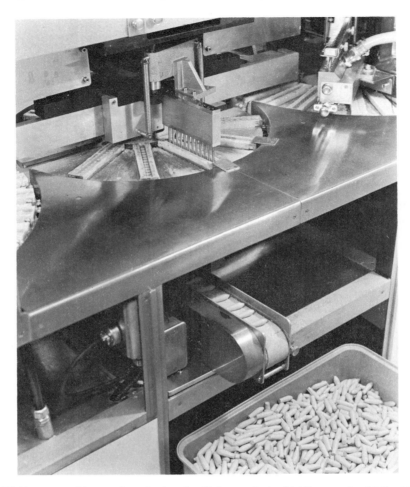

Fig. 11–4. *Highly automated large-scale production of molded suppositories. Molding operation (at the right) is followed by the removal of the suppositories from the molds, dropping them onto a conveyor belt and into a collection basket. (Courtesy of Wyeth-Ayerst Laboratories.)*

stance that he desires in each suppository, but he leaves the amount of base to the discretion of the pharmacist. Generally, in filling such prescriptions, the pharmacist calculates the amounts of materials needed for the preparation of one or two more suppositories than the number prescribed to compensate for the inevitable loss of some material and to ensure having enough material to prepare the last required suppository.

In determining the amount of base to be incorporated with the medicaments, the pharmacist must be certain that the required amount of drug is provided in each suppository. Because the volume of the mold is known (from the determined volume of the melted suppos-

itories formed from the base), the volume of the drug substances subtracted from the total volume of the mold will give the volume of base required. In instances in which the added amounts of medicaments are slight, they may be considered to be negligible, and no deduction from the total volume of base may be deemed necessary. However, if considerable quantities of substances are to be incorporated into the suppository, the volumes of these materials are important and should be used to calculate the amount of base actually required to completely fill the mold. The total volumes of these materials are subtracted from the volume of the mold, and the appropriate amount of base is added. Since the suppository bases are solids at room temperature, the volume of base determined may be converted to weight from the density of the material. For example, if 12 mL of cocoa butter are required to fill a suppository mold and if the medicaments in the formula have a collective volume of 2.8 mL, then 9.2 mL of the cocoa butter will be required. By multiplying 9.2 mL times the density of cocoa butter, 0.86 g/mL, it may be calculated that 7.9 g of cocoa butter will be required. After adjusting for the preparation of an extra suppository or two, the calculated amount is weighed.

Another method for the determination of the amount of base in the preparation of medicated suppositories requires the following steps: (a) weigh the active ingredient for the preparation of a single suppository; (b) dissolve it or mix it (depending upon its solubility in the base) with a portion of melted base insufficient to fill one cavity of the mold, and add the mixture to a cavity; (c) add additional melted base to the cavity to fill it completely; (d) allow the suppository to congeal and harden; and (e) remove the suppository from the mold and weigh it. The weight of the active ingredients present, subtracted from the weight of the suppository, yields the weight of the amount of base used. This amount of base multiplied by the number of suppositories to be prepared in the mold is the total amount of base required.

A third method involves the placing of all of the required medicaments for the preparation of the total number of suppositories (including one extra) in a calibrated beaker. To this is added a portion of the melted base and the drug substances incorporated. Then sufficient additional melted base is added until the volume of mixture is reached that is required for the preparation of the necessary suppositories, based on the original calibration of the volume of the mold.

PREPARING AND POURING THE MELT. Using the least possible heat, the weighed suppository base material is melted, generally over a water bath, since a great deal of heat is not usually required. A porcelain casserole, which is a dish having a pouring lip and a handle, is perhaps the best utensil to use, since it later permits the convenient pouring of the melt into the cavities of the mold. Medicinal substances are usually incorporated into a portion of the melted base by mixing on a glass or porcelain tile with a spatula. After incorporation, this material is added with stirring to the remaining base which

has been allowed to cool almost to its congealing point. Any volatile materials or heat labile substances should be incorporated at this point with thorough stirring.

It is generally best to chill the mold in the refrigerator before pouring the melt. Then, the melt is added carefully and continuously in the filling of each cavity in the mold. If any undissolved materials in the mixture art of greater density than the base so that they have a tendency to settle, constant stirring, even during pouring, is required, else the last filled cavity will contain a disproportionate share of the undissolved materials. The solid materials remain suspended if the pouring is performed just above the congealing point and not when the base is too fluid. The chilled mold encourages prompt congealing and discourages any settling of the materials within the mold's cavities. If the melt is not near the congealing point when poured, the solids may settle within each cavity of the mold to reside at the tips of the suppositories, with the result that the suppositories may be broken when removed from the mold. In filling each suppository cavity, the pouring must be continuous to prevent *layering*, which may lead to a product easily broken on handling. To ensure a completely filled mold upon congealing, the melt is poured excessively over each opening, actually rising above the level of the mold. The excessive material may actually form a continuous ribbon along the top of the mold above the cavities. This use of extra suppository material prevents the formation of recessed dips in the ends of the suppositories and justifies the preparation of extra suppository melt. When solidified, the excess material is evenly scraped off of the top of the mold with a spatula. The mold is usually placed in the freezer section of the refrigerator to hasten the hardening of the suppositories.

When the suppositories are hard, the mold is removed from the freezer, and slight pressure is exerted with the thumb on the ends of each suppository to loosen it in the mold. Then the sections of the mold are separated, and the suppositories are dislodged with the pressure being exerted principally on their ends and only if needed on the tips. Generally, little, if any, pressure is required, and the suppositories simply fall out of the mold when it is opened.

Preparation by Compression

Suppositories may be prepared by forcing the mixed mass of the suppository base and the medicaments into special molds using suppository-making machines. In preparation for compression into the molds, the suppository base and the other formulative ingredients are combined by thorough mixing, the friction of the process causing the base to soften into a paste-like consistency. On a small scale, mortar and pestle may be used. If the mortar is heated in warm water before use and then dried, the softening of the base and the mixing process is greatly facilitated. On a large scale, a similar process may be used, employing mechanically operated kneading mixers and a warmed mixing vessel.

The process of compression is especially suited for the making of suppositories containing medicinal substances that are heat labile and for suppositories containing a great deal of substances insoluble in the base. In contrast to the molding method, there is no likelihood of insoluble matter settling during the preparation of suppositories by compression. The disadvantage to the process is that the special suppository machine is required and there is some limitation as to shapes of suppositories that can be made from the available molds.

In preparing suppositories with the compression machine, the suppository mass is placed into a cylinder which is then closed, and pressure is applied from one end, mechanically, or by turning a wheel, and the mass is forced out of the other end into the suppository mold or die. When the die is filled with the mass, a movable end plate at the back of the die is removed and when additional pressure is applied to the mass in the cylinder, the formed suppositories are ejected. The end plate is returned, and the process is repeated until all of the suppository mass has been used. Various sizes and shapes of dies are available. It is possible to prepare suppositories of uniform circumference by extrusion through a perforated plate and by cutting the extruded mass to the desired length.

Preparation by Hand Rolling and Shaping

With the ready availability of suppository molds of accommodating shapes and sizes, there is little requirement for today's pharmacist to shape suppositories by hand. Hand rolling and shaping is a historic part of the art of the pharmacist; a description of the method may be found in the third edition of this text.

Rectal Suppositories

Examples of rectal suppositories are presented in Table 11–1. As noted earlier, drugs as aspirin given for pain, ergotamine tartrate for treating migraine headaches, theophylline as a smooth muscle relaxant in treating asthma, and chlorpromazine and prochlorperazine, which act as antiemetics and tranquilizers, are intended to be absorbed into the general circulation to provide systemic drug effects. The rectal route of administration is especially useful in instances in which the patient is unwilling or unable to take medication by mouth.

Suppositories are also intended to provide local action within the perianal area. Local anesthetic suppositories are commonly employed to relieve *pruritus ani* of various causes, and the pain sometimes associated with hemorrhoids. Many of the commercial hemorrhoidal suppositories contain a number of medicinal agents including astringents, protectives, anesthetics, lubricants, and others, intended to relieve the discomfort of the condition. Cathartic suppositories are contact-type agents which act directly on the colonic mucosa to produce normal peristalsis. Because the contact action is restricted to the colon, the motility of the small intestine is not appreciably affected. Cathartic suppositories are more rapid-acting than orally administered medication. Suppositories of bisacodyl are usually effective in 15 minutes to an hour, and glycerin suppositories usually within a few minutes following insertion.

Some commercially prepared suppositories are available for both adult and pediatric use. The difference is in the shape and drug content. Pediatric suppositories are more narrow and pencil-shaped than the typical bullet-shaped adult suppository. Glycerin suppositories are commonly available in each type.

The formula given in the USP for Glycerin Suppositories is as follows:

Glycerin.........................	91 g
Sodium Stearate.................	9 g
Purified Water	5 g
To make about................	100 g

In the preparation of this suppository, the glycerin is heated in a suitable container to about 120° F. Then the sodium stearate is dissolved with stirring in the hot glycerin, the purified water added, and the mixture immediately poured into the suppository mold. It is recommended that if the mold is of metal, that it

Table 11–1. Examples of Rectal Suppositories

Suppository	Corresponding Commercial Product	Active Constituent per Suppository	Type of Effect	Category and Comments
Bisacodyl Suppositories	Dulcolax Suppositories (Boehringer Ingelheim)	10 mg	Local	Cathartic. See text for additional discussion. Base: hydrogenated vegetable oil.
Chlorpromazine Suppositories	Thorazine Suppositories (Smith Kline & French)	25 and 100 mg	Systemic	Anti-emetic; tranquilizer. Base: glycerin, glyceryl monopalmitate and monostearate, and hydrogenated fatty acids of coconut and palm kernel oils.
Ergotamine Tartrate and Caffeine Suppositories	Cafergot Suppositories (Sandoz)	2 mg ergotamine tartrate and 100 mg caffeine	Systemic	Antiadrenergic; cental. Base: cocoa butter.
Indomethacin Suppositories	Indocin Suppositories (Merck Sharp & Dohme)	50 mg	Systemic	Nonsteroidal antiinflammatory analgesic indicated in various forms of arthritis. The rate of rectal absorption from suppositories is more rapid than from orally administered capsules. Base: polyethylene glycols 3350 and 8000.
Prochlorperazine Suppositories	Compazine Suppositories (Smith Kline & French)	2.5, 5, and 25 mg	Systemic	Anti-emetic. Base: glycerin, glyceryl monopalmitate and monostearate, and hydrogenated fatty acids of coconut and palm kernel oils.
Promethazine HCl Suppositories	Phenergan Rectal Suppositories (Wyeth-Ayerst)	12.5, 25, and 50 mg	Systemic	Antihistaminic, antiemetic and sedative actions: used to manage conditions of allergic origin; for preoperative or postoperative sedation or nausea and vomiting; and for motion sickness. Base: cocoa butter and white wax.

also be heated prior to the addition of the glycerin mixture. After cooling to solidification, the suppositories are removed. From the above formula, about fifty adult suppositories may be prepared.

Glycerin, a hygroscopic material, contributes to the laxative effect of the suppository by drawing water from the intestine and also from its irritant action on the mucous lining. The sodium stearate, a soap, is the solidifying agent in the suppository and may also contribute to the laxative action. Because of the hygroscopic nature of glycerin, the suppositories attract moisture and should be maintained in tight containers, preferably at temperatures below 25°F.

The pharmacist should relate several helpful items of information about the proper use of suppositories. If they must be stored in the refrigerator, suppositories should be allowed to warm to room temperature before insertion. The patient should be advised to rub cocoa butter suppositories gently with the fingers to melt the surface to provide lubrication for insertion. Glycerinated gelatin or polyethylene glycol suppositories should be moistened with water to enhance lubrication. If the polyetheylene glycol suppository formulation does not contain at least 20% water, dipping it into water just prior to insertion prevents moisture from being drawn from rectal tissues after insertion and decreases subsequent irritation. The shape of the suppository determines how it will be inserted. Bullet-shaped rectal suppositories should be inserted point-end first. When the patient is instructed to use one-half suppository, the patient should be told to cut the suppository in half lengthwise with a clean razor blade. Most suppositories are dispensed in paper, foil, or plastic wrappings, and the patient must be instructed to remove the wrapping thoroughly before insertion.

Vaginal Suppositories

Examples of vaginal suppository and tablets are presented in Table 11–2. These preparations are employed principally to combat infections occurring in the female genitourinary area, to restore the vaginal mucosa to its normal state, and for contraception. In combating vaginal infections, the usual pathogenic organisms involved are *Trichomonas vaginalis, Candida (Monilia) albicans* or other species, and *Hemophilus vaginalis*. Among the anti-infective agents found in commercial vaginal preparations are: nystatin, clotrimazole and miconazole (antifungals) and triple sulfas, sulfanilamide and oxytetra-

cycline (antibacterials). Nonoxynol-9, a spermicide, is employed for vaginal contraception. Estrogenic substances as dienestrol are found in vaginal preparations to restore the vaginal mucosa to its normal state.

In the preparation of vaginal suppositories, the most commonly used base consists of combinations of the various molecular weight polyethylene glycols. To this base is frequently added surfactants and preservative agents, commonly the parabens. Many of the vaginal suppositories and other types of vaginal dosage forms are buffered to an acid pH, usually around pH 4.5 which resembles that of the normal vagina. This acidity discourages pathogenic organisms and at the same time provides a favorable environment for eventual recolonization by the acid-producing bacilli normally found in the vagina.

The polyethylene glycol-based vaginal suppositories are water-miscible and are generally sufficiently firm for the patient to handle and insert without great difficulty. However, to make the task even easier, many manufacturers provide plastic insertion devices with their products which are used to hold the suppository or vaginal tablet during insertion for proper placement within the vagina (Fig. 11–5).

As noted earlier, pharmacists frequently are called upon to prepare progesterone vaginal suppositories. Formulas for the extemporaneous preparation of these suppositories have been presented in the professional literature.[5,6]

Table 11–2. Examples of Vaginal Suppositories and Tablets

Product/Manufacturer	Active Constituents	Category and Comments
AVC Suppositories (Merrell Dow)	sulfanilamide	For the treatment of *Candida albicans* infections.
Betadine Medicated Vaginal Suppositories (Purdue Federick)	povidone-iodine	For relief of vaginitis due to *Candida albicans, Trichomonas,* and *Gardnerella vaginalis*
Gyne-Lotrimin Vaginal Tablets (Schering)	clotrimazole	Treatment of vulvovaginal candidiasis.
Monistat 7 Suppositories (Ortho)	miconazole	Antifungal for treatment of localized vulvovaginal candidiasis (moniliasis).
Mycostatin Vaginal Tablets (Squibb)	nystatin	Local treatment of vulvovaginal candidiasis.
Semicid Vaginal Contraceptive Inserts (Whitehall)	nonoxynol-9	Non-systemic reversible method of birth control
Sultrin Vaginal Tablets (Ortho)	sulfathiazole, sulfacetamide, sulfabenzamide and urea	Treatment of *Haemophilus vaginalis* vaginitis.
Vagisec Plus Suppositories (Schmid)	aminoacridine, polyoxyethylene nonyl phenol, and docusate sodium	Treatment of vaginitis caused by *T. vaginalis* and mixed infections.

Fig. 11–5. *Dosage forms used intravaginally, including suppositories (top and middle), vaginal tablets packaged in foil (bottom), vaginal cream, and corresponding insert devices.*

Micronized progesterone powder is generally utilized in a base of polyethylene glycol, although in some formulas cocoa butter is employed. The suppositories are prepared by mixing the progesterone to a melt of the base and molding. Some representative formulas are:

Progesterone, micronized powder	q.s.
Polyethylene Glycol 400	60%
Polyethylene Glycol 8000	40%
Progesterone, micronized powder	q.s.
Polyethylene Glycol 1000	75%
Polyethylene Glycol 3350	25%
Progesterone, micronized powder	q.s.
Cocoa Butter	100%

The amount of progesterone prescribed per suppository ranges from 25 to 600 mg. The suppositories are used in treating luteal phase defect, premenstrual syndrome, luteal phase spotting, and in the preparation of the endometrium for implantation.[6]

The pharmacist should share several helpful hints with a woman who is about to use a vaginal suppository product. She should first be told to read the patient instructions included with the product. Throughout the entire course of therapy, the suppository should be inserted high into the vagina with the provided applicator. The patient should not discontinue therapy when the symptoms abate. Further, she should notify her physician if burning, irritation, or any signs of an allergic reaction occur. When vaginal inserts (i.e., compressed tablets) are prescribed, the pharmacist should instruct the woman to dip the tablet into water quickly

before insertion. Because these dosage forms are usually administered at bedtime and can be somewhat messy if formulated into an oleaginous base, the pharmacist should suggest that the woman wear a sanitary napkin to protect her nightwear and bed linens.

Packaging and Storage

Glycerin suppositories and glycerinated gelatin suppositories are generally packaged in tightly closed glass containers to prevent a moisture change in the content of the suppositories. Suppositories prepared from a cocoa butter base are usually individually wrapped or otherwise separated in compartmentalized boxes to prevent contact and adhesion. Suppositories containing light-sensitive drugs are generally individually wrapped in an opaque material such as a metallic foil. In fact, most commercially available suppositories are individually wrapped in either foil or a plastic material. Some are packaged in a continuous strip with suppositories being separated by tearing along perforations placed between suppositories. Suppositories are also commonly packaged in slide boxes or in plastic boxes.

Since suppositories are adversely affected by heat, it is necessary to maintain them in a cool place. Suppositories having cocoa butter as the base must be stored below 30°F, preferably in a refrigerator. Glycerinated gelatin suppositories are best stored at temperatures below 35°F. Suppositories made from a base of polyethylene glycol may be stored at usual room temperatures without the requirement of refrigeration.

Suppositories stored in environments of high humidity may absorb moisture and tend to become spongy, whereas suppositories stored in places of extreme dryness may lose moisture and become brittle.

Other Dosage Forms Used Rectally, Vaginally, and Urethrally

Tablets and Capsules

Vaginal tablets are more widely used nowadays than are vaginal suppositories. The tablets are easier to manufacture, more stable, and less messy to handle in use. Vaginal tablets, frequently referred to as *vaginal inserts*, are usually ovoid in shape and are accompanied in their packaging with a plastic inserter, a device for easy placement of the tablet within the vagina. Vaginal tablets contain the same types of anti-infective and hormonal substances as the vaginal suppositories. They are prepared by tablet compression, and are commonly formulated to contain lactose as the base or filler, a disintegrating agent, as starch, a dispersing agent, as polyvinylpyrrolidine, and a tablet lubricant, as magnesium stearate. The tablets are intended to disintegrate within the vagina releasing their medication. Examples of vaginal tablets are presented in Table 11–2.

Some vaginal inserts are capsules of gelatin containing medication to be released intravaginally. Capsules may also be used rectally, especially in pediatrics to administer medication to children unwilling or unable to tolerate the drug orally. Their insertion into the rectum is facilitated by first lightly wetting the capsule with water. Drugs are absorbed from the rectum, but frequently at unpredictable rates and in varying amounts as has been previously noted in this chapter. Drugs which do not dissolve rapidly and which are irritating to mucous membranes should not be placed in direct contact with such membranes.

Ointments, Creams, and Aerosol Foams

Rectal and vaginal ointments and vaginal creams are in common use. Rectal ointments are used primarily to allay local conditions as pruritus ani and to relieve the pain and discomfort associated with hemorrhoids. The drugs present are generally the same as previously discussed for rectal suppositories, including local anesthetics, analgesics, protectives, and anti-inflammatory agents. To facilitate the insertion of ointment into the rectum, each rectal ointment tube is accompanied with a special rectal insertion and delivery tip. This tip replaces the ordinary ointment cap prior to use. After placement of the rectal tip on the ointment tube, the tip is slowly and carefully inserted into the anus. The ointment tube is depressed to release the medication through the rectal tip and into the anal canal. After use, the tip should be removed from the ointment tube and replaced with the original cap. The rectal tip should be thoroughly cleaned following each use. During the product selection process, either by the physician or the patient with assistance from the pharmacist, consideration should be given to the product formulation base. Water-soluble bases are easier and less messy to clean from applicator tips than oleaginous bases.

Patients should be advised by the pharmacist not to interchange rectal tips from one product to another. Unfortunately, this is the means that some patients use to rectally insert, for example, over-the-counter hydrocortisone ointments that are really intended only for external use.

Vaginal ointments and creams are typically available containing anti-infective agents, estrogenic hormonal substances, and contraceptive agents. The anti-infective and hormonal substances used are the same as have previously been discussed for vaginal suppositories. Contraceptive creams and foams contain spermicidal agents such as nonoxynol 9 and octoxynol and are used alone or in combination with a cervical diaphragm to prevent conception. When used with a diaphragm, the cream is placed on the diaphragm surface in contact with the cervix and around the edges of the diaphragm. When used alone, the cream is first squeezed into the special inserter-applicator tube provided. This applicator is then inserted well into the vagina, the plunger of the applicator depressed and the cream deposited. The contraceptive creams are utilized just prior to intercourse.

Aerosol foams are commercially available containing estrogenic substances and contraceptive agents. The foams are used intravaginally in the same manner as that employed for creams. The aerosol package contains an inserter device which is filled with foam and the contents placed in the vagina through activation of the plunger. The foams are generally oil-in-water emulsions, resembling light creams. They are water-miscible and non-greasy.

There are some commercial preparations of rectal foams available which utilize rectal inserters for the presentation of the foam to the anal canal. One such product, proctoFoam (Reed & Carnrick), contains pramoxine hydrochloride and is used in relieving inflammatory anorectal disorders (Fig. 11–6).

Jellies and Gels

Jellies are a class of gels in which the structural coherent matrix contains a high proportion of liquid, usually water. Pharmaceutical jellies are usually formed by adding a thickening agent as tragacanth or carboxymethyl cellulose to an aqueous solution of a drug substance. The resultant product is usually clear and of a uniform semisolid consistency.

There are a number of commercially available contraceptive jellies and gels containing the same types of spermicidal agents and used in-

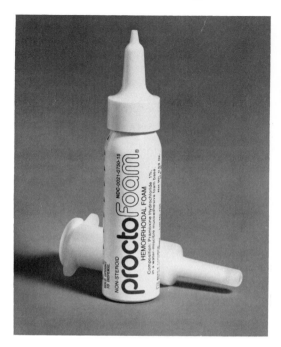

Fig. 11–6. *A product-example of a foam for anal and perianal use. To fill the applicator, the foam container is shaken vigorously, held upright, and the applicator tip placed on the container opening. With the plunger of the applicator drawn out all the way, pressure is exerted on the container cap and foam fills the applicator tube. (Courtesy of Reed & Carnrick)*

Fig. 11–7. *The Today ™ Vaginal Contraceptive Sponge (Courtesy of Whitehall Laboratories).*

travaginally in the same manner as previously discussed for contraceptive creams. Also, a number of antiseptic, anesthetic, and nonmedicated lubricant jellies are available, primarily for use by physicians in their rectal, urethral, and vaginal examination procedures.

Jellies are subject to bacterial contamination and growth and thus most are preserved with antimicrobial preservatives. The tubes of jellies should be tightly closed when not in use, as they have a tendency to lose water to the air and dry out.

Contraceptive Sponge

A vaginal contraceptive sponge (Today, Whitehall) passed the FDA new drug review process for safety and efficacy in 1983 and was placed on the market as an over-the-counter drug. The product, shown in Figure 11–7, consists of a resilient, hydrophilic, polyurethane foam sponge, impregnated during manufacture with nonoxynol-9, a spermicidal agent. Contraception occurs by the action of the spermicidal

agent, sperm absorption on the sponge, and by physical blockage by the sponge of the cervix.[7]

The contraceptive sponge is manufactured in a slightly concave, rounded form designed to fit snugly in the upper vagina (see Fig. 11–8). During manufacture, approximately 1 g of the spermicide nonoxynol-9 is incorporated into its structure. The spermicide is activated when the sponge is moistened with water and inserted into the vagina. The sponge is designed to provide contraceptive protection for a 24-hour period. The sponge is intended to remain in place for at least 6 hours following intercourse. A ribbon loop attached to the interior scrim facilitates removal.

Intrauterine Progesterone Drug Delivery System

The Progestasert Intrauterine Progesterone Contraceptive System (Alza Corporation)

Fig. 11–8. *Placement of the Today ™ Vaginal Contraceptive Sponge (Courtesy of Whitehall Laboratories).*

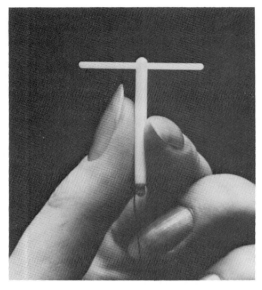

Fig. 11–9. *Progestasert Intrauterine Progesterone Contraceptive System enables the prevention of pregnancy in women for a year or more after each insertion. This small, flexible unit releases the natural hormone progesterone directly into the uterus. (Courtesy of Alza Corporation.)*

DRUG RESERVOIR

RATE CONTROLLING MEMBRANE

MONOFILAMENT THREAD

Fig. 11–10. *Schematic of the Progestasert intrauterine drug delivery system. (Courtesy of Alza Corporation.)*

shown in Figures 11–9 and 11–10 slowly releases progesterone for a period of 1 year after insertion. The continuous release of progesterone into the uterine cavity provides a local rather than a systemic action. Two hypotheses for the contraceptive action have been offered: progesterone-induced inhibition of sperm capacity or survival; and, alteration of the uterine milieu so as to prevent nidation.[8] The intrauterine device contains 38 mg of progesterone, a much smaller amount than would otherwise be taken by other routes over a year period for the same purpose. The intrauterine device is replaced annually for the maintenance of contraception.

Powders

Powders are used to prepare solutions for vaginal *douche*, that is, for the irrigative cleansing of the vagina. The powders themselves may be prepared and packaged in bulk or as unit packages. A unit package is designed to contain the appropriate amount of powder to prepare the specified volume of douche solution. The bulk powders are utilized by the teaspoonful or tablespoonful amounts in the preparation of the desired solution. The user simply adds the prescribed amount of powder to the appropriate

volume of warm water and stirs until dissolved. Among the components of douche powders are the following:

a. Boric acid or sodium borate.
b. Astringents, as potassium alum, ammonium alum, zinc sulfate.
c. Antimicrobials, as oxyquinoline sulfate, povidone-iodine.
d. Quaternary ammonium compounds, as benzethonium chloride.
e. Detergents, as sodium lauryl sulfate.
f. Oxidizing agents, as sodium perborate.
g. Salts, as sodium citrate, sodium chloride.
h. Aromatics, as menthol, thymol, eucalyptol, methyl salicylate, phenol.

Douche powders are generally employed for their hygienic effects. A few douche powders, containing specific therapeutic anti-infective agents as those mentioned previously in the discussion of vaginal suppositories, are employed against Monilial and Trichomonal infections.

Solutions

Vaginal Douches—Solutions may be prepared from powders as indicated above or from liquid solutions or liquid concentrates. In using liquid concentrates, the patient is instructed to add the prescribed amount of concentrate (usually a teaspoonful or bottle-capful) with a certain amount of warm water (frequently a quart). The resultant solution then contains the appropriate amount of chemical agents in proper strength.

Fig. 11–11. *Products for vaginal use, including solution concentrates, powder, and aerosol foam with insert device.*

The agents present are similar to the ones described above for douche powders. Examples are shown in Figure 11–11.

RETENTION ENEMAS. A number of solutions are administered rectally for the local effects of the medication (e.g., hydrocortisone) or for systemic absorption (e.g., aminophylline). In the case of aminophylline, the rectal route of administration minimizes the undesirable gastrointestinal reactions associated with oral therapy. Clinically effective blood levels of the agents are usually obtained within 30 minutes following rectal instillation.

Corticosteroids are administered as retention enemas or continuous drip as adjunctive treatment of some patients with ulcerative colitis.

EVACUATION ENEMAS. Rectal enemas are employed to cleanse the bowel. Commercially, many enemas are available in disposable plastic squeeze bottles containing a premeasured amount of enema solution. The agents present are solutions of sodium phosphate and sodium biphosphate, glycerin and docusate potassium, and light mineral oil.

Patient instruction from a pharmacist is advantageous to ensure that the patient correctly uses these products. The patient should be advised to gently insert the rectal tip of the product with steady pressure and be told that it is not absolutely necessary to squeeze all of the contents out of the disposable plastic bottle. Lastly, the patient should be told that the product will most probably work within 5 to 10 minutes.

Suspensions

Barium Sulfate for Suspension, USP, previously discussed in Chapter 7, may be employed

orally or rectally for the diagnostic visualization of the gastrointestinal tract. Meselamine (i.e., 5-aminosalicylic acid) suspension was introduced onto the market in 1988 as Rowasa (Reid-Rowell) for treatment of Crohn's disease, distal ulcerative colitis, proctosigmoiditis, and proctitis. Before its introduction, an extemporaneous formulation of this suspension was necessary.[9]

Selected Reading

Anschel, J., and Lieberman, H.A.: Suppositories: Part I. Bases. *Drug & Cosmetic Ind.*, 97:341, 1965; Part II. Formulation Problems. *ibid.*, 97:507, 1965.
Gibaldi, M., and Grundhofer, B.: Bioavailability of Aspirin from Commercial Suppositories. *J. Pharm. Sci.*, 64:1064–1066, 1975.
Lowenthal, W., and Borzelleca, J.F.: Drug Absorption from the Rectum. I. Suppository Bases: A Preliminary Report. *J. Pharm. Sci.*, 54:1790–1794, 1965.
Moolenaar, F., and Schoonen, A.J.M.: Biopharmaceutics of the Rectal Administration of Drugs. *Pharmacy International*, 1:144–146, 1980.
Parrott, E.L.: Influence of Particle Size on Rectal Absorption of Aspirin. *J. Pharm. Sci.*, 64:878–880, 1975.

Notes

1. According to Merkus, the derivation of the word "suppository" is from the Latin *supponere* meaning "to place under" as derived from *sub* (under) and *ponere* (to place). Thus, suppositories are meant linguistically and therapeutically to be placed "under" in the body, or, in the rectum. (Merkus, F.W.H.M.: The Correct Application of Suppositories. Editorial, *Pharmacy International*, December, 1980).
2. Adapted in part from Anschel, J., and Lieberman, H.A.: Suppositories. *Drug & Cosmetic Ind.*, 97:341, 1965, and, Moolenaar, F., and Schoonen, A.J.M.: Biopharmaceutics of the Rectal Administration of Drugs. *Pharmacy International* 1:144–146, 1980.
3. Gibaldi, M., and Grundhofer, B.: Bioavailability of Aspirin from Commercial Suppositories. *J. Pharm. Sci.*, 64:1064–1066, 1975.
4. Oleopalmitostearin has a molecule each of oleic, palmitic, and stearic acids esterified with the glycerin, and oleodistearin has one molecule of oleic acid and two of stearic acid esterified with glycerin.
5. Roffe, B.D., Zimmer, R.A., and Derewicz, H.J.: Preparation of Progesterone Suppositories. *Am. J. Hosp. Pharm.*, 34:1344, 1977.
6. Allen, L.V., and Stiles, M.L.: Progesterone Suppositories. *U.S. Pharmacist*, 13:16–19, 1988.
7. Product Literature, *Today* Vaginal Contraceptive Sponge, Whitehall Laboratories, New York.
8. Product literature, Alza Corporation, Palo Alto, CA, 1988.
9. Allen, L.V., and Stiles, M.L.: 5-ASA Colon Enema. *U.S. Pharmacist*, 13:78–79, 1988.

12 | *Aerosols, Inhalations, and Sprays*

Pharmaceutical Aerosols

Pharmaceutical aerosols are "pressurized dosage forms containing one or more active ingredients which upon actuation emit a fine dispersion of liquid and/or solid materials in a gaseous medium." Pharmaceutical aerosols are similar to other dosage forms in that they require the same types of considerations with respect to formulation, product stability, and therapeutic efficacy. However, they differ from most other dosage forms in their dependence upon the function of the container, its valve assembly, and an added component—the propellant—for the physical delivery of the medication in proper form.

The term *pressurized package* is commonly used when referring to the aerosol container or completed product. Pressure is applied to the aerosol system through the use of one or more liquefied or gaseous propellants. Upon activation of the valve assembly of the aerosol, it is the pressure exerted by the propellant which forces the contents of the package out through the opening of the valve. The physical form in which the contents are emitted is dependent upon the formulation of the product and the type of valve employed. Aerosol products may be designed to expel their contents as a fine mist, a coarse, wet or a dry spray, a steady stream, or as a stable or a fast-breaking foam. The physical form selected for a given aerosol is based on the intended use of that product. For instance, an aerosol intended for inhalation therapy, as in the treatment of asthma or emphysema, must present particles in the form of a fine liquid mist or as finely divided solid particles if the product is to be efficacious. It has been generally accepted that particles less than 6 μm will reach the respiratory bronchioles, and those less than 2 microns will reach the alveolar ducts and alveoli (see Fig. 12–1). However, when deposition in the trachea and the primary or secondary bronchioles is desired for localized effects, a particle range of 20 to 60 μm is indi-

Fig. 12–1. *Relationship of INTAL (cromolyn sodium, Fisons) particle size to airway penetration. (Courtesy of Fisons Corporation.)*

cated. In contrast, the particle size for a dermatologic spray intended for deposition on the skin would be more coarse and generally less critical to the therapeutic efficacy of the product. Some dermatologic aerosols present the medication in the form of a powder, a wet spray, a stream of liquid (usually a local anesthetic), or an ointment-like product. Other pharmaceutical aerosols include oral, vaginal and rectal foams.

Aerosols used to provide an airborne mist are termed *space sprays*. Room disinfectants, room deodorizers, and space insecticides characterize this group of aerosols. The particle size of the released product is generally quite small, usually below 50 μm, and must be carefully controlled so that the dispersed droplets or particles remain airborne for a prolonged period of time. A one-second burst from a typical aerosol space spray will produce 120 million particles, a substantial number of which will remain suspended in the air for an hour.

Aerosols intended to carry the active ingredient to a surface are termed *surface sprays* or *surface coatings*. The dermatologic aerosols can be placed in this group. Also included are a great many nonpharmaceutical aerosol products, as personal deodorant sprays, cosmetic hair lacquers and sprays, perfume and cologne sprays, shaving lathers, toothpaste, surface pesticide sprays, paint sprays, and various household products such as spray starch, waxes, polishers, cleaners, and lubricants. A number of veterinary and pet products have been put into aerosol form as have been such food products as dessert toppings and food spreads. Physically, some of these products are sprays; others, foams; and a few, paste-like products.

Advantages of the Aerosol Dosage Form

Some features of pharmaceutical aerosols that may be considered advantages over other types of dosage forms are as follows:

1. A portion of medication may be easily withdrawn from the package without contamination or exposure to the remaining material.
2. By virtue of its hermetic character, the aerosol container protects medicinal agents adversely affected by atmospheric oxygen and moisture. Being opaque, the usual aerosol container also protects drugs adversely affected by light. This protection persists during the use and the shelf-life of the product. If the product is packaged under sterile conditions, sterility may also be maintained during the shelf-life of the product.
3. Topical medication may be applied in a uniform, thin layer to the skin, without touching the affected area. This method of application may reduce the irritation that sometimes accompanies the mechanical (fingertip) application of topical preparations. The rapid volatilization of the propellant also provides a cooling, refreshing effect.
4. By proper formulation and valve control, the physical form and the particle size of the emitted product may be controlled which may contribute to the efficacy of a drug; e.g., the fine controlled mist of an inhalant aerosol. Through the use of *metered valves*, dosage may be controlled.
5. Aerosol application is a "clean" process, requiring little or no "wash-up" by the user.

The Aerosol Principle

An aerosol formulation consists of two component parts, the *product concentrate* and the *propellant*. The product concentrate is the active ingredient of the aerosol combined with the required adjuncts, such as antioxidants, surface-active agents, and solvents, to prepare a stable and efficacious product. The propellant is usually a liquefied gas or a mixture of liquefied gases which frequently serves the dual role of propellant and solvent or vehicle for the product concentrate. In certain aerosol systems, nonliquefied compressed gases, as carbon dioxide, nitrogen, and nitrous oxide, are employed as the propellant.

For many years, the liquefied gas propellants most used in the preparation of aerosols were the fluorinated hydrocarbons.[1] However, in 1977 the FDA in conjunction with the Consumer Product Safety Commission initiated a labeling requirement warning that fluorinated hydrocarbon propellants could harm the public health and environment by reducing ozone in the upper atmosphere. This labeling requirement was followed in 1978 with the prohibition to the use of these propellants in nearly all aerosol products. Most consumer products were reformulated to contain different propellants. However, some pharmaceutical products, as inhalant aerosols, were exempt from the ruling because suitable substitute propellants were not available. Among the chlorofluorocarbons used as propellants in pharmaceuticals were dichlorodifluoromethane, dichlorotetrafluoroethane, and trichloromonofluoromethane (see Table 12–1).

Fluorinated hydrocarbons are gases at room temperature. They may be liquefied by cooling below their boiling point or by compressing the gas at room temperature. For example, dichlorodifluoromethane ("Freon 12") gas will form a liquid when cooled to $-22°F$ or when compressed to 70 psig (pounds per square inch gauge) at 70°F. Both of these methods for liquefying gases are employed in aerosol packaging as will be discussed later in this section.

When a liquefied gas propellant or propellant mixture is sealed within an aerosol container with the product concentrate, an equilibrium is quickly established between that portion of propellant which remains liquefied and that which vaporizes and occupies the upper portion of the aerosol container (Fig. 12–2). The vapor phase exerts pressure in all directions—against the walls of the container, the valve assembly, and the surface of the liquid phase, which is composed of the liquefied gas and the product concentrate. It is this pressure which upon actua-

Table 12–1. Physical Properties of Some Fluorinated Hydrocarbon Propellants

Chemical Name	Chemical Formula	Numerical Designation[a]	Vapor Pressure (psia[b]) 70° F	Boiling Point (1 ATM) ° F	Liquid Density (g/mL) 70° F
Trichloromonofluoromethane	CCl_3F	11	13.4	74.7	1.485
Dichlorodifluoromethane	CCl_2F_2	12	84.9	-21.6	1.325
Dichlorotetrafluoroethane	$CClF_2CClF_2$	114	27.6	38.4	1.468
Chloropentafluoroethane	$CClF_2CF_3$	115	117.5	-37.7	1.29
Monochlorodifluoroethane	CH_3CClF_2	142b	43.8	15.1	1.119
Difluoroethane	CH_3CHF_2	152a	76.4	-11.2	0.911
Octafluorocyclobutane	$CF_2CF_2CF_2CF_2$	C318	40.1	21.1	1.513

[a]The numerical designations for fluorinated hydrocarbon propellants have been designed within the refrigeration industry to simplify communications when referring to these agents. The numerical designations are arrived at by the following method: (1) the digit at the extreme right refers to the number of fluorine atoms in the molecule; (2) the second digit from the right represents one *greater* than the number of hydrogen atoms in the molecule; (3) the third digit from the right is one *less* than the number of carbon atoms in the molecule; if this number is zero, it is omitted and a two-digit number is used; (4) a capital letter "C" is used before a number to indicate the cyclic nature of a compound; (5) the small letters following a number are used to indicate decreasing symmetry of isomeric compounds, with the "b" indicating less symmetry than the "a," and so forth. The number of chlorine atoms in a molecule may be determined by subtracting the total number of hydrogen and fluorine atoms from the total number of atoms which may be added to the carbon chain.

[b]psia is pounds per square inch absolute, which is equal to psig + 14.7.

Fig. 12–2. *Cross section sketches of contents and operation of a typical two-phase aerosol system. (Courtesy of Armstrong Laboratories, Inc., Division of Aerosol Techniques, Inc.)*

tion of the aerosol valve forces the liquid phase up the dip tube and out of the orifice of the valve into the atmosphere. As the propellant meets the air, it immediately evaporates due to the drop in pressure, leaving the product concentrate as airborne liquid droplets or dry particles, depending upon the formulation. As the liquid phase is removed from the container, equilibrium between the propellant remaining liquefied and that in the vapor state is reestablished. Thus even during expulsion of the product from the aerosol package, the pressure within remains virtually constant, and the product may be continuously released at an even rate and with the same propulsion. However, when the liquid reservoir is depleted, the pressure may not be maintained, and the gas may be expelled from the container with diminishing pressure until it is exhausted.

Aerosol Systems

The pressure of an aerosol is critical to its performance. It can be controlled by (1) the type and amount of propellant and (2) the nature and amount of material comprising the product concentrate. Thus, each formulation is unique unto itself, and a specific amount of propellant to be employed in aerosol products cannot be firmly stated. However, some general statements may be made within the context of this discussion. Space sprays generally contain a greater proportion of propellant than do aerosols intended for surface coating, and thus they are released with greater pressure, and the resultant particles are projected more violently from the valve. Space aerosols usually operate at pressures between 30 and 40 psig at 70°F and may contain as much as 85% propellant. Surface aerosols commonly contain 30 to 70% propellant with pressures between 25 and 55 psig at 70°F. Foam aerosols usually operate between 35 and 55 psig at 70°F and may contain only 6 to 10% propellant.

Foam aerosols may be considered to be emulsions, in that the liquefied propellant is partially emulsified with the product concentrate rather than being dissolved in it. Because the fluorinated hydrocarbons are nonpolar organic solvents having no affinity for water, the liquefied propellant does not dissolve in the aqueous formulation. The utilization of surfactants or emulsifiers in the formulation encourages the mixing of the two components to enhance the emulsion. Shaking of the package prior to use further

mixes the propellant throughout the product concentrate. When the aerosol valve is activated, the mixture is expelled to the atmosphere where the propellant globules vaporize rapidly, leaving the active ingredient in the form of a foam.

Blends of the various liquefied gas propellants are generally used in pharmaceutical aerosols to achieve the desired vapor pressure and to provide the proper solvent features for a given product. Some propellants are eliminated from use in certain products because of their reactivity with other formulative materials, or with the proposed container or valve components. For instance, trichloromonofluoromethane tends to form free hydrochloric acid when formulated with systems containing water or ethyl alcohol, the latter a commonly used cosolvent in aerosol systems. The free hydrochloric acid not only affects the efficacy of the product, but also exerts a corrosive action on some container components.

The physiologic effect of the propellant must also be considered in formulating an aerosol to assure safety of the product in its intended use. Even though an individual propellant or propellant blend and the active ingredient of a formulation are nontoxic when tested individually, the use of the combination in aerosol form may have undesirable features. For instance, when an active ingredient ordinarily used in a nasal or oral spray is placed in a fine aerosol mist, it may reach deeper into the respiratory tract than desired and may result in irritation. In other instances, as with new dermatologic, vaginal, and rectal aerosol products, the influence of the aerosol form of the drug on the recipient tissue membranes must be evaluated for irritating effects and changes in the absorption of the drug from the site of application. The absorption pattern of a drug may change due to an increased rate of solubility of the fine particles usually produced in aerosol products.

Although the fluorinated hydrocarbons have a relatively low order of toxicity and are generally nonirritating, certain individuals, who may be sensitive to the propellant agent and who utilize an inhalation aerosol, may exhibit cardiotoxic effects following rapid and repeated use of the aerosol product.[2]

TWO-PHASE SYSTEMS. As noted previously, the two-phase aerosol system is comprised of the liquid phase, containing the liquefied propellant and product concentrate, and the vapor phase.

THREE-PHASE SYSTEMS. This system is comprised of a layer of water-immiscible liquid propellant, a layer of highly aqueous product concentrate, and the vapor phase. Because the liquefied propellant usually has a greater density than the aqueous layer, it generally resides at the bottom of the container with the aqueous phase floating above it. As with the two-phase system, upon activation of the valve, the pressure of the vapor phase causes the liquid phase to rise in the dip tube and be expelled from the container. To avoid expulsion of the reservoir of liquefied propellant, the dip tube must extend only within the aqueous phase (product concentrate) and not down into the layer of liquefied propellant. The aqueous product is broken up into a spray by the mechanical action of the valve. If the container is shaken immediately prior to use, some liquefied propellant may be mixed with the aqueous phase and be expelled through the valve to facilitate the dispersion of the exited product or the production of foam, depending upon the formulation. The vapor phase within the container is replenished from the liquid propellant phase.

COMPRESSED GAS SYSTEMS. Compressed, rather than liquefied, gases may be used to prepare aerosols. The pressure of the compressed gas contained in the headspace of the aerosol container forces the product concentrate up the dip tube and out of the valve. The use of gases that are insoluble in the product concentrate, as is nitrogen, will result in the emission of a product in essentially the same form as it was placed in the container, because no gas will be emitted from the valve to induce particle dispersion or foaming. Thus, any particle size reduction on emission of the product would be a function of the type of valve employed. An advantage of nitrogen as a propellant is its inert behavior toward other formulative components and its protective influence on products subject to oxidation. Further, nitrogen is an odorless and tasteless gas and thus does not contribute adversely to the smell or taste of a product.

Other gases, such as carbon dioxide and nitrous oxide, which are slightly soluble in the liquid phase of aerosol products, may be employed in instances in which their expulsion with the product concentrate is desired to achieve spraying or foaming.

Unlike aerosols prepared with liquefied gas propellants, there is no reservoir of liquid propellant in compressed gas filled aerosols. Thus higher gas pressures are generally required in these systems, and the pressure in these aerosols progressively diminishes as the product is used.

The Aerosol Container and Valve Assembly

The effectiveness of a pharmaceutical aerosol is dependent upon achieving the proper combination of formulation, container, and valve assembly. The formulation must not chemically interact with the container or valve components so as to interfere with the stability of the formulation or with the integrity and operation of the container and valve assembly. The container and valve must be capable of withstanding the pressure required by the product, it must be corrosive-resistant, and the valve must contribute to the form of the product to be emitted.

CONTAINERS. Various materials have been used in the manufacture of aerosol containers, including (1) glass, uncoated or plastic coated; (2) metal, including tin-plated steel, aluminum, and stainless steel; and (3) plastics. The selection of the container for an aerosol product is based on its adaptability to production methods, compatibility with formulation components, ability to sustain the pressure intended for the product, the interest in design and aesthetic appeal on the part of the manufacturer, and cost.

Were it not for their brittleness and danger of breakage, glass containers would be preferred for most aerosols. Glass presents fewer problems with respect to chemical compatibility with the formula than do metal containers and is not subject to corrosion. Glass is also more adaptive to creativity in design. On the negative side, glass containers must be precisely engineered to provide the maximum in pressure safety and impact resistance. Plastic coatings are commonly applied to the outer surface of glass containers to render them more resistant to accidental breakage, and in the event of breaking, the plastic coating prevents the scattering of glass fragments. When the total pressure of an aerosol system is below 25 psig and no more than 50% propellant is used, glass containers are considered quite safe. When required, the inner surface of glass containers may be coated to render them more chemically resistant to formulation materials.

At the present time, tin-plated steel containers are the most widely used metal containers for aerosols. Because the starting material used is in the form of sheets, the completed aerosol cylinders are seamed and soldered to provide a sealed unit. When required, special protective coatings are employed within the container to prevent corrosion and interaction between the container and formulation. The containers must be carefully examined prior to filling to ensure that there are no flaws in the seam or in the protective coating that would render the container weak or subject to corrosion.

Most aluminum containers are manufactured by extrusion or by other methods that make them seamless. They have the advantage over the seam type of container in that there is greater safety against leakage, incompatibility, and corrosion. Stainless steel is employed to produce containers for certain small volume aerosols in which a great deal of chemical resistance is required. The main limitation of stainless steel containers is their high cost.

Plastic containers have met with varying success in the packaging of aerosols due to their inherent problem of being permeated by the vapor within the container. Also, certain drug-plastic interactions have been found to occur which affect the release of drug from the container and reduce the efficacy of the product.

VALVE ASSEMBLY. The function of the valve assembly is to permit the expulsion of the contents of the can in the desired form, at the desired rate, and, in the case of metered valves, in the proper amount or dose. The materials used in the manufacture of valves must be inert toward the formulations and must be approved by the Food and Drug Administration. Among the materials used in the manufacture of the various valve parts are plastic, rubber, aluminum, and stainless steel.

The usual aerosol valve assembly is composed of the following parts (Fig. 12–3):
1. *Actuator*—The actuator is the button which the user presses to activate the valve assembly for the emission of the product. The actuator permits the easy opening and closing of the valve. It is through the orifice in the actuator that the product is discharged. The design of the inner chamber and size of the emission orifice of the actuator contribute to the physical form (mist, coarse spray, solid stream, or foam) in which the product is discharged. The combination of the type and quantity of propellant used,

Fig. 12–3. *Sketch showing valve assembly components.*

and the actuator design and dimensions control the particle size of the emitted product. Larger orifices (and less propellant) are used for products to be emitted as foams and solid streams than for those intended to be sprays or mists.
2. *Stem*—The stem supports the actuator and delivers the formulation in the proper form to the chamber of the actuator.
3. *Gasket*—The gasket, placed snugly with the stem, serves to prevent leakage of the formulation when the valve is in the closed position.
4. *Spring*—The spring holds the gasket in place and also is the mechanism by which the actuator retracts when pressure is released, thereby returning the valve to the closed position.
5. *Mounting cup*—The mounting cup, which is attached to the aerosol can or container, serves to hold the valve in place. Because the underside of the mounting cup is exposed to the formulation, it must receive the same consideration as the inner part of the container, with respect to meeting criteria of compatibility. If necessary, it may be coated with an inert material (as an epoxy resin or vinyl) to prevent an undesired interaction.
6. *Housing*—The housing, located directly below the mounting cup, serves as the link

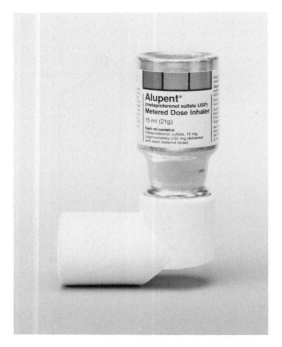

Fig. 12–4. *Example of metered dose inhaler. (Courtesy of Boehringer Ingelheim.)*

between the dip tube and the stem and actuator. With the stem, its orifice helps to determine the delivery rate and the form in which the product is emitted.

7. *Dip tube*—The dip tube, which extends from the housing down into the product, serves to bring the formulation from the container to the valve. The viscosity of the product and its intended delivery rate dictate to a large extent the inner dimensions of the dip tube and housing for a particular product.

The actuator, stem, housing, and dip tube are generally made of plastic, the mounting cup and spring of metal, and the gasket of rubber or plastic predetermined to be resistant to the formulation.

Metering valves are employed when the formulation is a potent medication, as in inhalation therapy (Fig. 12–4). In these metered valve systems, the amount of material discharged is regulated by an auxiliary valve chamber by virtue of its capacity or dimensions. A single depression of the actuator causes the evacuation of this chamber and the delivery of its contents. The integrity of the chamber is controlled by a dual valving mechanism. When the actuator valve is in the closed position, a seal is effected between the chamber and the atmosphere. However, in this position the chamber is permitted to fill with the contents of the container to which it is open. Depression of the actuator causes a simultaneous reversal of positions sealed; the chamber becomes open to the atmosphere, releasing its contents, and at the same time becomes sealed from the contents of the container. Upon release of the actuator, the system is restored for the next dose. The USP contains a test to determine quantitatively the amount of medication from a metered valve.

A unique translingual aerosol formulation of nitroglycerin has been developed (Nitrolingual Spray, Rorer) that permits a patient to spray droplets of nitroglycerin onto or under the tongue for acute relief of an attack, or for prophylaxis, of angina pectoris due to coronary artery disease. The product is not to be inhaled. At the onset of an attack, two metered spray emissions, each containing 0.4 mg of nitroglycerin, are administered. The product contains 200 doses of nitroglycerin in a propellant mixture of dichlorodifluoromethane and dichlorotetrafluoroethane.

Most aerosol products have a protective cap or cover that fits snugly over the valve and mounting cup. This protects the valve against contamination with dust and dirt. The cap, which is generally made of plastic or metal, also serves a decorative function.

Filling Operations

As explained earlier, fluorinated hydrocarbon gases may be liquefied by cooling below their boiling points or by compressing the gas at room temperature. These two features are utilized in the filling of aerosol containers with propellant.

COLD FILLING. In the cold method, both the product concentrate and the propellant must be cooled to temperatures of $-30°$ to $-40°F$. This temperature is necessary to liquefy the propellant gas. The cooling system may be a mixture of dry ice and acetone or a more elaborate refrigeration system. After the chilled product concentrate has been quantitatively metered into an equally cold aerosol container, the liquefied gas is added. The heavy vapors of the cold liquid propellant generally displace the air present in the container. However, in the process, some of the propellant vapors are also lost.

When sufficient propellant has been added, the valve assembly is immediately inserted and crimped into place. Because of the low temperatures required, aqueous systems cannot be filled by this process, since the water turns to ice. For nonaqueous systems, some moisture usually appears in the final product due to the condensation of atmospheric moisture within the cold containers.

PRESSURE FILLING. By the pressure method, the product concentrate is quantitatively placed in the aerosol container (Fig. 12–5), the valve assembly is inserted and crimped into place, and the liquefied gas, under pressure, is metered into the valve stem from a pressure burette (Fig. 12–6). The desired amount of propellant is allowed to enter the container under its own vapor pressure. When the pressure in the container equals that in the burette, the propellant stops flowing. Additional propellant may be added by increasing the pressure in the filling apparatus through the use of compressed air or nitrogen gas. The trapped air in the package may be ignored if it does not interfere with the quality or stability of the product, or it may

be evacuated prior to filling or during filling, using special apparatus. After filling the container with sufficient propellant, the valve actuator is tested for proper function. This spray testing also rids the dip tube of pure propellant prior to consumer use.

Pressure filling is used for most pharmaceutical aerosols. It has the advantage over the cold filling method in that there is less danger of moisture contamination of the product, and also less propellant is lost in the process.

When compressed gases are employed as the propellant in aerosol systems, the gas is transferred from large steel cylinders into the aerosol containers. Prior to filling, the product concentrate is quantitatively placed in the container, the valve assembly is crimped into place, and the air is evacuated from the container by a vacuum pump. The compressed gas is then passed into the container through a pressure reducing valve attached to the gas cylinder; when the pressure within the aerosol container is equal to the predetermined and regulated delivery pressure, the gas flow stops, and the aerosol valve is restored to the closed position. For

Fig. 12–5. *Filling the empty aerosol cans with the drug mixture. (Courtesy of Pennwalt Corp.)*

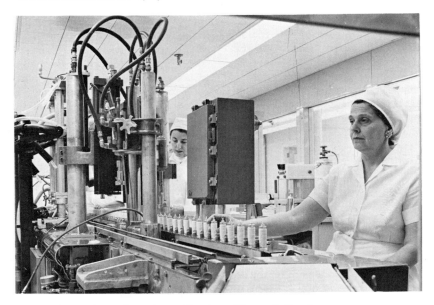

Fig. 12–6.   *Pressure filling of aerosol containers. (Courtesy of Pennwalt Corp.)*

gases like carbon dioxide and nitrous oxide, which are slightly soluble in the product concentrate, the container is manually or mechanically shaken during the filling operation to achieve the desired pressure in the headspace of the aerosol container.

Testing the Filled Containers

After filling by either the cold method or the pressure method, the aerosol container is tested under various environmental conditions for leaks or weakness in the valve assembly or container.

Filled aerosol containers are also tested for the proper function of the valve. The *valve discharge rate* is determined by discharging a portion of the contents of a previously weighed aerosol during a given period of time, and calculating, by the difference in weight, the grams of contents discharged per unit of time. As is deemed desirable, aerosols also may be tested for their spray patterns, for particle size distribution of the spray, and for accuracy and reproducibility of dosage when using metered valves.[3]

Packaging, Labeling, and Storage

A unique aspect of pharmaceutical aerosols compared to other dosage forms is that the product is actually packaged as part of the manufacturing process. With most other dosage forms, the product is completely manufactured and then placed in the appropriate container.

Medicinal aerosols that are to be dispensed only upon prescription usually may be labeled by the manufacturer with plastic peel-away labels or easily removed paper labels so that the pharmacist may easily replace the manufacturer's label with his label containing the directions for use specified by the prescribing practitioner. Most other types of aerosols have the manufacturer's label printed directly on the container or on firmly affixed paper. Aerosols should contain the following warning information:

Warning: Contents under pressure. Do not puncture or incinerate container. Do not expose to heat or store at temperatures above 120°F (49°C). Keep out of reach of children.
Warning: Avoid inhaling. Keep away from eyes or other mucous membranes.
(Note: warning not required for inhalation aerosols and those to be used on mucous membranes respectively)

For aerosols containing propellants of halocarbon or hydrocarbon:

Warning: Use only as directed; intentional misuse by deliberately concentrating and inhaling the contents can be harmful or fatal.

Aerosols should be maintained with the protective caps in place to prevent accidental activation of the valve assembly or its contamination by dust and other foreign materials.

Fig. 12–7. *Examples of some pharmaceutical aerosols.*

Pharmaceutical Aerosols

Examples of pharmaceutical aerosols are shown in Figure 12–7 and presented in Table 12–2.

Proper Administration and Use of Pharmaceutical Aerosols

The pharmacist should make every attempt to educate the patient about aerosol dosage forms, particularly for oral or nasal administration, because these are only effective when properly used. To complement verbal instructions the pharmacist should provide the patient with the written instructions found within the product package. It is difficult to predict what percentage of patients will read or even understand the printed instruction. Thus, the pharmacist must verbally transmit instruction for proper use. Using the oral, metered aerosols as a model, the pharmacist should demonstrate how the inhaler is assembled, stored and cleaned. The patient should be told whether the inhaler requires shaking before use and how to hold it between the index finger and thumb so that the aerosol canister is up-side-down. The patient should understand that coordination must be achieved between inhalation (after exhaling as completely as possible) and pressing down the inhaler to release one dose. The patient should be instructed to hold his breath for several seconds or as long as possible to gain the maximum benefit from the medication. The patient is told to then remove the inhaler from the mouth and exhale slowly through pursed lips.

Approximately 20% of patients are unable to use metered-dose inhalers properly. Thus, after a new prescription is dispensed, it is advisable for the pharmacist to follow up with the patient to make sure the patient is capable of using the inhaler. If the patient confides an inability to use the inhaler, it is advisable for the pharmacist to recommend to the patient or the patient's physician the use of an extender device with the inhaler. Extender devices or "spacers" were originally developed for patients who could not learn to coordinate release of the medication with inhalation. These are now considered an important therapeutic aid because they can effectively assist the delivery of medication despite improper patient inhalation technique. By placing an extender device between the metered-dose inhaler's mouthpiece and the patient's mouth, the patient is permitted to separate activation of the aerosol from inhalation by up to 3 to 5 seconds (a valve in the spacer opens when the patient inhales). Another advantage of the extender device is that aerosol velocity is reduced, and droplet size is decreased because there is time for evaporation of the fluorohydrocarbon propellant. Thus, extender devices also cause less deposition of medication in the oropharynx. Currently, at least four extender devices are available that can be adapted to most pressurized canisters, i.e., Aerochamber (Monoghan), Brethancer (Geigy), Inhal-Aid (Plough), and InspirEase (Plough).

To ensure continuity of therapy it is wise for the pharmacist to share with the patient ways to assess how much medication is left in the canister (see Fig. 10–8, p. 368). This is important to ensure continuity of therapy, especially for those who suffer from respiratory illness and may need their medication on a moment's notice.

For topical administration of aerosol dosage forms, the patient should be told to first clean the affected area gently and to pat it dry. Holding the canister with the nozzle pointing toward the body area and about 6 to 8 inches away, the patient should press down the button to deliver enough medication to cover the area. The patient should allow the spray to dry and not cover the area with a bandage or dressing unless instructed to do so by the physician. The patient should avoid accidently spraying the product into the eyes or mouth. If it is necessary to apply the product to a facial area, the patient should spray the product into the palm of the hand and apply it by this means.

Inhalations

Inhalations are drugs or solutions of drugs administered by the nasal or oral respiratory

Table 12–2. Examples of Aerosols

Aerosol	Some Representative Commercial Products	Category and Comments
Albuterol Aerosol	Proventil (Schering) Ventolin (Glaxo)	Sympathomimetic for the relief of bronchospasm in patients with reversible obstructive airway disease.
Beclomethasone Dipropionate Aerosol	Beclovent (Glaxo) Vanceril (Schering)	Adrenocortical steroid; aerosol for oral administration for control of bronchial asthma in patients requiring chronic treatment with corticosteroids with other therapy, e.g., xanthines, sympathomimetics.
	Beconase Nasal Inhaler (Glaxo) Vancenase Nasal Inhaler (Schering)	Adrenocortical steroid; aerosol for intranasal relief of symptoms of seasonal or perennial rhinitis in those cases poorly responsive to conventional treatment.
Betamethasone Dipropionate Topical Aerosol	Diprosone Aerosol (Schering)	Glucocorticoid; sprayed topically for anti-inflammatory, antipruritic, and vasoconstrictive actions.
Cromolyn Sodium Aerosol	Intal Aerosol (Fisons)	An antiasthmatic, antiallergic and mast cell stabilizer; aerosol for oral administration for prevention of exercise-induced bronchospasm, and for prevention of acute bronchospasm induced by environmental pollutants and known allergens.
Isoetharine Mesylate Inhalation Aerosol	Bronkometer (Breon)	Sympathomimetic for the temporary relief of bronchial asthma and other conditions of bronchospasm.
Metaproterenol Sulfate Aerosol	Alupent (Boehringer Ingelheim) Metaprel (Dorsey)	Sympathomimetic for the relief of bronchospasm in patients with reversible obstructive airway disease.
Povidone-Iodine Topical Aerosol Solution	Betadine (Purdue Frederick)	Local anti-infective; sprayed on affected area topically. The povidone-iodine is present as a 5% solution, equivalent to 0.5% of available iodine
Thimerosal Topical Aerosol	Merthiolate Aeropump (Lilly)	Local anti-infective; sprayed on affected area topically. Thimerosal is present as a 0.1% solution containing stabilizers and usually colorants to delineate the area of application. Merthiolate is incompatible with iodine, strong acids, and heavy metal salts, and these should be avoided in its manufacture, storage, and use.
Tolnaftate Topical Aerosol Powder	Tinactin Powder Aerosol (Schering)	Fungicidal; applied topically.
Crystallized Trypsin for Inhalation Aerosol	Granulex (Hickam)	Proteolytic; for debridement of eschar and other necrotic tissue.
Triamcinolone Acetonide Topical Aerosol	Kenalog Spray (Squibb)	Anti-inflammatory; applied topically to the affected area.

airflow

Plastic Slide

Capsule-Piercing Needle
Gelatin Capsule

Plastic Rotor Blade

Tapered Bearing

Plastic Mouthpiece

Powder Exit Holes

Cromolyn Sodium plus Lactose
(microfine particles)

Tubular Housing

Stainless Steel Shaft

Fig. 12–8. *Cross section of the SPINHALER turbo inhaler, used in the administration of INTAL (cromolyn sodium, Fisons). (Courtesy of Fisons Corporation.)*

Fig. 12–9. *An example of a nebulizer used in inhalation therapy. See text for description of operation. (Courtesy of The DeVilbiss Co.)*

route. The drugs may be administered for their local action on the bronchial tree or for their systemic effects through absorption from the lungs. Certain gases, as oxygen and ether, are administered by inhalation as are finely powdered drug substances and solutions of drugs administered as fine mists. Sterile Water for Inhalation, USP and Sodium Chloride Inhalation, USP may be used as vehicles for inhalation solutions.

As noted previously in Table 12–2, a number of drug substances are administered through pressure packaged *inhalation aerosols,* as the type shown in Figure 12–4. In order for the inhaled drug substance or solution to reach the bronchial tree, the inhaled particles must be just a few microns in size.

A unique form of powder administration involves the inhalation of a micronized powder directly into the lungs using a special breath-activated device (Fig. 12–8). The drug present in the inhaled powder is cromolyn sodium, an agent used in the management of patients with severe perennial asthma. The drug is supplied to the patient in hard gelatin capsules as a powder mixture with the inert substance lactose. The particles of lactose are designed to be larger (30 to 60 μ) than the particles of cromolyn sodium powder (1 to 10 μ) and upon inhalation the cromolyn sodium passes deeply into the respiratory tract, whereas the lactose particles are retained in the upper airways (Fig. 12–1). The powder in the capsule is prepared for inhalation by placing it in the special inhaler device.

When ready for medication the patient makes two perforations in the capsule by a piercing mechanism present in the inhaler-device. When the mouth is placed on the mouthpiece and air inhaled, the turbo-vibratory action of the propeller causes the powdered drug to be dispensed into the inspired air through the perforations in the capsule wall.

A widely used instrument capable of producing fine particles for inhalation therapy is the *nebulizer.* This apparatus, shown in Figure 12–9, contains an atomizing unit within a curved, glass, bulb-like chamber. A rubber bulb at the end of the apparatus is depressed and the medicated solution is drawn up a narrow glass tube and broken into fine particles by the passing airstream. The fine particles produced range between 0.5 and 5 microns. The larger, heavier droplets of the mist do not exit the apparatus but fall back into the reservoir of medicated liquid. The lighter particles do escape with the airstream and are inhaled by the patient who operates the nebulizer with the exit orifice in his mouth, inhaling as he depresses the rubber bulb.

The pharmacist should advise the patient on the proper technique to use the nebulizer and provide additional patient instructions, e.g., do not exceed physician's instructions and use the

Fig. 12–10. *An example of a commercially available vaporizer. (Courtesy of The DeVilbiss Co.)*

smallest amount of product necessary to afford relief. The pharmacist could also advise on how to cope with dryness of the mouth that might occur. Further, the pharmacist should emphasize the need to clean the nebulizer after its use and explain how to do it.

The common household *vaporizer*, as the one depicted in Figure 12–10, produces a fine mist of steam that may be used to humidify a room. When a volatile medication is added to the water in the chamber or to a special medication cup present in some models, the medication volatilizes and is also inhaled by the patient. *Humidifiers*, as shown in Figure 12–11, are employed to provide a cool mist to the air in a room. Moisture in the air is important to prevent mucous membranes of the nose and throat from becoming dry and irritated. Vaporizers and humidifiers are commonly used in the adjunctive treatment of colds, coughs, and chest congestion.

The pharmacist can help a patient select a vaporizer or humidifer depending upon one's

Fig. 12–11. *An example of a commercially available humidifier. (Courtesy of The DeVilbiss Co.)*

needs. Both devices have advantages and disadvantages. Manufacturing guidelines and legal regulations, e.g., lock tops, have made vaporizers more safe today than in the years past. So the possibility of scalding due to an overturned vaporizer is less with newer models. Further, the heat generated in a vaporizer kills the mold and bacteria that may be in the water tank. Humidifiers are more costly, but use less electricity than vaporizers. In addition, compared to vaporizers, humidifiers are noisier during operation, can leave a deposition of minerals on woodwork and furniture, and can effectively cool down a room by 1° to 3° (a problem with young children). The patient should learn about these subtle differences from the pharmacist.

Ultrasonic humidifiers are also available, and while they are effective and operate at an almost noiseless level, they apparently pose a health problem. While these are highly efficient at nebulizing water into fine droplets, they are also efficient at nebulizing up to 90% of water contaminants as well. These contaminants include mold, bacteria, lead, and dissolved organic gases, which could ultimately cause acute respiratory irritation to chronic lung problems in unsuspecting patients. Thus, patients should either be advised to run water through a high-grade demineralization filter before filling their ultrasonic humidifier, or buy a humidifier with a built-in filter that works.

Examples of Medicated Inhalations

As noted previously, a number of inhalations are pressure packaged as inhalation aerosols and are listed in Table 12–2. Several other inhalations used in medicine are solutions intended to be administered by nebulizer or other apparatus. Among these are: Isoetharine Hydrochloride Inhalation, and Isoproterenol Hydrochloride Inhalation, both used for the relief of bronchial spasms in the treatment of bronchial asthma and related conditions.

Inhalants

Inhalants are drugs or combinations of drugs that by virtue of their high vapor pressure can be carried by an air current into the nasal passage where they exert their effect. The device in which the drug or drugs is contained and from which they are administered is termed an *inhaler.*

Amyl Nitrite Inhalant

Amyl nitrite is a clear, yellowish, volatile liquid that acts as a vasodilator when inhaled. The drug is prepared in sealed glass vials which are covered with a protective gauze cloth (Fig. 12–12). Upon use, the glass vial is broken in the fingertips and the cloth soaks up the liquid which is then inhaled. The vials generally contain 0.3 mL of the drug substance. The effects of the drug are rapid and are used in the treatment of anginal pain.

Propylhexedrine Inhalant

Propylhexedrine is a liquid adrenergic (vasoconstrictor) agent that volatilizes slowly at room temperature. This quality enables it to be effectively used as an inhalant. The official inhalant consists of cylindrical rolls of suitable fibrous material impregnated with propylhexedrine, usually aromatized to mask its amine-like odor, and contained in a suitable inhaler. The vapor of the drug is inhaled into the nostrils when needed to relieve nasal congestion due to colds and hay fever. It may also be employed to relieve ear block and the pressure pain in air travelers.

Each plastic tube of the commercial product contains 250 mg of propylhexedrine with aromatics. The containers should be tightly closed after each opening to prevent loss of the drug vapors. The counterpart commercial product is Benzedrex Inhaler (SmithKline Consumer Products).

Sprays

Sprays may be defined as aqueous or oleaginous solutions in the form of coarse droplets or as finely divided solids to be applied topically, most usually to the nasal-pharyngeal tract or to the skin. Many commercially available sprays are used intranasally to relieve nasal congestion and inflammation and to combat infection and contain antihistamines, sympathomimetic agents, and antibiotic substances. Because of the noninvasive nature and quickness with which nasal sprays can deliver medication systemically, the future will demonstrate the administration of several drugs by this route that typically have been administered by other routes of administration. Most notably, insulin and glucagon will be administered in this fashion. Research has demonstrated that the administration of glucagon, for example, via a nasal spray can relieve hypoglycemic symptoms within 7 minutes, a definite advantage over conventional emergency intravenous glucose or intramuscular glucagon.

Other sprays are employed against sunburn and heat burn and contain local anesthetics, antiseptics, skin protectants, and antipruritics. Throat sprays containing antiseptics, deodorants, and flavorants may be effectively employed to relieve conditions such as halitosis, sore throat, or laryngitis. Other sprays may be employed to treat athlete's foot and other fungal infections. Numerous other medicinal and cosmetic uses of sprays are commonly available in pharmacies.

To achieve the breaking up of a solution into small particles so that it may be effectively sprayed or to facilitate the spraying of a powder, several mechanical devices have been developed and are commonly employed. The plastic spray bottle, which is gently squeezed to issue a spray of its contents, is familiar to most persons. It is commonly used for nasal decongestant sprays as well as cosmetically, especially for body deodorant products. Recently, one-way pump sprays have been developed to deliver medication into the nose. These sprays are used for both legend, e.g., Nasalide (Syntex), and nonlegend, e.g., Nostrilla (Boehringer-Ingelheim), medicines. The advantage of these over the conventional sprays is that its design prevents drawback contamination of nasal fluids into the bottle after administration, a definite advantage for someone trying to cope with viruses associated with the common cold. Pharmacists are familiar with medicinal *atomizers*, which are employed for the issuance of a medicated solution to the patient in the form of fine droplets (Fig. 12–13). One type of atomizer operates by the squeezing of a rubber bulb at the end of the apparatus, which causes a flow of air partially to enter the glass reservoir in which the solution is held and partially to exit from the opposite end of the system. The air forced into the reservoir causes the liquid to rise in a small dip tube, which is maintained below the level of the liquid, forcing the solution up and into the stream of air exiting the system. The

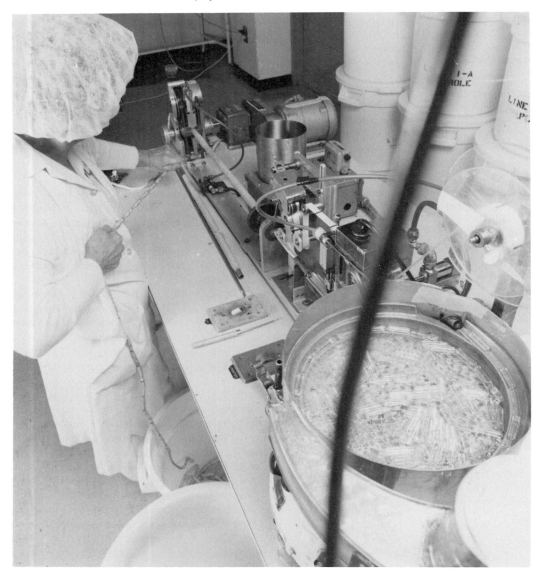

Fig. 12–12. *Silking operation in the production of amyl nitrate Vaporole. (Courtesy of Burroughs Wellcome Company.)*

air and the solution are forced through a jet opening and the liquid is broken up into a spray, the droplets being carried by the airstream. In other similar apparatuses, the stream of air caused by the depression of the bulb does not enter the reservoir of solution, but passes swiftly over it, creating a pressure change that causes a sucking up of the liquid into the dip tube and into the airstream in which it exits the system. In instances in which powdered substances are employed rather than solutions, a *powder blower* or a powder *insufflator* may be employed to produce a powder spray. Such an apparatus is similar to the atomizer for liquids; the squeezing of the rubber bulb causes a turbulence within the reservoir of powder, forcing some up the dip tube and out of the tip of the apparatus by the exiting airstream (Fig. 12–14).

Proper Administration and Use of Nasal Sprays

Before using the drops the patient should be advised to gently blow the nose to clear the

Fig. 12–13. *A common type of atomizer for the administration of a spray of liquid medication. The model shown has an adjustable tip for directing the spray upward or downward to reach otherwise inaccessible areas of the throat. (Courtesy of The DeVilbiss Co.)*

nostrils. The patient should be told not to shake the plastic squeeze bottle for use, but be sure to remove the plastic cap. While holding the head upright the patient should insert the nosepiece into the nostril, pointing it slightly backward, and close the other nostril with one finger. The patient should then spray the prescribed or recommended amount, squeezing the bottle sharply and firmly while sniffing through the nose. Sprays should always be administered with the patient in an upright position. Spraying medicine into the nostrils should not be performed with the head over the edge of a bed (the preferred procedure for administration of nasal drops) because it could result in the systemic absorption of the drug, rather than a local effect.

The patient should be advised not to overuse the product. For example, some decongestant medicines such as oxymetazoline and xylometazoline can predispose the patient to rebound congestion if used for more than three to five consecutive days. The patient should also understand the normal time frame in which to see results and be advised that after a certain number of days if relief if not achieved to consult the physician. Lastly, patients should realize not to share their medicated spray with another person to prevent the possibility of cross-contamination between individuals.

Examples of Medicated Sprays

A number of nasal solutions are commercially packaged in plastic spray-bottles for use as sprays. Among these are:

Flunisolide Nasal Solution [Nasalide (Syntex)]

Oxymetrazoline Hydrochloride Nasal Solution, USP [Afrin Nasal Spray (Schering)]

Phenylephrine Hydrochloride Nasal Solution, USP [Neo-Synephrine Hydrochloride Nasal Spray (Winthrop)]

Sodium Chloride Nasal Solution [Salinex Solution (Muro)]

Xylometazoline Hydrochloride Nasal Solution [Sine-Off (SmithKline)]

Selected Reading

Cascella, P.J., and Powers, J.E.: The Inhalation Route of Drug Administration, *US Pharmacist*, 13:44–57, 1988.

Goddard, R.F.: Inhalation Therapy for Infants and Children. *Mod. Med.*, 38:90, 1970.

Sciarra, J.J.: Pharmaceutical Aerosols. In *The Theory and Practice of Industrial Pharmacy*, 3rd Ed., L. Lachman, H.A. Lieberman, and J.L. Kanig, eds., Philadelphia, Lea & Febiger, 1986, pp. 589–618.

Sciarra, J.J.: Pharmaceutical and Cosmetic Aerosols, *J. Pharm. Sci.*, 63:1815–1837, 1974.

Self, T.H., and Fuentes, R.J.: Metered Dose Inhalers and Extender Devices, *US Pharmacist*, 10:36–44, 1985.

Fig. 12–14. *A general purpose insufflator, used in the application of powdered substances to the nose, throat, ear, tooth sockets, or to body surfaces. (Courtesy of The DeVilbiss Co.)*

Notes

1. Many of these propellants are products of the Dupont Company, marketed as "Freon" propellants or refrigerants. They are also available as "Genetrons" from the General Chemical Division, Allied Chemical Corporation, or as "Ucons" from Union Carbide Chemicals Company, Division of Union Carbide Corporation.

2. Chiou, W.L.: Aerosol Propellants: Cardiac Toxicity and Long Biological Half-Life, *JAMA*, 227:658, 1974.

3. These and other tests are described in detail by J.J. Sciarra in *The Theory and Practice of Industrial Pharmacy*, 3rd Ed. Edited by L. Lachman, H.A. Lieberman, and J.L. Kanig. Philadelphia, Lea & Febiger, 1986, pp. 595–597.

13 | *Miscellaneous Preparations*

Tinctures, Fluidextracts, Extracts[1]

Certain pharmaceutical preparations are prepared by the process of *extraction*—that is, by the withdrawal of desired constituents from crude drugs through the use of selected solvents in which the desired constituents are soluble. *Crude drugs* are vegetable or animal drugs that have undergone no other processes than collection and drying. Because each crude drug contains a number of constituents that may be soluble in a given solvent, the products of extraction, termed *extractives*, do not contain just a single constituent but rather varying numbers of constituents, depending upon the drug used and the conditions of the extraction. *Tinctures, fluidextracts* and *extracts* are the pharmaceutical products most commonly prepared from extractives.

Plant materials are composed of heterogeneous mixtures of constituents, some of which are pharmacologically active and others that are pharmacologically inactive and considered inert. Among the varied plant constituents are sugars, starches, mucilages, proteins, albumins, pectins, cellulose, gums, inorganic salts, fixed and volatile oils, resins, tannins, coloring materials, and a number of very active constituents such as alkaloids and glycosides. The solvent systems used in extraction are selected on the basis of their capacity to dissolve the maximum amount of desired active constituents and the minimum amount of undesired constituents.

In many instances the active constituents of a plant drug are of the same general chemical type, have similar solubility characteristics and can be simultaneously extracted with a single solvent or a single solvent-mixture. The process of extraction concentrates the active constituents of a crude drug and removes from it the extraneous matter. In drug extraction, the solvent or solvent-mixture is referred to as the *menstruum*, and the plant residue, which is exhausted of active constituents, is termed the *marc*.

The Menstruum

The selection of the menstruum to use in the extraction of a crude drug is based primarily upon the relative solubility in it of the active constituents. Although water and alcohol and, to a lesser extent, glycerin are probably the most frequently employed solvents in drug extraction, acetic acid and organic solvents like ether may be used for special purposes.

Because of its ready availability, cheapness, and good solvent action for many plant constituents, water has some use in drug extraction, particularly in combination with other solvents. However, as a sole solvent it has many disadvantages and is infrequently used alone. For one thing, most active plant constituents are complex organic chemical compounds that are less soluble in water than in alcohol. Although water has a great solvent action on such plant constituents as sugars, gums, starches, coloring principles, and tannins, most of these are not particularly desirable components of an extracted preparation. Water also tends to extract plant principles which upon standing in the extractive later separate leaving an undesired residue. Finally, unless preserved, aqueous preparations serve as excellent growth media for molds, yeasts, and bacteria. When water alone is employed as the menstruum, alcohol is frequently added to the extractive or to the final preparation as an antimicrobial preservative.

Hydroalcoholic mixtures are perhaps the most versatile and most widely employed menstruums. They combine the solvent effects of both water and alcohol, and the complete miscibility of these two agents permits a flexible combining of the two agents to form solvent mixtures most suited to the extraction of the active principles from a particular drug. A hydroalcoholic menstruum generally provides inherent protection against microbial contamination and helps to prevent the separation of extracted material on standing. Alcohol is used alone as a menstruum only when necessary because it is more expensive than hydroalcoholic mixtures.

Glycerin, a good solvent for many plant substances, is occasionally employed as a cosolvent with water or alcoholic menstruums because of its ability to extract and then prevent inert materials from precipitating upon standing. It is especially useful in this regard in preventing the separation of tannin and tannin oxidation products in extractives. Because glycerin has preservative action, depending upon its concentration in the final product, it may contribute to the stability of a pharmaceutical extractive.

Methods of Extraction

The principal methods of drug extraction are maceration and percolation. Generally, the method of extraction selected for a given drug depends on several factors, as the nature of the crude drug, its adaptability to each of the various extraction methods, and the interest in obtaining complete or near-complete extraction of the drug. The nature of the crude drug is the primary factor to be considered in selecting the method of extraction. Certain drugs simply do not lend themselves to the process of percolation, which demands that they be capable of being reduced to a uniform powder and packed firmly and evenly in the percolation apparatus. Other drugs, although packable in a percolator, may yield their active constituents so readily to a solvent that they simply need to be soaked in it to provide a satisfactory extractive. They may be extracted by maceration rather than by percolation. The process of percolation requires a greater skill on the part of the operator than does maceration, and of the two processes, percolation is more expensive to conduct, because it requires specialized equipment and a great deal of the operator's time.

Frequently a combination of maceration and percolation is actually employed in the extraction of a crude drug. The drug is macerated first to soften the plant tissues and to dissolve much of the active constituents, and the percolation process is then conducted to achieve the separation of the extractive from the marc.

Maceration

The term "maceration" comes from the Latin *macerare*, meaning "to soak." It is a process in which the properly comminuted drug is permitted to soak in the menstruum until the cellular structure is softened and penetrated by the menstruum and the soluble constituents are dissolved.

In the maceration process, the drug to be extracted is generally placed in a wide-mouth container with the prescribed menstruum, the vessel is stoppered tightly, and the contents are agitated repeatedly over a period usually ranging from 2 to 14 days. The agitation permits the repeated flow of fresh solvent over the entire surface area of the comminuted drug. An alternative to this repeated shaking is to place the drug in a porous cloth bag that is tied and suspended in the upper portion of the menstruum, much the same as a tea bag is suspended in water in the preparation of a cup of tea. As the soluble constituents dissolve in the menstruum, they tend to settle to the bottom because of an increase in the specific gravity of the liquid due to its added weight. Fresh menstruum then comes to the top and the process continues in a cyclic manner. Occasional dipping of the drug bag may facilitate the speed of the extraction. The extractive is separated from the marc by expressing the bag of drug and washing it with additional fresh menstruum, the washings being added to the extractive. If the maceration is performed with an unbagged drug, the marc may be removed by straining and/or filtration, with the marc being washed free of extractive by the additional passage of menstruum through the strainer or filter into the total extractive.

For drugs containing little or no cellular material, such as benzoin, aloe and tolu, which dissolve almost completely in the menstruum, maceration is the most efficient method of extraction.

Maceration is usually conducted at a temperature of between 15° to 20°C for a period of 3 days or until the soluble matter is dissolved.

Percolation

The term *percolation*, from the Latin *per*, meaning "through," and *colare*, meaning "to strain," may be described generally as a process in which a comminuted drug is extracted of its soluble constituents by the slow passage of a suitable solvent through a column of the drug. The drug is packed in a special extraction apparatus termed a *percolator*, with the extractive collected called the *percolate*. Most drug extractions are performed by percolation.

In the process of percolation the flow of the

menstruum over the drug column is generally downward to the exit orifice, drawn by the force of gravity as well as the weight of the column of liquid. In certain specialized and more sophisticated percolation apparatus, additional pressure on the column is exerted with positive air pressure at the inlet and suction at the outlet or exit.

Percolators for drug extraction vary greatly as to their shape, capacities, composition, and, most important, their utility. Percolators employed in the large-scale industrial preparation of extractives are generally made of stainless steel or are glass-lined large metal vessels that vary greatly in size and in operation. Percolators used to extract leaves, for instance, may be 6 to 8 feet in diameter and 12 to 18 feet high (Fig. 13–1). Percolators employed to extract other vegetable parts like seeds that are greater in density than leaves and would pack too tightly in percolators of such large dimensions are extracted in much smaller percolators. Some special industrial percolators are designed to percolate with hot menstruums; in others pressure is utilized to force the menstruum through the drug columns.

Percolation on a small scale generally involves the use of glass percolators of various shapes for extraction of small amounts (perhaps up to 1000 g) of crude drug. The shape of percolators in common laboratory and small-scale use are generally (a) cylindrical, with little if any taper except for the lower orifice; (b) cylindrical-like, but with a definite taper downward; and (c) conical, or funnel-shaped. Each type has a special utility in drug extraction.

The cylindrical percolator is particularly suited to the complete extraction of drugs with a minimal expenditure of menstruum. By the passage of the menstruum over the drug contained in a high, narrow column (rather than in a lower, wider column), each drug particle is more repeatedly exposed to passing solvent. A funnel-shaped percolator is useful for the percolation of drugs that swell a great deal during the maceration process, since the large upper surface permits the expansion of the drug column with little risk of a too tightly packed column or breakage of a glass percolator.

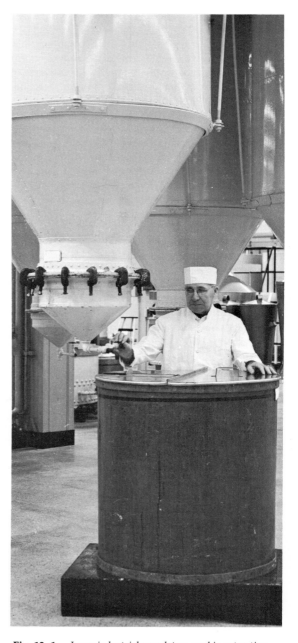

Fig. 13–1. *Large industrial percolators used in extracting crude drugs to make fluidextracts, tinctures, and powdered extracts. (Courtesy of the Upjohn Company.)*

Tinctures

Tinctures are alcoholic or hydroalcoholic solutions prepared from vegetable materials or from chemical substances. They vary widely in their method of preparation, the strength of their active ingredient, their alcoholic content, and their intended use in medicine or pharmacy. When they are prepared from chemical substances (e.g., iodine, thimerosal, etc.) tinctures are prepared by simple solution of the chemical agent in the solvent and their concentrations vary widely. Tinctures prepared from crude vegetable drugs are termed "compound" if they are prepared by extracting more than a single drug (e.g., compound benzoin tincture, which contains the extractive from benzoin, aloe, storax and tolu balsam). There is no set strength for tinctures; they vary with the particular preparation. Depending upon the amount of soluble active constituents in a crude drug, the quantity of active constituents in the resultant tincture will vary considerably. For example, Belladonna Tincture, which is prepared by percolating belladonna leaf, contains between 0.027 and 0.033% of active constituents (the alkaloids of the leaf) in contrast to compound benzoin tincture, which contains in each 100 mL nearly all of the 24 g of solid starting material exposed to alcohol in the process of maceration.

Depending upon the preparation, tinctures contain alcohol in amounts ranging from approximately 15 to 80%. The alcoholic content protects against microbial growth and keeps the alcohol-soluble extractives in solution. In addition to alcohol, other solvents, as glycerin, may be employed. The solvent mix of each tincture is important in maintaining the integrity of the product. Tinctures cannot generally be mixed successfully with liquids too diverse in solvent character without the likelihood of inducing the precipitation of the solute. For example, compound benzoin tincture, prepared with alcohol as the sole menstruum, contains alcohol-soluble principles that are immediately expelled from solution upon the addition of water.

Because of the alcoholic content, tinctures must be tightly stoppered and not exposed to excessive temperatures. Also, because many of the constituents found in tinctures undergo a photochemical change upon exposure to light, many tinctures must be stored in light-resistant containers and protected from sunlight.

Examples of Tinctures

Medicated tinctures taken orally are becoming a thing of the past. For one thing, they are bad-tasting. A person requiring oral medication nowadays would prefer to take a tablet or capsule or a pleasant-tasting elixir or syrup. Secondly, physicians prefer to prescribe single drugs and not preparations of plant extractives which contain many plant constituents, both active and inactive. Thirdly, since tinctures generally have a rather high alcoholic content, some physicians and patients alike prefer other forms of medication.

Examples of tinctures are presented in Table 13–1.

Fluidextracts

Fluidextracts are liquid preparations of vegetable drugs, containing alcohol as a solvent or as a preservative, or both, and so made that each mL contains the therapeutic constituents of 1 g of the standard drug that it represents. Because of their concentrated nature, many fluidextracts are considered too potent to be taken safely in self-administration by the patient and their use *per se* is almost nonexistent in medical practice. Also, many fluidextracts are simply too bitter tasting or otherwise unpalatable to be accepted by the patient. Therefore, most fluidextracts today are either modified by the addition of flavoring or sweetening agents before use, or are used pharmaceutically as the drug source component of other liquid dosage forms, such as syrups.

Fluidextracts are prepared by percolation, the menstruum used in each case determined on an individual basis. The selection of the menstruum is based primarily on achieving a complete but economical extraction of the active constituents from a plant drug while keeping to a minimum the extraction of inactive materials. These inactive materials frequently have a tendency to deposit from solution upon standing, and although this does not generally affect the potency or therapeutic efficacy of the product, it does render it unsightly and pharmaceutically unattractive. To avoid this occurrence the manufacturer of a fluidextract generally permits a period of aging before final packaging to allow any insoluble material to settle out so that it may be removed by filtration before distribution.

Specific methods for the preparation of fluidextracts may be found in the third edition of this text or in other references.

Table 13–1. Examples of Tinctures

Tincture	Method of Preparation	Use and Comments
Belladonna Tincture	Percolation	Prepared from belladonna leaves with a hydroalcoholic menstruum. Contains 30 mg of belladonna alkaloids in each 100 mL. Used as an anticholinergic primarily to overcome intestinal spasm and check secretions.
Compound Benzoin Tincture	Maceration	Topical protectant. Contains benzoin, aloe, storax and tolu balsam in alcohol.
Green Soap Tincture	Solution	Topical detergent. Contains green soap, and lavender oil in alcohol.
Iodine Tincture	Solution	Topical antiinfective. Contains 2% iodine and 2.4% sodium iodide in 50% alcohol.
Opium Tincture	Percolation	Contains 1% anhydrous morphine. Alcoholic content is 17 to 21%. Tincture formerly called Laudanum. Used orally as an analgesic and antiperistaltic with a usual dose of 0.3 to 1.0 mL. Also used in the preparation of paregoric.
Paregoric	Maceration/ Solution	Analgesic and antiperistaltic with an oral dose of 5 to 10 mL one to four times daily. Preparation contains 40 mg of anhydrous morphine per 100 mL, and about 0.4% each of anise oil, camphor and benzoic acid, 4% of glycerin and about 45% of alcohol. Paregoric is also called Camphorated Opium Tincture. It is commonly used to relieve diarrhea and as an analgesic in menstrual cramps.
Thimerosal Tincture	Solution	Topical antiinfective. Contains 0.1% thimerosal in a mixture of alcohol, acetone, water, ethylenediamine and monoethanolamine. (Commercial Product: Merthiolate Tincture, Lilly).
Tolu Balsam Tincture	Maceration	Flavoring tincture. Used in the preparation of Tolu Balsam Syrup.
Vanilla Tincture	Maceration/ Percolation	Flavoring tincture prepared from vanilla, sucrose, alcohol and water.

Examples of fluidextracts are presented in Table 13–2.

Extracts

Extracts are concentrated preparations of vegetable or animal drugs obtained by removal of the active constituents of the respective drugs with suitable menstrua, evaporation of all or nearly all of the solvent, and adjustment of the residual masses or powders to the prescribed standards.

Extracts are potent preparations, usually between two and six times as potent on a weight basis as the crude drug used as the starting material. They contain primarily the active constituents of the crude drug, with a great portion of the inactive constituents and structural components of the crude drug having been removed. Their function is to provide in small amounts and in convenient, stable physical form the medicinal activity and character of the more bulky plants that they represent. As such, they have use in product formulation.

In the manufacture of most extracts, percolation is employed to remove the active constituents from the drug, with the percolates generally being reduced in volume by evaporation of the solvent by distillation under reduced pressure, the latter being used to reduce the degree of heat and to protect the drug substances against thermal decomposition. The extent of the removal of the solvent determines the final physical character of the extract. Extracts are made into three forms: (a) *semiliquid extracts* or those of a syrupy consistency prepared without the intent of removing all or even most of the menstruum, (b) *pilular* or *solid extracts* of a plastic consistency prepared with nearly all of the menstruum removed, and (c) *powdered extracts* prepared to be dry by the removal of all of the menstruum insofar as is feasible or practical. Pilular and powdered extracts differ only by the slight amount of remaining

Table 13–2. Examples of Fluidextracts and Extracts

Fluidextract or Extract	Method of Preparation	Use and Comments
Aromatic Cascara Sagrada Fluidextract	Maceration/ Percolation	Cathartic taken orally in doses of about 5 mL. Magnesium oxide is macerated with the cascara sagrada prior to percolation to neutralize and prevent the extraction of some bitter tasting principles from the drug. The preparation is sweetened with saccharin and flavored with Pure Glycyrrhiza Extract and various oils to taste like licorice.
Cascara Sagrada Fluidextract	Percolation	Bitter tasting cathartic most commonly used as the source of the cathartic principles in the preparation of other products. Fluidextract prepared with boiling water as the menstruum to extract water-soluble active constituents. Alcohol added as a preservative.
Senna Fluidextract	Percolation	Cathartic used primarily in the preparation of Senna Syrup.
Eriodictyon Fluidextract	Percolation	Flavoring fluidextract used primarily in the preparation of Aromatic Eriodictyon Syrup.
Belladonna Extract	Percolation	Belladonna extract is used in both pilular and powdered forms. Each type is required to contain about 1.25 g of belladonna alkaloids per 100 g of extract. The extract is about forty times as concentrated as the tincture of belladonna. The extract is used as the source of the alkaloids in preparing other products, particularly Belladonna Extract Tablets. These tablets commonly contain 15 mg of the extract for its anticholinergic action in reducing gastrointestinal spasms.
Cascara Sagrada Extract	Percolation	A powdered extract used primarily to prepare proprietary tablets and capsules for use as cathartics.
Pure Glycyrrhiza Extract	Percolation	A pilular extract prepared with boiling water as the menstruum. The sweet licorice taste of the extract is used to mask bitter tasting drugs, most notably in Aromatic Cascara Sagrada Fluidextract.

solvent in the former preparation, but each has its pharmaceutical advantage because of its physical form. For instance, the pilular extract is preferred in compounding a plastic dosage form such as an ointment or paste or one in which a pliable material facilitates compounding, whereas the powdered form is preferable in the compounding of such dosage forms as powders, capsules, and tablets.

Examples of extracts are presented in Table 13–2.

Aromatic Waters[1]

Aromatic waters are clear, aqueous solutions generally saturated with volatile oils or other aromatic or volatile substances. Aromatic waters are no longer in widespread use. In years past, aromatic waters were prepared from a number of volatile substances including the following: orange flower oil, peppermint oil, rose oil, anise oil, spearmint oil, wintergreen oil, camphor and chloroform. Naturally, the odors

and tastes of aromatic waters are of the volatile substances from which they are prepared. The aromatic waters most recently official in the USP/NF are those of orange flower, rose and peppermint.

Most of the aromatic substances in the preparation of aromatic waters have very low solubilities in water, and even though a water may be saturated, its concentration of aromatic material is still rather small. Aromatic waters may be used for perfuming and/or flavoring.

Diluted Acids

Diluted acids are aqueous solutions prepared by diluting the corresponding concentrated acids with purified water. The strength of a diluted acid is generally expressed on a per cent weight-to-volume (% w/v) basis, that is, the weight in grams of solute per 100 mL of solution, whereas the strength of a concentrated acid is generally expressed in terms of per cent weight-to-weight (% w/w), which indicates the number of grams of solute per 100 g of solution. In order to prepare a diluted acid from a concentrated one, it is first necessary to calculate the amount of solute required in the diluted product. Then, the amount of concentrated acid required to supply the needed amount of solute can be determined.

To illustrate, concentrated hydrochloric acid, contains not less than 35 g and not more than 38 g of solute (absolute HCl) per 100 g of acid and therefore is considered to be, on the average, 36.5% w/w in strength. Diluted hydrochloric acid contains between 9.5 and 10.5 g of solute per 100 mL of solution and is therefore considered to be approximately 10% w/v in strength. If, for example, one wished to prepare 100 mL of the diluted acid from the concentrated acid, he would require 10 g of solute. The amount of concentrated hydrochloric acid required to supply this amount of solute may be calculated by the following proportion:

$$\frac{36.5 \text{ g (solute)}}{100 \text{ g (conc. acid)}} = \frac{10 \text{ g (solute)}}{x \text{ (g conc. acid)}}$$

solving for x:

$$36.5x = 1000 \text{ g}$$
$$x = 27.39 \text{ g (conc. acid)}$$

Thus, 27.39 g of concentrated acid are required to supply 10 g of solute needed for the preparation of 100 mL of the diluted acid. Although the required amount of concentrated acid may be accurately weighed, it is a cumbersome task, and as a rule pharmacists prefer to measure liquids volumetrically. Therefore, in the preparation of diluted acids, the calculations are generally carried one step further to determine the *volume* of concentrated acid that corresponds with the calculated weight. Because this additional step requires the use of the concentrated acid's specific gravity, a brief review of specific gravity seems appropriate.

By definition, specific gravity is a ratio, expressed decimally, of the weight of a substance to the weight of an equal volume of a standard, both substances having the same temperature or the temperature of each being known. Water is used as the standard for liquids and solids; hydrogen or air, for gases. In pharmacy, specific gravity calculations mainly involve liquids and solids, and water is an excellent choice for a standard, because it is readily available and easily purified.

At 4°C, the density of water is 1 g per cubic centimeter (cc). Because the USP states that 1 mL may be considered the equivalent of 1 cc, in pharmacy, water is assumed to weigh 1 g per mL. By the following equation, used to calculate specific gravity, a substance having a density the same as water would have a specific gravity of 1.0:

$$\text{sp gr} = \frac{\text{weight of a substance}}{\text{weight of an equal volume of water}}$$

In solving this equation, the same units of weight must be used in each part of the ratio. These units cancel out, and the ratio is expressed decimally.

Specific gravity indicates the relative weight of a substance compared to an equal volume of water. For example, if 10 mL of a liquid weigh 20 g, an equal volume of water would weigh 10 g, and the ratio in the equation would be 20 g/10 g yielding a specific gravity of 2.0. This would indicate that the liquid is twice as heavy as water in equal volume. By the same token, a liquid having a specific gravity of 0.5 would be half as heavy as water; a liquid with a specific gravity of 0.8 would be eight-tenths as heavy as water, etc.

If both the volume of a liquid and its specific gravity are known, its weight may be calculated. For instance, if concentrated hydrochloric acid has a specific gravity of 1.17, it is that number times as heavy as water, and 100 mL of the acid would weigh 1.17 times as much as 100 mL of water. Since 100 mL of water weigh 100 g, 100 mL of the acid would weigh 1.17 times that or 117 g.

If one knows the weight of a liquid and its specific gravity, the volume of the liquid may be determined. For example, a liquid that is twice as heavy as water would have a specific gravity of 2.0 and would occupy half the volume that an equal weight of water would occupy. If one had 100 g of this liquid and substituted in the above equation as indicated below, the volume of the liquid could be arrived at:

$$2.0 = \frac{100 \text{ g}}{\text{weight of an equal volume of water}}$$

$$\text{weight of an equal volume of water} = \frac{100 \text{ g}}{2.0}$$
$$= 50 \text{ g}$$

Since 50 g is the weight of an equal volume of water, it follows that the water must measure 50 mL. Since the volume of the water is an "equal volume" to the other liquid, that liquid must also measure 50 mL.

The volume represented by 27.39 g of the concentrated hydrochloric acid may be similarly determined by dividing the specific gravity of the concentrated acid into its weight and equating the answer of weight of an equal volume of water to the volume of the acid:

$$\frac{27.39 \text{ g}}{1.17} = 23.41 \text{ g, weight of equal volume of water.}$$

Thus, because 23.41 g of water measures 23.41 mL and because it is equal in volume to the concentrated acid, the latter also measures 23.41 mL and would be required to prepare 100 mL of the 10% w/v diluted acid.

Once the aforementioned is thoroughly understood, the following simplified formula can be used to calculate the amount of a concentrated acid required in the preparation of a specific volume of the corresponding diluted acid:

$$\frac{\text{Percentage strength (w/v) of diluted acid} \times \text{Volume of diluted acid to be prepared}}{\text{Percentage strength (w/w) of concentrated acid} \times \text{Specific gravity of concentrated acid}}$$

= Volume of concentrated acid to use

Recalculating the preparation of 100 mL of diluted hydrochloric acid from the concentrated acid gives the following:

$$\frac{10 \times 100 \text{ mL}}{36.5 \times 1.17} = 23.41 \text{ mL of concentrated acid to use.}$$

Most diluted acids have a strength of 10% w/v, with the exception of diluted acetic acid which is 6% w/v. The strengths of these acids are commensurate with the concentrations generally used for medicinal or pharmaceutical purposes. The concentrations of the corresponding concentrated acids vary widely from one acid to another, depending upon various properties of the solute such as solubility, stability, and ease of preparation. For instance, concentrated sulfuric acid is generally between 95 and 98% w/w, nitric acid between 69 and 71% w/w, and concentrated phosphoric acid between 85 and 88% w/w. As a result, the amounts of each concentrated acid required to prepare the corresponding diluted acid vary widely and must be calculated on an individual basis.

Examples of Diluted Acids

Diluted Acetic Acid

Diluted acetic acid is an aqueous solution containing approximately 6% of CH_3COOH. It is prepared by diluting either acetic acid, approximately a 36.5% acid, or the more concentrated glacial acetic acid, which is not less than 99.4% in strength and which is itself diluted to prepare the acetic acid. Glacial acetic acid is so named because of its solid glassy appearance when congealed, an event that occurs at various temperatures depending upon the concentration of the acid. For example, an acid of 99.4% strength will congeal at a temperature of 15.47°C, whereas acids of a lesser concentration will require colder temperatures to reach their congealing points. Diluted acetic acid is used as a pharmaceutical aid (solvent). Medicinally, acetic acid is bactericidal to many types of microorganisms and finds application in 1% solutions in surgical dressings, as an irrigating solution to the bladder in 0.25% concentration, and also as a spermatocidal in some proprietary contraceptive preparations. The concentrated acids are useful to the pharmaceutical chemist in the preparation of acetate salts and esters of numerous drugs.

Diluted Hydrochloric Acid

Diluted hydrochloric acid is a 10% solution of HCl prepared by adding 234 mL of the concentrated acid (about 36.5% w/w) with a sufficient amount of purified water to make a liter of solution. The concentrated acid was first prepared commercially by distilling sea salt with sulfuric acid, and for this reason, it has become widely known as muriatic acid, a name derived from the Latin *murea* for salt and meaning the acid from salt. The diluted acid has been used medicinally in the treatment of achlorhydria, a condition generally associated with pernicious anemia and characterized by failure of the gastric secretion to produce gastric acid. The diluted acid is categorized as a pharmaceutic aid (acidifying agent).

Diluted Phosphoric Acid

Diluted phosphoric acid is a 10% preparation of H_3PO_4 made by diluting the concentrated acid (about 85 to 88% w/w). The concentrated phosphoric acid is a rather heavy liquid with a specific gravity of 1.71 and a syrupy consistency, which is responsible for its synonym, "syrupy phosphoric acid." Both the diluted and the concentrated acids are mainly pharmaceutical necessities as chemical reagents and in the preparation of various phosphate salts.

Spirits[1]

Spirits are alcoholic or hydroalcoholic solutions of volatile substances. Generally, the alcoholic concentration of spirits is rather high, usually over 60%. Because of the greater solubility of aromatic or volatile substances in alcohol than in water, spirits can contain a greater concentration of these materials than the corresponding aromatic waters. When mixed with water or with an aqueous preparation, the volatile substances present in spirits generally separate from solution and form a milky preparation.

Spirits may be employed pharmaceutically as flavoring agents and medicinally for the therapeutic value of the aromatic solute. As flavoring agents they are used to impart the flavor of their solute to other pharmaceutical preparations. For medicinal purposes, spirits may be taken orally, applied externally, or used by inhalation, depending upon the particular preparation. When taken orally, they are generally mixed with a portion of water to reduce the pungency of the spirit. Depending upon the materials utilized, spirits may be prepared by simple solution, solution by maceration, or distillation. The spirits most recently official in the USP/NF were aromatic ammonia spirit, camphor spirit, compound orange spirit, and peppermint spirit.

Effervescent Salts

Effervescent salts, as previously defined in Chapter 5, are prepared by two general methods: (1) the *wet method,* and (2) the *dry or fusion method.* Irrespective of the method used, the initial step is the determination of the proper formula for the preparation that will result in effective effervescence, efficient utilization of the acids and base present, a stable granulation, and a pleasant tasting and efficacious product.

Effervescent salts are usually prepared from a combination of citric and tartaric acids rather than from a single acid because the use of either acid alone presents difficulties. When tartaric acid is the sole acid, the resulting granules lose their firmness readily and crumble. Citric acid alone results in a sticky mixture difficult to granulate. Granulation is due to the presence of one molecule of water of crystallization in each molecule of citric acid, a feature that is taken advantage of and utilized in the preparation of granules by the fusion method using the combination of acids and sodium bicarbonate. Although the proportion of acids may be varied, so long as the total acidity is maintained and the bicarbonate completely neutralized, a general guideline of usual proportions of these materials can be shown from the formula of the only remaining official effervescent salt, Effervescent Sodium Phosphate, USP. The formula for this preparation is as follows:

Dried Dibasic Sodium Phosphate,
    dried and powdered . . . . 200 g
Sodium Bicarbonate, in dry powder . . . 477 g
Tartaric Acid, in dry powder . . . . 252 g
Citric Acid, monohydrate . . . . 162 g
    To make about   1000 g

From this formula it can be observed that of the effervescence-producing agents, about 53% of the mixture is sodium bicarbonate, 28% is tartaric acid, and about 19% is citric acid. The reactions between citric and sodium bicarbonate (1) and tartaric acid and sodium bicarbonate (2) may be shown as follows:

(1) $\underset{\text{citric acid}}{H_3C_6H_5O_7 \cdot H_2O} + \underset{\text{sodium bicarbonate}}{3NaHCO_3} \rightarrow$

$\underset{\text{sodium citrate}}{Na_3C_6H_5O_7} + \underset{\text{water}}{4H_2O} + \underset{\text{carbon dioxide}}{3CO_2}$

(2) $\underset{\text{tartaric acid}}{H_2C_4H_4O_6} + \underset{\text{sodium bicarbonate}}{2NaHCO_3} \rightarrow$

$\underset{\text{sodium tartrate}}{Na_2C_4H_4O_6} + \underset{\text{water}}{2H_2O} + \underset{\text{carbon dioxide}}{2CO_2}$

It should be noted that it requires 3 molecules of sodium bicarbonate to neutralize 1 molecule of citric acid (1) and 2 molecules of sodium bicarbonate to neutralize 1 molecule of tartaric acid (2). In preparing a pharmaceutical formula of an effervescent salt from these components, one can determine the precise amounts of reactants to employ. For instance, using the official formula for Effervescent Sodium Phosphate, USP, one can calculate from information of the above reactions and the molecular weights of the three reactants the amount of sodium bicarbonate required to neutralize 252 g of tartaric acid and 162 g of uneffloresced citric acid:

(1) For the amount of sodium bicarbonate required to neutralize 162 g of citric acid:

$$\frac{162 \text{ g citric acid}}{210.13 \text{ g m.w. citric acid}}$$

$$= \frac{\times \text{ g sodium bicarbonate}}{(252.03 \text{ g m.w. sodium bicarbonate}}$$
(84.01) times 3 (molecules)
x = *194.3 g of sodium bicarbonate*

(2) For the amount of sodium bicarbonate required to neutralize 252 g of tartaric acid:

$$\frac{252 \text{ g tartaric acid}}{150.09 \text{ g m.w. tartaric acid}}$$

$$= \frac{\times \text{ g sodium bicarbonate}}{168.02 \text{ g m.w. sodium bicarbonate}}$$
(84.01) times 2 (molecules)
x = *282.1 g of sodium bicarbonate*
Total: 194.3 + 282.1
= *476.4 g of sodium bicarbonate*

The amount of medicinal agent in effervescent preparations is determined by the intended dose of the medication. Generally the dose of the drug is contained in a teaspoonful or two of the dry effervescent salt. After the formula has been determined, the powders are uniformly mixed, being certain that the powders are dry to avoid premature chemical reaction. Then the granules are prepared.

FUSION METHOD. In the fusion method, the one molecule of water present in each molecule of citric acid acts as the binding agent for the powder mixture. Just before mixing the powders, the citric acid crystals are powdered and then mixed with the other powders (previously passed through a number 60 sieve) to ensure uniformity of the mixture. The sieves and the mixing equipment should be made of stainless steel or other material resistant to the effect of the acids. The mixing of the powders is performed as rapidly as is practical, preferably in an environment of low humidity to avoid the absorption of moisture from the air by the chemicals and a premature chemical reaction. After mixing, the powder is placed on a plate or glass or a suitable dish in an oven (or other suitable source of heat) previously heated to between 93°F and 104°F. During the heating process, an acid-resistant spatula is used to turn the powder. The heat causes the release of the water of crystallization from the citric acid, which in turn dissolves a portion of the powder mixture, setting of the chemical reaction and the consequent release of some carbon dioxide. This causes the softened mass of powder to become somewhat spongy, and when of the proper consistency (as bread dough), it is removed from the oven and rubbed through an acid-resistant sieve to produce granules of the desired size. A No. 4 sieve may be used to produce large granules, a No. 8 sieve to produce medium size granules, and a No. 10 sieve to prepare small granules. When all of the mass has passed through the sieve, the granules are immediately dried at a temperature not exceeding 54° and immediately transferred to containers which are then promptly and tightly sealed.

The fusion method is used in the preparation of most commercial effervescent powders and in the preparation of the official Effervescent Sodium Phosphate, USP.

WET METHOD. The wet method differs from the fusion method in that the source of binding agent is not necessarily the water of crystallization from the citric acid but may be water added to the nonsolvent (such as alcohol), which is employed as the moistening agent, to form the pliable mass of material for granulation. In this method all of the powders may be anhydrous so long as water is added to the moistening liquid. Just enough liquid is added (in portions) to prepare a mass of proper consistency; then the granules are prepared and dried in the same manner as described above.

Divided Powders

Divided powders, as previously defined in Chapter 5, are prepared as follows.

Depending upon the potency of the drug substance, the pharmacist decides whether to weigh each portion of powder separately before enfolding in a paper or to approximate each portion by using the so-called *block-and-divide method*. By this method, used only for nonpotent drugs, the pharmacist places the entire amount of prepared powder on a flat surface such as a porcelain or glass plate or pill tile or a large sheet of paper on the prescription counter and with a large spatula forms a rectangular or square-shaped block of powder having a uniform depth. Then, using the spatula, he partially cuts into the powder vertically and horizontally to delineate the appropriate number of smaller, uniform blocks, each representing a dose or unit of medication. Each of the smaller blocks is then separated from the main block with the spatula and transferred to a powder paper and wrapped.

The powder papers may be of any convenient size to hold the amount of powder issued, but the most popular sizes are commercially available and include 2¾ × 3¾ inches, 3 × 4½ inches, 3¾ × 5 inches, and 4½ × 6 inches. The papers may be (1) simple bond paper, white or colored; (2) vegetable parchment, a thin, semiopaque paper having limited moisture-resistant qualities; (3) glassine, a glazed, transparent paper, also having limited moisture-resistant qualities; and (4) waxed paper, a transparent, waterproof paper. The selection of the type of paper is based primarily on the nature of the powder. If the powder contains hygroscopic or deliquescent materials, a waterproof or a waxed paper should be used. In practice, such powders are double-wrapped in waxed paper, and then for aesthetic appeal they are finally wrapped in bond paper. Glassine and vegetable parchment papers may be used when only a limited barrier against moisture is necessary. Powders containing volatile components should be wrapped in waxed or in glassine papers. Powders containing neither volatile components nor ingredients adversely affected by air or moisture are usually wrapped in white bond paper.

A certain degree of expertise is required in the folding of a powder paper, and the student should practice until he becomes proficient at preparing neat and uniform papers. Basically the steps in the folding of a powder paper are as follows:

1. Place the paper flat on a hard surface and fold toward you a uniform flap of about ½ inch of the long side of the paper. To ensure uniformity of all of the papers, this step should be performed on all the required papers concurrently, using the first folded paper as the guide (Fig. 13–2A).
2. With the flap of each paper away from you and pointing upward, place the weighed or divided amount of powder in the center of each paper.
3. Being careful not to disturb the powder excessively, bring the lower edge of the paper upward, and place it proximate to the crease of the flap (Fig. 13–2B).
4. Grasp the flap, press it down upon the tucked-in bottom edge of the paper and fold again toward you an amount of paper equal to the size of the original flap (½ inch) (Fig. 13–2C).
5. Pick the paper up with the flap upward and facing you, being careful not to disturb the position of the powder, and place the partially folded paper over the open powder box (to serve as the container) so that the ends of the paper extend equally beyond the sides (lengthwise) of the open container. Then, press the sides of the box slightly inward and the ends of the paper gently downward along the sides of the box to form a crease on each end of the paper. Lift the paper from the box and fold the ends of the paper along each crease sharply so that the powder cannot escape (Fig. 13–2D).
6. The folded papers are then each placed in the box so that the double-folded flaps are at the top, facing the operator, and the ends are folded away from the operator (Fig. 13–2E).

Papers folded properly should fit snugly in the box, have uniform folds, and should be of uniform length and height. There should be no powder in the folds, and none should be capable of escape with moderate agitation. Powder boxes, which are generally pasteboard and of the hinged type, should close easily without coming in contact with the tops of the papers. The label for the powders may be placed on the container, but some pharmacists affix a label of directions to each individual paper.

For convenience and uniformity of appearance, some pharmacists use commercially available cellophane or plastic envelopes to enclose individual doses or units of powders rather than folding individual papers. These envelopes are usually moisture resistant, and their use results in handsome and efficacious products.

Fig. 13–2. *Steps in the folding of powder papers.*

Molded Tablet Triturates

Molded tablet triturates, as previously defined in Chapter 5, are prepared as follows.

The Mold

The mold used in the preparation of molded tablets is usually made of hard rubber, metal, or a hard plastic composition, and it consists of two parts, the upper part, or the *die* portion, and the lower part containing the squat, flat punches. The die portion is simply a plate of the thickness of the desired tablets and generally having from 50 to 200 uniformly drilled and spaced circular holes (Fig. 13–3). The lower part of the mold contains punches corresponding in number, position, and diameter with the holes of the die. When the two parts of the mold are joined, the punches fit precisely in the holes of the upper plate. When the die is filled with the material to be tableted and the die is placed upon the lower portion of the mold, the punches gently lift the fill material from the holes to rest openly on the flat punches for drying. In assembling the two parts of the mold,

the pharmacist must make certain that the upper plate is right side up and facing in the proper direction in order that the punches may be properly directed and fit snugly in the holes. To assist the pharmacist, the mold manufacturers generally make the two parts of the mold each with one slightly rounded end and one squared end which are each placed in the same direction when the two parts are joined. The upper plate also usually bears a number which corresponds to the number of the bottom of the mold to identify the two parts as a unit. In positioning the upper plate, the number usually faces upwards for the proper fit on the punches.

Preparing the Tablet Formulation for Molding

The base for tablet triturates is generally a mixture of finely powdered lactose alone or in combination with an amount of powdered sucrose varying from about 5 to 20% of the base. The addition of sucrose results in the production of tablets that are less brittle than when lactose alone is employed. The greater the proportion of sucrose added, the harder will be the

Fig. 13–3.   *A tablet triturate mold.*

resulting tablet triturates. To the base is added the amount of drug substance required to prepare the desired number of tablets of the desired drug strength. It should be pointed out that the medicinal agent is generally added to the base by geometric dilution, since the drug is generally a potent substance.

The molding of the tablets is effected by the solvent action of a liquid *excipient* used to moisten the powder mixture preparative to molding. The excipient is usually a mixture of alcohol and water in equal proportions. The water portion of the excipient exerts the solvent action on a portion of the base, effecting the binding action on drying. The alcoholic portion of the excipient speeds the drying process. If a large proportion of the powder formulation is very rapidly soluble in water, it is usually desirable to use an excipient of a greater alcoholic content than the mixutre described above. Care must also be exercised in selecting the proper excipient with respect to chemical interaction or drug destruction (as from hydrolysis) due to an interaction between a part of the excipient and the drug. For drugs adversely affected by alcohol, the alcoholic content of the excipient must therefore be reduced or eliminated. Similarly, for drugs adversely affected by water, an excipient of

greater than usual alcoholic strength may be preferred.

The amount of excipient used to dampen the powder mixture is largely determined by experience, but it may be said that the powder mixture should be damp but not wet. The particles of powder should have the tendency to cling together when pressed slightly between the fingers.

The moistened powder is added to the mold by placing the upper part of the mold flatly on a glass or porcelain plate and forcing the moistened material into the openings of the mold by a rubbing motion with a steel spatula. The spatula should be moved so that the fill in each opening is complete and flat with the surface. The underside of the mold should be inspected to make certain that the fill is complete on that side also. It is permissible to work both sides with the spatula until the mold is evenly and completely filled. After the mold has been filled, it is placed upon the lower punch of the mold, and the tablets are ejected for drying.

Standardizing the Mold

Since the upper plate of the mold is capable of holding different weights of materials depending upon the densities of the materials, each mold must be "standardized" by the pharmacist in terms of weight for each formulation that is molded into tablets. It is advisable for him to maintain a record of such standardizations for each mold so that they need not be repeated the next time the same formula is prepared into tablets. Although several methods for standardizing the mold have been presented, perhaps the most efficient in terms of preparing the proper amount to fill completely all of the perforations with the proper amount of drug and base is the following method:

1. Weigh the proper amount of medicinal substance for the preparation of the desired number of tablets which corresponds to the number of openings in the mold.
2. Mix the medicinal substance with an amount of base known to be insufficient to fill the mold completely.
3. Moisten the mixture and place it in the openings as far as it will go, spending little time trying to achieve uniform distribution.
4. Moisten an additional amount of base (with no medicinal agent present) and use this to finish filling the mold, being careful not to remove any of the medicated base from the openings.
5. Punch out the tablets, remove them from the punches, and remix thoroughly to obtain a uniform distribution of the medicinal substance.
6. Refill the mold with the thoroughly blended mixture and punch out the tablets and allow them to dry.

The final weight of the dry tablets should be taken and recorded as the standard weight for that mold for that particular formulation. On the next occasion that formulation is prepared, the identical mold and same formula may be employed. This of course assumes that the same degree of manual pressure is used in each occasion in packing the mold.

Radiopharmaceuticals

A *radiopharmaceutical* is a chemical containing a radioactive isotope for use in humans for the purpose of diagnosis, mitigation, or treatment of a disease. It should be recalled from general chemistry that substances that have the same number of protons but have varying numbers of neutrons are called *isotopes*. Isotopes may be stable or unstable; those that are unstable are radioactive because their nuclei undergo a re-arrangement while changing to a stable state, and energy is given off.

All of the atoms of an unstable isotope do not completely rearrange at the same instant. The time required for a radioisotope to decay to 50% of its original activity is termed its radioactive half-life. Isotopes vary widely in their half-life; carbon-14 has a radioactive half-life of some 5730 years, whereas that for sodium-24 is only 15 hours.

The activity of a radioactive material is expressed as the number of nuclear transformations per unit time. The fundamental unit of radioactivity is the *curie* (Ci), defined as 3.700×10^{10} nuclear transformations per second. The *millicurie* (mCi), *microcurie* (μCi), and *nanocurie* (nCi) are commonly used subunits:

$$1 \text{ millicurie} = 10^{-3} \text{ curie}$$

$$1 \text{ microcurie} = 10^{-6} \text{ curie}$$

$$1 \text{ nanocurie} = 10^{-9} \text{ curie}$$

The Becquerel is the international unit of radioactivity and is equal to one disintegration per second, i.e., 1 mCi = 37 MBq. The amount of radiation absorbed by body tissue in which a radioactive substance resides is called the "radiation dose." Traditionally, this is measured in units of rads (i.e., radiation *a*bsorbed *d*ose): 1 rad = 100 ergs of energy absorbed by 1 g of tissue. The Gray is the international unit of absorbed dose and equal to 1 joule of energy absorbed in 1 kg of tissue (i.e., 1 Gy = 100 rads).

The three types of radiation most frequently emitted from radioactive nuclei are *alpha, beta,* and *gamma* radiations. Alpha particles, which constitute alpha radiation, consist of two protons and two neutrons, thus being identical with the helium nucleus. As an alpha particle loses energy, its velocity decreases. It then attracts electrons and becomes a helium atom. Most alpha particles are unable to pierce the outer layers of skin or penetrate a thin piece of paper. Beta particles may be either electrons with negative charge, *negatrons,* or positive electrons, *positrons.* These two particles, β- and β+ have a range of over 10 feet in air and up to about 1 mm in tissue. Nuclear medicine depends mostly on radiopharmaceuticals that decay by gamma (γ) emission. Gamma rays are electromagnetic vibrations comparable with light but of much shorter wavelength. Because of their short wavelength and high energy, they are very penetrating.

The optimum dosage of radiopharmaceuticals is that which allows the acquisition of the desired information with the least amount of radiation dose or exposure to the patient. Thus, the clinical utility of a radiopharmaceutical is determined by the radionuclide's physical properties (e.g., radiation, energy, half life). Thus, the best diagnostic images at the lowest radiation dose are attained if the radionuclide has a short half-life and emits only gamma radiation of low energy. Technetium-99m is a prime example of a radionuclide with these properties. Its half life is 6 hours and gamma emission is of the nature of 140 keV, efficiently detected by the gamma camera. For therapeutic use, however, radionuclides should emit particulate radiation (i.e., beta particles), which deposits the radiation within the target organ. Iodine-131 is a prime example and used for hyperthyroidism and eradication of metastatic disease of the thyroid gland. But because iodine-131 emits both beta and gamma radiation, it can be used diagnostically (gamma rays) and therapeutically (beta rays).

The majority of radiopharmaceuticals are produced by the process of nuclear activation in a nuclear reactor. In such a reactor, stable atoms are bombarded with excess neutrons present in the rector. The resulting neutron additions to the stable atoms produce unstable atoms and radioactive isotopes. The facilities for the production, use, and storage of radioactive pharmaceuticals are subject to licensing by the Nuclear Regulatory Commission, or in certain instances to appropriate state agencies. As for all pharmaceuticals, the Federal Food and Drug Administration enforces strict adherence to good manufacturing practice and proper labeling and use of the products. The Federal Department of Transportation regulates the conditions of shipment of the radiopharmaceuticals, as do state and local agencies.

Radiopharmaceuticals are used to diagnose the presence of disease or evaluate the progression of disease following specific therapy intervention. Radiopharmaceuticals can also be used to evaluate drug-induced toxicity, and to a less extent have been utilized to treat diseased tissue with radiation.

The distribution pattern of radiopharmaceuticals can be used for imaging purposes to attain diagnostic information about organs or various body systems. Imaging procedures are classified either as *dynamic* or *static*. The dynamic study provides useful information through the rate of accumulation and removal of the radiopharmaceutical from a specific organ. A static study merely provides morphological information, i.e., organ size, shape, position, presence of space occupying lesions.

Every radiopharmaceutical is formulated with the intent to localize it within a target organ. Sodium iodide, I-131, is actively taken up by thyroid cells following its absorption into the bloodstream after oral administration from either a capsule or a solution dosage form. The extent of the uptake of the dose by the gland helps assess thyroid function, or an image of the gland can be obtained after administration to visualize, i.e., static imaging, thyroid morphology. Alternatively, if I-131 is labeled to orthoiodohippuric acid and intravenously injected, kidney tubules will actively secrete this agent into urine. Measuring the time course of activity over the kidney with a gamma camera and plotting the rate of radioactivity accumulation and removal *versus* time, yields a measure of kidney function. Such a dynamic study is termed a *renogram,* a particularly useful procedure to assess renal function in patients with transplanted kidneys.

Radiopharmaceuticals also are useful to evaluate a patient's response to drug therapy and surgery. These agents can detect early changes in physiologic function which come before morphologic or biochemical endpoints. An example is perfusion lung imaging using Tc-99 macroaggregated albumin particles to detect pulmonary embolism. Once the embolism is confirmed and thrombolytic and/or anticoagulant therapy initiated, this lung perfusing agent can be readministered to evaluate its resolution with drug therapy. Cardiac radionuclide ventriculograms utilizing Tc-99m labeled red blood cells are performed to assess left ventricular function (e.g., ejection fraction, regional wall motion) to evaluate the effect of surgery (e.g., coronary artery bypass graft, valve repair) or the response to drug therapy (e.g., beta-blocking agents, calcium channel blocking agents).

Radiopharmaceuticals also find utility to help monitor drug therapy inclusive of toxicity. For example, the ability of doxorubicin to cause irreversible drug-induced heart failure is well known and the cumulative dosage of this drug should not exceed 550 mg/m^2. Because there is much variability in the individual response to this drug, serial determinations of left ventricular ejection fraction using Tc-99m radiopharmaceuticals are useful to determine on an individual basis the risk of developing doxorubicin-induced heart failure.

To a limited degree, radiopharmaceuticals can be used therapeutically. Thyroid disease can be treated with sodium iodide, I-131, polycythemia vera can be treated with sodium phosphate, P-32, and peritoneal effusions can be treated with chromic phosphate, P-32. The intent is to use the beta radiation of the radiopharmaceutical to selectively destroy diseased tissue in which it resides. Thus, a minimum, sufficient dosage must be administered. In the case of I-131, the therapeutic dosage is between 1000 to 10000 times greater than the diagnostic dosage used to assess organ function. The major indications for radioiodine therapy include hyperthyroidism (e.g., diffuse toxic goiter [Graves' disease], toxic multinodular goiter) and eradication of metastatic disease (i.e., thyroid cancer).

At present radiolabeled antibodies are being investigated for the diagnosis and treatment of cancer. There are a group of scientists who envision monoclonal antibodies as the "magic bullets" or "guided missiles" that will bring the detection and treatment mechanisms necessary to make the next significant advancement in the management of many types of cancer. Many current modalities lack the specificity for tumor cells, but monoclonal antibodies have the potential to provide the targeting of tumor cells.

Two new areas of nuclear medicine are emerging, i.e., detection of disease localization, treatment, using monoclonal antibody technology. Radioimmunodetection (RID) and radioimmunoguided surgery (RIGS) are used to identify the tumor externally and during surgery to enhance complete removal of the cancer and improve patient prognosis. Radioimmunodetection involves external imaging of the distribution of the radiolabeled antibodies.

Radiopharmaceuticals

Examples of some radiopharmaceuticals are presented below. The category for each indicates the types of cells or tissues for which the isotope has an affinity.

Cyanocobalamin Co 57 Capsules—Diagnostic aid (pernicious anemia)

Iodinated I 125 Serum Albumin Injection—

Diagnostic aid (blood volume determination)

Iodohippurate Sodium I 131 Injection—Diagnostic aid (renal function)

Sodium Chromate Cr 51 Injection—Diagnostic aid (blood volume determination)

Sodium Iodide I 131 Capsules—Diagnostic aid (thyroid function); thyroid inhibitor

Sodium Iodide I 131 Solution—Diagnostic aid (thyroid function); thyroid inhibitor

Sodium Pertechnetate Tc 99m Injection—Diagnostic aid (brain scanning; thyroid scanning)

Sodium Phosphate P 32 Solution—Antipolycythemic; diagnostic aid (ocular tumor localization)

Technetium Tc 99m Albumin Aggregated Injection—Diagnostic aid (lung scanning)

Technetium Tc 99m Sulfur Colloid Injection—Diagnostic aid (liver scanning)

Technetium Tc-99m labeled red blood cells—Diagnostic aid (cardiac blood pool imaging)

Technetium Tc-99m methylene diphosphonate (MDP)—Diagnostic aid (bone imaging)

Technetium Tc-99m pyrophosphate (PYP)—Diagnostic aid (cardiac infarct imaging)

Technetium Tc-99m sulfur colloid cooked in scrambled eggs—Diagnostic aid (gastric emptying imaging)

Positron Emission Tomography

An interesting new area within nuclear pharmacy is positron emission tomography (PET). It is a method for quantitative imaging of regional function and chemical reactions within various organs of the living human body. Basically, this procedure allows the physician and pharmacist to obtain a patient image that is essentially a low-resolution "autoradiograph" showing the regional concentration of a positron-emitting nuclide inside of the living body. In fact no other technology can image body chemistry with such sensitivity, so that the moment-to-moment change in concentration of a tracer in the blood or tissue can be determined in absolute units. Other imaging modalities, such as x ray computed tomography (CT) and magnetic resonance imaging (MRI), provide predominantly anatomic information. CT scanning is based on the portrayal of the distribution of attenuation of x rays passing through the body. MRI exploits the variation in regional concentrations of hydrogen and nuclear relaxation parameters to generate image contrast and to provide information about free water content, relative blood flow and the concentration of contrast agents.

Chemical changes occur prior to anatomic changes in most disease states, and PET offers the advantage of being capable to detect functional abnormalities before anatomic changes have occurred. It has already been introduced in epilepsy, Huntington's disease, cerebrovascular disease, coronary artery disease and recently as a means to assess estrogen receptors in primary and metastatic breast cancers. In epilepsy, PET and surface electroencephalography (EEG) are used in concert with clinical assessment of symptoms and signs to try to localize areas of the brain that are the foci of epileptic seizures when surgical intervention is the only remaining method to prevent the seizures.

In tissue, a positron travels only about 1 mm before it encounters a negative electron. Their interaction results in the simultaneous emission of two photons, each having a specific energy and emitted at an angle of exactly 180° from each other. Thus, if two scintillation detectors are placed, one on either side of the tissue in which the isotope is located, and detectors connected to a coincident circuit which provides an output only when a certain level of gamma ray radiation can be simultaneously detected by both, the result is a low background detector, highly specific for the particular isotope used and also giving excellent resolution.

The major production source of isotopes for PET are in-house cyclotrons, a very expensive proposition. Thus, PET is conducted primarily in large medical centers. Another consideration is that PET nuclides have short half lives (e.g., 2 to 20 minutes) which makes their availability from commercial sources almost nonexistent. By the time the nuclear pharmacist would receive the nuclide it would already be gone. Out of necessity the production facility must be on site and after rapid synthesis, the pharmaceutical needs to be purified. Thus, research at present focuses upon noncyclotron, e.g., radionuclide generators, sources of PET nuclides that would allow PET technology in community-based nuclear medicine/pharmacy environments.

It is anticipated that studies of new drug en-

tities in the future will include pharmacokinetic determination using PET technology. Further, PET will allow the manufacturer actually to quantify how much of the drug reaches a specific drug receptor. Thus, comparative PET studies will shed light on which drug, for example, within a therapeutic category attains the most optimal distribution and concentration at the intended receptor site. It is also conceivable that PET technology will open new vistas for the interpretation of drug interactions, particularly where there is competition by two drugs for one receptor site.

The following is an abbreviated listing of some positron-emitting radiopharmaceuticals used for common PET imaging procedures:

[^{15}O]-O$_2$—Cerebral oxygen extraction and metabolism
[^{11}C]-n-butanol—Cerebral blood flow
[^{11}C]-glucose—Cerebral glucose metabolism
[^{13}N]-ammonia—Cerebral and myocardial blood flow
[^{18}F]-fluorodeoxyglucose—Cerebral and myocardial glucose metabolism
[^{18}F]-16-alpha-fluoro-17-beta-estradiol—Estrogen receptor binding
[^{68}Ga]-citrate/transferrin—Plasma volume

The Practice of Nuclear Pharmacy

Nuclear pharmacy is a patient-oriented service that embodies the scientific knowledge and professional judgment required to improve and promote health through the assurance of the safe and efficacious use of radioactive drugs for diagnosis and therapy. The pharmacist is expected to understand nuclear medicine procedures, their advantages and disadvantages, when used for diagnostic or therapeutic purposes. The practice is composed of the following general areas: the procurement of radiopharmaceuticals, the compounding of radiopharmaceuticals, the performance of routine quality control procedures, the dispensing and distribution of radiopharmaceuticals, the implementation of basic radiation protection procedures and practices, the consultation and education to the nuclear medicine community, e.g., patients, health professionals, general public, and research and development of new formulations.

In a typical nuclear pharmacy environment the daily routine of the nuclear pharmacist begins with the elution of the Technetium Tc-99m generator, preparation of Tc-99m labeled radiopharmaceuticals for the day's studies, performing quality control tests on these agents and on radiation measuring instruments and receiving prepared radiopharmaceuticals from commercial manufacturers. Because most radiopharmaceuticals are administered intravenously, the nuclear pharmacist must also take precaution to ensure the sterility of these products against microbial and foreign contamination, as well as for personal protection against radiation exposure.

Prior to administration to the patient, the nuclear pharmacist reviews the prescription or hospital order that has been signed by the authorized nuclear medicine physician. Radioactive decay calculations are made, and the required dosage is prepared and radioassayed to assure the correct amount of radioactivity. The drug product is then labeled and appropriately shielded prior to release for patient use.

The nuclear pharmacist must also be prepared to handle encountered questions about the clinical use of radiopharmaceuticals. Much like inquiries about non-radioactive drugs questions center on the pharmacokinetic properties of radiopharmaceuticals, adverse effects encountered with radiopharmaceuticals, dosing questions (e.g., pediatric, pregnancy), and alternative routes of administration.

Nuclear pharmacy was the first specialty in pharmacy recognized by the Board of Pharmaceutical Specialties (BPS). In 1978, BPS approved a petition submitted by the American Pharmaceutical Association of Pharmacy Practice (APP) Section on Nuclear Pharmacy and recognized nuclear pharmacy as a specialty in pharmacy practice. A Specialty Council on Nuclear Pharmacy was appointed and given the charge to develop a certification program for this specialty and over 100 pharmacists are now Board Certified in Nuclear Pharmacy through an examination procedure.

Notes

1. Because of the diminished use nowadays of tinctures, fluidextracts, extracts, aromatic waters, and spirits, these sections have been greatly reduced from those in the previous editions. Readers interested in additional details regarding these pharmaceutical preparations should refer to the third edition of this text.

Selected Readings

ACNP/SNM Task Force on Clinical PET. Positron Emission Tomography: Clinical Status in the United States in 1987. *J. Nucl. Med.*, 29:1136–1143, 1988.

Chilton, H.M. and Witcofski, R.L.: *Nuclear Pharmacy: An Introduction to the Clinical Application of Radiopharmaceuticals*, Philadelphia, Lea & Febiger, 1986.

Green, M.A. and Welch, M.J.: *Radiopharmaceuticals for Positron Emission Tomography*, in *Principles and Practice of Nuclear Medicine*, Sodee, P.B., Ed., C.V. Mosby Company (IN PRESS).

Kowalsky, R.J. and Perry, J.R.: *Radiopharmaceuticals in Nuclear Medicine Practice*, Appleton and Lange, Los Altos, CA, 1987.

Mintun, M.A. *et al*: Breast Cancer: PET imaging of Estrogen Receptors. *Radiology*, 169:45–48, 1988.

Nuclear Pharmacy Certification Examination Candidate's Guide, Board of Pharmaceutical Specialities, C/O American Pharmaceutical Association, Washington, DC.

Positron Emission Tomography—A New Approach to Brain Chemistry. The Report of the Positron Emission Tomography Panel, Jacobson, H.G., Section Editor, *JAMA*, 260:2704–2710, 1988.

Yonekura, Y., Tamaki, N., Senda, M. et al: Detection of coronary artery disease with ^{13}N-ammonia and high-resolution positron-emission computed tomography. *Am. Heart J.*, 113:645–654, 1987.

Appendix I

Definitions of Selected Drug Categories*

Abradent—an agent that removes an external layer, such as dental plaque. (Pumice)

Absorbent—a drug that takes up other chemicals into its substance, used to reduce the free availability of toxic chemicals. (Polycarbophil, gastrointestinal absorbent)

ACE Inhibitor—see Angiotensin Converting Enzyme Inhibitor.

Acidifier, Systemic—a drug that lowers internal body pH, useful in restoring normal pH in patients with systemic alkalosis. (Ammonium Chloride)

Acidifier, Urinary—a drug that lowers the pH of the renal filtrate and urine. (Sodium Dihydrogen Phosphate)

Adrenergic—a drug that activates organs innervated by the sympathetic nervous system; a sympathomimetic drug. (Epinephrine)

Adrenocorticosteroid, Anti-inflammatory—an adrenal cortex hormone that regulates organic metabolism and inhibits inflammatory response; a glucocorticoid. (Prednisolone)

Adrenocorticosteroid, Salt-regulating—an adrenal cortex hormone that regulates sodium/potassium balance in the body; a mineralocorticoid. (Desoxycorticosterone Acetate)

Adrenocorticotropic Hormone—a hormone that

stimulates the adrenal cortex to produce glucocorticoids. (Corticotropin)

Adsorbent—a drug that binds other chemicals onto its surface, used to reduce the free availability of toxic chemicals. (Kaolin, gastrointestinal adsorbent)

Agonist—a drug that reacts with and activates physiologic receptors, and induces the associated biological response. (Morphine, opiate receptor agonist; Isoproterenol, beta adrenergic receptor agonist)

Alcohol-Abuse Deterrent—a drug that alters physiology so that unpleasant symptoms follow ingestion of ethanol-containing products. (Disulfiram)

Alkalinizer, Systemic—a drug that raises internal body pH, useful in restoring normal pH in patients with systemic acidosis. (Sodium Bicarbonate)

Alkylating Agent—an antineoplastic drug that attacks malignant cells by reacting covalently with their DNA. (Chlorambucil)

Alpha Receptor Agonist—a drug that activates sympathetic nervous system alpha receptors, e.g., to induce vasoconstriction. (Norepinephrine)

Alpha Receptor Antagonist—a drug that reacts asymptomatically with sympathetic nervous system alpha receptors and prevents their endogenous activation, e.g., to induce vasodilation. (Phentolamine)

---

*Prepared by H. Douglas Johnson, Ph.D., Professor of Pharmacology/Toxicology, College of Pharmacy, University of Georgia.

Anabolic Steroid—an androgen analogue with relatively greater anabolic activity, used to treat catabolic disorders. (Methandrostenolone)

Analeptic—a central nervous system stimulant, sometimes used to stimulate respiration during severe CNS depression. (Doxapram)

Analgesic—a drug that suppresses pain perception (nociception) without inducing unconsciousness. (Morphine Sulfate, narcotic analgesic; Aspirin, nonnarcotic analgesic)

Androgen—a hormone that stimulates and maintains male reproductive function and sex characteristics. (Testosterone)

Anesthetic, General—a drug that eliminates pain perception by inducing unconsciousness. (Ether, inhalation anesthetic; Thiopental Sodium, intravenous anesthetic)

Anesthetic, Local—a drug that eliminates pain perception in a limited body area by local action on sensory nerves. (Procaine)

Anesthetic, Topical—a local anesthetic that is effective upon application to mucous membranes. (Tetracaine)

Angiotensin Converting Enzyme Inhibitor—a drug that inhibits biotransformation of Angiotensin I into vasoconstricting Angiotensin II, used to treat hypertension. (Captopril)

Anorexic—a drug that suppresses appetite, usually by elevating mood. (Phenmetrazine)

Antacid—a drug that neutralizes excess gastric acid. (Aluminum Hydroxide Gel)

Antagonist—a drug that reacts asymptomatically with physiologic receptors and prevents their endogenous activation. (Naloxone, opioid receptor antagonist; Propranolol, beta adrenergic receptor antagonist)

Anthelmintic—a drug that eradicates intestinal worm infestations. (Thiabendazole)

Antiacne Agent—a drug that combats the lesions of acne vulgaris. (Tretinoin)

Antiadrenergic—a drug that inhibits response to sympathetic nerve impulses and adrenergic drugs; a sympatholytic drug. (Phentolamine, alpha adrenergic antagonist; Propranolol, beta adrenergic antagonist)

Antiamebic—a drug that kills or inhibits protozoan parasites such as *Entamoeba histolytica*, causative agent of amebiasis. (Metronidazole, intestinal antiamebic; Chloroquine, extraintestinal antiamebic)

Antiandrogen—a drug that inhibits response to androgenic hormones. (Cyproterone)

Antianginal—a coronary vasodilator useful in preventing or treating attacks of angina pectoris. (Nitroglycerin)

Antiarrhythmic—a cardiac depressant useful in suppressing rhythm irregularities of the heart. (Procainamide)

Antiarthritic—a drug that reduces the joint inflammation of arthritis. (Prednisolone, glucocorticoid; Indomethacin, NSAID)

Antibacterial—a drug that kills or inhibits pathogenic bacteria. (Penicillin G, systemic antibacterial; Nitrofurantoin, urinary antibacterial; Bacitracin, topical antibacterial)

Anticholesterol Agent—a drug that lowers plasma cholesterol level. (Colestipol)

Anticholinergic—a drug that inhibits response to parasympathetic nerve impulses and cholinergic drugs; a parasympatholytic drug. (Atropine)

Anticholinesterase Antidote—a drug that reactivates cholinesterase enzyme after its inactivation by organophosphate poisons. (Pralidoxime)

Anticoagulant Antagonist—a drug that opposes overdosage of anticoagulant drugs. (Phytonadione, supplies vitamin K to oppose vitamin K-antagonist anticoagulants)

Anticoagulant, Systemic—a drug administered to slow clotting of circulating blood. (Warfarin)

Anticoagulant, for Storage of Whole Blood—a nontoxic agent added to collected blood to prevent clotting. (Anticoagulant Citrate Dextrose Solution)

Anticonvulsant—an antiepileptic drug administered prophylactically to prevent seizures, or a drug that arrests convulsions by inducing general CNS depression. (Phenytoin, antiepileptic prophylactic; Diazepam, CNS depressant anticonvulsant)

Antidepressant—a centrally acting drug that induces mood elevation, useful in treating mental depression. (Amitriptyline)

Antidiabetic—a drug that supplies insulin, or stimulates secretion of insulin, useful in treating diabetes mellitus. (Insulin Injection, supplies insulin; Tolbutamide, stimulates insulin secretion)

Antidiarrheal—a drug that inhibits intestinal peristalsis, used to treat diarrhea. (Diphenoxylate)

Antidiuretic—a drug that promotes renal water reabsorption, thus reducing urine volume, used to treat neurogenic diabetes insipidus. (Desmopressin)

Antianemic—a drug used to treat anemia; see Hematopoietic, Hematinic.

Antibiotic—a drug, originally of microbial origin, used to kill or inhibit bacterial and other infections. (Penicillin, Tetracycline)

Antidote, General Purpose—a drug that reduces the effects of ingested poisons (or drug overdoses) by adsorpting toxic material. (Activated Charcoal)

Antidote, Specific—a drug that reduces the effects of a systemic poison (or drug overdose) by a mechanism that relates to the particular poison. (Dimercaprol, specific antidote for arsenic, mercury and gold poisoning)

Antieczematic—a topical drug that aids in control of chronic exudative skin lesions. (Coal Tar)

Antiemetic—a drug that suppresses nausea and vomiting. (Prochlorperazine)

Antienuretic—a drug that aids in control of bedwetting (enuresis). (Imipramine)

Antiepileptic—a drug that prevents epileptic seizures upon prophylactic administration. (Ethosuximide)

Antiestrogen—a drug that inhibits action of estrogenic hormones. (Tamoxifen)

Antifibrinolytic—a drug that promotes hemostasis by inhibiting clot dissolution (fibrinolysis). (Aminocaproic Acid)

Antifilarial—a drug that kills or inhibits pathogenic filarial worms. (Diethylcarbamazine)

Antiflatulent—a drug that reduces gastrointestinal gas. (Simethicone)

Antifungal, Systemic—a drug that kills or inhibits pathogenic fungi. (Griseofulvin)

Antifungal, Topical—a drug applied externally to kill or inhibit pathogenic fungi. (Tolnaftate)

Antiglaucoma Agent—a drug that lowers intraocular fluid pressure, used to treat glaucoma. (Methazolamide reduces fluid formation; Isofluorophate promotes fluid drainage)

Antigonadotropin—a drug that inhibits anterior pituitary secretion of gonadotropins, used to suppress ovarian malfunction. (Danazol)

Antigout Agent—a drug that reduces tissue deposits of uric acid in chronic gout, or suppresses the intense inflammatory reaction of acute gout. (Allopurinol for chronic gout; Indomethacin for acute gout)

Antihemophilic—a drug that replaces blood clotting factors absent in the hereditary disease hemophilia. (Antihemophilic Factor)

Antiherpes Agent—a drug that inhibits replication of *Herpes simplex* virus, used to treat genital herpes. (Acyclovir)

Antihistaminic—a drug that antagonizes histamine action at H-1 histamine receptors, useful in suppressing the histamine-induced symptoms of allergy. (Chlorpheniramine)

Antihyperlipidemic—a drug that lowers plasma cholesterol and lipid levels. (Clofibrate)

Antihypertensive—a drug that lowers arterial blood pressure, especially the elevated diastolic pressure of hypertension. (Guanethidine)

Antihypocalcemic—a drug that elevates plasma calcium level, useful in treating hypocalcemia. (Parathyroid Injection)

Antihypoglycemic—a drug that elevates plasma glucose level, useful in treating hypoglycemia. (Glucagon)

Anti-infective, Topical (or Local)—a drug that kills or inhibits pathogenic microorganisms and is suitable for sterilizing skin and wounds. (Hexachlorophene Liquid Soap)

Anti-inflammatory—a drug that inhibits physiologic response to cell damage (inflammation). (Prednisolone, adrenocorticosteroid; Ibuprophen, nonsteroid)

Antileishmanial—a drug that kills or inhibits pathogenic protozoa of the genus *Leishmania.* (Hydroxystilbamidine Isethionate)

Antileprotic—a drug that kills or inhibits *Mycobacterium leprae,* causitive agent of leprosy. (Dapsone)

Antimalarial—a drug that kills or inhibits protozoa of the genus *Plasmodium,* causitive agents of malaria. (Chloroquine)

Antimanic—a drug that suppresses the excitement phase (mania) of manic-depressive psychosis. (Lithium Carbonate)

Antimetabolite—a drug that attacks malignant cells or pathogenic cells by serving as a nonfunctional substitute for an essential metabolite. (Fluorouracil, antineoplastic antimetabolite)

Antimigraine Agent—a drug that reduces incidence or severity of migraine vascular headaches. (Methylsergide)

Antimotion Sickness Agent—a drug that suppresses motion-induced nausea, vomiting, and vertigo. (Dimenhydrinate)

Antimuscarinic—an anticholinergic drug that inhibits symptoms mediated by acetylcholine receptors of visceral organs (muscarinic receptors). (Atropine)

Antinauseant—a drug that suppresses nausea and vomiting; an antiemetic. (Triethylperazine)

Antineoplastic—a drug that attacks malignant (neoplastic) cells in the body. (Chlorambucil, alkylating agent)

Antiparasitic—a drug that eradicates parasitic arthropods, helminths, protozoa, etc. (Lindane for scabies; Thiabendazole for intestinal worms; Metronidazole for amebic dysentary)

Antiparkinsonian (antidyskinetic)—a drug that suppresses the neurologic disturbances and symptoms of Parkinsonism. (Levodopa)

Antiperistaltic—a drug that inhibits intestinal motility; an antidiarrheal drug. (Diphenoxylate)

Antiplatelet Agent—a drug that inhibits aggregation of blood platelets, used prophylactically to prevent heart attack. (Aspirin)

Antiprotozoal—a drug that kills or inhibits pathogenic protozoa. (Metronidazole)

Antipruritic—a drug that reduces itching (pruritus). (Trimeprazine, systemic antipruritic; Menthol, topical antipruritic)

Antipsoriatic—a drug that suppresses the lesions and symptoms of psoriasis. (Methotrexate, systemic antipsoriatic; Anthralin, topical antipsoriatic)

Antipsychotic—a drug that suppresses symptoms of psychoses of various diagnostic types. (Haloperidol)

Antipyretic—a drug that restores normal body temperature in the presence of fever. (Acetaminophen)

Antirachitic—a drug with vitamin D activity, useful in treating vitamin D deficiency and rickets. (Cholecalciferol)

Antirheumatic—an anti-inflammatory drug used to treat arthritis and rheumatoid disorders. (Indomethacin)

Antirickettsial—a drug that kills or inhibits pathogenic microorganisms of the genus *Rickettsia.* (Chloramphenicol)

Antischistosomal—a drug that kills or inhibits pathogenic flukes of the genus *Schistosoma.* (Oxamniquine)

Antiscorbutic—a drug with vitamin C activity, useful in treating vitamin C deficiency and scurvy. (Ascorbic Acid)

Antiseborrheic—a drug that aids in the control of seborrheic dermatitis (dandruff). (Selenium Sulfide)

Antispasmodic—a drug that inhibits motility of visceral smooth muscles. (Atropine)

Antithyroid Agent—a drug that reduces thyroid hormone action, usually by inhibiting hormone synthesis. (Methimazole)

Antitreponemal—a drug that kills or inhibits *Treponema pallidum,* causitive agent of syphilis. (Penicillin)

Antitrichomonal—a drug that kills or inhibits

pathogenic protozoa of the genus *Trichomonas*. (Metronidazole)

Antitubercular—a drug that kills or inhibits *Mycobacterium tuberculosis*, causitive agent of tuberculosis. (Isoniazid)

Antitussive—a drug that suppresses coughing. (Dextromethorphan)

Antiviral—a drug that kills or inhibits viral infections. (Idoxuridine, Ophthalmic Antiviral)

Antiviral, Prophylactic—a drug useful in preventing (rather than treating) viral infections. (Amantadine, prophylactic for influenza)

Antixerophthalmic—a drug with vitamin A activity, useful in treating vitamin A deficiency and xerophthalmia. (Vitamin A)

Anxiolytic—a drug that suppresses symptoms of anxiety. (Diazepam)

Astringent—a drug used topically to toughen and shrink tissues. (Aluminum Acetate Solution)

Astringent, Ophthalmic—a mild astringent suitable for use in the eye. (Zinc Sulfate)

Barbiturate—a sedative-hypnotic drug that contains the barbituric acid moiety in its chemical structure. (Pentobarbital)

Belladonna Alkaloid—a plant principle derived from *Atropa belladonna* and related species, with anticholinergic action. (Atropine)

Benzodiazepine—a sedative-anxiolytic-muscle relaxant drug that contains the benzodiazepine moiety in its chemical structure. (Diazepam)

Beta Receptor Agonist—a drug that activates sympathetic nervous system beta receptors, e.g., to induce bronchodilation. (Isoproterenol)

Beta Receptor Antagonist—a drug that reacts asymptomatically with sympathetic nervous system beta receptors and prevents their endogenous activation, e.g., to oppose sympathetic stimulation of the heart. (Propranolol)

Bone Metabolism Regulator—a drug that slows calcium turnover in bone, used to treat Paget's disease. (Edidronate)

Bronchodilator—a drug that expands bronchiolar airways, useful in treating asthma. (Isoproterenol, adrenergic bronchodilator; Oxytriphylline, smooth muscle relaxant bronchodilator)

Calcium Channel Blocker—an antianginal drug that acts by impairing function of transmembrane calcium channels of vascular smooth muscle cells. (Verapamil)

Carbonic Anhydrase Inhibitor—a drug that inhibits the enzyme carbonic anhydrase, the therapeutic effects of which are diuresis and reduced formation of intraocular fluid. (Acetazolamide)

Cardiac Depressant, Antiarrhythmic—a drug that depresses myocardial function, useful in treating cardiac arrhythmias. (Procainamide)

Cardiac Glycoside—a plant principle derived from *Digitalis purpurea* and related species, with cardiotonic action. (Digoxin)

Cardiotonic—a drug that increases myocardial contractile force, useful in treating congestive heart failure. (Digoxin)

Catecholamine Synthesis Inhibitor—a drug that inhibits biosynthesis of catecholamine neurotransmitters such as norepinephrine. (Metyrosine)

Cathartic—a drug that promotes defecation, usually considered stronger in action than a laxative. (Danthron)

Caustic—a topical drug that destroys tissue on contact, useful in removing skin lesions. (Toughened Silver Nitrate)

Centrally Acting Drug—a drug that produces its therapeutic effect by action on the central nervous system, usually designated by type of therapeutic action (sedative, hypnotic, anticonvulsant, etc.)

Cephalosporin—an antimicrobial drug that contains the cephalosporin moiety in its chemical structure. (Cefotaxime)

Chelating Agent—a complexing agent that binds metal ions into stable ring structures (chelates), useful in treating poisoning. (Edetate Calcium Disodium, chelating agent for lead)

Cholelitholytic—a drug that promotes dissolution of gallstones. (Ursodoxycholic acid)

Choleretic—a drug that increases bile secretion by the liver. (Dehydrocholic Acid)

Cholinergic—a drug that activates organs innervated by the parasympathetic nervous system; a parasympathomimetic drug. (Neostigmine, systemic cholinergic; Pilocarpine, ophthalmic cholinergic)

Chrysotherapeutic—a drug containing gold, used to treat rheumatoid arthritis. (Auranofin)

Coagulant—see Hemostatic, Systemic.

Contraceptive, Oral—an orally administered drug that prevents conception. Currently available oral contraceptives are for use by females. (Norethindrone Acetate and Ethinyl Estradiol Tablets)

Contraceptive, Topical—a spermicidal agent used topically in the vagina to prevent conception. (Nonoxynol-9)

Cycloplegic—an anticholinergic drug used topically in the eye to induce paralysis of accommodation (cycloplegia) and dilation of the pupil. (Cyclopentolate)

Decongestant, Nasal—an adrenergic drug used orally or topically to induce vasoconstriction in nasal passages. (Phenylpropanolamine)

Demulcent—a bland viscous liquid, usually water-based, used to coat and soothe damaged or inflamed skin or mucous membranes. (Methylcellulose)

Dental Caries Prophylactic—a drug applied to the teeth to reduce the incidence of cavities. (Stannous Fluoride)

Dentin Desensitizer—a drug applied to the teeth to reduce the sensitivity of exposed sub-enamel dentin. (Zinc Chloride)

Depigmenting Agent—a drug that inhibits melanin production in the skin, used to induce general depigmentation in certain splotchy depigmented conditions (e.g., vitiligo). (Hydroquinone)

Detergent—an emulsifying agent used as a cleanser. (Hexachlorophene Liquid Soap, anti-infective detergent)

Diagnostic Aid—a drug used to determine the functional state of a body organ, or to determine the presence of disease. (Peptavlon, gastric secretion indicator; Fluorescein Sodium, corneal trauma indicator)

Digestive Aid—a drug that promotes digestion, usually by supplementing a gastrointestinal enzyme. (Pancreatin)

Disinfectant—an agent that destroys microorganisms on contact and suitable for sterilizing inanimate objects. (Formaldehyde Solution)

Diuretic—a drug that promotes renal excretion of electrolytes and water, useful in treating generalized edema. (Furosemide, loop diuretic; Hydrochlorothiazide, thiazide diuretic; Triamterene, potassium-sparing diuretic)

Dopamine Receptor Agonist—a drug that activates dopamine receptors, e.g., to inhibit anterior pituitary secretion of prolactin. (Bromocryptine)

Emetic—a drug that induces vomiting, useful in expelling ingested but unabsorbed poisons. (Ipecac Syrup)

Emollient—a topical drug, especially an oil or fat, used to soften the skin and make it more pliable. (Cold Cream)

Ergot Alkaloid—a plant principle derived from the fungus *Claviceps purpurea* grown on rye or other grains. (Ergonovine, uterine contractant; Ergotamine, migraine therapy)

Estrogen—a hormone that stimulates and maintains female reproductive organs and sex characteristics, and functions in the uterine cycle. (Ethinyl Estradiol)

Expectorant—a drug that increases respiratory tract secretions, lowers their viscosity and promotes removal. (Potassium Iodide)

Fecal Softener—a drug that promotes defecation by softening the feces. (Docusate)

Fertility Agent—a drug that promotes ovulation in women of low fertility, or spermatogenesis in men of low fertility. (Clomiphene)

Fibrinolytic-proteolytic—an enzyme drug used topically to hydrolyze exudates of infected and inflammatory lesions. (Fibrinolysin and Desoxyribuonuclease, Bovine)

Galactokinetic—a drug used to initiate lactation after childbirth. (Oxytocin Nasal Spray)

Glucocorticoid—an adrenocortical hormone that regulates organic metabolism and inhibits inflammatory response. (Betamethasone)

Gonadotropin—a drug that supplies the gonad-stimulating actions of follicle-stimulating hormone (FSH) and/or luteinizing hormone (LH), used to promote fertility. (Menotropins contains FSH and LH; Human Chorionic Gonadotropin has LH-like activity)

Growth Hormone, Human—a drug that duplicates endogenous growth hormone, used in children to treat growth failure due to growth hormone lack. (Somatrem)

Heavy Metal Antagonist—a drug used to antidote poisoning with toxic metals such as arsenic, mercury, etc. (Dimercaprol)

Hematopoietic—a vitamin that stimulates formation of blood cells, useful in treating vitamin-deficiency anemia. (Cyanocobalamin)

Hematinic—a drug that promotes hemoglobin formation by supplying iron. (Ferrous Sulfate)

Hemorheologic Agent—a drug that improves the flow properties of blood by reducing viscosity. (Pentoxyfylline)

Hemostatic, Local—a drug applied to a bleeding surface to promote clotting or to serve as a clot matrix. (Thrombin, clot promoter; Oxidized Cellulose, clot matrix)

Hemostatic, Systemic—a drug that stops bleeding by inhibiting systemic fibrinolysis. (Aminocaproic Acid)

Histamine H-1 Receptor Antagonist—a drug used to combat the histamine-induced symptoms of allergy; an antihistaminic (Chlorpheniramine)

Histamine H-2 Receptor Antagonist—a drug that inhibits histamine-mediated gastric acid secretion, used to treat peptic and duodenal ulcers. (Cimetidine)

Hormone—a drug that duplicates action of a physiologic cell regulator (hormone). (Insulin, Estradiol, Thyroxine)

Hydantoin—an antiepileptic drug that contains the hydantoin moiety in its chemical structure. (Phenytoin)

Hydrolytic, Injectible—an enzyme drug that promotes the diffusion of other injected drugs through connective tissues. (Hyaluronidase)

Hyperglycemic—a drug that elevates blood glucose level. (Glucagon)

Hypnotic—a central nervous system depressant used to induce sleep. (Flurazepam)

Hypotensive—see Antihypertensive.

Immune Globulin—Antibody proteins derived from blood serum, used to confer passive immunity to infectious diseases. (See Immunizing Agent, Passive)

Immunizing Agent, Active—an antigen that induces antibody production against a pathogenic microorganism, used to provide permanent but delayed protection against infection. (Tetanus Toxoid)

Immunizing Agent, Passive—a drug containing antibodies against a pathogenic microorganism, used to provide immediate but temporary protection against infection. (Tetanus Immune Globulin, Rabies Immune Globulin)

Immunosuppressant—a drug that inhibits immune response to foreign materials, used to suppress rejection of tissue grafts. (Azathioprine)

Inotropic Agent—a drug that increases the contractile strength of heart muscle; a cardiotonic. (Digitoxin, Dopamine)

Ion Exchange Resin—a drug that in the gastrointestinal tract takes up ions present in a toxic amount with equivalent release of nontoxic ions. (Sodium Polystyrene Sulfonate, takes up potassium ions with release of sodium ions)

Irritant, Local—a drug that reacts weakly and nonspecifically with biological tissue, used topically to induce a mild inflammatory response. (Camphor)

Keratolytic—a topical drug that softens the superficial keratin-containing layer of the skin and promotes desquamation. (Salicylic Acid)

Keratoplastic—a topical drug that toughens and protects skin. (Compound Benzoin Tincture)

Laxative—a drug that promotes defecation, usually considered milder in action than a cathartic. (Methylcellulose, bulk laxative; Mineral Oil, lubricant laxative; Sodium Phosphates Oral Solution, saline laxative)

Leprostatic—see Antileprotic

Loop Diuretic—a diuretic with renal site of action in the thick ascending loop of Henle. (Furosemide)

MAO Inhibitor—see Monoamine Oxidase Inhibitor.

Metal Complexing Agent—a drug that binds metal ions, useful in treating metal poisoning. (Dimercaprol, complexing agent for arsenic, mercury, and gold)

Mineralocorticoid—an adrenocortical hormone that regulates sodium/potassium balance in the body. (Desoxycorticosterone Acetate)

Miotic—a cholinergic drug used topically in the eye to induce constriction of the pupil (miosis). (Pilocarpine)

Monoamine Oxidase Inhibitor—an antidepressant drug that inhibits the enzyme monoamine oxidase, thereby increasing catecholamine levels of neurons. (Isocarboxazid)

Monoclonal Antibody—a highly specific immunoglobulin produced by cell culture cloning. (Muromonab-CD3, inactivates T-lymphocytes that reject tissue grafts)

Mucolytic—a drug that hydrolyzes mucoproteins, useful in reducing the viscosity of pulmonary mucus. (Acetylcysteine)

Muscle Relaxant, Skeletal—a drug that inhibits contraction of voluntary muscles. (Dantrolene, Succinylcholine)

Muscle Relaxant, Smooth—a drug that inhibits contraction of visceral smooth muscles. (Aminophylline)

Mydriatic—an adrenergic drug used topically in the eye to induce dilation of the pupil (mydriasis). (Phenylephrine)

Narcotic—a drug that induces action by reacting with opioid receptors of the central nervous system, or a drug legally classified as a narcotic with regard to prescribing regulations.

Narcotic Antagonist—a drug that reacts with opiate receptors asymptomatically, used to terminate the action of narcotic drugs. (Naloxone)

Neuromuscular Blocking Agent—a drug that paralyzes skeletal muscles by preventing transmission of neural impulses to them. (Succinylcholine)

Nonsteroidal Anti-inflammatory Drug—an analgesic, anti-inflammatory drug that inhibits prostaglandin synthesis. (Indomethacin)

NSAID—see Nonsteroidal Anti-inflammatory Drug.

Opiate—see Narcotic.

Opiate Antagonist—see Narcotic Antagonist.

Oxytoxic—a drug that stimulates uterine motility, used in obstetrics to initiate labor or to control postpartum hemorrhage. (Oxytocin)

Parasympatholytic—a drug that inhibits response to parasympathetic nerve impulses and to parasympathomimetic drugs; an anticholinergic drug. (Atropine)

Parasympathomimetic—a drug that activates organs innervated by the parasympathetic nervous system; a cholinergic drug. (Neostigmine)

Pediculicide—an insecticide suitable for eradicating louse infestations (pediculosis). (Lindane)

Penicillin Adjuvant—a drug that extends systemic duration of penicillin by inhibiting its renal excretion. (Probenecid)

Phenothiazine—an antipsychotic drug or an antidepressant drug that contains the phenothiazine nucleus in its chemical structure. (Chloropromazine, antipsychotic; Imipramine, antidepressant)

Photosensitizer—a drug that increases cutaneous response to ultraviolet light, used with ultraviolet light to treat certain skin diseases (e.g., psoriasis). (Methoxsalen)

Pigmenting Agent—a drug that promotes melanin synthesis in the skin. (Trioxsalen, oral pigmenting agent; Methoxsalen, topical pigmenting agent)

Posterior Pituitary Hormone, Antidiuretic—a hormone that promotes renal reabsorption of water, useful in treating diabetes insipidus. (Vasopressin Injection)

Potassium-sparing Diuretic—a diuretic that does not induce systemic potassium depletion as a side effect. (Triamterene)

Potentiator—an adjunctive drug that enhances the action of a primary drug, the total response being greater than the sum of the individual actions. (Hexafluorenium, potentiator for Succinylcholine)

Progestin—a progesterone-like hormone that stimulates the secretory phase of the uterine cycle. (Norethindrone)

Prostaglandin—a drug from the classes of cell-regulating hormones cyclized from arachidonic acid. (Alprostadil, maintains ductus arteriosus patency in newborn infants pending corrective surgery for congenital heart defects)

Prostaglandin Synthetase Inhibitor—a drug that inhibits prostaglandin synthesis and prostaglandin-induced symptoms such as inflammation; a nonsteroidal anti-inflammatory drug. (Ibuprofen)

Protectant—a topical drug that provides a physical barrier to the environment. (Zinc Gelatin, skin protectant; Methylcellulose, ophthalmic protectant)

Proteolytic, Injectable—an enzyme drug for injection into herniated lumbar intervertebral discs to reduce interdiscal pressure. (Chymopapain)

Prothrombogenic—a drug with vitamin K activity, useful in treating the hypoprothrombinemia of vitamin K deficiency or overdosage with a vitamin K antagonist. (Phytonadione)

Psychedelic—a drug (especially a street drug) that induces vivid sensory phenomena and hallucinations. (Mescaline)

Psychotherapeutic—A drug used to treat abnormal mental or emotional processes. (Chlorpromazine, Haloperidol)

Rauwolfia Alkaloid—a plant principle derived from *Rauwolfia serpentina* and related species, with antihypertensive and antipsychotic actions. (Reserpine)

Radiographic Agent—see X-Ray Contrast Medium.

Radiopharmaceutical—a drug containing a radioactive isotope, used for diagnostic or therapeutic purposes. (Iodinated Albumen, with I-125 or I-131)

Resin, Electrolyte Removing—see Ion Exchange Resin.

Rubefacient—a topical drug that induces mild skin irritation with erythema, and used as a toughening agent. (Rubbing Alcohol)

Salt Substitute—a sodium-free alternative to NaCl used for flavoring foods. (Potassium Chloride)

Scabicide—an insecticide suitable for eradication of the itch mite *Sarcoptes scabiei* (scabies). (Lindane)

Sclerosing Agent—an irritant drug suitable for injection into varicose veins to induce their fibrosis and obliteration. (Morrhuate Sodium Injection)

Sedative—a central nervous system depressant used to induce mild relaxation. (Phenobarbital)

Specific—a drug specially adapted to its indicated use, usually because of a functional relationship between drug mechanism and disease pathophysiology.

Stimulant, Central—a drug that increases the functional state of the central nervous system, sometimes used in convulsive therapy of mental disorders. (Flurothyl)

Stimulant, Respiratory—a drug that selectively stimulates respiration, either by peripheral initiation of respiratory reflexes, or by selective central nervous system stimulation. (Carbon Dioxide, reflex respiratory stimulant; Ethamivan, central respiratory stimulant)

Sun Screening Agent—a skin protectant that absorbs light energy at wave-lengths that cause sunburn. (Aminobenzoic Acid)

Sulfonylurea—an oral antidiabetic drug that contains the sulfonylurea moiety in its chemical structure. (Tolazamide)

Suppressant—a drug that inhibits the progress of a disease but does not cure it.

Sympatholytic—a drug that inhibits response to sympathetic nerve impulses and to sympathomimetic drugs; an antiadrenergic drug. (Phentolamine, alpha sympatholytic; Propranolol, beta sympatholytic)

Sympathomimetic—a drug that activates organs innervated by the sympathetic nervous system; an adrenergic drug. (Epinephrine)

Systemically Acting Drug—a drug administered so as to reach systemic circulation, from which the drug diffuses into all tissues, including the site of therapeutic action.

Thiazide Diuretic—a diuretic that contains the benzothiadiazide (thiazide) moiety in its chemical structure. (Hydrochlorothiazide)

Thrombolytic—an enzyme drug administered parenterally to solubilize blood clots. (Urokinase)

Thyroid Hormone—a hormone that maintains metabolic function and normal metabolic rate of tissues. (Levothyroxine)

Topically Acting Drug—a drug applied to the body surface for local therapeutic action.

Toxoid—a modified antigen from an infectious organism used as a vaccine. (Tetanus Toxoid)

Tranquilizer, Minor—an old term for an anxiolytic drug.

Tranquilizer—a drug (such as an antipsychotic) used to suppress an acutely disturbed emotional state. (Trifluoperazine, antipsychotic)

Tricyclic Antidepressant—an antidepressant that contains the tricyclic phenothiazine nucleus in its chemical structure. (Imipramine)

Tuberculostatic—see Antitubercular.

Uricosuric—a drug that promotes renal excretion of uric acid, useful in treating chronic gout. (Probenecid)

Uterine Contractant—an obstetric drug used after placenta delivery to induce sustained uterine contraction to reduce bleeding. (Methylergonovine)

Uterine Contraction Inhibitor—a drug that inhibits uterine muscle contraction, used in preterm labor to prolong gestation. (Ritodrine)

Vaccine—an antigen-containing drug used to induce active immunity against an infectious disease. (Hepatitis B Vaccine, Rabies Vaccine)

Vasoconstrictor—a drug that narrows arterioles, usually to elevate blood pressure. See Vasopressor.

Vasodilator, Coronary—a drug that expands blood vessels in the heart and improves coronary blood flow, useful in treating angina pectoris; an antianginal drug. (Nitroglycerin)

Vasodilator, Peripheral—a drug that expands peripheral blood vessels and improves blood flow to the extremities of the body. (Minoxidil)

Vasopressor—an adrenergic drug administered to constrict arterioles and elevate arterial blood pressure. (Norepinephrine)

Vinca Alkaloid—a plant principle derived from *Vinca rosea* and related species, with antineoplastic action. (Vincristine)

Vitamin—an organic chemical essential in small amounts for normal metabolism, used therapeutically to supplement the vitamin content of foods.

Xanthine Alkaloid—a plant principle chemically related to xanthine, with central nervous system stimulant, smooth muscle relaxant, and diuretic actions. (Caffeine)

X-Ray Contrast Medium—a drug opaque to x rays that assists visualization of an internal organ during radiographic examination. (Barium Sulfate, Iopanoic Acid)

Appendix II

Pharmaceutical Systems and Techniques of Measurement

The pharmacist's knowledge and application of accurate pharmaceutical measurement are essential to his practice of pharmacy. Whether practicing in the community or institutional pharmacy or in the large industrial pharmaceutical manufacturing firm, accuracy of measurement is a prime requisite in the preparation of medications.

Pharmaceuticals prepared industrially pass numerous inspections and assays during the course of their manufacture to ensure conformance to standards of quality and quantity. However, prescriptions and medication orders filled extemporaneously in the community and institutional pharmacy usually lack the advantage of such control by assay, and the pharmacist must be absolutely certain that his calculations and measurements are accurate. He should double check his work, and when possible he should have a colleague check it as well. An error in the placement of a decimal point, for instance, represents an error of a *minimum* factor of ten.

The student must have a working knowledge of the systems of pharmaceutical measurement as presented in this appendix, including factors of conversion between the systems used, and the methods of applying these systems in pharmaceutical measurement.

Systems of Pharmaceutical Measurement

In pharmacy today, three systems of measurement have common application. They are the *metric system,* the *apothecary system,* and the *avoirdupois system.* The metric and apothecary systems include units of weight and volume measure with the metric system additionally having units of linear measure. The pharmacist utilizes these systems in his pharmaceutical measurements. The avoirdupois system is the common commercial system of weight used in the United States that is slowly being replaced by the metric system. The avoirdupois system is used by the pharmacist in his purchase of bulk chemicals and commercial packages from manufacturers.

The Metric System

The metric system is the most widely used system in pharmacy. It is the system used by the official compendia and in the labeling of most of the commercial pharmaceutical products. Most of the prescriptions and medication orders written today are in the metric system.

In the metric system, the *gram* is the main unit of weight, the *liter* the main unit of volume, and the *meter* the main unit of length. Subunits and multiples of these basic units are indicated by the following prefix notations and symbols shown in Table A–1.

The following are most commonly used in pharmaceutical measurement:

units of weight, expressed in terms of the kilogram (kg), gram (g), milligram (mg), or microgram (μg).

units of liquid measure, expressed in terms of the liter (L) or milliliter (mL).

units of linear measure, expressed in terms of the

Table A–1.   Metric System Unit Prefixes*

Multiplication Factor		Prefix	Symbol	Term (USA)
1 000 000 000 000 000 000	$= 10^{18}$	exa	E	one quintillion
1 000 000 000 000 000	$= 10^{15}$	peta	P	one quadrillion
1 000 000 000 000	$= 10^{12}$	tera	T	one trillion
1 000 000 000	$= 10^{9}$	giga	G	one billion
1 000 000	$= 10^{6}$	mega	M	one million
1 000	$= 10^{3}$	kilo	k	one thousand
100	$= 10^{2}$	hecto	h	one hundred
10	$= 10$	deka	da	ten
0.1	$= 10^{-1}$	deci	d	one tenth
0.01	$= 10^{-2}$	centi	c	one hundreth
0.001	$= 10^{-3}$	milli	m	one thousandth
0.000 001	$= 10^{-6}$	micro	μ	one millionth
0.000 000 001	$= 10^{-9}$	nano	n	one billionth
0.000 000 000 001	$= 10^{-12}$	pico	p	one trillionth
0.000 000 000 000 001	$= 10^{-15}$	femto	f	one quadrillionth
0.000 000 000 000 000 001	$= 10^{-18}$	atto	a	one quintillionth

*Adapted from *Metric Editorial Guide,* 4th Ed., American National Metric Council, Washington, D.C., 20005. The table is based on The International System of Units ("SI," from the French "Le Systeme International System of Unites"), as modified for use in the United States by the Secretary of Commerce.

meter (m), centimeter (cm), or millimeter (mm).

units of area measure, expressed in terms of the square meter (m²) or square centimeter (cm²).

The "metric weight scale" in Figure A–1 is intended to depict the relationship between the units of weight in the metric system and to provide an example of an easy method of converting from one unit to another. In the example, 1.23 kilograms (kg) are to be converted to grams (g). On the scale, the gram position is three decimal positions from the kilogram position. Thus, the decimal point is moved three places toward the right. In the other example, the conversion from milligrams (mg) to grams also requires the movement of the decimal point three

DECIMAL MOVEMENT

◉► TO CONVERT FROM LARGER TO SMALLER UNITS

◄◉ TO CONVERT FROM SMALLER TO LARGER UNITS

Fig. A–1. *Metric Weight Scale*

places, but this time to the left. The same method may be used to convert metric units of volume or length.

Table of Metric Weight:

1 kilogram (Kg or kg)	=	1000.000 grams
1 hektogram (Hg or hg)	=	100.000 grams
1 dekagram (Dg or dg)	=	10.000 grams
1 gram (Gm, gm or g)	=	1.000 gram
1 decigram (dg)	=	0.100 gram
1 centigram (cg)	=	0.010 gram
1 milligram (mg)	=	0.001 gram
1 microgram (μg or mcg)	=	0.000,001 gram
1 nanogram (ng)	=	0.000,000,001 gram

or

1 gram = 0.001 kilogram

= 0.010 hektogram

= 0.100 dekagram

= 10 decigrams

= 100 centigrams

= 1000 milligrams

= 1,000,000 micrograms

= 1,000,000,000 nanograms

Table of Metric Volume:

1 kiloliter (Kl or kl)	=	1000.000 liters
1 hektoliter (Hl or hl)	=	100.000 liters
1 dekaliter (Dl)	=	10.000 liters
1 liter (L or l)	=	1.000 liter
1 deciliter (dl)	=	0.100 liter
1 centiliter (cl)	=	0.010 liter
1 milliliter (mL)	=	0.001 liter
1 microliter (μL)	=	0.000,001 liter

or

1 liter = 0.001 kiloliter

= 0.010 hektoliter

= 0.100 dekaliter

= 10 deciliters

= 100 centiliters

= 1000 milliliters

= 1,000,000 microliters

Table of Metric Length:

1 kilometer (Km or km)	=	1000.000 meters
1 hektometer (Hm)	=	100.000 meters
1 dekameter (Dm)	=	10.000 meters
1 meter (M or m)	=	1.000 meter
1 decimeter (dm)	=	0.100 meter
1 centimeter (cm)	=	0.010 meter
1 millimeter (mm)	=	0.001 meter
1 micrometer (μm)	=	0.000,001 meter
1 nanometer (nm)	=	0.000,000,001 meter

or

1 meter = 0.001 kilometer

= 0.010 hektometer

= 0.100 dekameter

= 10 decimeters

= 100 centimeters

= 1000 millimeters

= 1,000,000 micrometers

= 1,000,000,000 nanometers

The Apothecary System

The apothecary system provides for the measurement of both weight and volume. The tables of the system are presented below.

TABLES OF APOTHECARY SYSTEM

Table of Apothecaries' Fluid Measure:

60 minims (♏)	= 1 fluidrachm (f℥ or ℥)*
8 fluidrachms (480 minims)	= 1 fluidounce (f℥ or ℥)*
16 fluidounces	= 1 pint (pt or O)
2 pints (32 fluidounces)	= 1 quart (qt)
4 quarts (8 pints)	= 1 gallon (gal or C)

Table of Apothecaries' Measure of Weight:

20 grains (gr)	= 1 scruple (℈)
3 scruples (60 grains)	= 1 drachm (℥)
8 dram (480 grains)	= 1 ounce (℥)
12 ounces (5760 grains)	= 1 pound ℔

The Avoirdupois System

The avoirdupois system is used in commerce generally in the supplying of drugs, chemicals,

---

*When there is no doubt that the material referred to is a liquid, the *f* is usually omitted from this symbol. *Drachm* is also spelled *dram*.

and other materials by weight. The pharmacist who purchases bulk or prepackaged amounts of chemicals, as sodium bicarbonate powder or epsom salts, purchases them in the avoirdupois system. When he resells them "over the counter" in their original packages, he likewise sells them in the avoirdupois system. The "grain" in each of the apothecary and avoirdupois systems are equivalent. The other units (ounce and pound) are of different weights. It should also be noted that the symbols for the ounce and pound are different in the two systems.

*Table of Avoirdupois Measure
of Weight*

437.5 grains (gr)	= 1 ounce (oz)
16 ounces (7000 grains)	= 1 pound (lb)

Intersystem Conversion

It is sometimes advantageous or convenient for the pharmacist to convert the weight, volume, or dimensions of length from one system to another. Depending upon the circumstances and requirements of accuracy, conversion equivalents of different exactness may be used. The following is a table of those equivalents commonly used in prescription practice. They are not the exact equivalents, but are over 99% accurate and suffice nicely for most pharmaceutical measurements. Exact equivalents may be found in the USP.

Conversion Equivalents of Weight

1 g	= 15.432 gr
1 Kg	= 2.2 Avoirdupois lb
1 gr	= 0.0648 g or 64.8 or 65 mg
1 ℥	= 31.1 g
1 oz (Avoir)	= 28.35 g
1 ℔ (Apoth)	= 373.2 g
1 lb (Avoir)	= 453.6 or 454 g

Conversion Equivalents of Volume

1 mL	= 16.23 minims
1 minim	= 0.06 mL
1 f℥	= 3.69 mL
1 ℥	= 29.57 mL
1 pt	= 473 mL
1 gal (U.S.)	= 3785 mL
1 gal (British Imperial)	= 4546 mL

Conversion Equivalents of Length

1 inch	= 2.54 cm
1 meter	= 39.37 inches

Approximate Dose Equivalents

Oftentimes in communicating medication information to one another, health professionals may utilize "approximate equivalents." For instance, in ordering commercially prepared tablets, a physician may indicate "60 mg tablets." The pharmacist may find the commercial tablets labeled to contain "65 mg" or "1 gr." According to the Food and Drug Administration, when such prepared dosage forms are prescribed in the metric system, the pharmacist may dispense the corresponding "approximate dose equivalent" in the apothecary system, and vice versa, for drugs prescribed in the apothecaries' system.

The approximate or prescribing equivalents are not intended for use by the pharmacist in his calculations involving the compounding of prescriptions or the manufacture of pharmaceutical products.

Among the approximate dose equivalents listed in the *United States Pharmacopeia* are the following:

Liquid Measure

1000 mL	=	1 quart
500 mL	=	1 pint
30 mL	=	1 fluidounce
4 mL	=	1 fluid dram
1 mL	=	15 minims
0.06 mL	=	1 minim

Weight

30 g	=	1 Apothecary ounce
1 g	=	15 grains
60 mg	=	1 grain
30 mg	=	½ grain
15 mg	=	¼ grain
1 mg	=	$1/60$ grain
0.6 g	=	$1/100$ grain
0.4 mg	=	$1/150$ grain

Common Household Measure

Liquid and powdered medications which are not packaged in unit dose systems are usually measured at home by the patient with common household measuring devices as the teaspoon, tablespoon, and various cooking measure utensils. Although the household teaspoon may vary in volume capacity from approximately 3 to 8 mL, the American Standard Teaspoon has been established as having a volume of 4.93 ± 0.24 mL by the American National Standards Institute. For practical purposes, most pharmacy practitioners and pharmacy references utilize 5 mL as the capacity of the teaspoon. This is approximately equivalent to 1⅓ fluid drams although physicians commonly utilize the dram symbol (3) to indicate a teaspoonful in their prescription directions to be transcribed by the pharmacist to the patient. The tablespoon is considered to have a capacity of 15 mL, equivalent to three teaspoonfuls or approximately one-half fluid ounce.

Occasionally the pharmacist will dispense a special medicinal spoon which the patient may use in measuring this medication. These spoons are available in half-teaspoon, teaspoon, and tablespoon capacities. Some manufacturers provide specially designed devices to be used by the patient in measuring his medication. These include specially calibrated droppers, oral syringes, measuring wells or tubes, and calibrated bottle caps. In health care institutions, disposable measuring cups and unit-dose containers are commonly employed in administering liquid medication. Examples of measuring devices are shown in Fig. A–2.

Weighing and the Prescription Balance

In weighing materials, the selection of the instrument to use is based on the amount of material involved and the accuracy desired. In the large scale manufacture of pharmaceuticals, large industrial *scales* of varying capacity and sensitivity are employed, and later, highly sensitive analytical balances are utilized in the quality control and analytical work.

In the hospital and community pharmacy, most weighings are made on the *prescription balance*. Two examples of these balances are shown in Figure A–3. Prescription balances are divided into two classes, *Class A* and *Class B* prescription balances, which meet the prescribed standards of the National Bureau of Standards. Every prescription department is required by law to have a Class A prescription balance, which is the more sensitive of the two. The sensitivity of a balance is usually represented by the term *sensitivity requirement* (SR) which is defined as the maximum change in load that will cause a specified change, one subdivision on the index plate, in the position of rest of the indicating element(s) of the balance.[1] A Class A balance has an SR of 6 mg with no load as well as with 10 g on each pan. This means that under the

Fig. A–2. *Examples of medicinal spoons of various shapes and capacities, calibrated medicine droppers, an oral medication tube, and a disposable medication cup.*

Fig. A–3.   *Examples of commonly used Class A prescription balances. On left is the Troemner Model 800 Prescription Balance (Courtesy of Henry Troemner, Inc.); on right, the Model DRX2 Torsion balance (Courtesy of Torsion Balance Company.).*

above conditions, the addition of 6 mg of weight to one pan of the balance will disturb the equilibrium and move the balance pointer one division marking on the scale.

The USP directs that to avoid errors in weighing of 5% or greater, which may be due to the limits of accuracy of the Class A prescription balance, one must weigh a minimum of 120 mg (approximately 2 grains) of any material in each weighing (5% of 120 mg being the 6 mg SR or error inherent with the balance). If a smaller weight of material is desired, it is directed that the pharmacist mix a larger, calculated weight of the ingredient (120 mg or over), dilute it with a known weight of an inert dry diluent (as lactose), mix the two uniformly, and weigh an aliquot portion of the mixture (again 120 mg or over) calculated to contain the desired amount of agent. The Class A balance which has a capacity of 120 g should be used for all weighings required in prescription compounding.

The Class B prescription balance has an SR of 30 mg and a 120 g capacity. It must not be used for weighing loads of less than 600 mg. Both the Class A and Class B balance must be distinctively marked as to its class on the balance itself. The Class B balance is only rarely found and used in pharmacies.

Weights

Pharmacies usually have two sets of weights for use, one metric set and one apothecary set. Some commercial sets contain both systems of weights in a single container. Prescription weights meet the National Bureau of Standards' specifications for analytical weights. Metric weights of 1 g and greater, and apothecaries' weights of 1 scruple and greater, are generally conical in shape with a narrow neck and head which allows them to be easily grasped and picked up with a small forceps. Most of these weights are made of polished brass, with some coated with nickel or chromium or other materials to resist corrosion. Fractional gram weights are made of aluminum and are generally square-shaped and flat with one raised end or corner for picking up with the forceps (Fig. A–4). Apothecaries' weights of one-half scruple are frequently coin-shaped brass and those of 5 grains and less are usually bent aluminum wires, with each straight side representing 1 grain of weight. The half-grain weight is usually a smaller gauge wire bent in half.

To prevent the deposit of moisture and oils from the fingertips being deposited on the weights, all weights should be transferred with the forceps provided in each weight set.

Care and Use of a Prescription Balance

First and foremost, the prescription balance should be located in a well-lighted location, placed on a firm, level counter approximately

Fig. A–4. *Examples of some metric weights, showing their shape and markings.*

waist-high to the operator. The area should be as free from dust as is possible and in an area that is draft-free. There should be no corrosive vapors present nor high humidity or vibration. When not in use, the balance should be clean and covered with the balance cover. Any agent spilled on the balance during use should be wiped off immediately with a soft brush or cloth. When not in use, the balance should always be maintained with the weights off and the beam in the fixed or locked (arrested) position.

Before weighing an article, the balance must be made level. This is accomplished with the leveling screws on the bottom of the balance, according to the instructional materials accompanying the balance. The balance should be level, front-to-back and side-to-side, as indicated by the leveling bubble of the balance.

In using a prescription balance, neither the weights nor the substance to be weighed should be placed on the balance while the beam is in the *un*arrested position and free to oscillate. Before weighing, powder papers of equal size should be placed on both pans of the balance and the equilibrium of the balance tested by releasing the arresting knob. If the balance is unbalanced due to differences in the weight of the powder papers, additional weight may be added to the "light pan" by adding small tearings of powder papers. When balanced, the balance is placed in the arrested position and the desired weight added to the right-hand pan. Then, an amount of substance, considered to be approximately the desired weight, is carefully placed on the left hand pan, with the assistance of a spatula. The beam should then be slowly released by means of the locking device in the front of the balance. If the substance is in excess, the beam is fixed again and a small portion of the substance removed with the spatula. The process is continued until the two pans

balance, as indicated by central position of the balance pointer. If the amount of weight on the balance is initially too little, the reverse process is undertaken. The powder paper used on the left hand pan, intended to hold the substance to be weighed, is usually folded either diagonally or with the edges of the sides folded upwards to contain the material being weighed.

In transferring material by spatula, the material may be lightly tapped from the spatula when the correct amount to be measured is approached. Usually this is done by holding the spatula with a small amount of material on it in the right hand, and tapping the spatula with the forefinger. As material comes off the spatula, the left hand is working the balance arresting mechanism and the status of the weight observed alternately with the tappings of the spatula. Most balances have a "damping" mechanism which slows down the balance oscillations and permits more rapid determinations of the balance or imbalance positions of the pans.

Once the material has been weighed, the balance beam is again put in the fixed position and the paper holding the weighed substance carefully removed. If more than a single weighing is to be performed, the paper is usually marked with the name of the substance it holds. After the final weighing, all weights are removed with the forceps and the balance cleaned, closed, and the balance cover placed over the balance.

Most prescription balances contain built-in mechanisms whereby external weights are not required for weighings under 1 gram. Some balances utilize a rider, which may be shifted from the zero position toward the right side of the balance to add increments of weight marked on the scale in 10-mg units, up to 1 g. Another type of balance uses a centrally located dial, calibrated in 10-mg units, to add weight up to 1 gram. Both types of devices add the weight internally to the right-hand pan. In each case, the pharmacist may use a combination of the internal weights and external weights in his weighings. For instance, if 1.2 g are to be weighed, the pharmacist can place a 1-g weight on the right hand pan and place the rider or adjust the dial to add 0.2 g additionally. Care must always be exercised to bring the rider or dial to zero between weighings to avoid the inadvertent weighing of rider- or dial-amounts on subsequent weighings.

Most weighings on the prescription balance involve the weighing of powders or semisolid materials, as ointments. However, liquids may also be weighed through the use of tared (weighed) vessels of appropriate size, by placing the liquid inside of the vessel. The pharmacist must always be certain that he has accounted for the weight of the vessel in calculating the amount of liquid weighed.

Materials should never be "downweighed;" that is, substances should never be placed on the pan with the balance in the unarrested position forcing the pan to drop suddenly and forcefully as the excess material is placed on it. The sudden slamming down of the pan can do serious damage to the balance, affecting its sensitivity and the accuracy of subsequent weighings.

The two most popular types of prescription balances are the compound lever balance and the torsion balance. The former type operates through the use of a series of knife edges held in delicate contact and suspension. The torsion type operates on the tension of taut wires, which when twisted through the addition of weight, tend to twist back to the original balance position. The compound lever principle is the basis for the Troemner balance and the torsion principle is applied in the Torsion Balance (Fig. A–3).

Measuring Volume

The common instruments for pharmaceutical measurement are presented in Figure A–5. Two types of graduates are used in pharmacy, those which are *conical* in shape and those which are *cylindrical.* Cylindrical graduates are generally calibrated in metric units, whereas conical graduates may be graduated in both the metric and apothecaries' units (dual scale) or with a single scale of either of the systems. Graduates of both shapes are available in a wide variety of capacities, ranging from 5 to 1000 mL or more. Most graduates in use are made of a good quality, heat-treated glass, although graduates of polypropylene are also available. In measuring small volumes of liquids, as less than 1.5 mL, the pharmacist should utilize a pipet as the one shown in Figure A–5. The bulb-like device shown with the pipet is a pipet filler, used for drawing acids or other toxic solutions into the pipet without the necessity of using the mouth. The device, without being removed from the

pipet, also allows for the accurate delivery of the liquid.

In measuring volumes of liquids, the pharmacist should select the measuring device most appropriate to the volume of liquid to be measured and the degree of accuracy desired. It should be recognized that in measuring liquids, the more narrow the column of liquid, the more accurate is likely to be the measurement. Figure A–6 demonstrates this point. A reading error of the same dimension will produce a small volume-error when using a pipet, a greater volume-error when using a cylindrical graduate, and the greatest volume-error when using a conical graduate. The greater the flair in the design of the conical graduate, the greater is the volume-error due to an error in reading.

In reading the level of liquid in a graduate, it is important to recognize the error which could result due to the error of parallax. Figure A–7 depicts this point. A liquid in a graduate tends to be drawn to the inner surface of the graduate and rises slightly against that surface and above its true meniscus. If one measured looking downward, it would appear as though the meniscus of the liquid is at this upper level, whereas it is slightly lower, at the actual level of the liquid within the center of the graduate. Thus, measurements of liquids in graduates should be taken with the eyesight level with the liquid in the graduate.

If a pharmacist was in error in his reading of a graduate, the *percentage of error* of his measurement would be affected by the volume of liquid that he was measuring. According to the USP, an acceptable 10-mL graduate cylinder with an internal diameter of 1.18 cm contains 0.109 mL of liquid in each 1 mm of column. A reading error of 1 mm in magnitude would cause a percentage error in the measurement of only 1.09% when 10 mL were being measured, 2.18% when 5 mL were being measured, 4.36% when 2.5 mL were being measured, and 7.26% when 1.5 mL were being measured. It is apparent that the greatest percentage error occurs when the smallest amount is being measured. Thus, the rule of thumb for measuring liquids in graduates is that a graduate should be used having a capacity *equal to or just exceeding* the volume to be measured.

According to Goldstein and Mattocks,[2] based on a deviation of 1 mm from the mark and an allowable error of 2.5%, the smallest amounts that should be measured in the following size

Fig. A–5. *Typical equipment for the pharmaceutical measurement of volume. On the left are conical graduates and on the right, cylindrical graduates. In the front is a pipet for the measurement of small volumes. Behind the pipet is a pipet filler, used instead of the mouth to draw acids and other dangerous liquids into the pipet.*

Fig. A–6. *Drawing showing the difference in the volume-error occurring with the same reading-error in measuring devices of different diameters.*

cylindrical graduates having the stated internal diameters are as follows:

Graduate Cylinder Size	Internal Diameter	Deviation in Actual Volume	Minimum Volume Measurable
5 mL	0.98 cm	0.075 mL	3.00 mL
10 mL	1.18 cm	0.109 mL	4.36 mL
25 mL	1.94 cm	0.296 mL	11.84 mL
50 mL	2.24 cm	0.394 mL	15.76 mL
100 mL	2.58 cm	0.522 mL	20.88 mL

For a 5% error, the minimum volumes measurable would be one-half of those stated. It is apparent that for accuracy, one should not select a graduate for use when the measurement involves utilization of only the bottom portion of the scale.

In using graduates, the pharmacist pours the liquid into the graduate slowly, observing the level as he proceeds. In measuring viscous liquids, adequate time must be allowed for the liquid to settle in the graduate, as some may run slowly down the inner sides of the graduate. It is best to attempt to pour such liquids

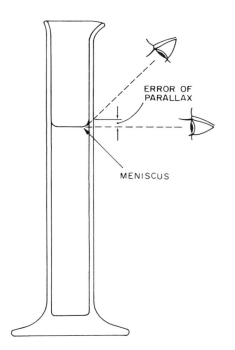

Fig. A–7. *Drawing depicting the error in the reading of the meniscus of a liquid in a graduate cylinder when the reading is made from above the level of the liquid rather than at the same level.*

toward the center of the graduate, avoiding contact with the sides. In emptying the graduate of its measured contents, adequate drain time should be allowed.

When pouring liquids from bottles, it is considered good pharmaceutical technique to keep the label on the bottle facing upwards; this avoids the possibility of drops of liquid running down the label as the bottle is righted after use. Naturally, the bottle orifice should be wiped clean after each use.

Notes

1. The *sensitivity requirement* (SR) of a balance is determined in the following manner: (1) level the balance, (2) determine the rest point, (3) place a 6-mg weight on one of the empty pans, (4) the rest point is shifted *not less than* one division on the index plate. The entire operation is repeated with a 10-g weight placed in the center of each balance pan.
2. Goldstein, S.W., and Mattocks, A.M.: How to Measure Accurately, *J. Am. Pharm.*, 12:421, 1951.

Index

Numbers in *italics* refer to illustrations; numbers followed by "t" indicate tables.